Management of Common Problems in Obstetrics and Gynecology

Edited by

Daniel R. Mishell Jr., M.D.
Professor and Chairman

and

Paul F. Brenner, M.D.
Associate Professor

Department of Obstetrics and Gynecology
University of Southern California
School of Medicine, Los Angeles

Joseph A. Carvelli

MEDICAL ECONOMICS BOOKS
Oradell, New Jersey 07649

Library of Congress Cataloging in Publication Data

Main entry under title:

Management of common problems in obstetrics and
    gynecology.

    Spine title: Common problems in obstetrics and
gynecology.
    Includes bibliographies and index.
    1. Pregnancy, Complications of.   2. Generative organs,
Female—Diseases.   I. Mishell, Daniel R.   II. Brenner,
Paul F.   III. Title: Common problems in obstetrics and
gynecology.   [DNLM: 1. Pregnancy complications—Therapy.
2. Genital diseases, Female—Therapy.   3. Genital
neoplasms, Female—Therapy.   4. Infertility, Female—
Therapy.   5. Fetal diseases—Therapy.   6. Family planning.
7. Endocrine diseases—Therapy.   WP 140 M266]
RG571.M23   1983   618   83-993
ISBN 0-87489-306-2

ISBN 0-87489-306-2

Medical Economics Company Inc.
Oradell, New Jersey 07649

Printed in the United States of America

CONTENTS

CONTRIBUTORS

Raul Artal, M.D.
Assistant Professor
Department of Obstetrics and Gynecology
University of Southern California
  School of Medicine
Los Angeles

Charles A. Ballard, M.D.
Professor
Department of Obstetrics and Gynecology
University of Southern California
  School of Medicine
Los Angeles

Thomas J. Benedetti, M.D.
Associate Professor
Department of Obstetrics and Gynecology
University of Washington
  School of Medicine
Seattle

Gerald S. Bernstein, Ph.D., M.D.
Professor
Department of Obstetrics and Gynecology
University of Southern California
  School of Medicine
Los Angeles

Paul F. Brenner, M.D.
Associate Professor
Department of Obstetrics and Gynecology
University of Southern California
  School of Medicine
Los Angeles

Andrew I. Brill, M.D.
Associate Clinical Instructor
Department of Obstetrics and Gynecology
Stanford University Medical School
Stanford, Calif.

Samuel L. Bruce, M.D.
Assistant Professor
Department of Obstetrics and Gynecology
University of Southern California
  School of Medicine
Los Angeles

Robert C. Corlett Jr., M.D.
Assistant Clinical Professor
Department of Obstetrics and Gynecology
University of Southern California
  School of Medicine
Los Angeles

David B. Cotton, M.D.
Assistant Professor
Department of Obstetrics and Gynecology
University of Texas Medical School
Houston

Val Davajan, M.D.
Professor
Department of Obstetrics and Gynecology
University of Southern California
  School of Medicine
Los Angeles

Maurice Druzin, M.D.
Assistant Professor
Department of Obstetrics and Gynecology
Cornell Medical School
New York

Otis Gaddis Jr., M.D.
Assistant Professor
Department of Obstetrics and Gynecology
University of Southern California
  School of Medicine
Los Angeles

William E. Gibbons, M.D.
Assistant Professor
Department of Obstetrics and Gynecology
Baylor College of Medicine
Houston

Uwe T. Goebelsmann, M.D.
Professor and Chief
Section of Reproduction Biology
Department of Obstetrics and Gynecology
University of Southern California
  School of Medicine
Los Angeles

Steven H. Golde, M.D.
Assistant Professor
Department of Obstetrics and Gynecology
University of Southern California
  School of Medicine
Los Angeles

Lester T. Hibbard, M.D.
Professor
Department of Obstetrics and Gynecology
University of Southern California
  School of Medicine
Los Angeles

Charles W. Hohler, M.D.
Director of Perinatology
  and Perinatal Ultrasound Services
St. Joseph's Hospital and Medical Center
Phoenix, Ariz.

John E. Holmes, M.D.
Associate Professor
Department of Neurology
University of Southern California
  School of Medicine
Los Angeles

Robert Israel, M.D.
Associate Professor
Department of Obstetrics and Gynecology
University of Southern California
  School of Medicine
Los Angeles

Oscar A. Kletzky, M.D.
Professor
Department of Obstetrics and Gynecology
University of Southern California
  School of Medicine
Los Angeles

Kee Seng Koh, M.D.
Assistant Clinical Professor
Department of Obstetrics and Gynecology
University of Southern California
  School of Medicine
Los Angeles

Marc R. Lebed, M.D.
Director of Maternal-Fetal Medicine
Huntington Memorial Hospital
Pasadena, Calif.

Rogerio A. Lobo, M.D.
Assistant Professor
Department of Obstetrics and Gynecology
University of Southern California
  School of Medicine
Los Angeles

Charles M. March, M.D.
Assistant Professor and Chief
Section of Gynecology
Department of Obstetrics and Gynecology
University of Southern California
  School of Medicine
Los Angeles

Richard P. Marrs, M.D.
Assistant Professor
Department of Obstetrics and Gynecology
University of Southern California
  School of Medicine
Los Angeles

Frank C. Miller, M.D.
Assistant Professor
Department of Obstetrics and Gynecology
University of Southern California
  School of Medicine
Los Angeles

Daniel R. Mishell Jr., M.D.
Professor and Chairman
Department of Obstetrics and Gynecology
University of Southern California
  School of Medicine
Los Angeles

Martin Montoro, M.D.
Assistant Clinical Professor
Department of Obstetrics and Gynecology
University of Southern California
  School of Medicine
Los Angeles

C. Paul Morrow, M.D.
Professor and Chief
Section of Gynecologic Oncology
Department of Obstetrics and Gynecology
University of Southern California
  School of Medicine
Los Angeles

Richard H. Nalick, M.D.
Associate Professor of Clinical Obstetrics
  and Gynecology
Department of Obstetrics and Gynecology
University of Southern California
  School of Medicine
Los Angeles

Richard H. Paul, M.D.
Professor and Chief
Section of Maternal-Fetal Medicine
Department of Obstetrics and Gynecology
University of Southern California
  School of Medicine
Los Angeles

Jeffrey P. Phelan, M.D.
Assistant Professor
Department of Obstetrics and Gynecology
University of Southern California
  School of Medicine
Los Angeles

Lawrence D. Platt, M.D.
Associate Professor
Department of Obstetrics and Gynecology
University of Southern California
  School of Medicine
Los Angeles

Subir Roy, M.D.
Associate Professor
Department of Obstetrics and Gynecology
University of Southern California
  School of Medicine
Los Angeles

Barry S. Schifrin, M.D.
Professor
Department of Obstetrics and Gynecology
University of Southern California
  School of Medicine
Los Angeles

John B. Schlaerth, M.D.
Assistant Professor
Department of Obstetrics and Gynecology
University of Southern California
  School of Medicine
Los Angeles

Suzanne Trupin, M.D.
Director
Department of Obstetrics and Gynecology
University of Illinois
  School of Clinical Medicine
Urbana-Champaign

J. Peter Van Dorsten, M.D.
Assistant Professor
Department of Obstetrics and Gynecology
Medical University of South Carolina
Charleston

Joyce M. Vargyas, M.D.
Assistant Professor
Department of Obstetrics and Gynecology
University of Southern California
  School of Medicine
Los Angeles

Sze-ya Yeh, M.D.
Associate Professor
Department of Obstetrics and Gynecology
University of Southern California
  School of Medicine
Los Angeles

Margaret Lynn Yonekura, M.D.
Assistant Professor
Department of Obstetrics and Gynecology
University of Southern California
  School of Medicine
Los Angeles

PREFACE

The clinical practice of obstetrics and gynecology has changed dramatically in the past decade. The monitoring of labor, the inhibition of premature labor, the assessment of fetal well-being, the treatment of dysmenorrhea, the evaluation of stress urinary incontinence, the staging and management of gynecologic malignancies, the diagnosis and treatment of infertility, in vitro fertilization, and the assessment of gynecologic endocrinopathies are just a few of the areas in which the quality of care has been greatly improved.

This book has been written for all physicians who treat obstetric or gynecologic problems. This encompasses not only the obstetrician-gynecologist, but also many physicians with postgraduate training in other fields, such as family medicine, emergency medicine, internal medicine, and general surgery, who also frequently deal with such disorders.

Management of Common Problems in Obstetrics and Gynecology consists of concise, clinically oriented chapters that provide the clinician with the latest diagnostic and therapeutic methods for the management of the most commonly encountered obstetric and gynecologic disorders. The contributing authors are current or former members of the Department of Obstetrics and Gynecology of the University of Southern California School of Medicine, located at Women's Hospital, Los Angeles County/University of Southern California Medical Center, Los Angeles. This 320-bed institution is the largest women's hospital in the United States.

In 1982 more than 15,000 women gave birth at Women's Hospital, and more than 3,500 gynecologic operations were performed. In addition, more than 35,000 emergency room consultations, 35,000 obstetric outpatient visits, and 15,000 gynecology outpatient visits took place.

As a result of this large volume of patients, a great deal of experience with newly developed diagnostic and therapeutic modalities has been accumulated over a relatively short time. Results of the faculty's experience have been synthesized in the easily readable chapters that will enable the reader to use the most recent diagnostic and therapeutic techniques in patient management.

The editors would like to express their sincere appreciation to the publisher for innovative suggestions and cooperation in the preparation of this book and to the departmental secretaries who typed the several drafts of each chapter.

Daniel R. Mishell Jr., M.D.
Paul F. Brenner, M.D.

PUBLISHER'S NOTES

Daniel R. Mishell Jr., M.D., is Professor and Chairman of the Department of Obstetrics and Gynecology, University of Southern California School of Medicine, and Chief of Professional Services, Women's Hospital, Los Angeles County/USC Medical Center, Los Angeles. He is Editor-in-Chief of *Contraception*, has published more than 250 papers in professional journals, and is co-editor of *Reproductive Endocrinology, Infertility and Contraception* (F.A. Davis Co., 1979; second edition to be published by Medical Economics Books in 1984). Dr. Mishell is also editor of *Advances in Fertility Research* (Raven Press, 1981) and is on the Editorial Boards of the *Journal of Reproductive Medicine* and *Core Journals in Obstetrics and Gynecology.* He is a Fellow of the American College of Obstetricians and Gynecologists.

Paul F. Brenner, M.D., is Associate Professor of Obstetrics and Gynecology and Pediatrics, University of Southern California School of Medicine. He has contributed numerous scientific papers to professional journals in the areas of reproductive endocrinology, contraception, menopause, gynecology, radioimmunoassay of steroids, and pediatric gynecology. He is a consultant for the following journals: *Contraception, American Journal of Obstetrics and Gynecology, International Journal of Gynaecology and Obstetrics, Analytical Biochemistry, Fertility and Sterility,* and the *Journal of the American Medical Association.* Dr. Brenner is a Fellow of the American College of Obstetricians and Gynecologists.

Medical Economics Books thanks F.A. Davis Company for permission to use portions of *Reproductive Endocrinology, Infertility and Contraception*, first edition, 1979, edited by Daniel R. Mishell Jr., M.D., and Val Davajan, M.D.

O N E

OBSTETRICS

1

Drugs in Pregnancy

SZE-YA YEH, M.D.

INTRODUCTION

Sir William Osler once said: "The desire to take medicine is, perhaps, the greatest feature that distinguishes man from animals." This applies to both the nonpregnant and the pregnant. There have been various reports documenting the drug intake habits of pregnant women, and the results are always striking. Forfar's survey in Edinburgh (1973) reported that, excluding iron preparations, drugs were prescribed for 82% of pregnant women with an average of four drugs each, and 65% took drugs not prescribed by their physicians.

But despite the enormous amounts of drugs ingested by pregnant women, proven untoward effects are relatively few. Most of the reports of ill effects are isolated, anecdotal, and descriptive. It is extremely difficult to prove the direct effects of drugs from these types of reports.

When a pregnant woman is given medication, two patients are being treated simultaneously, because almost all pharmacologic substances pass through the placenta. The fetal response to drugs is generally different from the maternal response, usually resulting in greater toxicity or irreversible changes. Therefore, it is mandatory for physicians to understand the nature of drugs and their effects on the fetus before prescribing them to the pregnant woman. Unfortunately, most of this information is not readily available.

In 1980, the Food and Drug Administration required that all prescription drugs be labeled as to teratogenic effects in pregnancy. The FDA established five categories (A, B, C, D, X) to indicate a drug's potential for causing birth defects. They are defined as follows:

1. *Category A* applies to drugs for which well-controlled studies in women fail to demonstrate a risk to the fetus.
2. *Category B* indicates that either (a) animal studies have not demonstrated a fetal risk but no adequate studies have been done in humans; or (b) animal studies have uncovered some risk that has not been confirmed in controlled studies in humans.
3. *Category C* also has two meanings: (a) animal studies have revealed adverse fetal effects but no adequate controlled studies have been done in humans; or (b) studies in humans and animals are not available.
4. *Category D* applies to drugs associated with birth defects in humans, but with potential benefits that may outweigh their known risks.

5. *Category X* indicates drugs for which abnormalities have been demonstrated in animal or human studies. The potential risks of the drugs in this category clearly outweigh their potential benefits. Such drugs are contraindicated in pregnancy.

MECHANISMS OF PLACENTAL TRANSFER

The six mechanisms by which substances cross the placenta are: (1) simple diffusion, (2) facilitated diffusion, (3) active transport, (4) metabolic conversion of transferred substrate, (5) physical disruption of placental membranes, and (6) pinocytosis.

The great majority of drugs are transferred by simple diffusion. The most significant factors influencing such transfer are concentration gradient, lipid solubility, degree of ionization, and molecular weight. Simple diffusion merely moves a substance from a medium or area of higher concentration to one of lower concentration. The greater the concentration gradient and lipid solubility, or the lower the degree of ionization, the greater will be the diffusion. Drugs with a molecular weight greater than 1,000 will not permeate the placental barrier.

TERATOGENICITY

The most significant drug effect in pregnancy is teratogenicity. To understand this effect, it is important to first understand basic human embryology. There are three basic periods in human fetal development: (1) the fertilization and implantation period, (2) the embryonic period, and (3) the fetal period.

The first period covers from conception to about the 17th day of gestation. During this time, toxic agents will interfere with cell development and cause an abortion. The embryonic period, from 18 to 55 days after conception, is the time organogenesis occurs. Various developing organs show extreme sensitivity to teratogenic agents at this stage; exposure could result in functional and/or morphologic malformations. The third period ranges from the 56th day to delivery. It is the time of fetal growth, and although teratogenic changes may appear, they are much less common.

Only a handful of drugs have been conclusively proven teratogenic in humans. They are: thalidomide, folic acid antagonists, diethylstilbestrol (DES), and synthetic progestins. Thalidomide was widely prescribed for treatment of vomiting in pregnancy, and was the proven cause of amelia and phocomelia in many infants before it was removed from the market. When the folic acid antagonists methotrexate and aminopterin were used for cancer treatment in pregnant women, they caused major cranial and skeletal deformities in the offspring. DES, once widely used for threatened abortion, has been proven to be related to vaginal adenosis at adolescence in many young women exposed in utero. Some of these women eventually developed adenocarcinoma of the vagina. Synthetic progestins are used primarily as oral contraceptives. When given in pregnancy, they have been shown to cause masculinization of the female fetus.

ADVERSE DRUG EFFECTS IN THE FIRST TRIMESTER

The major adverse drug effect during the first trimester is teratogenicity. The following drugs are contraindicated in the first trimester because their risks outweigh their benefits: thalidomide, serotonin, tolbutamide, methotrexate, aminopterin, meclizine, LSD, amphetamines, progestins, coumarins, podophyllin, and acetazolamide.

Also in this group are drugs that cause side effects in the fetus: Streptomycin causes eighth-nerve damage; tetracycline causes inhibition of bone growth and discoloration of the teeth; iodine causes congenital goiter; chloroquine causes eighth-nerve and retinal damage; DES causes clear-cell vaginal tumors in female offspring; and ethanol causes fetal alcohol syndrome.

Risk-to-benefit ratios are questionable for the following drugs: gentamicin, lithium, benzodiazepines, propylthiouracil, barbiturates, diazoxide, and phenytoin. These medications should be used only with proper medical judgment and supervision.

The potential benefits of the following drugs outweigh their risks: general anesthetics, sulfonamides, rifampin, and insulin. The majority of the teratogenic effects reported for these drugs have occurred in animal studies only. Drugs without any reports on teratogenic potential may also be used in pregnancy if, in the judgment of the physician, their benefits outweigh their risks.

ADVERSE DRUG EFFECTS IN THE SECOND AND THIRD TRIMESTERS

Drugs toxic to the fetus during the second and third trimesters generally produce their effects by direct action on the fetus. These drugs—listed with their possible effects—include: (1) aspirin—fetal bleeding, prolonged gestation, increased maternal bleeding with labor and delivery; (2) indomethacin—premature closing of the ductus arteriosus; (3) chloramphenicol—gray baby syndrome; (4) nitrofurantoin—fetal hyperbilirubinemia, hemolytic anemia; (5) tetracycline—depression of fetal bone growth, tooth discoloration; (6) cytotoxic drugs—intrauterine growth retardation, hypoplastic gonads; (7) reserpine—increased neonatal respiratory tract secretion, CNS depression, galactorrhea; (8) thiazides—fetal or neonatal jaundice, thrombocytopenia; (9) lithium—neonatal goiter, electrolyte imbalance; (10) narcotics—respiratory depression; (11) iodides—neonatal goiter, hypothyroidism; (12) warfarin—fetal hemorrhage, increased risk of fetal death, increased maternal bleeding.

ADVERSE DRUG EFFECTS DURING LACTATION

Most drugs taken by breast-feeding mothers will reach their neonates through the milk. Therefore, drug safety during lactation is also an important issue.

The following drugs—listed with their possible effects on the newborn—may cause problems when given to lactating mothers: (1) tetracycline—permanent staining of the teeth, reversible depression of bone growth; (2) chloramphenicol—gray baby syndrome; (3) sulfonamides—hyperbilirubinemia; (4) aspirin—hemorrhage; (5) diazepam—sedation; (6) lithium—electrolyte imbalance; (7) anticonvulsants—hemorrhage; (8) warfarin—hemorrhage; (9) reserpine—nasal obstruction, thermal instability, CNS depression; (10) thiazides—hypokalemia; thrombocytopenia; (11) oral hypoglycemics—hypoglycemia; (12) ergotamine—vomiting, diarrhea; (13) anticholinergics—inhibited maternal lactation; (14) nitrofurantoin—hemolytic anemia.

CONCLUSION

Before any drug is prescribed to a pregnant or lactating woman, its potential therapeutic value must be weighed against its potential adverse effects on the fetus or newborn. Unfortunately, our knowledge of drug teratogenicity in humans is limited, and is characterized by suspected, potential, and theoretical risks with little proof. To *guarantee* safety to all fetuses, we would have to deny all drug therapy to pregnant women. This is clearly not practical. Therefore, the benefit/risk decision must be based on existing knowledge and the best possible medical judgment for each given case.

Due to space limitations, only some commonly used drugs are listed in this chapter. Further details or information on drugs not listed here may be obtained from the sources listed in the Suggested Reading section, which follows. The Howard and Hill article concluded with two important points: (1) all over-the-counter drugs should be considered contraindicated in pregnancy; and (2) every drug taken by a pregnant woman must be documented in her antepartum chart—an essential precaution that will help us expand our knowledge of drug effects in pregnancy.

SUGGESTED READING

Berkowitz RL, Coustan DR, Mochizuki TK: *Handbook for Prescribing Medications During Pregnancy*. Boston: Little, Brown, 1981

Forfar JO, Nelson MN: Epidemiology of drugs taken by pregnant women. *Clin Pharmacol Ther* 14:632, 1973

Hill RM, Craig JP, Chaney MD, Tennyson LM, McCulley LB: Utilization of over-the-counter drugs during pregnancy. *Clin Obstet Gynecol* 20:381, 1977

Howard FM, Hill JM: Drugs in pregnancy. *Obstet Gynecol Surv* 34:643, 1979

Pitkin RM: Drugs in pregnancy. In Quilligan EJ, Kretchmer N, eds: *Fetal and Maternal Medicine*. New York: Wiley, 1980, pp 385-402

Yaffe SJ: Drugs and pregnancy. In Rathi M, Kumar S, eds: *Perinatal Medicine, Clinical and Biochemical Aspects*, vol 2. Washington, DC: Hemisphere, 1982, pp 151-168

2

Management of the Incompetent Cervix

RAUL ARTAL, M.D.

The etiology of the incompetent cervix is multifactorial, including any combination of traumatic, functional, and congenital factors. The reported incidence varies from 1:1,930 to 1:140 pregnancies.

The events leading to spontaneous abortion in cervical incompetence have been classically described as follows: The patient experiences an uneventful first trimester of pregnancy. In the mid- or late second trimester, there is bloodless and painless effacement and dilation of the cervix. A watery vaginal discharge accompanied by vague abdominal pressure is noticed. Then a sudden rupture of the membranes occurs. Most patients do not experience any uterine contractions until the last moment of membrane rupture, though some perceive regular contractions similar to labor pains prior to rupture. Soon after, the products of conception are aborted.

DIAGNOSIS

The most important diagnostic tool is a careful obstetric history. The classic history includes one or multiple spontaneous abortions or deliveries between 16 and 28 weeks' gestation, preceded by premature rupture of the membranes without bleeding and with few or no uterine contractions. Many, but not all, women with an incompetent cervix report such a history. In the majority of cases, there has been previous cervical trauma from surgical manipulation, traumatic delivery, therapeutic abortion, diagnostic D&C, or placenta previa.

Any history of second-trimester abortion in successive pregnancies strongly suggests the diagnosis of incompetent cervix. Serial vaginal examinations indicating rapid effacement of the cervix in the second trimester of pregnancy may confirm the diagnosis. (Cervical effacement usually occurs over 6-8 days.) But at that stage, it may be too late to intervene.

In the nonpregnant patient, the hysterogram and Hegar test are useful diagnostic adjuvants. A luteal phase hysterogram demonstrating an internal os width of 1 cm or greater when intrauterine pressure does not exceed 100 mm Hg confirms the diagnosis of incompetent cervix. If a No. 8 Hegar dilator can be passed beyond the internal os without resistance, or a pediatric Foley catheter with a 3-cc inflated bulb can be withdrawn through the internal os without resistance, the diagnosis is also confirmed.

MANAGEMENT

The incompetent cervix is managed surgically. The Lash procedure (designed for the nonpregnant patient) is no longer used; it causes permanent scarring of the cervix, frequently resulting in infertility or the need for cesarean section. Very rarely, maternal death has resulted.

The Shirodkar procedure originally utilized strips of fascia lata. They were inserted into the mucosa of the cervix at the level of the internal os, and then tied. But the McDonald cerclage procedure is currently the most commonly used method. With the availability of improved suture materials, such as Mersilene bands, the McDonald procedure has clear and distinct advantages. Compared with the Shirodkar procedure, it is simpler, faster, and less traumatic.

Timing of the Surgical Procedure

The optimal time for cervical cerclage is between 14 and 16 weeks' gestation. By 14 weeks, first-trimester spontaneous abortions have already occurred, and the possibility of performing a cerclage on a genetically defective pregnancy is markedly reduced. Conversely, if performed later than 20 weeks, the success of cerclage is very limited. In general, the earlier cerclage is performed, the greater will be the number of successes.

With the availability of real-time ultrasound, fetal movements and activity can be monitored very early in pregnancy. This can help ensure the presence of a normal pregnancy and allow cerclage to be performed as early as 12-13 weeks. An occasional patient will benefit from such an early procedure.

Contraindications and Complications

Contraindications, absolute or relative, to surgical cerclage are: (1) hyperirritability of the uterus with bulging membranes, (2) cervical dilation > 4 cm, (3) suspected fetal malformation, (4) suspected intrauterine fetal death, and (5) premature rupture of the membranes.

Complications of surgery include puncture of the chorioamniotic membranes during surgery, premature labor, amnionitis, and cervical lacerations from the suture. Occasionally, patients will have increased uterine irritability necessitating treatment. Magnesium sulfate and ritodrine hydrochloride (Yutopar) have both been found very effective in controlling it. Following the Shirodkar procedure, about 50% of patients experience vaginal infections that require treatment. Leukorrhea is rare following McDonald cerclage.

Postoperative Precautions

Following surgery, the patient should remain at bed rest for at least 24 hours, and the uterus should be observed for any unusual activity. Following the McDonald operation, patients are advised to abstain from intercourse for 4 weeks and to avoid strenuous physical activity for the remainder of the pregnancy. Patients are seen at frequent intervals, and a careful speculum examination is performed at each visit.

Excessive uterine irritability is the predominant cause of failure of surgical cerclage. Uterine activity can be suppressed with magnesium sulfate or ritodrine, as mentioned above. Patients exhibiting uterine irritability, when evaluated later, may or may not have anatomic uterine defects. The McDonald cerclage procedure is successful in 75% or more of properly selected patients, when performed at the correct gestational age.

Suture Removal

In the past, it was suggested that existing cervical sutures be left in place for future pregnancies, with elective cesarean sections performed to effect delivery. This approach should be abandoned. The simplicity of the McDonald procedure and the benefits of vaginal delivery outweigh the risks of complications associated with abdominal delivery. Other possible complications of leaving the sutures in place include granulomatous changes and foreign-body tissue reactions. Their consequences are unknown.

We advocate elective suture removal at 38-39 weeks' gestation. This approach results in a planned delivery and avoids possible lacerations of the cervix secondary to the dilating mechanism of labor.

Once the suture is removed, one-third of patients go into immediate labor. (Any patient showing cervical dilation > 4 cm will go into labor immediately after suture removal.) In the other two-thirds, pregnancy usually continues to term. This is explained by the formation of a fibrotic band that mechanically serves the function of the cerclage.

Labor and Delivery Following Suture Removal

Each stage of labor is usually shortened in these patients. The deceleration phase is absent, and the acceleration phase is shorter than usual. A prolonged latent phase may occur in patients with a fibrotic band in the cervical matrix. The cervix will usually remain dilated to 3-4 cm for 6-8 hours. Then the acceleration phase and delivery will occur suddenly within a period of 30 minutes. The incidence of complications and cesarean section is no greater than in control populations.

Alternatives to Surgical Cerclage

Synthetic gestagens have been used in the past because they have a quiescent effect on the uterus. But they are no longer used and are considered contraindicated in early pregnancy. Smith-Hodge pessaries have also been used. They usually shift the axis of intrauterine pressure from the cervix to the lower uterine segment, preventing cervical dilation. But the preferred treatment today for cervical incompetence is surgery.

SUGGESTED READING

Artal R, Shachar Y, Insler V, Serr DM: Course of delivery following cerclage for cervical incompetence. *Harefuah* 81:65, 1971

Artal R, Shachar Y, Insler V, Serr DM: Course of pregnancy following cerclage for cervical incompetence. *Harefuah* 81:63, 1971

Baden WF, Baden EE: Cervical incompetence, current therapy. *Am J Obstet Gynecol* 79:545, 1960

Kirkley WH, Gilbert JC, McDaniel GC: Pathologic examination of a postpartum uterus containing Dacron used for cerclage. *Obstet Gynecol* 20:626, 1962

Lash AF, Lash SR: Habitual abortion: The incompetent internal os of the cervix. *Am J Obstet Gynecol* 59:68, 1950

McDonald IA: Suture of the cervix for inevitable abortion. *J Obstet Gynecol Eur* 64:346, 1957

Raphael SI: Incompetent internal os of the cervix. *Obstet Gynecol* 28:438, 1966

Shirodkar VN: Long term results with operative treatment of habitual abortion. *Triangle* 8:123, 1967

3

Hydrocephalus

FRANK C. MILLER, M.D., and MARC R. LEBED, M.D.

Hydrocephalus is the result of an excessive accumulation of cerebrospinal fluid (CSF) within the brain. The excessive accumulation of CSF can be due to its overproduction by a papilloma of the choroid plexus or, more commonly in the fetus and newborn, to an obstruction of CSF flow. Table 3-1 summarizes common factors in the etiology of hydrocephalus.

Congenital hydrocephalus occurs in approximately 1:2,000 live births. About 3% of mothers who previously delivered a hydrocephalic infant have another with this defect. Isolated hydrocephalus—that is, without a neural tube defect—varies from 0.39 to 0.87:1,000 live births. Hydrocephalus can occur as an X-linked recessive trait with a 50% recurrence rate in male fetuses. The true incidence of this type of hydrocephalus is unknown, although it is estimated to comprise 2% of all cases of isolated hydrocephalus in the newborn.

Women with a history of having delivered an infant with hydrocephalus should have the following evaluation during any subsequent pregnancy:

1. Serologic evaluation for infectious teratogens, such as cytomegalovirus, *Toxoplasma gondii* (agent of toxoplasmosis), and the rubella virus
2. Sonography before the 20th week of pregnancy to determine the size of the fetal lateral ventricles and cerebral hemisphere and to explore the fetal spine for defects
3. Amniocentesis for α-fetoprotein and chromosome analysis at 16-18 weeks
4. Parental karyotyping.

Hydrocephalus during the second trimester is usually diagnosed as a result of genetic counseling and the associated ultrasound scan and amniocentesis. It is important to remember that prior to 24 weeks' gestation ventricular enlargement can occur before an increase in biparietal diameter. Johnson et al reported that fetuses with hydrocephalus developed dilation of the occipital horns of the lateral ventricles, followed by enlargement of the lateral ventricular width and cerebral hemisphere width, before an increase in the biparietal diameter.

The normal range of ventricular size and ventricular/cortical ratios is quite large during the second trimester. Where questionable abnormalities exist,

TABLE 3-1. ETIOLOGY OF FETAL HYDROCEPHALUS

Genetic
  Failure of any part of the CSF pathway to develop
  Stenosis of the aqueduct of Sylvius
  Cerebellar agenesis
  Spina bifida cystica
  Chromosomal abnormalities, such as trisomy 13
Nongenetic
  Obstructing tumor
  Postinflammatory fibrosis secondary to viral infection and encephalitis
    (rubella, cytomegalovirus, possibly mumps) or protozoal infection

Adapted from Habib.

especially in relation to ventricular dilation, serial ultrasound scans and additional consultation should be obtained before a diagnosis is established. The diagnosis of mild hydrocephalus does not necessarily result in a severely handicapped infant. The determination of management must involve typing of the disorder, the extent of anatomic involvement, and the experience of the neonatal personnel who will care for the infant.

Diagnosis of hydrocephalus becomes easier as gestation advances. Always be cautious in making the diagnosis in a large fetus, because a large normal infant may have a biparietal diameter and/or head circumference at the upper limit of the normal range. Generally the diagnosis is obvious from widely dilated ventricles and/or other intracranial abnormalities. A word of caution about ultrasound equipment and imaging: Because the brain is homogeneous, ultrasound images from some of the older equipment will appear dark and may be mistaken for large, fluid-filled areas. If there is any question about the diagnosis, obtain consultation from an expert in fetal ultrasound.

Because of the rapidly expanding experience with ventricular shunting (even in utero), management of a pregnancy with a hydrocephalic fetus is changing almost daily. One of the most widely accepted prognostic criteria for hydrocephalus has been the thickness of the cortex at the time of ultrasound scan. An established guideline has been that a 1-cm rim of cortex justifies atraumatic delivery (cesarean section) for fetal salvage, provided there are no additional CNS lesions. Unfortunately, these criteria have failed to predict long-term outcome consistently. The decision on management is best made in consultation with the neurosurgeon and neonatologist. Their experience in dealing with these infants will strongly influence obstetric management.

Atraumatic delivery of a hydrocephalic fetus probably reduces the risk of intrapartum and neonatal intracranial hemorrhage and thus gives a better outcome. This is the preferred route of delivery of an infant who is a candidate for shunting. The decision to decompress the fetal head in cases of severe hydrocephalus or in cases with associated CNS lesions is always a difficult one.

Technically, the insertion of a large-bore needle into a dilated ventricle is not difficult. If done vaginally, an endoscope should be used to provide direct vision. The CNS fluid either can be allowed to drain off or can be aspirated. Transabdominal and vaginal insertion can also be aided by visualization with ultrasound to guide the needle to the correct position.

The emotional impact on the parents is often quite staggering, whether the diagnosis is made in midpregnancy or at term. They must be fully counseled regarding the eventual prognosis, plans for management during labor, the method of delivery, and plans for care of the newborn, and allowed to participate fully in the decisions that will affect their child.

There are still no acceptable antepartum criteria for long-term prognosis, except for grossly affected fetuses. Until a formula is determined, management of the fetus must be individualized on the basis of the following:

1. The type of anomaly/abnormality
2. The extent of anatomic involvement (including thalamic and brain stem involvement)
3. Neonatal support available during the immediate neonatal period
4. Parental input.

SUGGESTED READING

DeVore GR, Hobbins JC: Ultrasound diagnosis of congenital birth defects. In Sciarra JJ, ed: *Gynecology and Obstetrics.* Hagerstown, Md: Harper & Row Loose Leaf Reference Service, 1982, p 1

Freeman RK, McQuown DS, Secrist LJ, Larson EJ: The diagnosis of fetal hydrocephalus before viability. *Obstet Gynecol* 49:109, 1977

Habib Z: Genetics and genetic counselling in neonatal hydrocephalus. *Obstet Gynecol Surv* 36:529, 1981

Holmes LB, Nash A, Zurheim GM, Levin M, Opitz JM: X-linked aqueductal stenosis: Clinical and neuro-pathological findings in two families. *Pediatrics* 51:697, 1973

Johnson ML, Dunne MG, Mack LA, Rashbaum CL: Evaluation of fetal intracranial anatomy by static and real-time ultrasound. *J Clin Ultrasound* 8:311, 1980

Shulman K: Hydrocephaly. In Bergsma D, ed: *Birth Defects Compendium,* ed 2. New York: Alan R Liss, 1979, p 534

4

Acquired Anemia in Pregnancy

SZE-YA YEH, M.D.

During pregnancy, profound changes occur in the maternal hematologic system, allowing it to adjust to the newly formed maternal-fetal unit. In addition, requirements for certain nutrients essential for hemopoiesis, such as iron and folic acid, increase due to expanding blood volume and cell mass, and fetal growth. Therefore, as expected, anemia is relatively common in pregnancy.

Values diagnostic of anemia are generally lower in pregnancy than in the nonpregnant state. In general, hemoglobin levels lower than 10 gm/dl and hematocrit lower than 30% indicate anemia in pregnancy. Patients with such values must be carefully evaluated to establish the specific cause, to initiate treatment, and to prevent a more severe anemia.

The direct effect of anemia on the fetus is not clear. When anemia is mild, no apparent fetal effects can be found. But when anemia becomes profound, the oxygen-carrying capacity of the maternal blood will be affected. Severe anemia is associated with an increased incidence of abortion, stillbirth, premature birth, and growth retardation. Most important, anemic women cannot tolerate hemorrhage or blood loss from the process of delivery.

PHYSIOLOGIC ALTERATIONS IN PREGNANCY

The major hematologic change in pregnancy is a proportionate increase in plasma volume exceeding that of cell volume. This results from the need for increased circulation to the vascular placenta and growing breast mass. Numerous studies in the 1960s indicated that plasma volume increases 45% or 1,000 ml, starting at the third month of gestation and reaching a peak during the ninth month. It returns to normal by the third week postpartum. Placental lactogen, which causes an increase in aldosterone secretion, may cause the increase in plasma volume.

Total red blood cell volume and hemoglobin mass increase 25% or 300-350 ml, starting at 6 months' gestation and reaching a peak at term. These values return to normal by the sixth week postpartum. This increase may result from the interrelation between placental lactogen, progesterone, estrogen, and the increased levels of erythropoietin in pregnancy. Thus, pregnancy itself produces a certain dilution effect on hemoglobin concentration, which is markedly higher during the second trimester than during the third.

CAUSES OF ANEMIA IN PREGNANCY

In addition to the normal physiologic changes, some pathologic conditions may result in anemia during pregnancy. They can be divided into two groups: acquired and hereditary. This chapter will deal with only acquired anemias.

Acquired types of anemia in pregnancy are:

1. Iron-deficiency anemia
2. Anemia caused by blood loss
3. Anemia associated with infection
4. Megaloblastic anemia
5. Acquired hemolytic anemia
6. Aplastic or hypoplastic anemia.

The first two are the most common.

Iron-Deficiency Anemia

Iron requirements increase considerably during pregnancy. In a gestation with a single fetus, total additional need for iron is approximately 1,000 mg, of which 300 mg go to the fetus and placenta and 500 mg are used to expand the maternal hemoglobin mass. The other 200 mg are lost during the process of delivery. The majority of adult women have some iron stores, primarily in the liver, spleen, and bone marrow. But the amount stored is usually below 300 mg during the reproductive years, which is insufficient for the additional requirements in pregnancy. Patients with poor diets will be more likely to rapidly develop marked anemia during pregnancy.

Signs and symptoms of iron-deficiency anemia vary from asymptomatic cases to general malaise, anorexia, palpitation, ankle edema, and fever of unknown origin. The characteristic blood smear shows hypochromic and microcytic red blood cells. Reticulocyte count will be low for the degree of anemia unless iron supplementation has been given. These morphologic changes may not occur until the hematocrit has fallen far below normal levels.

The first result of iron deficiency is depletion of iron stores in the liver, spleen, and marrow, followed by a decrease in serum iron and an increase in total serum iron-binding capacity. A serum iron (Fe) level below 60 μg%, total iron-binding capacity (TIBC) greater than 350 μg/dl, and an Fe/TIBC ratio (transferrin saturation) less than 16%, are diagnostic of iron-deficiency anemia. If a serum ferritin assay is available, a value of 12 ng/ml or lower is indicative of subnormal iron storage.

Once a diagnosis of iron-deficiency anemia is established, proper treatment should begin as soon as possible. The treatment of choice is oral iron supplementation, which should continue throughout gestation. Other types of treatment, such as parenteral iron and blood transfusion, are indicated only rarely—for rapid correction of anemia when delivery is near or for marked anemia when oral iron therapy is not adequate.

Iron absorption from the small intestine is very poor, especially after iron therapy is instituted. In most cases of iron-deficiency anemia, at least 200 mg of elemental iron are required daily, and treatment should be continued for at least 6 months. Elemental iron constitutes only $\frac{1}{9}$-$\frac{1}{3}$ of most iron preparations. For example, a 325-mg tablet of ferrous sulfate contains 60-65 mg of elemental iron; a 325-mg tablet of ferrous gluconate contains 37-39 mg of elemental iron. Iron absorption is slightly improved in an acid environment; therefore, simultaneous ingestion of ascorbic acid may enhance absorption.

Side effects of iron therapy include gastric distress, eructation, and constipation. These problems can be minimized by taking iron tablets with meals or using tablets containing added ingredients, such as laxatives.

Because most iron-deficiency anemia is due to poor dietary habits, dietary review and improvement are the most important measures in treatment. Animal sources of iron (meat, liver, fish, etc.) are usually better absorbed than vegetable sources, and thus are more effective in improving anemic conditions. Milk interferes with iron absorption; patients should be advised not to take iron tablets and milk simultaneously. A rise in hemoglobin concentration of about 0.2 gm/dl/week indicates the patient is responsive to the therapy.

Anemia Caused by Blood Loss

Anemia resulting from recent hemorrhage is not an uncommon problem in obstetrics. Hemorrhage due to abortion, placenta previa, abruptio placentae, trauma, or complicated delivery often causes hypovolemia and severe anemia. Under these circumstances, fluid replacement and blood transfusion may be necessary.

It is always important to remember that a blood transfusion is not a totally benign procedure. In addition to exposing the patient to the risk of hepatitis infection, it increases the possibility of sensitization to certain blood type antigens. A patient with stable vital signs and no orthostatic changes may be a candidate for restoration of blood volume with substances other than whole blood or packed cells, such as lactated Ringer's solution or dextrans, followed by long-term iron therapy.

In certain underdeveloped areas of the world, severe anemia can be caused by chronic blood loss due to parasitic infection. When this condition is suspected, investigation and proper treatment should be provided.

Anemia Associated With Infection

Subacute and chronic infections sometimes produce moderate or severe anemia, usually with normocytic or slightly microcytic erythrocytes. This type of anemia is thought to be caused by alterations in reticuloendothelial function and iron metabolism. If the underlying infection is not corrected, anemia will persist despite long-term administration of iron and folic acid. Therefore, this type of anemia is also called "refractory anemia of pregnancy." This anemia is treated by eliminating the underlying infection and giving iron and folic acid supplementation.

Chronic renal disease, suppurative granulomatous infections, malignancies, and rheumatoid arthritis may also cause this type of anemia.

Megaloblastic Anemia

The major causes of megaloblastic anemia are folic acid deficiency and vitamin B_{12} deficiency. Both folic acid and vitamin B_{12} are important in the biosynthesis of purine molecules essential for the formation of DNA. Vitamin B_{12}-deficiency anemia, or pernicious anemia, is extremely rare in pregnancy. Women with this type of anemia are usually infertile.

Folic acid is found in only a few types of food, and the normal storage can last only a few weeks when intake is limited and/or the need is increased. In the nonpregnant state, 50-100 μg of folic acid are required daily, but in pregnancy the requirement increases to 300 μg/day. This is due to decreased folic acid absorption and increased need due to fetal growth. Only green vegetables and some organ meats are rich in folic acid. Therefore, the most common cause of folic acid deficiency in pregnancy is inadequate dietary intake.

Signs and symptoms of folic acid deficiency vary according to the degree and duration of the deficiency. After 3 weeks of deprivation, a decrease in the serum folate level can be detected. This is followed by hypersegmentation of neutrophils at 7 weeks. Macrocytosis, bone marrow megaloblastosis, and severe anemia do not occur until the 18th to 19th week.

The most important diagnostic test for folic acid deficiency is the serum folate level: 4 ng/ml or less is considered deficient. Other available tests may also be useful. A blood smear may be tested for the presence of macrocytic erythrocytes and hypersegmentation of neutrophils. (But if iron deficiency is also present, the red blood cells may show microcytic, normocytic, or mixed patterns.) Following histidine loading, elevated levels of formiminoglutamic acid (FIGLU) in urine indicate folate deficiency. However, pregnancy may cause both false-positive and false-negative results, making this test unreliable for pregnant women. Megaloblastic bone marrow changes are seen in severe folic acid deficiency.

The treatment for folic acid deficiency in pregnancy is supplementation. Usually, 1 mg of folic acid daily is sufficient.

Folic acid-deficiency anemia may be precipitated by certain conditions associated with increased requirements or altered folic acid metabolism. These include: acute infections, hemolytic anemia, and prolonged use of drugs such as sulfonamides, anticonvulsants, and oral contraceptives.

Acquired Hemolytic Anemia

Drug-induced hemolytic anemia is the most significant type of anemia in this category. It occurs in patients with a specific, inherited deficiency of the enzyme glucose-6-phosphate dehydrogenase (G6PD). About 2% of black women are homozygous for this deficiency; 10-15% of black women are heterozygous for it, with a lesser degree of deficiency. Several oxidant drugs may induce massive hemolysis in these women. Among the more common ones are antimalarial agents such as primaquine and quinine, several sulfonamides, nitrofurans, analgesics, and antipyretics such as aspirin and phenacetin. Infection and acidosis intensify the drug-induced hemolysis.

Other forms of acquired hemolytic anemia include idiopathic autoimmune hemolytic anemia, hemolysis complicating preeclampsia/eclampsia, and hemolysis caused by the exotoxin of *Clostridium perfringens*. Patients with autoimmune hemolytic anemia often demonstrate a positive direct Coombs test and are responsive to steroid therapy. Hemolysis in preeclampsia is thought to be related to disseminated intravascular coagulation. Elimination of the toxemia will stop the process of hemolysis. *Clostridium* infection is very rare, but is very often fatal; therefore, active and aggressive treatment is necessary.

Aplastic or Hypoplastic Anemia

This is a rare and serious occurrence in pregnancy. Diagnosis is relatively easy, but the treatment is extremely difficult because none of the erythropoietic agents can produce remission. Corticosteroid therapy may be of some value. Blood transfusion will maintain the blood count, but will not produce a cure. Hemorrhage due to thrombocytopenia and infection related to leukopenia are serious potential complications.

CONCLUSION

During pregnancy, the blood hemoglobin concentration is diluted, and requirements increase for various nutrients. Therefore, anemia is one of the most common complications of pregnancy. A complete blood count should be performed at the first prenatal visit. Patients with low hemoglobin and hematocrit values should be given anemia work-ups. The work-up should include measurements of serum iron and folate levels, G6PD levels, and total iron-binding capacity, as well as blood smear examination and hemoglobin electrophoresis. Treatment, especially the iron therapy, should be instituted as early as possible, for it takes several months for the hemoglobin level to return to normal.

SUGGESTED READING

Chesley LC: Plasma and red cell volumes during pregnancy. *Am J Obstet Gynecol* 112:440, 1972

DeLeeuw NKM, Lowenstein L, Hsieh YS: Iron deficiency and hydremia in normal pregnancy. *Medicine* 45:291, 1966

Kitay DZ: Folic acid deficiency in pregnancy. *Am J Obstet Gynecol* 104:1067, 1969

McFee JG: Anemia in pregnancy—A reappraisal. *Obstet Gynecol Surv* 28:769, 1973

Pritchard JA, MacDonald PC: *Williams Obstetrics,* ed 16. New York: Appleton-Century-Crofts, 1980, pp 712-720

Puolakka J: Serum ferritin as a measure of iron stores during pregnancy. *Acta Obstet Gynecol Scand Suppl* 95:1, 1980

5

Seizure Disorders in Pregnancy

SUZANNE TRUPIN, M.D., and JOHN E. HOLMES, M.D.

Seizure disorders are the most common neurologic complication of pregnancy. About 1:1,000 pregnant women will have a seizure disorder.

TYPES

Seizure disorders may be classified as generalized or focal and as idiopathic or organic. *Generalized* seizures are either grand mal or petit mal. Petit mal seizures are the "absence" attacks or brief lapses of consciousness without falling or convulsive movements. Grand mal seizures involve loss of consciousness and symmetrical tonic or clonic movements of the musculature, with a generalized discharge from all parts of the cortex as recorded on the EEG, hypoxia, tongue biting, urinary-fecal incontinence, and a prolonged after-stage (postictal period) of confusion and somnolence. A grand mal seizure may last many minutes, but is usually about 1 minute in duration.

Focal seizures originate in the cortex and should be considered symptomatic of a focal brain lesion. The symptoms of the seizure reflect the area of the brain involved. For example, there may be convulsive movements of one side or one limb, one-sided sensory symptoms, or bizarre behavior. The latter would suggest a temporal lobe focus. In such cases, the patient will have some degree of confusion during the attack and amnesia afterwards, but can be conscious throughout.

Idiopathic seizures are not associated with any demonstrable brain pathology. These seizures may also be either grand mal or petit mal. The attacks usually begin in childhood and persist into adulthood. The term "epilepsy" refers to this type of disorder.

Seizures beginning in adulthood should be considered symptomatic of *organic* disease. A search for the underlying etiology should be made. In a pregnant woman, the first etiology to consider is eclampsia.

Other organic causes of seizures are:
1. Head injuries
2. Vascular disease; in young women, usually a malformation (arteriovenous malformation, aneurysm)
3. Infections—meningitis, encephalitis, brain abscess
4. Metabolic disorders, such as hypoxia, cardiac arrhythmia or arrest, urinary or liver failure, hypoglycemia, hypocalcemia

5. Toxic causes—usually associated with drug withdrawal, commonly from alcohol or barbiturates
6. Brain tumors
7. Miscellaneous diseases of the brain, such as multiple sclerosis, hereditary disorders, and some dementias.

ANTICONVULSANT THERAPY DURING PREGNANCY

Half of patients with a prior history of seizures will have difficulty with seizure control during pregnancy. There will be a tendency toward recurrence and increased frequency or severity of seizures that may necessitate an increase in medication. Blood levels of anticonvulsant drugs drop during pregnancy. This is thought to be related to increases in blood volume, liver metabolism, and glomerular filtration rate (GFR). Folic acid administration has been shown to lower serum phenytoin (Dilantin) levels.

Pregnant patients with an increased frequency of seizures need increased dosages of anticonvulsant medication. Seizures pose a more serious risk to the mother and fetus than any known toxic effects of anticonvulsant drugs. Despite associated teratogenic risks, it is unwise to stop anticonvulsant medication in pregnant, seizure-free patients because of the risk of recurrent seizures and the possible precipitation of status epilepticus.

In the well-controlled, seizure-free patient, medication dosage should not be increased merely to achieve therapeutic blood levels; this may require very high doses. The important principle is to prevent seizures, not to conform to an arbitrary laboratory standard. But when a seizure occurs in a treated pregnant patient, a determination of anticonvulsant blood levels is helpful in deciding whether to increase dosage or add another drug.

If a pregnant woman is taking an anticonvulsant, the risk of a major malformation in her infant is roughly doubled. The most common abnormalities are cleft lip, cleft palate, and congenital heart defects. A "Dilantin syndrome" (or "phenytoin syndrome") has been described that includes these defects, plus wide-set eyes, low forehead, flat nose, small and low-set ears, and short digits. A "Tridione syndrome" (or "trimethadione syndrome") has also been described. In some series, patients with seizures who were not on anticonvulsant drugs also had an increased incidence of infant malformations. On the basis of currently available reports, it appears that phenytoin carries a higher risk of teratogenicity than phenobarbital. Thus, phenobarbital is the primary drug of choice in the treatment of seizure disorders in pregnancy.

All known anticonvulsants cross the placenta. A withdrawal syndrome in the infant has been reported for phenobarbital. Bleeding tendencies, secondary to phenytoin use, have produced fetal vitamin K deficiency.

If a nonpregnant patient with a seizure disorder contemplates pregnancy, an attempt should be made to control the seizures on phenobarbital alone. Dosage should be adjusted to the lowest level that is effective in preventing seizures. If the patient has a seizure or an aura (indicating impending seizure), phenobarbital dosage should be increased.

We do not recommend changes in anticonvulsant medication other than dosage adjustments during pregnancy. Early in pregnancy, anticonvulsant blood levels should be obtained, since it may be necessary to increase dosage. It is preferable to try increasing the medication the patient is already taking before adding another medication.

If a seizure occurs in a pregnant patient, etiology should be determined. If eclampsia is excluded, phenobarbital 30 mg tid should be started at once. If symptoms recur, dosage should be increased. If potentially toxic levels of phenobarbital are reached but seizures continue, the dosage should be lowered and phenytoin added. The starting dose of phenytoin is 100 mg tid. If any doubt exists as to whether the "blackout" or other bizarre event reported by the patient was actually a seizure, another etiology, such as syncope or hyperventilation, must be considered.

In status epilepticus, the patient has a seizure, remains comatose throughout the postictal period, and has another seizure without waking up. This condition is rare and nearly always associated with a severe, often lethal, disease such as intracranial hemorrhage, meningitis, or drug withdrawal.

ACUTE SEIZURE MANAGEMENT

Seizures always stop. Treatment is not necessary to stop an attack, but to prevent injury to the patient during the attack. In the postictal period, the dangers to the patient are airway obstruction, apnea, and coma.

When a seizure occurs, blood should be drawn for drug levels, glucose, and calcium. Then a bolus of 50 ml of 50% glucose is given if hypoglycemia is present, and drug therapy can proceed. Therapy alternatives for acute seizure control include: 10 mg of diazepam (Valium), 500 mg (10-15 mg/kg) of phenytoin, or 300 mg (5 mg/kg) of phenobarbital. Phenobarbital and diazepam may be given by intravenous push, but phenytoin must be given slowly (over 30 minutes) in a normal saline infusion, since it precipitates in glucose. Diazepam is effective, but wears off in an hour. If convulsions continue, not enough medication has been given. The maximum acceptable phenytoin dosage is 500 mg. High doses of phenobarbital and diazepam in combination will generally be successful in controlling acute attacks. If unsuccessful, surgical anesthesia may be used as ultimate therapy.

SUMMARY

Seizure disorders are associated with a slightly increased risk to the pregnant woman and her infant. With careful management of the illness, a successful outcome can be anticipated.

SUGGESTED READING

Aminoff MJ: Neurological disorders and pregnancy. *Am J Obstet Gynecol* 132:325, 1978

Annegers FJ: Do anticonvulsants have a teratogenic effect? *Arch Neurol* 31:364, 1974

Bjerkedal T, Bahna SL: The course and outcome of pregnancy in women with epilepsy. *Acta Obstet Gynecol Scand* 52:245, 1973

Knight AW, Rhind EG: Epilepsy and pregnancy: A study of 153 pregnancies in 59 patients. *Epilepsia* 16:99, 1975

McClure JH: Idiopathic epilepsy in pregnancy. *Am J Obstet Gynecol* 70:296, 1955

Montouris GD, Fenichel GM, McLain W Jr: The pregnant epileptic. *Arch Neurol* 36:601, 1979

6

Heart Disease in Pregnancy

DAVID B. COTTON, M.D., and THOMAS J. BENEDETTI, M.D.

Heart disease is present in approximately 1:100 pregnancies, and its incidence has been decreasing in recent years. The types of heart disease have also been changing. Because of the decreasing frequency of rheumatic fever and the advances in cardiovascular surgery, fewer patients with rheumatic heart disease and more with congenital heart disease are now entering the childbearing years. At present, nearly 25% of all pregnant cardiac patients have congenital heart disease, either corrected or uncorrected.

An understanding of the usual cardiovascular adjustments to pregnancy will aid in providing optimal care to pregnant patients with cardiac problems. The following section discusses the changes seen in normal pregnancies.

CARDIOVASCULAR CHANGES IN PREGNANCY

Cardiac output is elevated significantly by 12 weeks' gestation, reaches a 50% increase at 29-32 weeks, and remains elevated at this level until labor begins. The resting heart rate increases 10-15 beats per minute (bpm) above baseline level at term.

Blood volume increases rapidly during the first 20-30 weeks and continues to expand until term. The expansion ranges from 20-100% with a mean of 40-50% in normal pregnancies. Plasma volume expands more rapidly than red cell volume, accounting for the physiologic anemia of pregnancy. Twin pregnancies are associated with greater increases in blood volume, and patients with preeclampsia and chronic hypertension have lesser increases than normotensive patients.

Position, labor, and anesthesia all influence the cardiovascular status during pregnancy. The supine position, leading to uterine compression of the inferior vena cava and aorta, can lead to decreased cardiac output. Uterine contractions have a more pronounced effect on cardiac output in this position than in the lateral recumbent position.

Analgesics blunt the tachycardiac response to pain. Careful conduction anesthesia further limits the progressive rise in cardiac output during labor to a greater extent than pudendal or paracervical anesthesia, although more careful monitoring is required with this mode of anesthesia because of the risk of maternal hypotension.

During maternal bearing down in the second stage of labor, rapid fluctuations in venous return to the heart are encountered. The immediate effect is rapid inflow of blood from the lungs to the left atrium, with elevated mean arterial pressure. With the release of held breath, mean arterial pressure transiently falls as the pulmonary vascular bed refills with blood.

During delivery and in the immediate puerperium, there is an increase in cardiac output. This is thought to be secondary to the release of obstruction to venous return and the return of blood to the heart from venous channels in the uterus.

These normal physiologic adjustments are usually well tolerated by a person with a young, healthy heart. However, patients with diseased hearts may have serious difficulties during pregnancy, and especially during labor and delivery.

HEART DISEASE PROBLEMS IN PREGNANCY

Heart disease is conveniently classified using the New York Heart Association's standards. Patients with class I disease (59%) have no limitation in physical activity as a consequence of their heart disease. Patients with class II disease (34%) have dyspnea with strenuous physical activity. Patients with class III disease (6%) have no symptoms at rest, but have to limit themselves to minimal physical activity because of dyspnea. Finally, class IV patients (1%) have symptoms at rest and present a tremendous therapeutic challenge.

The risk of maternal morbidity and mortality is directly related to heart disease classification. In patients with class I and II heart disease, the risk of cardiac failure during pregnancy is 10% or less, and the incidence of maternal mortality is 0.3% or less. With class III heart disease, the risk of failure during pregnancy is 80%, and maternal mortality may be as high as 7%. With class IV heart disease, failure is present in all patients, and maternal mortality may reach 25%. Fetal mortality is increased if heart failure or atrial fibrillation complicates pregnancy. In this group, unexplained intrauterine fetal demise and prematurity account for the majority of fetal deaths. Bed rest and antepartum surveillance may help to reduce the increased perinatal mortality.

The identification of pregnant patients with heart disease can be quite difficult in the absence of a history of heart disease or previous cardiac surgery. Even normal pregnant patients may complain of many symptoms characteristic of heart failure. A systolic flow murmur and S_3 gallop are common findings that should arouse suspicions in a particular patient. However, four clinical findings should serve to alert the physician: (1) diastolic murmur, (2) cardiac enlargement on x-ray, (3) systolic murmur, grade III or greater, and (4) cardiac arrhythmias (atrial fibrillations, atrial flutter, or heart block).

If heart disease is strongly suspected, noninvasive cardiac evaluation by echocardiography and phonocardiography is indicated. Cardiac catheterization is best reserved for the nonpregnant state. The most common lesion of rheumatic heart disease is mitral stenosis. Atrial septal defect is the most common lesion of congenital heart disease.

ANTEPARTUM MANAGEMENT

Antepartum care of the pregnant cardiac patient should be by a team approach, involving both an obstetrician and an internist. Patients should be seen every 1-2 weeks depending on severity of the cardiac disease. (Generally, class I and II patients are seen every other week; class III patients every week.) Class IV patients usually spend the majority of the pregnancy in the hospital.

The two most important parameters used to monitor the status of the pregnant cardiac patient are heart rate and weight. Heart rate greater than 100 bpm or rapid weight gain are often signs of impending cardiac failure. A liberal policy of hospitalization should be used when these signs appear. Bed rest at home should also be encouraged, as this is the easiest and most reliable way to decrease cardiac work load for the mother and, at the same time, increase uteroplacental blood flow.

In patients with rheumatic heart disease, benzathine penicillin G (Bicillin) is given each month as prophylaxis against recurrent episodes of rheumatic fever. The usual dose is 1.2 million units IM. An acceptable alternative is potassium penicillin V (Pen•Vee K), 250 mg orally twice daily. In patients allergic to penicillin, erythromycin, 250 mg orally twice daily, will suffice.

In patients with cardiac lesions that increase the incidence of thromboembolism, prophylactic heparin, 5,000 units subcutaneously every 12 hours, may be used. Digoxin, 0.25-0.375 mg orally per day, should be used in patients who show evidence of cardiac failure. Prophylactic digitalization may be used in selected patients when atrial fibrillation poses a significant risk. In this instance, it is used for its negative chronotropic effect rather than its positive inotropic effect.

All patients should be allowed to go into spontaneous labor unless fetal indications necessitate early delivery or maternal condition deteriorates while at bed rest in the hospital.

INTRAPARTUM MANAGEMENT

Intrapartum management of the heart disease patient can be challenging. Prophylactic antibiotics should be used for the intrapartum period and for 72 hours postpartum. Aqueous crystalline penicillin G, 2.0 million units intramuscularly or intravenously every 8 hours; or gentamicin, 80 mg intramuscularly or intravenously every 8 hours, may be used.

Rapid fluctuations in heart rate are hazardous and should be avoided by appropriate analgesia and anesthesia. Conduction anesthesia (epidural and caudal) will limit cardiovascular fluctuations, but caution must be used to avoid hypotension. Therefore, it is best to use a local anesthetic. Many authors have suggested the lateral recumbent position be used for labor and the Sims position for delivery. These positions may be associated with the least stress to the maternal cardiovascular system.

The second stage of labor should be shortened if possible. However, midforceps procedures may pose a significant risk to mother and fetus. Some clinicians have found the vacuum extractor to be safer under these circumstances. Another alternative is to await descent of the fetal head after complete dilation without Valsalva maneuvers. With this strategy, midforceps delivery may often be avoided in favor of low forceps or spontaneous delivery.

Immediately postpartum, cardiac output may increase and precipitate acute pulmonary edema. This is especially characteristic of mitral stenosis.

CONTRACEPTION IN HEART DISEASE

Postpartum sterilization, if desired by the patient, is best delayed until the cardiovascular system has readjusted to the nonpregnant state—a process that usually takes approximately 6 weeks.

Patients on anticoagulants may experience excessive menstrual bleeding and intraperitoneal hemorrhage from ruptured corpus luteum cysts. Patients with organic heart disease who require anticoagulants are advised to select oral contraception. This is a highly effective method and also reduces the chance of intraperitoneal bleeding by suppressing ovulation. The concomitant use of anticoagulants diminishes the risk of thromboembolic disease related to oral contraceptives. In patients with a history of thromboembolism, hypertension, and/or a cardiac lesion that predisposes to an increased risk of thromboembolism, oral contraceptives are contraindicated unless anticoagulant therapy is also being given.

Barrier methods of contraception (diaphragm; foam and condom) may be offered to women with organic heart disease. But reduced efficacy of these methods limits their use in women for whom pregnancy presents a life-threatening challenge.

Finally, some clinicians have suggested that the IUD is an acceptable form of contraception for patients with organic heart disease.

SUGGESTED READING

Brenner PF, Mishell DR Jr: Contraception for the woman with significant cardiac disease. *Clin Obstet Gynecol* 18:155, 1975

Spielman FJ, Popio KA: Pregnancy and Heart Disease. Key References (155). *Circulation* 65:831, 1982

7

Hypothyroidism in Pregnancy

MARTIN MONTORO, M.D.

Pregnancy in women with hypothyroidism is considered to be very rare. In fact, until 1980 a review of the literature back to 1897 revealed only 36 reasonably well-documented cases. However, in most of the cases the diagnosis of hypothyroidism was based on clinical grounds alone. Only in the few more recent reports was the clinical suspicion confirmed by measurement of thyroid hormone levels. These recent reports are seldom mentioned except to illustrate how rarely pregnancy occurs in hypothyroidism. The outcome of these pregnancies was generally good (86% live births) and without excessive complications (8% stillbirths and 6% abortions).

But most obstetric and endocrinologic literature refers to older reports from the last 20-30 years describing frequent poor outcomes of those pregnancies that did occur in hypothyroid women: twice the average incidence of abortions, 20% perinatal mortality, high incidence of congenital anomalies (10-20% or more), and, above all, impaired mental and somatic development in 50-60% of the surviving children.

However, close scrutiny reveals that the exact thyroid status of the women described is unclear. Diagnoses were generally based on what is described as hypothyroxinemia, or failure of the protein-bound or butanol-extractable iodines to increase as expected during pregnancy. Neither TSH (thyroid-stimulating hormone) concentrations nor other more accurate determinations of thyroid status were obtained. And the authors did not suggest any explanations for the mechanisms causing the severe complications they described.

Thus, the literature contains controversial data on the effects of hypothyroidism on gestation and offspring. There are a few isolated reports of reasonably well-documented hypothyroidism without excessive complications and more extensive reports with many complications but no good evidence that they were caused by hypothyroidism.

A RECENT STUDY

At the University of Southern California, we had the opportunity to study 11 hypothyroid women during 13 pregnancies and follow the infants for up to 3 years so far. This is the largest series reported to date in which the diagnosis of hypothyroidism is unequivocally documented by currently available, accurate determinations of thyroid function. Based on the number of infants delivered at our institution during the 5 years of study, the frequency was approximately 1:5,000 pregnancies.

All our patients had primary hypothyroidism. In 8 of the 13 pregnancies, the patients first presented untreated after the 24th week. The remainder were first seen after the first trimester. They had a similar incidence of signs and symptoms of hypothyroidism as reported for larger series of nonpregnant hypothyroid patients: 3 were asymptomatic, 5 had several signs and symptoms, and the remainder of the patients presented with most of the classic signs and symptoms.

The incidence of types of hypothyroidism was also similar to that seen among nonpregnant hypothyroid patients: 5 had iatrogenic hypothyroidism (4 remote thyroidectomy, 1 remote ^{131}I therapy), 2 Hashimoto's thyroiditis, and 4 idiopathic primary hypothyroidism.

In the 2 patients with Hashimoto's thyroiditis, who were the only ones with a palpable goiter, the diagnosis was made during pregnancy. The past medical history was the clue to the diagnosis in the asymptomatic patients without goiter. The other patients' diagnosis was known, but no thyroid hormone replacement had been taken for at least 6-8 months before conception.

In 4 patients, gestation was completed without treatment. The remaining patients, after evaluation, received L-thyroxine 0.15 mg/day PO, or higher doses depending on individual clinical response and measurement of plasma T_4 and TSH.

In the 13 pregnancies we studied, outcome was as follows: 1 first-trimester spontaneous abortion, 1 stillbirth at 29 weeks in the only patient who developed preeclampsia, and 11 live births of infants of normal weight with Apgar scores of 9. All placentas were normal. The 11 infants were clinically and biochemically euthyroid and without goiter. Only one infant was born with anomalies: Down's syndrome and an ostium primum with common atrioventricular canal. The mother's age was 41.

The children have been followed for up to 3 years. Except for the child with Down's syndrome, they are developing normally and have normal thyroid function. The child with Down's syndrome has severe developmental delay, but his thyroid function remains normal.

In all these cases conception, embryogenesis, and most of the fetal development occurred in the presence of maternal hypothyroidism. But the incidence of complications was much lower than is usually reported.

However, our results are in agreement with current research. It is now well accepted that the placenta is practically impermeable to T_4, T_3, and TSH. But the fetal hypothalamic-pituitary-thyroid axis seems to develop and function independently from the mother and does not need maternal thyroid hormone for support. The fact that the infants of our hypothyroid mothers were euthyroid at birth supports that view. It thus appears that if maternal hypothyroidism affects the fetus at all, it must do so indirectly and in ways that have yet to be demonstrated.

Although longer follow-up of the children is needed, the information thus far justifies some optimism. Based on our own data and on the few other well-documented cases, we do not think that pregnant hypothyroid women should be discouraged from carrying their pregnancies to term.

THYROID REPLACEMENT THERAPY

Treatment should be instituted once the diagnosis is made, as in any patient with hypothyroidism. Since most pregnant women are young and without cardiovascular disease, therapy can usually be started with 0.075-0.1 mg of oral L-thyroxine per day. Though we prefer L-thyroxine, equivalent doses of desiccated thyroid can be used. After 2 weeks, the dosage can be increased to 0.15 mg, according to the response and plasma levels of T_4 and TSH.

In patients with severe hypothyroidism of long duration or associated cardiovascular disease, replacement should be instituted more slowly, as would be done in older patients. Therapy is started with 0.025-0.05 mg PO daily, with biweekly increments of 0.025-0.05 mg until the usual replacement dose is reached, generally 0.15 mg/day.

Some women may require higher doses during pregnancy; to determine this, thyroid hormones and TSH should be monitored. Ideally, T_4 should be kept in the upper normal range, with the free-T_4 index and TSH levels normal. Therapy should be continued during pregnancy in patients with a history of hypothyroidism who are already receiving adequate replacement. If there is any question about the diagnosis of hypothyroidism and the need for thyroid replacement, proper investigation should wait until after delivery.

SUGGESTED READING

Echt CR, Doss JF: Myxedema in pregnancy: Report of three cases. *Obstet Gynecol* 22:615, 1963

Fisher DA, Klein AH: Thyroid development and disorders of thyroid function in the newborn. *N Engl J Med* 304:702, 1981

Jones WS, Man EB: Thyroid function in human pregnancy. VI. Premature deliveries and reproductive failure of pregnant women with low butanol extractable iodines. *Am J Obstet Gynecol* 104:909, 1969

Man EB: Maternal hypothyroxinemia, development of a 4 and 7 year old offspring. In Fisher DA, Burrow GN, eds: *Perinatal Thyroid Physiology and Disease*. New York: Raven Press, 1975, pp 117-132

Montoro M, Collea JV, Frasier D, Mestman JH: Successful outcome of pregnancy in women with hypothyroidism. *Ann Int Med* 94:31, 1981

Refetoff S: Thyroid hormone therapy. *Med Clin North Am* 59:1147, 1975

8

Rh Erythroblastosis Fetalis: Diagnosis

ANDREW I. BRILL, M.D., and LAWRENCE D. PLATT, M.D.

HISTORY

Although erythroblastosis fetalis was probably first recorded by Hippocrates in 400 B.C., its etiology remained without convincing elucidation until the discovery of the Rh blood group system in 1940 by Landsteiner and colleagues. Shortly thereafter, Levine and co-workers demonstrated the central role of Rh-antigen incompatibility in a reported pregnancy complicated by maternal transfusion reaction that ended in hydropic stillbirth. A modern concept of maternal immunologic intolerance for a foreign fetal blood-cell antigen then emerged. Despite conceptual insight, however, perinatal mortality remained at 40-50%.

Wallerstein, in 1946, introduced the use of exchange transfusion. This nearly halved the neonatal mortality. His original use of the sagittal sinus for transfusion was later modified by Diamond, who successfully used umbilical vessels for cannulation.

The actual relationship between hyperbilirubinemia from fetal hemolysis and subsequent newborn kernicterus was demonstrated by Allen in 1950. This helped explain how exchange transfusion improved neonatal outcome.

Despite these advances, there still remained no help for the erythroblastotic infant doomed to die of hydrops fetalis before term. Starting in 1954, induction of labor at as early as 32 weeks' gestation was instituted, based on either high maternal Rh-antibody titers or the poor outcome of previously affected pregnancies. Mortality rates were further reduced to less than 20%. However, correct prediction of actual severity of disease based on titer and history alone was accurate only 62% of the time.

Critical work by Bevis in 1956, using spectrophotometric analysis of fluids obtained by amniocentesis, established the inseparable relationship between amniotic fluid bilirubin concentration and the severity of disease in utero. This provided the first reliable tool for antenatal assessment of potentially hydropic fetuses.

In 1957, Kleihauer and Betke developed a differential staining technique to identify and quantitate fetal red blood cells in the maternal circulation. Beyond its immediate clinical applicability, this technique served to cement the thesis of transplacental passage of fetal red blood cells.

Using established techniques, in the early 1960s Liley developed a graphic means of evaluating normal versus abnormal amniotic fluid bilirubin trends in affected pregnancies. He then reported the first successful intrauterine transfusion: After accidentally puncturing the fetal abdomen during amniocentesis, he injected blood into the fetus. With intrauterine transfusion, overall mortality dropped to nearly 10%.

Based on a thoroughly investigated pathogenetic model for erythroblastosis fetalis, and data obtained using Kleihauer-Betke staining that detected most fetal cells passing into maternal circulation, independent American and British teams set forth to develop preventive, passive immunization for Rh-sensitization. In 1966, Freda et al reported successful prevention of sensitization by administration of an anti-Rh antibody preparation following delivery. It was released for general use in 1968, under the trade name RhoGAM.

Bowman and co-workers in Canada have now demonstrated further reduction of maternal sensitization by prophylactic administration of RhoGAM in the late second and early third trimesters of pregnancy. Recently, this treatment has been gaining wider acceptance in the United States.

Thus, after a relatively short period of distinguished efforts, the enigma of erythroblastosis fetalis was unraveled. Its clinical description has long been well known. The newer discoveries about its pathogenesis, which became the basis for its prevention, broke down into three prerequisite principles: (1) the existence of a maternal-fetal red-cell-antigen incompatibility; (2) the maternal ability to develop a specific and potentially destructive antibody against this foreign antigen; and (3) the entrance of this maternal antibody into the fetal circulation, causing hemolysis and subsequent hydrops.

Unhindered, this biologically determined cycle would fatally affect up to 50% of infants from sensitized pregnancies. The implementation of early delivery, prenatal analysis, and finally intrauterine transfusion cut this staggering mortality to nearly 10%. With the introduction of RhoGAM, along with a heightened clinical consciousness, the sensitized woman is fortunately becoming an infrequent clinical problem.

SENSITIZATION AND INCIDENCE

In the classic case, the unsensitized Rh-negative pregnant woman is exposed to Rh-positive cells by fetal transplacental hemorrhage. The Kleihauer-Betke technique has provided a sensitive method for detecting its incidence and relative magnitude. Nearly 50% of studied cases demonstrate evidence of transplacental hemorrhage during pregnancy or immediately postpartum. The incidence increases as gestation progresses: Up to 7% in the first trimester, 16% by the second, and 30% by the third trimester show positive evidence of fetal cells in the maternal circulation.

Fetal-maternal hemorrhage may be increased with antepartum bleeding, cesarean section, manual removal of the placenta, tumultuous labor, midforceps delivery, and toxemia. Significant fetal-maternal hemorrhage may occur with ectopic pregnancy and abortion. Amniocentesis is not without risk; it is well known to be another cause of fetal-maternal hemorrhage. Retrospective analysis of second-trimester genetic amniocentesis in our institution revealed a net sensitization rate of 5.4% at term in fetuses at risk. In addition to pregnancy-related events, sensitization may occur from incompatible transfusions of blood or blood products, or immunizations when human serum is used.

Naturally, the amount of transplacental hemorrhage influences the risk of isoimmunization. In 8% of Rh-negative women, demonstrable sensitization occurs within 6 months postpartum after the first Rh-positive, ABO-compatible pregnancy. Most often, primary exposure to a foreign antigen during pregnancy results in little antibody production, but significant immunologic memory. A subsequent Rh-incompatible pregnancy will usually provoke an anamnestic response, and also carry a general risk of 8%. Thus, the overall risk is 16%. As parity increases, the anamnestic response may diminish, reaching an acme of risk of 50% by the fifth Rh-incompatible pregnancy.

In contrast, ABO incompatibility of the Rh-positive fetus confers some protection against sensitization, probably by somehow interfering with immunologic recognition of Rh-antigen sites on the red blood cell membrane. Here, the overall risk is reduced to nearly 2%.

And, finally, up to 2% of first Rh-positive pregnancies in Rh-negative women will result in sensitization during gestation or within 3 days postpartum.

DETECTION OF THE AFFECTED PREGNANCY

Management of isoimmunization is critically dependent upon identifying mothers at risk and detecting sensitization. The first prenatal visit requires a blood sample for blood grouping and antibody screening. Approximately 17% of a mixed Caucasian population will lack the Rh antigen. In sharp contrast, most Orientals are Rh-positive. All Rh-negative women with negative antibody screens are at risk for isoimmunization during pregnancy.

It is essential to determine both the identity and nature of any blood group antibody. Although 98% of reported cases of erythroblastosis fetalis involve either ABO or Rh incompatibilities, there are at least 30 other irregular blood group antigens associated with this disease. Thus, the presence of a non-Rh antibody does not preclude the development of hydrops fetalis.

Rh-positive patients deserve to be rescreened at least once during pregnancy in order to eliminate any possible laboratory error. In confirmed Rh-positive patients with no irregular antibodies, only normal prenatal follow-up is required.

Rh-negative mothers without detectable Rh or irregular antibodies require monthly rescreening after 22 weeks to rule out developing sensitization. (A paternal blood sample is also essential and should be submitted for blood grouping and Rh genotype.) Patients without detectable antibodies should be expected to deliver without complication at term. The development of a detectable maternal Rh-antibody titer indicates sensitization and requires further diagnostic attention. Rh-positive mothers with detectable non-Rh-associated antibody should be treated with equivalent precautions.

The reported titer is often dependent upon laboratory technique, and, thus, may vary between different centers. The obstetrician must become familiar with both the methods used and the significance of values reported by the laboratory doing the testing.

In our own laboratory, in a first sensitized pregnancy, or in subsequent pregnancies when prior ones required no exchange transfusion, an albumin titer of 1:8 or less has not been associated with a stillbirth. On the other hand, with a titer of 1:16 or greater, or a previous history of affected fetuses, the risk of hydrops becomes very real. These cases should be managed according to the technique described in the next chapter.

SUGGESTED READING

Allen FH Jr, Diamond LK, Vaughan VC III: Erythroblastosis fetalis. VI. Prevention of kernicterus. *Am J Dis Child* 80:779, 1950

Bevis, DCA: Blood pigments in haemolytic disease of the newborn. *J Obstet Gynaecol Br Emp* 63:68, 1956

Bowman JM, Pollock JM: Antenatal prophylaxis of Rh isoimmunization: 28-weeks'-gestation service program. *Can Med Assoc J* 118:627, 1978

Diamond LK: Erythroblastosis foetalis or haemolytic disease of the newborn. *Proc R Soc Med* 40:546, 1947

Freda VJ, Gorman JG, Pollack W: Rh factor: Prevention of isoimmunization and clinical trial on mothers. *Science* 151:828, 1966

Hill LM, Platt LD, Kellog B: Rh sensitization after genetic amniocentesis. *Obstet Gynecol* 56:459, 1980

Kleihauer E, Braun M, Betke K: Demonstration von foetalen Haemoglobin in den Erythrocyten eines Blutausstrichs. *Klin Wochenschr* 35:637, 1957

Landsteiner K, Wiener A: An agglutinable factor in human blood recognized by immune sera for Rhesus blood. *Soc Exp Biol NY* 43:223, 1940

Levine P, Katzin P, Burnham L: Isoimmunization in pregnancy. *JAMA* 116:825, 1941

Liley AW: Liquor amnii analysis in management of pregnancy complicated by rhesus sensitization. *Am J Obstet Gynecol* 82:1359, 1961

Queenan JT, ed: *Modern Management of the Rh Problem*, ed 2. Hagerstown, Md: Harper & Row, 1977

Scott JR: Isoimmunization in pregnancy. *Clin Obstet Gynecol* 25:241, 1982

Wallerstein H: Treatment of severe erythroblastosis by simultaneous removal and replacement of the blood of the newborn infant. *Science* 103:583, 1946

9

Rh Erythroblastosis Fetalis: Management

ANDREW I. BRILL, M.D., and LAWRENCE D. PLATT, M.D.

DETERMINING FETAL STATUS

Since fetal status is reflected by bilirubin components measurable in the surrounding amniotic fluid, amniocentesis provides the best estimate, although static, of fetal intravascular hemolysis. In our institution, amniocentesis for amniotic fluid analysis is considered mandatory when the maternal albumin titer is 1:16 or greater. This first tap may be performed as early as 20 weeks when intrauterine transfusion is technically feasible. Regardless of titer, women with obstetric histories of previous stillbirth, intrauterine transfusion, or the need for neonatal exchange transfusion also deserve analysis this early in gestation. We recommend that amniocentesis be done under ultrasound guidance to reduce the incidence of traumatic taps. In a study at our institution, we have shown that real-time, B-scan-directed amniocentesis successfully accomplishes this goal.

Once obtained, the amniotic fluid is centrifuged and filtered to remove debris, and placed in a brown bottle to prevent photo-oxidation of the bilirubin. A separate aliquot is set aside for pulmonary maturity studies. Using a spectrophotometer, optical densities are then measured over a range of 350-700 mμ and recorded on graph paper (see Fig. 9-1). Normally, a smooth sloping curve appears with increasing absorbance of incident light at shorter wavelengths. Affected pregnancies demonstrate a characteristic rise, or hump, in optical density peaking at 450 mμ, secondary to bilirubin and associated hemoglobin breakdown products. This rise from the curve may be used as a reliable indicator of the degree of fetal disease.

The deviation from normal is then quantitated by drawing a straight line tangent to the curve connecting points at 375 and 525 mμ, and measuring the vertical distance (in units of optical density) between the line and the peak of the hump at 450 mμ. The value obtained is referred to as the ΔOD 450.

Using the Liley method, the ΔOD 450 is plotted on a graph where the vertical axis is logarithmic and in units of optical density, while the horizontal axis is linear and in units of weeks of gestation. Thus, successive ΔOD 450 measurements are plotted against weeks of estimated gestational age.

FIGURE 9-1

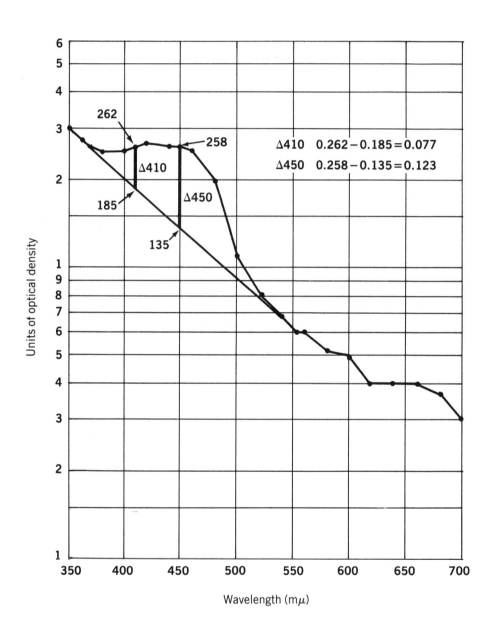

Plot of optical density against wavelength, showing peak around 450 mμ due to bilirubin and associated hemoglobin breakdown products in amniotic fluid.

The graph is divided into three oblique zones of prognostic significance with downward sloping parallel lines from left to right. Values falling in the upper zone (zone 3) are usually ominous and signify impending death. Those falling in the intermediate zone (zone 2) usually indicate moderate disease. Values falling in the upper 80% of zone 2 are more worrisome; lower values are more reassuring. Values falling in the lower 20% of zone 2 or in zone 1 may reflect either a normal infant or one who will require exchange transfusion after delivery.

Although single values on the Liley graph may be predictive, a series of examinations and plottings on the graph establishes a valuable trend. The trend indicates the course of intrauterine disease more reliably than an individual value. In our institution, amniocentesis is repeated in 3 weeks when the plots remain in zone 1; 2 weeks if in low zone 2; 1 week if in high zone 2 with a downward trend; and sooner with a rising trend in high zone 2. Plots in zone 3 are ominous and require immediate plans for either intrauterine transfusion or delivery of the fetus.

ANTEPARTUM AND INTRAPARTUM MANAGEMENT

Some authors recommend that intrauterine transfusion be considered for trends in high zone 2 if the gestational age is less than 30 weeks. When the trend remains in low zone 2 or in zone 1, the pregnancy is generally allowed to go to term. With a mature L/S ratio and a trend rising to high zone 2 or into zone 3 at 34 weeks, delivery is instituted. With an immature L/S ratio, intrauterine transfusion is considered.

Intrauterine transfusion may be repeated up to every 2 weeks. The risk to the fetus increases with the number of procedures; overall fetal risk is 10-15%. Success is poor in the presence of fetal ascites. In place of fluoroscopy, we now use real-time B-scan to aid in the actual transfusion. This technique reduces antenatal exposure to x-rays and lowers fetal risk. Since the introduction of antenatal corticosteroids for acceleration of fetal lung maturation, in many centers steroids are administered to mothers of severely affected fetuses and early delivery is instituted. With this procedure, the significant risks of intrauterine transfusion are avoided.

After intrauterine transfusion, delivery is dependent upon a number of interrelated variables, including pulmonary maturity, reliability of estimated gestational age, the outcome of previously affected pregnancies, the Liley graphic trend, and the presence or absence of hydrops. Consideration must be given to whether vaginal delivery might exert undue stress upon an affected fetus. We have elected to deliver patients by cesarean section to ensure optimal conditions and pediatric attendance at delivery. Ultimately, early delivery with maximum surveillance is desired.

Adequate preparation for delivery demands communication with an alerted pediatric team, and available frozen type O, Rh-negative, buffy-coat-free, packed red blood cells, crossmatched with maternal serum, in case neonatal transfusion is needed in the delivery suite.

PREVENTION

Since the availability of RhoGAM, the incidence of Rh-isoimmunization has fallen dramatically. The protective effect is dose-dependent. A single dose of 300 μg appears to suppress the immune response to up to 30 ml of whole Rh-positive blood or 15 ml of packed cells. Transplacental hemorrhage greater than this occurs in approximately 1:300 pregnancies at risk, leading to a net failure rate of only 0.3%. The Kleihauer-Betke or Fetaldex stain may be used to help assess suspected large transplacental hemorrhage. Since the Rh antigen has been detected in the fetus as early as 38 days after conception, the risk of sensitization from abortion in the first trimester or later is real and estimated to range from 2% to 4%. The presence of the Rh antigen group variant, D^u, in an Rh-negative mother may protect her from sensitization.

In our institution, indications for RhoGAM administration include: (1) completion of any term pregnancy in which the mother lacks both Rh and D antigens and has no previous history of exposure, and the infant is Rh-positive and/or D-positive with a negative direct Coombs test; (2) ectopic pregnancy in an Rh-negative woman; (3) amniocentesis performed on an Rh-negative woman whose husband is not known to be Rh-negative; (4) abortion in an Rh-negative woman; (5) antepartum transplacental hemorrhage in an Rh-negative woman as demonstrated by the Kleihauer-Betke method; and (6) incompatible transfusion of Rh-positive blood or blood products. It should be emphasized that the Rh-negative mother with an atypical antibody is still a RhoGAM candidate. Naturally, previous exposure and sensitization make attempted prophylaxis useless in any case.

Reduced doses of RhoGAM have been successfully used in preventing sensitization from abortion. (Vials containing only 50 μg are commercially available under the trade name MICRhoGAM.) Nevertheless, if bleeding is felt to be excessive, quantitative staining techniques should be done, and extra RhoGAM given as indicated. Optimally, RhoGAM should be administered within the first 72 hours postpartum.

Canadian studies have recently demonstrated that antenatal administration of Rh immune globulin at 28 weeks is remarkably effective in preventing sensitization. This recommendation, although not universally accepted as without risk to mother or fetus, has become part of the official recommendation of the American College of Obstetricians and Gynecologists for the use of Rh immune globulin. Those few unsensitized women developing antibodies during gestation are the potential beneficiaries.

Active research has recently begun into oral desensitization by the creation of an intestinal IgA antibody that supersedes the endogenous IgG antibody. This enterically induced immunologic tolerance method may prove to be quite beneficial for the patient with severe sensitization.

CONCLUSION

Given the high mortality of fetal hydrops prior to 22 weeks' gestation, the morbidity of intrauterine transfusion, and the inherent inaccuracies in present modes of prediction, further reduction in overall mortality from erythroblastosis fetalis can come only through eradication of Rh-isoimmunization. This attendant burden must therefore rest upon every physician who is associated with the care of women. Ideally, the virtual elimination of erythroblastosis fetalis is in sight.

SUGGESTED READING

Bierme C, Blanc M, Abbal M, Bournier A: Oral treatment for severely immunized mothers. *Lancet* 1:604, 1979

Liley AW: Intrauterine transfusion of foetus in hemolytic disease. *Br Med J* 21:1107, 1963

Liley AW: Liquor amnii analysis in management of pregnancy complicated by rhesus sensitization. *Am J Obstet Gynecol* 82:1359, 1961

Lim OW, Fleisher AA, Ziel HK: Reduction of Rho(o) sensitization. A cost effective analysis. *Obstet Gynecol* 59:477, 1982

Mauth JC, Brekken AL, Pollack W: Plasmapheresis as an adjunct to management of Rh isoimmunization. *Obstet Gynecol* 57:132, 1981

Platt LD, Keegan KA, Druzin MD, Gauthier RJ, Everlsu LR, Manning FA: Intrauterine transfusion utilizing linear array real time B-scan. A preliminary report. *Am J Obstet Gynecol* 135:1115, 1979

Queenan JT, ed: *Modern Management of the Rh Problem*, ed 2. Hagerstown, Md: Harper & Row, 1977

Scott JR: Isoimmunization in pregnancy. *Clin Obstet Gynecol* 25:241, 1982

10

Thrombophlebitis and Pulmonary Embolism in Pregnancy: Diagnosis

MARGARET LYNN YONEKURA, M.D.

The diagnosis and management of deep venous thrombosis, thrombophlebitis, and pulmonary embolism in pregnancy remain controversial subjects even today. Yet therapeutic decisions can have a significant impact; as maternal deaths from hemorrhage, eclampsia, and sepsis have decreased, pulmonary embolism has become a leading cause of maternal mortality in many obstetric services.

INCIDENCE

Fortunately, thrombophlebitis and pulmonary embolism are rare in pregnancy. The incidence of antepartum deep venous thrombophlebitis varies from 0.018% to 0.29% of deliveries. Postpartum, the incidence of thrombophlebitis increases to 0.1-1.0% of deliveries; hence 70-80% of cases occur postpartum. More important, approximately 24% of antepartum patients with deep venous thrombophlebitis will develop pulmonary embolism if they are not treated, and this is associated with a maternal mortality rate of 15-18%. In patients receiving anticoagulants, the incidence of embolism decreases to 4.5%, and the maternal mortality rate falls to 0.7%.

PATHOGENESIS

The pathogenesis of thrombophlebitis and pulmonary embolism in pregnancy is still not completely understood. However, certain physiologic changes of pregnancy predispose to thrombosis. There is increased venous stasis in the lower extremities, particularly in late pregnancy. This is brought about by both hormonal effects causing increased venous distensibility and the mechanical effect of the gravid uterus impeding venous return. The increased bed rest often recommended in pregnancy may also augment venous stasis.

Pregnancy is associated with significant changes in circulating clotting factors. In particular, the levels of fibrinogen and factors VII, VIII, and X show a substantial rise; antithrombin III levels decrease; and the plasma shows an increased capacity to neutralize heparin in late pregnancy. Fibrinolytic activity in the circulating blood is also decreased in late pregnancy, and the amount of plasminogen activator that can be released from the venous endothelium is greatly reduced. Moreover, in the early puerperium there is a further increase in fibrinogen and factors VII, IX, and X, as well as activation of the fibrinolytic system. All these effects return to normal by the third or fourth week postpartum.

Hence, it is easy to understand why pregnancy is associated with a hypercoagulable state. But it remains a mystery why the majority of cases of thrombophlebitis and pulmonary embolism occur during the puerperium rather than antepartum. Perhaps various intrapartum events produce alterations or damage to venous intima, thus completing Virchow's triad of factors predisposing to venous thrombosis (i.e., venous stasis, hypercoagulability, and endothelial injury). For example, it has been shown that cesarean section, instrumental delivery, and prolonged elevation of the legs in stirrups all predispose to venous thrombosis and/or pulmonary embolism. In addition, lactation suppression with estrogen compounds has been shown to cause a 10-fold increase in the incidence of thromboembolism in postpartum women.

DIAGNOSIS OF VENOUS THROMBOSIS

The diagnosis of deep venous thrombosis during pregnancy is often difficult and requires a high index of suspicion and the use of confirming laboratory tests. The normal discomforts of pregnancy may mimic the symptoms of leg vein thrombosis. Leg cramps, swelling of the ankles, slight cyanosis of the legs on standing, and increased prominence of the superficial veins are often seen, especially in late pregnancy. However, venous thrombosis will almost invariably cause more symptoms in one leg than in the other. The diagnosis of deep venous thrombosis is almost certain when there is *unilateral* calf tenderness, swelling, and increased warmth of the extremity, associated with a positive Homans' sign. Examination of the legs should include the comparison of specific measurements of the calves and thighs at points equidistant bilaterally from the patella. A difference of 2 cm or more at identical sites should be regarded as significant.

The greatest diagnostic problem occurs with patients in whom these clinical signs are either absent or equivocal. Moreover, studies have shown that up to 50% of patients with an almost certain clinical diagnosis of deep venous thrombosis have entirely normal venograms. Therefore, it is mandatory that, whenever possible, an objective diagnostic technique be used to confirm the suspected diagnosis.

The most accurate and precise diagnostic test for deep venous thrombosis is ascending phlebography, commonly known as venography. When performed by a skilled radiologist, phlebography detects at least 95% of peripheral thrombi, and can provide information not only about the presence of a thrombus, but also its exact position, size, and whether it is loose or adherent to the vein wall. At our institution, 1,000 cc of dilute (50-60%) Renografin are injected into a vein on the dorsum of the foot; and the whole venous system of the leg, including the external and common iliac veins, is examined. When the mother's abdomen is shielded with a lead apron, contrast phlebography presents minimal radiation risk to the fetus and may prove to be very beneficial to the mother, especially if no thrombus is found and anticoagulation therapy can be avoided.

Leg scanning using [^{125}I]fibrinogen, the most reliable method for detecting developing calf thrombi, is contraindicated in pregnancy because the radioactive iodine crosses the placenta and is concentrated in the fetal thyroid. In addition, [^{125}I]fibrinogen given in the puerperium will result in secretion of radioactive iodine in the breast milk and lochia. For these reasons, [^{125}I]fibrinogen has rarely been used in pregnancy and the puerperium.

Two noninvasive techniques, Doppler ultrasonography and impedance plethysmography, are currently being used in some centers to diagnose deep venous thrombosis. However, these techniques accurately demonstrate only thrombi obstructing larger veins, such as the femoral and iliac veins. They are completely unable to detect calf vein thrombosis. Therefore, we recommend that one of these noninvasive techniques be used initially, as a screening test. Venograms will then be necessary only in patients with negative studies to rule out calf vein thrombosis.

DIAGNOSIS OF PULMONARY EMBOLISM

The clinical diagnosis of pulmonary embolism during pregnancy can be equally difficult. The immediate effects of an embolus can vary from a total absence of symptoms to sudden death, depending on the size of the embolus and the patient's underlying state of health.

The classic symptoms of massive pulmonary embolism are sudden collapse, chest pain, and air hunger. The predominant clinical signs are tachypnea associated with dyspnea, cyanosis, and jugular vein distension. Hemoptysis, pleuritic chest pain, cough, and friction rub are not usually features of massive embolism, but are more likely from small emboli causing peripheral pulmonary infarction. Unfortunately, as many as 50-80% of pulmonary emboli present without premonitory signs of peripheral venous thrombosis, even though 75% arise from thrombi in veins of the lower extremities.

As with deep venous thrombosis, the clinical diagnosis of pulmonary embolism is subject to error. Therefore, whenever pulmonary embolism is suspected, arterial blood gases, a chest x-ray with the abdomen shielded, an electrocardiogram, and a ventilation-perfusion lung scan should be obtained.

Although measurement of arterial blood gases is a nonspecific test, it is extremely unusual for a patient with a significant pulmonary embolus to have an arterial $pO_2 > 80$ mm Hg on room air. The chest x-ray may be normal. But it also may show diminished vascular markings in the area of the embolus, or early evidence of pulmonary infarction with an infiltrate, elevation of the diaphragmatic dome, and pleural effusion.

Major embolism is associated with characteristic ECG changes consistent with acute right heart strain, the $S_1Q_3T_3$ pattern. However, the ECG may be normal if the embolus is small, or it may reveal only sinus tachycardia.

A combination ventilation-perfusion lung scan is the most accurate method for diagnosing or excluding pulmonary embolism, particularly when the chest x-ray is normal. The lung scan is performed using microspheres or albumin macroaggregates labeled with technetium. The biologic half-life of ^{99m}Tc is about 6 hours. The dose required for the scan results in extremely low radiation exposure to the fetus, since the material is held in the lung and very little crosses the placenta. A dose of 1 millicurie given to the mother results in an estimated fetal exposure of 0.002 rad, equivalent to that of a single abdominal x-ray. One millicurie is sufficient for a quality lung scan.

The definitive diagnostic technique for pulmonary embolism is pulmonary angiography. But experience with this technique in pregnancy is limited, and most authors recommend its use only if surgical therapy, i.e., embolectomy, is indicated.

SUGGESTED READING

Aaro LA, Juergeno JL: Thrombophlebitis associated with pregnancy. *Am J Obstet Gynecol* 109:1128, 1971

Barnes RW, Russell HE, Wu KK, et al: Accuracy of Doppler ultrasound in clinically suspected venous thrombosis of the calf. *Surg Gynecol Obstet* 143:425, 1976

Bergquist A, Bergquist D, Hallbook T: Acute deep vein thrombosis after cesarean section. *Acta Obstet Gynecol Scand* 58:473, 1979

Bonnar J: Venous thrombo-embolism and pregnancy. In Stallworthy J, Bourne G, eds: *Recent Advances in Obstetrics and Gynaecology, No. 13*. New York: Churchill Livingstone, 1979, p 173

Clarke-Pearson DL, Creasman WT: Diagnosis of deep vein thrombosis in obstetrics and gynecology by impedance phlebography. *Obstet Gynecol* 58:52, 1981

Flessa HC, et al: Thromboembolic disorders in pregnancy: Pathophysiology, diagnosis, and treatment with emphasis on heparin. *Clin Obstet Gynecol* 17:195, 1974

Henderson SR, et al: Antepartum pulmonary embolism. *Am J Obstet Gynecol* 93:142, 1965

Laros RK, Alger LS: Thromboembolism and pregnancy. *Clin Obstet Gynecol* 22:871, 1979

Sashara AA: Clinical and physiological studies in pulmonary thromboembolism. *Am J Cardiol* 20:10, 1967

Villasanta U: Thromboembolic disease in pregnancy. *Am J Obstet Gynecol* 93:142, 1965

11

Thrombophlebitis and Pulmonary Embolism in Pregnancy: Management

MARGARET LYNN YONEKURA, M.D.

The management goals in cases of deep venous thrombosis and/or pulmonary embolism are to improve venous flow in the lower extremities and to prevent clot propagation or further embolization.

ACUTE MANAGEMENT

Venous flow in the legs can be improved by initial bed rest in the Trendelenburg position until the acute symptoms of thrombophlebitis subside. Elevation of just the leg causes flexion of the leg at the thigh, promoting stasis in the femoral vein and possible progression of phlebitis. For this reason, elevation of the foot of the bed 6-8 inches without flexion of the bed at the patient's knees or thighs is desirable.

Exercise of the affected leg should be restricted only by the symptom of pain. Mobilization and leg exercises are of vital importance in opening up collateral venous channels, thereby preventing long-term venous insufficiency. During effective anticoagulation therapy, active mobilization in order to reduce venous stasis is no longer regarded as causing an increased risk of thromboembolism. Support panty hose designed for use during pregnancy or specially designed Jobst stockings should also be used to help promote venous return.

Anticoagulation will prevent initial or recurrent embolization in the majority of patients with deep venous thrombosis or pulmonary embolism. Most authorities agree that the initial pharmacologic approach should be with continuous intravenous heparin. Its high molecular weight of approximately 12,000 and its high anionic charge prevent heparin from crossing the placenta or from being secreted in breast milk. Hence, it appears to be the safest anticoagulant to use during pregnancy.

Heparin interferes with coagulation at several sites. However, its primary action is believed to be enhancement of the effects of a plasma alpha$_2$ globulin known as heparin cofactor (probably identical to antithrombin III), which blocks the conversion of fibrinogen to fibrin. This heparin cofactor also inhibits activated factor X, blocking the conversion of prothrombin to thrombin.

Because activation of factor X is the common link between the intrinsic and extrinsic pathways, a slight decrease in the rate of formation of activated factor X effectively blocks the synthesis of large amounts of later reaction products. This is the rationale for low-dose heparin therapy, discussed later.

For the treatment of deep venous thrombophlebitis, an initial bolus of 5,000 units of heparin is given by IV push, followed by a continuous infusion of heparin in D5/W at a rate of 1,000-2,000 units/hour. The infusion rate is adjusted to maintain the partial thromboplastin time (PTT) at $2-2\frac{1}{2}$ times the control value or to maintain the plasma heparin level at 0.05-0.3 IU/ml. The risk of clot propagation and embolization will remain until endothelialization of the thrombus has occurred. Since it takes 7-10 days for a thrombus to become adherent to the vessel wall and to be covered with endothelium, continuous heparin therapy should be given for at least this period.

We do not use intermittent bolus injections of heparin because of the wide fluctuations in heparin levels and seven-fold greater incidence of bleeding associated with this method, even when compared with continuous intravenous infusion.

For initial anticoagulation of a patient with a pulmonary embolus, a higher loading dose of 10,000-15,000 units of heparin is often administered. There is evidence that this helps to alleviate some of the bronchoconstriction and pulmonary vasoconstriction that is associated with a large embolus. Following the loading dose, the patient is maintained on a continuous infusion of heparin in D5/W at 1,000-2,000 units/hour, adjusted to maintain adequate anticoagulation as outlined above.

LONG-TERM ANTICOAGULATION

When venous thrombosis or pulmonary embolism occurs in early pregnancy, the patient must be considered at risk for propagation of the thrombus or recurrence of embolism until at least 6 weeks after delivery. Antepartum, long-term anticoagulation is achieved by giving 150-250 units/kg of subcutaneous heparin sodium every 12 hours. The dose is adjusted over the first few days to maintain the midinterval activated PTT (determined 6 hours after injection) at $1\frac{1}{2}$ times the control value. An alternative procedure is to give $\frac{2}{3}$ of the total daily IV heparin dose needed to keep the PTT therapeutic in three divided doses subcutaneously (q8h).

A concentrated aqueous solution of 25,000 units/ml should be used. The patient is taught to self-administer the drug prior to discharge from the hospital. A tuberculin-type syringe with a 25- or 26-gauge needle, 1.5 cm long, is used. A fold of skin is gently raised on the lateral aspect of the anterior abdominal wall—this is facilitated by bending forward; the skin is cleansed; and the needle is inserted to full depth at a right angle to the skin. The hub of the needle is held firmly between the thumb and index finger as the exact dose of heparin is injected. The needle is removed at the same angle as insertion. The injection site must be routinely rotated to prevent tissue necrosis. Subcutaneous heparin is best avoided in the arms and legs.

To monitor anticoagulation, a weekly PTT should be measured 6 hours after subcutaneous injection. The platelet count should also be monitored weekly, as some patients develop thrombocytopenia on heparin therapy. A gradual increase in dosage may be needed, particularly during the third trimester, to maintain adequate anticoagulation.

At our institution, we do *not* use oral anticoagulants at any time during pregnancy. Warfarin (Coumadin, Panwarfin), a vitamin K antagonist, readily crosses the placenta and is a recognized teratogen during the first trimester, producing a syndrome of hypoplastic nose, stippled epiphyses, frontal bossing, optic atrophy or cataracts, and mental retardation. The elevated levels of coagulation factors in pregnancy contrast sharply with the low levels of factors II, VII, IX, and X in the fetus and newborn. Though the mother may be within therapeutic range on warfarin, the fetus is likely to be considerably overdosed because of immature liver enzymes and low levels of vitamin K-dependent clotting factors.

Recently, birth defects have been reported in children whose mothers received warfarin only during the second and third trimesters. Common findings in these children include microcephaly, bifrontal narrowing, mental retardation, and ophthalmologic abnormalities including blindness. The presumed cause of these defects is fetal intracranial hemorrhage. In addition, a number of studies have documented the danger of continuing oral anticoagulation until term; stillbirth or neonatal death can result from perinatal fetal/neonatal hemorrhage.

During the intrapartum period, patients on heparin can be managed in one of two ways. Heparin may be withheld at the onset of labor and resumed 2-4 hours postpartum. Or the heparin dose can be reduced to 5,000 units given subcutaneously every 12 hours and continued during labor. The latter approach is preferable for certain high-risk patients, such as those with prosthetic heart valves or recent or recurrent pulmonary embolism. Because of the risk of local bleeding, spinal or epidural anesthesia is best avoided in patients on heparin therapy. Immediately postpartum, there will usually be a dramatic reduction in the amount of heparin required for adequate anticoagulation. Care must be taken to adjust the heparin dosage according to either the PTT or plasma heparin level.

Postpartum, oral warfarin is started while subcutaneous heparin is continued. Once adequate anticoagulation (as determined by PTT) is achieved with warfarin, heparin is discontinued and the patient may be discharged from the hospital on oral anticoagulant therapy alone. Warfarin enters the breast milk in only minute amounts; therefore, breast-feeding is not contraindicated during warfarin therapy.

Duration of anticoagulant therapy depends on the indication, but it should be continued for at least 6 weeks postpartum. The puerperium is the period of highest risk for deep venous thrombosis and embolization. If the patient has had a pulmonary embolus, the recommended length of therapy varies from 3-6 months postpartum.

In a patient with a previous history of thromboembolism, whether in a previous pregnancy or unrelated to pregnancy, we recommend prophylactic heparin therapy throughout pregnancy and therapeutic warfarin during the puerperium. The subcutaneous heparin *sodium* dosage utilized is 5,000-7,500 units every 12 hours. Low-dose heparin accelerates the rate of neutralization of activated factor X by antithrombin III, retarding the accumulation of sufficient amounts of activated factor X to provoke venous thrombus formation. The dose of heparin that is needed to inhibit activated factor X is much lower than the dose that is needed to prevent clotting once a thrombus has already been formed.

If anticoagulant therapy must be neutralized because of hemorrhage or other problems, heparin can simply be discontinued. The effects will clear within a few hours. When the situation is urgent, the heparin effect can be reversed immediately with protamine sulfate. For every 100 units of heparin in the circulation, 1 mg of protamine sulfate should be given IV. Excessive amounts of protamine should be avoided; large amounts inhibit the thrombin-fibrinogen reaction and act as an anticoagulant.

If the anticoagulant effect of warfarin must be reversed immediately, an infusion of 1-2 units of fresh frozen plasma should be given. Oral or intravenous vitamin K will reverse the effect of warfarin within 24 hours, but this may render the patient resistant to further oral anticoagulant therapy for about 2 weeks.

Heparin therapy is not without its complications. The primary risk is, of course, hemorrhage. Other problems are rare, but do occur occasionally. These include thrombocytopenia, alopecia, and allergic reactions. Osteoporosis has been related to prolonged therapy (i.e., therapy lasting longer than 6 months).

SUMMARY

With a high index of clinical suspicion, appropriate use of diagnostic procedures, and the prompt institution of appropriate therapy when indicated, we should be able to further reduce the morbidity and mortality associated with thromboembolic disease in pregnancy. Moreover, the identification of patients at high risk for complications and the institution of prophylactic heparin therapy, particularly in the early puerperium, should reduce the overall incidence of thromboembolic complications in pregnancy.

SUGGESTED READING

Bloomfield DK: Fetal deaths and malformations associated with the use of coumarin derivatives in pregnancy. *Am J Obstet Gynecol* 107:883, 1970

Gallus AS, Hirsh J, Tuttle R, et al: Small subcutaneous doses of heparin in prevention of venous thrombosis. *N Engl J Med* 288:545, 1973

Hirsh J, Cade J, Gallus AS: Anticoagulants in pregnancy: A review of indications and complications. *Am Heart J* 83:301, 1972

Hull R, Delmore T, Carter C, et al: Adjusted subcutaneous heparin versus warfarin sodium in the long-term treatment of venous thrombosis. *N Engl J Med* 306:189, 1982

Orme M, Lewis PJ, DeSwiet M, et al: May mothers given warfarin breast feed their infants? *Br Med J* 1:1564, 1977

Rosenberg R: Actions and interactions of antithrombin and heparin. *N Engl J Med* 292:146, 1975

Spearing G, Fraser I, Turner G, Dixon G: Long-term self-administered subcutaneous heparin in pregnancy. *Br Med J* 1:1457, 1978

12

Urinary Tract Infections in Pregnancy: Diagnosis

J. PETER VAN DORSTEN, M.D.

Urinary tract infection is the most common type of bacterial infection in females in developed countries. Obstetricians have long recognized the significance of urinary tract infections in pregnancy. Acute pyelonephritis remains the most common medical complication of pregnancy, with an overall incidence of 1-2%. Morbidity from pyelonephritis affects both mother and fetus. The mother is at risk for sepsis, recurrent pyelonephritis in the same pregnancy, and subsequent development of chronic renal disease. The fetus is jeopardized by the potential ill-effects of maternal fever, antibiotic administration, and premature labor.

Asymptomatic bacteriuria in pregnancy can lead to acute pyelonephritis. A number of randomized studies have shown that the diagnosis and treatment of asymptomatic bacteriuria can virtually eliminate the threat of pyelonephritis in pregnancy.

DEFINITIONS

Asymptomatic bacteriuria is defined as the presence of pathogens with a colony count of $\geq 10^5$/ml in urine from an asymptomatic patient. Acute cystitis is significant bacteriuria (colony count $\geq 10^5$/ml) in a patient complaining of frequency, urgency, and dysuria, but without fever or costovertebral-angle tenderness. Acute pyelonephritis is the presence of significant bacteriuria with associated symptoms of chills, fever, and costovertebral-angle tenderness; lower tract symptoms are also frequently present.

Several facts suggest that asymptomatic bacteriuria usually antedates the pregnancy. If the initial urine culture in the first trimester is negative, there is only a 1% chance that a subsequent urine culture later in pregnancy will be positive. Furthermore, the incidence of asymptomatic bacteriuria in the non-pregnant state is similar to its incidence in pregnancy. Pregnancy, therefore, plays little, if any, role in the acquisition of bacteriuria. On the other hand, the physiologic changes of pregnancy (decreased ureteral and bladder tone and ureteral compression) render the pregnant patient much more likely to develop pyelonephritis if asymptomatic bacteriuria is present. Untreated, the patient with asymptomatic bacteriuria has a 20-40% risk of developing pyelo-nephritis during the same pregnancy.

URINE COLLECTION

Several methods of urine collection are used during pregnancy. The most common is the clean-catch, midstream collection. If one specimen is positive for a pathogen with a $\geq 10^5$ colony count, there is a 91% chance that the next specimen will also be positive; if two specimens are positive, there is a 96% chance that the third will be positive. An even more accurate method is ure-thral catheterization, where a colony count of $\geq 10^5$ is 95% accurate on a single collection. Pure cultures of pathogen with 10^3 and 10^4 colony counts may also be significant when collected by catheterization. Because there is a risk of introducing bacteria into an otherwise sterile bladder at the time of the procedure, this method is not recommended for routine screening, but is re-served for special circumstances: suspected pyelonephritis and resolution of confusing clean-catch specimens. The most accurate method is suprapubic aspiration, but it is rarely necessary because of the accuracy of the other two methods.

It is important that collected urine not be allowed to stand at room tem-perature for more than 30 minutes because of potential false-positives in both urinalysis and culture. If not examined or plated within 30 minutes, the urine should be stored at 4°C.

DIAGNOSTIC STUDIES

A number of diagnostic studies can be performed on the urine specimen. Al-though some authors have recommended microscopic urinalysis (using spun or unspun urine) or the nitrite test as inexpensive and reliable alternatives to urine culture, the latter is more accurate. The object of microscopic urinalysis is the detection of either bacilluria or pyuria. Though microscopic urinalysis is cheaper and quicker, one study found that it was not very sensitive in predict-ing positive urine cultures; bacilluria was present in only 61% of positive cul-tures and pyuria, in 67%. Additionally, there was a false-positive rate of 11% and 15%, respectively; this would lead to unnecessary treatment in such pa-tients. More important, the false-negative rate (39% and 33%, respectively), would preclude the diagnosis of asymptomatic bacteriuria and render these patients at risk for pyelonephritis.

The nitrite test is done with a colorimetric dipstick (commercially available with simultaneous testing for proteinuria and glycosuria) that detects nitrites in urine. Pathogenic bacteria convert nitrates, which are normally present in urine, to nitrites, which are normally absent. If positive, the test is virtually 100% predictive of a positive culture. Unfortunately, the false-negative rate is high; the test predicts only 22% of positive cultures. The nitrite test, howev-er, is cheap, easily performed, and allows early treatment if positive.

We believe that none of these tests is sensitive enough to warrant its use as the sole screening test. The office urine culture kit has been found to be an accurate and inexpensive method of diagnosing significant bacteriuria. If the colorimetric test indicates a significant colony count, the specimen is sent for routine culture and sensitivity. The most accurate, but also the most expensive, method for detecting significant bacteriuria is still quantitative culture by the calibrated bacteriologic loop or the pour-plate dilution technique.

Other tests are also helpful in evaluating the urinary tract. In acute pyelonephritis, 27% of patients have a creatinine clearance less than 80 cc/minute, with a return to normal in 3 to 8 weeks. Altered renal function in patients with pyelonephritis is also suggested by a high incidence of hypokalemia (53%) and hyponatremia (32%).

Various tests have been devised to differentiate bladder from renal bacteriuria. Direct methods, such as ureteral catheterization, renal biopsy, and bladder washout, and indirect methods, such as fluorescent-coated antibody, urine concentrating ability, and serum antibody titer, have all been used. The direct methods are now considered too invasive for pregnancy, and the indirect methods too unreliable for routine use.

Radiography, with its potential for fetal damage, is rarely indicated in pregnancy. The single-exposure, delayed, 20-minute intravenous pyelogram (IVP) is indicated only in unresponsive pyelonephritis or unresolving lithiasis; it is done to rule out obstruction by either urinary calculus or anomaly. Postpartum IVPs, however, should be routinely obtained in patients with pyelonephritis or persistent or recurrent asymptomatic bacteriuria in pregnancy. The optimal time is 3 months postpartum, when the physiologic urinary tract alterations have returned to normal.

PATHOGENS

The causative organisms are usually aerobic gram-negative bacilli, with *E. coli* accounting for 85% of the cultured pathogens; *Klebsiella, Enterobacter, Proteus,* and *Staphylococcus* make up the remainder. The enterococcus has been incriminated as a urinary pathogen; however, several studies have failed to detect it. Its pathogenicity in the urinary tract currently remains suspect. Approximately one-fourth of these pathogens are resistant to ampicillin; half are also resistant to cephalosporins. Resistance to nitrofurantoins is rare, and to aminoglycosides, almost unheard of.

CULTURE REPORTS

Interpretation of the clean-catch urine culture report can be perplexing. Cultures showing a 10^3 or 10^4 colony count and contaminated cultures should be repeated without treatment; one study found 69% of 10^4, 22% of 10^3, and 26% of contaminated cultures positive on follow-up culture. If the second culture is also confusing, we suggest an in-and-out catheterization for clarification.

ASYMPTOMATIC BACTERIURIA

Asymptomatic bacteriuria is present in 4-7% of the obstetric population. Among indigent patients, the rate is 6-10%; among private patients, 2-3%.

The rate is doubled in patients with sickle cell trait. The incidence increases with age, parity, and sexual activity just as it does in the nonpregnant state.

Patients with asymptomatic bacteriuria are not a homogeneous group. In 40%, positive ureteral cultures are found; 45% are unable to appropriately concentrate their urine; 25% have renal involvement on bladder washout; fluorescent-coated antibody, indicative of upper tract disease, is present in 46%. In other words, 25-46% of patients with asymptomatic bacteriuria have "silent pyelonephritis," and these patients with upper tract disease are more likely to develop acute symptomatic pyelonephritis in pregnancy.

In a 10- to 12-year follow-up of patients with asymptomatic bacteriuria in pregnancy, 27% were found to have persistent bacteriuria, and 10-15% to have evidence of chronic pyelonephritis. Patients with upper tract disease during pregnancy are the ones at risk for persistent bacteriuria, even if it was appropriately treated during pregnancy. Postpartum pyelograms reveal an 8-33% incidence of abnormalities; the risk is highest in patients who had evidence of upper tract disease accompanying asymptomatic bacteriuria, or who had persistent or recurrent bacteriuria. The relationship between asymptomatic bacteriuria during pregnancy and the future development of chronic renal disease is not apparent; pregnancy probably only provides an opportunity to detect renal disease that was present prior to pregnancy, and to institute follow-up to prevent chronic end-stage renal disease.

If asymptomatic bacteriuria is not treated in pregnancy, 28% of patients can be expected to develop acute pyelonephritis in the same pregnancy. Only 2-3% of treated patients will develop pyelonephritis. If patients with asymptomatic bacteriuria are promptly diagnosed and treated early in pregnancy, acute pyelonephritis in pregnancy can virtually be eliminated. The goal is to eradicate bacteriuria during pregnancy.

PYELONEPHRITIS

It is hoped that aggressive therapy of asymptomatic bacteriuria and cystitis will prevent the development of acute symptomatic pyelonephritis, a more serious complication of pregnancy. The diagnosis of acute pyelonephritis in pregnancy is usually quite easy. Most patients complain of chills, fever, back pain, and dysuria. Some also have associated contractions; the diagnosis of pyelonephritis should always be entertained in patients with premature labor. Objective findings usually include an oral temperature of 101°F or greater, costovertebral-angle tenderness, and a positive microscopic urinalysis with both pyuria (>5 white blood cells/hpf) and bacilluria (numerous motile rods). The diagnosis is often delayed if the patient is afebrile. About 9% of patients with pyelonephritis will be afebrile early in the course of the disease. Back pain associated with costovertebral-angle tenderness in the pregnant patient should be assumed to be due to pyelonephritis until proven otherwise. Systemic signs and symptoms will soon follow if therapy is delayed.

The following chapter deals with the management of urinary tract infections in pregnancy.

SUGGESTED READING

Brumfitt W, Davies EI, Rosser EI: Urethral catheter as a cause of urinary tract infection in pregnancy and puerperium. *Lancet* 2:1059, 1961

Cunningham FG, Morris GB, Mikal A: Acute pyelonephritis of pregnancy: A clinical review. *Obstet Gynecol* 42:112, 1973

Fairly KF, Whitworth JA, Radford HJ, et al: Pregnancy bacteriuria. The significance of site of infection. *Med J Aust* 2:424, 1973

Harris RE, Gilstrap LC: Prevention of recurrent pyelonephritis during pregnancy: *Obstet Gynecol* 44:637, 1974

Harris RE, Thomas VL, Shelokov A: Asymptomatic bacteriuria in pregnancy: Antibody-coated bacteria, renal function, and intrauterine growth retardation. *Am J Obstet Gynecol* 126:20, 1976

Kaitz AL: Urinary concentrating ability in pregnant women with asymptomatic bacteriuria. *J Clin Invest* 40:1331, 1961

Kass EH: Asymptomatic infections of the urinary tract. *Trans Assoc Am Physicians* 69:56, 1956

Kass EH: Should bacteriuria be treated? *Med J Aust* (suppl) 1:38, 1973

Kunin CM: Asymptomatic bacteriuria. *Ann Rev Med* 17:383, 1966

Kunin CM: Epidemiology of bacteriuria and its relationship to pyelonephritis. *J Infect Dis* 120:1, 1969

Kunin CM, De Groot JE: Self-screening for significant bacteriuria: Evaluation of the dip-strip combination nitrite/culture test. *JAMA* 231:1349, 1975

Lenke RR, Van Dorsten JP: The efficacy of the nitrite test and microscopic urinalysis in predicting urine culture results. *Am J Obstet Gynecol* 147:427, 1981

Lenke RR, Van Dorsten JP, Schifrin BS: Pyelonephritis in pregnancy: A prospective randomized controlled trial evaluating suppressive therapy with nitrofurantoin in preventing recurrent disease. *Obstet Gynecol* (in press)

Norden CW, Kass EH: Bacteriuria of pregnancy—A critical appraisal. *Ann Rev Med* 19:431, 1968

Parker J, Kunin C: Pyelonephritis in young women: A 10-20 year follow-up. *JAMA* 224:585, 1973

Sweet RL: Bacteriuria and pyelonephritis during pregnancy. *Semin Perinatol* 1:25, 1977

Turck M, Goffe BS, Petersdorf RG: Bacteriuria of pregnancy: Relation to socioeconomic factors. *N Engl J Med* 266:857, 1962

Van Dorsten JP, Lenke RR, Schifrin BS: Pyelonephritis in pregnancy: The role of in-hospital management and nitrofurantoin suppression on subsequent urine culture. *Am J Obstet Gynecol* (in press)

Whalley PJ: Bacteriuria of pregnancy. *Am J Obstet Gynecol* 97:723, 1967

Whalley PJ, Cunningham FG: Short-term vs. continuous antimicrobial therapy for asymptomatic bacteriuria in pregnancy. *Obstet Gynecol* 49:262, 1977

Whalley PJ, Cunningham FG, Martin FG: Transient renal dysfunction associated with acute pyelonephritis of pregnancy. *Obstet Gynecol* 46:174, 1974

Whalley PJ, Martin F, Peters P: Significance of asymptomatic bacteriuria detected during pregnancy. *JAMA* 193:879, 1965

Zinner SH, Kass EH: Long-term (10-14 years) follow-up of bacteriuria of pregnancy. *N Engl J Med* 285:820, 1971

13

Urinary Tract Infections
in Pregnancy: Management

J. PETER VAN DORSTEN, M.D.

ASYMPTOMATIC BACTERIURIA

Some authors recommend two consecutive positive urine cultures before instituting treatment. However, we initiate therapy on the basis of a single positive culture, because we believe that the benefits of early treatment compensate for the few false-positives that are treated unnecessarily.

Antibiotic selection is based on sensitivity testing. Though bacteriostatic, nitrofurantoin is appropriate in most cases and has been proven effective. Short-term therapy (100 mg PO qid for 10 days) has been shown to be as effective as continuous therapy. Nitrofurantoin is excreted mainly in the urine, and its rapid gastrointestinal absorption prevents emergence of resistant coliforms. Theoretically, nitrofurantoins should be avoided in the 2-3% of black patients with G6PD (glucose-6-phosphate dehydrogenase) deficiency; practically, this has been no problem.

Occasionally, gastrointestinal side effects require switching from nitrofurantoin to a short-acting sulfonamide (1 gm qid for 10 days). But sulfa drugs should be avoided in the last month of pregnancy, as they compete with bilirubin for binding sites in the fetus and theoretically could cause neonatal kernicterus. Though ampicillin and the cephalosporins are bactericidal and equally effective, urinary pathogens are usually less susceptible to them. The prescriber should be familiar with antibiotic susceptibility patterns in his own practice or institution, and choose specific drugs accordingly.

Rarely, parenteral agents such as aminoglycosides must be used to treat unusually resistant bacteria. These agents can be used on an outpatient basis (IM bid for 5 days), as nephrotoxicity is not a concern in short-term therapy.

Test-of-cure urine cultures should be performed 7 days after completion of therapy. Follow-up cultures should then be obtained: (1) monthly until delivery; (2) at the 6-week postpartum exam; and (3) at least annually thereafter. Patients with recurrent bacteriuria should be treated with a second short-term course of antibiotics based on sensitivity testing. Patients with a second recurrence may benefit from long-term suppression (nitrofurantoin, 100 mg at bedtime). In persistent bacteriuria, a 6- to 8-week course of treatment with a bactericidal agent is indicated. If such prolonged treatment fails to eradicate bacteriuria, consideration should be given to a single-shot intravenous pyelo-gram (IVP) to rule out renal or ureteral calculi.

Patients with recurrent or persistent bacteriuria should have cultures more often (every 2 weeks) for the remainder of pregnancy, as well as in the puerpe-rium and at the 6-week postpartum exam. Intravenous pyelography (a com-plete study) should be performed at 3 months postpartum, since such patients are at high risk for abnormalities (chronic pyelonephritis, renal or ureteral calculi, or anomalies).

ACUTE CYSTITIS

Acute cystitis is less common in pregnancy, but an incidence of 1-2% is re-ported. Since acute cystitis produces obvious symptoms, patients are usually treated promptly, thereby averting ascending infection. Our management of acute cystitis in pregnancy is similar to our management of asymptomatic bac-teriuria. Although these patients are not at significant risk for abnormal IVPs, those with recurrent episodes should be given postpartum IVPs.

PYELONEPHRITIS

Once the diagnosis of pyelonephritis is made or strongly suspected, the pa-tient should be hospitalized immediately. Because of the risk of maternal sep-sis, premature labor, and fetal loss, outpatient therapy is considered inappro-priate. Parenteral antibiotic administration is necessary not only for adequate urinary levels, but also to produce the serum and tissue levels needed to treat renal parenchymal infection and bacteremia. A urine specimen should be ob-tained by in-and-out catheterization prior to initiating therapy so that an accu-rate culture and sensitivity report can be available should manipulation of antibiotics be indicated.

Bactericidal agents are preferred. *E. coli* accounts for 85% of cases; antibiot-ic selection should be made accordingly. The traditional choice has been am-picillin (2 gm IV q6h), but a 20-25% incidence of resistance has made cephalo-sporin therapy more popular.

Within 24 to 48 hours, culture and sensitivity results should be available. If the organism is resistant, or even intermediately resistant, to the initial anti-biotic, we switch to an appropriate one; 40-50% of follow-up cultures will be positive if antibiotics are not switched (irrespective of clinical response). A 3% incidence of septic shock makes prompt sterilization of the urine mandatory. Clinical response should not be used as the only barometer, as most patients will be afebrile in 72 hours regardless of the appropriateness of antibiotic se-lection. In the natural course of pyelonephritis, improvement will occur sim-ply with bed rest and hydration.

Occasionally, an aminoglycoside will be necessary because of an unusually resistant organism. Aminoglycosides are potentially nephrotoxic agents. Since creatinine clearance is reduced in patients with pyelonephritis, dosages must be lowered accordingly. Hypokalemia and hyponatremia are also frequent findings, but potassium supplementation and adequate hydration soon correct these problems.

Intravenous antibiotics are traditionally stopped after the patient has been afebrile for 24 hours. After an additional 24 hours on an appropriate oral antibiotic, the patient is discharged to complete a 10- to 14-day course of oral therapy. Using this regimen, we have discovered that, despite appropriate therapy and negative follow-up cultures in the hospital, one-third of patients have positive cultures on clinic follow-up 7-14 days later. Our data suggest that a 5-day course of intravenous antibiotics in the hospital may be more advantageous.

Most patients are afebrile within 72 hours after institution of appropriate therapy. If fever persists at 96 hours, obstruction (usually ureteral or renal calculi) should be suspected. A single-shot intravenous pyelogram is probably indicated at this point.

Some authors have recommended chronic suppressive therapy in patients who have had acute pyelonephritis in pregnancy. We recently concluded a randomized prospective study comparing patients on chronic antibiotic suppression (nitrofurantoin 50 mg PO tid) with controls, and found no difference in likelihood of recurrent pyelonephritis. Overall, recurrent pyelonephritis occurred in only 8% of our patients and was always associated with either inappropriate antibiotic management or poor compliance (failed clinic appointments). Our results indicate that while suppressive therapy does reduce the incidence of positive cultures, it does not eliminate the need for close follow-up and repeat cultures.

Since both the treated and untreated groups require intensive surveillance with frequent cultures, the value of suppression is questionable. Instead, we recommend that patients have urine cultures every 2 weeks with appropriate intermittent treatment as indicated. With such surveillance, we had only one recurrence of pyelonephritis in 102 patients. Clinic follow-up with cultures every 2 weeks will virtually eliminate recurrent pyelonephritis in pregnancy.

Patients with a history of pyelonephritis in pregnancy have a high incidence (50%) of abnormal IVPs. The risk is especially great if the pyelonephritis was left-sided or bilateral. (Nearly all pyelonephritis in pregnancy is right-sided.) We recommend an IVP at 3 months postpartum to detect chronic pyelonephritis, calculus, or anomaly. Patients with a history of pyelonephritis should continue to have periodic cultures and renal function studies to prevent development of chronic renal disease.

SUGGESTED READING

Hanley HG: Pyelonephritis of pregnancy. *Brit J Urol* 37:53, 1965

Harris RE, Gilstrap LC: Prevention of recurrent pyelonephritis during pregnancy. *Obstet Gynecol* 44:637, 1974

Kincaid-Smith P, Bullen M: Bacteriuria in pregnancy. *Lancet* 1:395, 1965

Lenke RR, Van Dorsten JP, Schifrin BS: Pyelonephritis in pregnancy: A prospective randomized controlled trial evaluating suppressive therapy with nitrofurantoin in preventing recurrent disease. *Obstet Gynecol* (in press)

Mead PJ, Harris RE: Incidence of group B beta-hemolytic streptococcus in antepartum urinary tract infections. *Obstet Gynecol* 49:262, 1977

Norden CW, Kass EH: Bacteriuria of pregnancy—A critical appraisal. *Ann Rev Med* 19:431, 1968

Staney TA, Condy M, Mihara G: Prophylactic efficacy of nitrofurantoin macrocrystals and trimethoprim-sulfamethoxazole in urinary infections. Biological effects on the vaginal and rectal flora. *N Engl J Med* 296:780, 1977

Sweet RL: Bacteriuria and pyelonephritis during pregnancy. *Semin Perinatol* 1:25, 1977

Van Dorsten JP, Lenke RR, Schifrin BS: Pyelonephritis in pregnancy: The role of in-hospital management and nitrofurantoin suppression on subsequent urine culture. *Am J Obstet Gynecol* (in press)

Whalley PJ, Cunningham FG: Short-term vs. continuous antimicrobial therapy for asymptomatic bacteriuria in pregnancy. *Obstet Gynecol* 49:262, 1977

Whalley PJ, Cunningham FG, Martin FG: Transient renal dysfunction associated with acute pyelonephritis of pregnancy. *Obstet Gynecol* 46:174, 1974

14

Current Approach to the Care of the Pregnant Diabetic

RAUL ARTAL, M.D.

Our current ability to manage the pregnant diabetic is one of the major achievements of modern obstetrics. Significant recent changes in management schemes have had a profound impact on outcome.

SCREENING FOR DIABETES

Due to the significant maternal and infant morbidity and mortality that have been associated with diabetes in pregnancy, extensive screening programs have been instituted in the past. These programs have been guided by historical and clinical clues, including family history of diabetes, poor obstetric history, age over 30, obesity, accelerated fetal growth, and hydramnios.

In 1973, O'Sullivan completed a study that involved prospective screening of 18,812 pregnant women. He found that 56.2% of patients diagnosed as diabetic had no historical or clinical clues suggesting diabetes. This study has caused some to suggest that *every* pregnant woman should be screened for diabetes and challenged with carbohydrates at least once during pregnancy, preferably after 28-30 weeks' gestation.

The use of one of the following oral or IV loading tests has been recommended for detection of glucose intolerance in pregnancy: (1) a 50-gm glucose load given at random, with a 1-hour postload plasma glucose determination (positive if glucose concentration $\geq$ 150 mg/dl); (2) a 75-gm glucose load given at random, with a 2-hour capillary finger-stick determination (positive if glucose concentration $\geq$ 120 mg/dl); or (3) a 100-gm glucose load given fasting, with a 2-hour plasma glucose determination (positive if glucose concentration $\geq$ 140 mg/dl). If the screening test is positive, a 3-hour glucose tolerance test, using a 100-gm glucose load, should be done. Patients with normal fasting blood glucose, but an abnormal glucose tolerance test, are class A diabetics under the White classification system.

In our institution, we use the 100-gm glucose load and recommend screening every pregnant woman. Based on our experience, about 25% of infants of class A (non-insulin-requiring) mothers experience perinatal morbidity, the same incidence as infants of overtly diabetic mothers. We also recognize that about 10% of class A diabetics develop insulin-dependent diabetes in pregnancy. Consequently, we provide intensive follow-up for all class A patients, and attempt to individualize care for patients at added risk of complications, ultimately managing them obstetrically in a manner similar to overt diabetics.

Pregnant women with insulin-dependent diabetes are also classified in the White system, and are grouped according to age of onset, duration of disease, and presence or absence of vascular complications.

ANTEPARTUM MANAGEMENT

Class A patients, once identified, are given information about diabetes in general and the possible complications associated with pregnancy. They are advised to follow a balanced diet of 30 calories/kg of ideal weight and to avoid concentrated carbohydrates.

Class A patients are given weekly fasting blood glucose determinations, and are usually allowed to go to term. If pregnancy continues past term and the cervix is unripe, or if dates are uncertain, patients are monitored with twice-weekly nonstress tests (NSTs), and contraction stress tests (CSTs) as necessary. Pregnancies are not permitted to continue past 42 weeks if estimated fetal weight exceeds 4,000 gm and fetal lung maturity is documented. If the cervix is inducible, oxytocin is administered. Otherwise, a primary cesarean delivery is performed.

In our approach to the care of insulin-dependent diabetics, we are guided not only by the White classification and experience, but also by the European experience, specifically, that of Pedersen. The Pedersen prognostic indicator classification takes into account the presence or absence of complications, such as clinical pyelonephritis, precoma or severe acidosis, pregnancy-induced hypertension, and patient neglectfulness. Such complications are prevented, or treated promptly if they occur. Emphasis is also placed on detection of retinal changes reflecting vascular disease.

Goals of metabolic management include prevention of ketoacidosis, maintenance of normal glycemia, and achievement of appropriate fetal growth for gestational age. Goals of obstetric management include early detection of intrauterine distress, prevention of iatrogenic prematurity, and prevention of birth injuries.

In our institution, we hospitalize patients identified as insulin-dependent diabetics for 3-4 days. During hospitalization, we educate the patients, carefully date their pregnancies, and establish laboratory baseline data, such as creatinine clearance and urine culture. We also carefully look for signs of pregnancy-induced hypertension, and provide ophthalmologic examinations.

Patients are instructed in the use of insulin and of home devices for monitoring blood glucose, and advised to follow a diabetic dietary regimen. After discharge, patients are seen weekly through 37 weeks' gestation. During this period, patients test their urine four times daily for glucose and acetone and check their blood daily for glucose (fasting, 11:00 AM, 4:00 PM, and 8:00 PM). If any complications appear, hospitalization is promptly resumed.

At 32-34 weeks' gestation, fetal antepartum testing is instituted, including twice-weekly NSTs. (The NST has proven to be a reliable method of fetal surveillance in the pregnant diabetic.) Daily determinations of plasma unconjugated estriols are somewhat inconvenient for outpatients, but daily blood samples can be stored, if practical, and assayed all at once when necessary. Patients are instructed to monitor fetal activity, keeping records of fetal movements for 1 hour three times daily—after breakfast, lunch, and dinner. If fetal activity decreases, or other doubts arise about fetal condition, we usually rely on monitoring fetal heart rate, repeat NSTs, and CSTs as necessary.

Ultrasound is used at the first visit, at 28-32 weeks, and prior to amniocentesis at 37-38 weeks to assess fetal growth. The amniocentesis at 37 weeks permits assessment of fetal lung maturity. In our experience, lecithin-sphingomyelin (L/S) ratios in excess of 3:1 or the presence in amniotic fluid of phosphatidylglycerol in excess of 2% indicates lung maturity.

INSULIN THERAPY

There may be a significant reduction in insulin requirements during the first half of pregnancy and a significant increase in the second half, possibly diminishing again near term. Insulin should be given to maintain the fasting and 4:00 PM plasma glucose levels below 90 mg/dl. Many patients can be maintained with one dose of long-acting insulin administered in the morning.

When a patient is receiving about 40 units of NPH insulin in the morning, with fasting plasma glucose levels higher than 120 mg/dl and 4:00 PM levels of 90 mg/dl or lower, split doses may facilitate control. In such cases, we usually recommend administering $\frac{2}{3}$ of the total insulin dose in the morning, and the remaining $\frac{1}{3}$ in the evening. Of the morning dose, $\frac{2}{3}$ is NPH and $\frac{1}{3}$ is CZI (crystalline-zinc insulin). Of the evening dose, $\frac{1}{2}$ is NPH and $\frac{1}{2}$ is CZI.

Insulin requirements invariably drop significantly in the immediate postpartum period. About 50% of patients do not require any insulin in the intrapartum and immediate postpartum periods.

INTRAPARTUM MANAGEMENT

The timing of delivery should be individualized. We generally advocate delivery at about 38 weeks' gestation, if fetal lung maturity has been documented.

Intrapartum management should be carefully planned. The duration of induced labor should not exceed 8-10 hours, since long, exhausting inductions can adversely affect the metabolic control of both mother and fetus. All patients scheduled for labor induction should be brought to the labor area early in the day. Every possible attempt should be made to establish an efficient and judicious induction of labor, e.g., with early rupture of membranes and adequate oxytocin administration. An IV with half D5/W and half normal saline should be set up, and blood glucose values should be obtained at frequent intervals, preferably every hour. Insulin should be adjusted to maintain plasma glucose levels under 90 mg/dl. About 50% of patients require no insulin at all during labor; the remainder require 1-2 units/hour.

In circumstances where insulin infusion cannot be used, the patient should be given either all or a portion of the usual morning dose of NPH, usually $\frac{1}{3}$-$\frac{2}{3}$ of the usual dose, depending on anticipated length of labor. Regular blood glucose determinations should be used to detect hyperglycemia, and doses of regular insulin should be given as indicated.

After vaginal delivery, a prompt return to the prepregnancy diabetic diet is recommended. Insulin requirements in the postpartum period can usually be determined by symptomatology and plasma glucose values. Following cesarean delivery, postoperative blood glucose levels should be measured every 6 hours, and regular insulin should be administered as required. Once oral diet has been established, patients will gradually return to the prepregnancy treatment plan. Initially, only $\frac{1}{3}$ of the prepregnancy dosage of insulin will be required.

NEONATAL OUTCOME

Despite significant reduction in perinatal mortality, neonatal morbidity in infants of diabetic mothers is still excessively high. The most common complications are hypoglycemia, hyperbilirubinemia, hypocalcemia, polycythemia, transient respiratory distress, and congenital malformations. Though most of these complications are mild and transitory, they require the attendance of skilled pediatricians and a well-equipped nursery.

Malformations occur twice as often in infants born to diabetic mothers as in the general population. Improved diabetic control starting at the time of conception may reduce this incidence. The most common abnormalities are cardiac, and include transposition of the great vessels and ventricular septal defects. A much rarer anomaly, and one that is specific to infants of diabetic mothers, is the caudal regression syndrome (hypoplasia of the sacrum and lower extremities). CNS malformations such as anencephaly and neural tube defects occasionally occur.

SUMMARY

Intensive obstetric observation of pregnant women with diabetes results in fewer perinatal deaths. Delivery near term and documentation of lung maturity result in delivery of mature infants. Less metabolic variation in the mother results in less morbidity in the infant.

SUGGESTED READING

Abell DA, Beischer NA, Wood C: Routine testing for gestational diabetes, pregnancy hypoglycemia and fetal growth retardation, and results of treatment. *J Perinat Med* 4:197, 1976

Freinkel N, Josimovich J: Symposium on gestational diabetes: Summary and recommendations. *Diabetes Care* 3:499, 1980

Jorge CD, Artal R, Paul RH, et al: Antepartum fetal surveillance in diabetic pregnant patients. *Am J Obstet Gynecol* 141:641, 1981

Miller E, Hare SW, Coherty SP, et al: Elevated maternal hemoglobin AIC in early pregnancy and major congenital anomalies in infants of diabetic mothers. *N Engl J Med* 304:331, 1981

O'Sullivan JB, Mahan CM, Charles D, et al: Screening criteria for high-risk gestational diabetic patients. *Am J Obstet Gynecol* 116:895, 1973

Pedersen J, Molsted-Pedersen L, Andersen B: Assessors of fetal perinatal mortality in diabetic pregnancy. *Diabetes* 23:302, 1974

Spellacy WN, Cohn JE: Human placental lactogen levels and daily insulin requirements in patients with diabetes mellitus complicating pregnancy. *Obstet Gynecol* 42:330, 1973

15

Pregnancy-Induced Hypertension

SAMUEL L. BRUCE, M.D.

Pregnancy-induced hypertension (PIH) remains one of the leading causes of maternal death in the United States. At least 250 maternal and about 25,000 fetal and neonatal deaths occur each year as a result of PIH.

The general incidence in the United States is about 8%. Many poor areas of the world report a many-fold higher incidence.

A. **Etiology:** The basic etiology of PIH is still unknown, but some of the implicated causes include:
   1. Uteroplacental ischemia
   2. Disseminated intravascular coagulation
   3. Poor nutrition
   4. Immunological disturbance.
B. **Predisposing factors to the development of PIH:**
   1. Multiple gestation
   2. Hydramnios
   3. Diabetes mellitus
   4. Prior history of chronic hypertension or vascular diseases (e.g., essential hypertension; lupus erythematosus and other collagen diseases)
   5. Hydatidiform mole, onset in second trimester.
C. **Some facts about PIH:**
   1. It is primarily a disease of the primigravida.
   2. It is more common among the poor.
   3. It is more prevalent as term approaches.
   4. It is more prevalent in certain geographic areas.
   5. The disease resolves completely by 6 weeks postpartum.
   6. It is associated with increased perinatal and maternal morbidity and mortality.
D. **Diagnosis of mild PIH:** Mild PIH is defined as hypertension, proteinuria, and/or edema after 20 weeks of gestation. Hypertension is defined as blood pressure of 140/90 mm Hg or a 30 mm Hg rise in systolic pressure (above prepregnant level) or 15 mm Hg rise in diastolic pressure, measured on at least two occasions, 6 or more hours apart.
E. **Diagnosis of severe PIH:** The patient is considered to have severe PIH if any of the following is present:

1. Blood pressure of 160/110 mm Hg or more on two occasions, 6 hours apart
2. Proteinuria: 3+ or 4+ on dipstick or 5 gm or more in 24-hour urine collection
3. Oliguria: 500 cc or less in 24-hour collection
4. Cerebral or visual disturbances
5. Epigastric pain
6. Pulmonary edema or cyanosis
7. Jaundice
8. Intrauterine growth retardation
9. HELLP syndrome (H—hemolytic anemia-microangiopathic anemia; EL—elevated liver enzymes; LP—low platelets).

F. **Diagnosis of eclampsia:** The patient with PIH who has convulsions not due to any prior neurological disease is presumed to have eclampsia. The incidence of eclamptic seizure is about 1:700 to 1:1,000 pregnancies.

G. **Pathophysiology:** The basic underlying pathophysiology of PIH is vasospasm or arteriolar constriction. This causes an increase in total peripheral resistance and leads to hypertension. The deviation in blood pressure, specifically in diastolic pressure, is the most reliable prognostic sign. The higher the diastolic pressure, the worse the prognosis.

H. **Laboratory assessment:** Patients with PIH should have the following performed on admission:
   1. CBC, differential, and platelet count
   2. Serum electrolytes and uric acid
   3. Liver profile (bilirubin, SGOT, SGPT, alkaline phosphatase)
   4. Coagulation profile (fibrinogen, fibrin split products), PT (prothrombin time), PTT (partial thromboplastin time); in severe preeclampsia, repeated every 12 hours
   5. Type and crossmatch for whole blood
   6. Urinalysis (specific gravity)
   7. Intravenous infusion of D5/W or lactated Ringer's solution at 125-150 cc/hour. Because of vasospasm and resulting decrease in vascular space, pulmonary edema can develop easily. Therefore, a strict fluid input and output record must be maintained. An appropriate adjustment in the fluid administered must be made in the presence of oliguria or anuria.

I. **Antepartum management:** It is generally agreed that the only definitive therapy for PIH is termination of the pregnancy. Termination is indicated in patients with either mild PIH and a mature fetus or severe PIH or eclampsia regardless of gestational age.

   In patients with mild preeclampsia and a premature fetus, however, a conservative approach is in order. Hospitalization and bed rest are indicated. The patient should be kept in the left lateral recumbent position to facilitate blood return to the heart, which leads to an increase in cardiac output, and kidney and uterine perfusion. This must be accompanied by both fetal assessment, using twice weekly fetal heart rate testing (non-stress test and contraction stress test), and assessment of maternal vital signs, coagulation competence, liver function, and kidney function. If the mother's condition improves and the fetal condition remains stable, pregnancy can be prolonged. If the mother's condition deteriorates (meets the criteria for severe PIH) or fetal surveillance tests predict jeopardy, delivery is in order. In the patient with an unfavorable cervix, premature fetus, and/or breech presentation, cesarean section should be performed. Otherwise, labor may be induced with oxytocin.

J. **Intrapartum management:** The definitive treatment for PIH is delivery after control of hypertension and prevention of convulsions.

1. *Objectives.*
   a. Prevention of convulsions
   b. Control of blood pressure
   c. Prevention of complications:
      1) Cerebrovascular hemorrhage
      2) Pulmonary edema
      3) Renal failure
      4) Fetal and/or maternal death.
   d. Delivery of a surviving neonate to a surviving mother.

2. *Prevention of convulsions:* Although magnesium sulfate is not the best available anticonvulsant, it is the drug of choice in this setting for the following reasons:
   a. The patient is usually alert and awake. This would not be true if barbiturates, tranquilizers (e.g., diazepam), or narcotics were used.
   b. Airway problems and aspiration of gastric contents are less likely.
   c. Fetal depression is avoided, and neonatal adjustments are not severely obtunded, although neonatal hypermagnesemia and hypotonia have been described.
   d. Magnesium sulfate is very easily managed.

3. *Administration of magnesium sulfate.*
   a. Intravenous: This is by far the best way to administer the drug. The main advantages are: therapeutic levels are attained rapidly; and the amount of drug given is known. Disadvantages include: the patient must be watched closely; and overdose is more likely.

      Dosage: An initial IV loading dose of 2-4 gm of $MgSO_4$ in 10% solution is followed by a maintenance dose of 1.5-2 gm/hour (depending on maternal renal function) via continuous infusion pump.
   b. Intramuscular: Advantages include: less demand on nurse and physician; less likelihood of overdose. Disadvantages include: pain at injection site; potential damage to sciatic nerve from injection; delay in attaining therapeutic levels, especially in obese patients.

      Dosage: An initial IM loading dose of 10 gm $MgSO_4$ in 50% solution (20 ml) is divided into 2 doses of 5 gm each, and injected deep in each buttock. This is followed by 5 gm IM (10 ml) every 4 hours.

c. Combination: Initially, 2-4 gm $MgSO_4$ are given slowly IV to attain therapeutic levels rapidly. This is followed by 10 gm IM. Then a maintenance dose of 5 gm is given IM every 4 hours.

K. Mode of action of magnesium sulfate: Magnesium sulfate is a neuromuscular blocker, similar to other nondepolarizing agents such as succinylcholine and curare. It prevents or blocks the release of acetylcholine at the neuromuscular junction. In addition, it has a mild, but transient, hypotensive effect when given as a bolus intravenously. (It should not be given as a bolus.)

1. *Precautions.*

   a. Magnesium sulfate is excreted unchanged via the urinary tract. Dosage should be reduced in anuria or oliguria. Therefore, assessment of urinary output is mandatory. Output must exceed 100 ml/4 hours.

   b. Patellar reflexes should be checked every 2-4 hours during $MgSO_4$ administration. Absence of patellar reflex is the first sign of $MgSO_4$ toxicity (blood level of 10 mEq/l or higher).

   c. Respiratory rate should be monitored, since respiratory depression occurs late.

2. *Toxicity.* The normal physiologic blood level of $MgSO_4$ is 1.5-2.5 mEq/l. The anticonvulsant level is approximately 4-7.5 mEq/l. Disappearance of patellar reflexes (the first sign of toxicity) occurs at a blood level of about 10 mEq/l. Respiratory paralysis is induced at 15 mEq/l, and total paralysis is produced at 25 mEq/l or greater.

3. *Antidote.* Calcium gluconate is used to treat magnesium sulfate toxicity. As a precaution, 10 ml of 10% calcium gluconate solution should be drawn and ready at the bedside of every patient receiving $MgSO_4$. This dose should be given slowly IV over 3-5 minutes after blood has been drawn to measure the magnesium level.

L. Eclamptic seizure: Seizure activity can vary from simple twitching of the face to full-blown grand mal seizure. The etiology is presumed to be cerebral edema or hemorrhage. A review of the world literature shows maternal mortality in eclampsia ranging from 0-10% and fetal mortality of about 33%. These figures emphasize the need to prevent eclamptic seizures or manage them appropriately when they occur.

M. Management of eclamptic seizure: Pritchard's method of managing eclampsia has become the standard in this country. The patient with convulsion prior to admission is given:

1. 4 gm $MgSO_4$ IV in not less than 3 minutes.

2. Continuous IV infusion of 1.5-2 gm/hour of $MgSO_4$.

3. If a convulsion follows in a few minutes, a repeat dose of 2-4 gm $MgSO_4$ is given IV.

4. If this fails to stop the convulsions, sodium amobarbital, 250 mg IV, should be given slowly. The patient may need to be intubated for respiratory depression.

5. $MgSO_4$ maintenance dosage is continued.

6. If all else fails (this happens rarely), diazepam (Valium) should be given IV to stop the convulsions. Then $MgSO_4$ maintenance is continued.

In the patient admitted without prior history of eclamptic seizure who has a seizure after receiving loading and maintenance doses of $MgSO_4$, management should be as follows:

1. Obtain blood sample for $MgSO_4$ level.

2. Give 4 gm $MgSO_4$ IV over 3 minutes.

3. Continue maintenance dosage of 1.5-2 gm/hour.

4. If seizure activity continues, consider sodium amobarbital IV as described above.

5. If seizure continues, use diazepam (Valium) IV to stop the seizure; then continue $MgSO_4$ maintenance.

Diazepam and sodium amobarbital cause profound depression of the mother and the neonate. These should be used only in the rare cases where adequate doses of $MgSO_4$ fail to control maternal seizures.

N. Control of blood pressure: Antihypertensive therapy (to prevent maternal cerebrovascular accident) is indicated when maternal diastolic pressure exceeds 110 mm Hg. The drug of choice in this situation is hydralazine (Apresoline), a mild vasodilator. This drug is preferred because it does not lower blood pressure precipitously; and it increases cardiac output and renal and uterine perfusion. Hydralazine may cause maternal tachycardia.

1. *Administration of hydralazine.*

  a. Intermittent intravenous method: 5 mg hydralazine (test dose) is given IV. Then blood pressure is checked every 5 minutes. If there is no response within 20 minutes, the dose is increased in 5-mg increments (10, 15, 20), and the procedure is repeated. A 20-minute interval between injections is recommended because hydralazine's maximal effect is seen in 20-30 minutes. The 20-minute interval prevents overdosage and severe hypotension that can occur with multiple doses. This procedure is repeated until the desired effect is achieved. Usually, 5- to 10-mg doses are sufficient. The drug effect lasts 4-6 hours.

  b. Continuous infusion method: 20 mg hydralazine in 250 ml D5/W solution is infused via continuous infusion pump and titrated to desired blood pressure.

2. *Other drugs.*

  a. Diazoxide, a potent vasodilator, is a thiazide derivative with no diuretic properties. It is rapidly protein-bound and, thus, must be given intravenously as a bolus (300 mg). It causes a precipitous drop in blood pressure and severe maternal hypotension; and decreases cardiac output, renal perfusion, and uterine perfusion. It should not be used as first-line treatment.

  b. Nitroprusside is also a vasodilator. Its drawback is that blood pressure rebounds immediately after cessation of the infusion. It is metabolized to cyanide; if large doses are required, this drug should not be used because of the potential for cyanide poisoning.

   c. Diuretics are generally contraindicated in the management of pre-eclampsia/eclampsia, regardless of severity of the edema or the disease. They should be used only in cases complicated by congestive heart failure or pulmonary edema. Diuretics aggravate the already present hypovolemia, decrease cardiac output, and cause electrolyte imbalances and thrombocytopenia in both mother and fetus.

It must be emphasized that antihypertensive therapy is not to be given for long periods antepartum. If antihypertensive agents are necessary, the pregnancy should be terminated regardless of gestational age.

O. Delivery: Delivery is the definitive therapy for PIH, and the method of delivery is based upon obstetric indications. If no contraindication to vaginal delivery exists, labor is induced with oxytocin. In the eclamptic patient, the delivery process is initiated after the patient becomes oriented to time and place.

P. Anesthesia: General anesthesia is preferred for cesarean section. Pudendal or local perineal and vaginal infiltration can be used for vaginal delivery. Conduction anesthesia such as spinal, epidural, or caudal is not recommended; severe hypotensive episodes have been associated with conduction anesthesia in preeclampsia, due to contracted blood volume.

Q. Postpartum management:

   1. *Mild preeclampsia.* Magnesium sulfate infusion is stopped after delivery, and the patient is observed for a few hours. If no signs of severe preeclampsia ensue, no further medication is necessary.

   2. *Severe preeclampsia.* Magnesium sulfate infusion is continued for 24 hours postpartum, since the majority of eclamptic seizures occur in this interval. Blood pressure is controlled with hydralazine, as necessary. Monitoring of maternal vital signs, fluid input and output, hematocrit, coagulation competency, and magnesium level is continued. Any abnormality noted is treated immediately. After 24 hours, the $MgSO_4$ is stopped, and the patient is given 60 mg phenobarbital IM, followed by 60 mg orally tid. After 72 hours, the phenobarbital dosage is changed to 30 mg tid for a few days, then stopped. In a few patients, blood pressure remains elevated (diastolic > 90 mm Hg) for several days. In such cases, methyldopa (Aldomet) is given, 250 mg orally tid, with dosage adjustments as needed to maintain diastolic pressure < 90. Some patients are discharged on methyldopa, and treatment is continued for a short period.

SUGGESTED READING

Kraus GW, Marchese JR, Yen SSC: Prophylactic use of hydrochlorothiazide in pregnancy. *JAMA* 198:1150, 1966

Pritchard JA: The use of magnesium sulfate in preeclampsia-eclampsia. *J Reprod Med* 23:107, 1979

Pritchard JA, Cunningham FG, Mason RA: Coagulation changes in eclampsia: Their frequency and pathogenesis. *Am J Obstet Gynecol* 124:855, 1976

Pritchard JA, Pritchard SA: Standardized treatment of 154 cases of eclampsia. *Am J Obstet Gynecol* 123:543, 1975

Pritchard JA, Stone SR: Clinical and laboratory observations on eclampsia. *Am J Obstet Gynecol* 99:754, 1967

Shoemaker ES, Gant NF, Madden JD, MacDonald PC: The effect of thiazide diuretics on placental function. *Tex Med* 69:109, 1973

Weinstein L: Syndrome of hemolysis, elevated liver enzymes, and low platelet count: A severe consequence of hypertension in pregnancy. *Am J Obstet Gynecol* 142:159, 1982

Zuspan FP: Treatment of severe preeclampsia and eclampsia. *Clin Obstet Gynecol* 9:954, 1966

Zuspan FP, Talledo OE: Factors affecting delivery in eclampsia: Condition of the cervix and uterine activity. *Am J Obstet Gynecol* 100:672, 1968

Zuspan FP, Ward MC: Improved fetal salvage in eclampsia. *Obstet Gynecol* 26:893, 1965

16

Appendicitis in Pregnancy

LESTER T. HIBBARD, M.D.

Appendicitis is the most common acute surgical condition of pregnancy and is encountered during every trimester as well as the puerperium. Its frequency is the same as in the nonpregnant population, for an incidence of roughly 1:2,000 births.

DIAGNOSIS

The signs and symptoms of appendicitis in pregnancy are similar to those that occur in the nonpregnant patient. But they tend to be masked by symptoms and physical changes of pregnancy, making the diagnosis more difficult and likely to be delayed. Some of the confusing factors are the nausea, vomiting, and abdominal discomfort of early pregnancy, displacement of the appendix by the growing uterus, laxity of the abdominal wall, round ligament spasm, physiologic leukocytosis, and an elevated sedimentation rate.

The initial pain of appendicitis is visceral and usually referred to the epigastrium or paraumbilical area. Its onset is gradual and often colicky, denoting an element of obstruction. In early pregnancy, pain localizes to McBurney's point as the overlying parietal peritoneum becomes involved in the inflammatory process. Past the fourth month of pregnancy, the appendix is displaced upward and laterally by the expanding uterus. By the sixth month the point of maximal tenderness is above the iliac crest, and by the eighth month it rises to the level of the right costal margin. Anorexia, nausea, and vomiting usually begin 1 or 2 hours following the onset of pain and are variable in severity. In the majority of cases there will be right lateral tenderness on rectal examination, and in about half the cases there will be appreciable abdominal signs of muscle spasm or guarding. Movement of the uterus may cause increasing pain in the appendiceal area. Pain of uterine origin can often be distinguished when the area of maximal abdominal wall tenderness diminishes or disappears as the uterus falls away from the examining fingers when the patient lies on her left side.

The patient's temperature may range from normal to 101°F. Because of the physiologic leukocytosis of pregnancy, the white blood count is of more significance if it rises over a period of time or there is an increasing left shift. A urinalysis should be negative unless the appendix is lying in a retrocecal position in close proximity to the ureter. There are no characteristic x-ray findings. A culdocentesis may demonstrate inflammatory fluid either before or after perforation.

If the appendix should rupture, the uterus may become the median wall of an abscess cavity, leading to abortion or premature labor. The incidence of abortion and premature labor is increased when appendicitis occurs in pregnancy, and dramatically increased if appendiceal perforation and peritonitis occur. As pregnancy continues, the uterus expands outside the pelvis, displacing bowel and omentum upward and laterally. If the appendix should rupture at that stage, effective walling-off of an abscess is less likely. Widespread peritonitis can result. Finally, emptying of the uterus by birth or abortion leads to rupture of any formed abscess cavity with resulting peritonitis.

Maternal mortality and morbidity are directly related to the duration of the infection and the stage of gestation. Peritonitis in the third trimester of pregnancy is associated with a very grave prognosis. Fetal mortality is about 15%.

For these reasons, it is important to make an early diagnosis and to operate on all suspicious cases. It is better to remove a normal appendix than to expose the patient to the risks of perforation.

In the first trimester of pregnancy the differential diagnosis includes salpingitis, ectopic pregnancy, corpus luteum accidents, and renal calculi. As pregnancy progresses, other differential diagnoses include pyelonephritis, round ligament pain, placental accident, degenerating myomata, twisted cyst, pancreatitis, and cholecystitis. Appendicitis is also masked by labor and confused with myoparametritis during the puerperium.

In early pregnancy, there is some advantage to using laparoscopy in doubtful cases before proceeding to laparotomy. As pregnancy advances, laparoscopy becomes technically more difficult and less rewarding because of the bulk of the enlarging uterus.

MANAGEMENT

While some authorities advocate a vertical incision for suspected appendicitis, we prefer a transverse muscle-splitting (or Rocky-Davis) incision over the point of maximal tenderness. This approach almost always gives adequate surgical exposure and can easily be extended if more space is required.

If the appendix has not ruptured, the incision can be closed primarily without using either an abdominal drain or a drain to the surgical incision. Neither tocolytic agents nor antibiotics are necessary, and abortion or premature labor is unlikely.

If the appendix has ruptured, the patient should receive triple antibiotic therapy, including an agent effective against anaerobic organisms. If an abscess has formed or peritonitis is well established, it may be necessary to employ suction drainage of the abdominal cavity through a flank incision. Cul-de-sac drainage is to be avoided. Cesarean section is also to be avoided unless some compelling obstetric indication exists. The surgical incision may be drained by means of a vertical Penrose drain extending from the midpoint of the skin incision through the lateral muscles of the abdominal wall to the external surface of the peritoneal closure. Or the skin may be left open, to be closed in a secondary procedure after 3 or 4 days. Should labor ensue, the surgical incision will not disrupt.

With modern care, the overall maternal mortality in appendicitis in pregnancy is less than 1%, but the incidence of complications—spontaneous abortion, premature labor, and perinatal mortality—is still significant.

SUGGESTED READING

Babaknia A, et al: Appendicitis in pregnancy. *Obstet Gynecol* 50:40, 1977

Cunningham FG, McCubbin JH: Appendicitis in pregnancy. *Obstet Gynecol* 45:415, 1975

Gomez A, Wood M: Acute appendicitis in pregnancy. *Am J Surg* 137:180, 1979

Mohammed JA, Oxhorn H: Appendicitis in pregnancy. *Can Med Assoc J* 112:1187, 1975

Townsend JM, et al: Appendicitis in pregnancy. *South Med J* 69:1161, 1976

17

Multiple Pregnancy

CHARLES W. HOHLER, M.D.

Multiple gestation, defined as the development of more than one fetus in utero, is associated with a perinatal mortality rate that is three to six times that of singleton pregnancies. Consequently, every patient who presents with a multiple gestation should be considered "high-risk" and receive the best medical care possible.

INCIDENCE

The incidence of multiple gestation is reported as 1:90 pregnancies for twins, 1:8,000 for triplets, and 1:700,000 for quadruplets. Quintuplets are extremely rare and rarely survive. In general, the greater the number of fetuses, the greater the perinatal morbidity and mortality.

The incidence of monozygotic (MZ) twins is about 3.5:1,000 pregnancies and is constant throughout the world. The incidence of dizygotic (DZ) twins varies by geographic region, race, and maternal age. DZ twinning seems to be related to levels of gonadotropin produced by the maternal pituitary. MZ twins are reported to have a three-fold greater incidence of perinatal mortality than DZ twins.

ASSOCIATED RISKS

Compared to women with singleton gestations, women with multiple gestations are at greater risk for pregnancy-induced hypertension, placenta previa, abruptio placentae, hydramnios, and postpartum hemorrhage. Of greatest concern to obstetricians and neonatologists, however, is the increased incidence of premature labor resulting in delivery of low-birth-weight infants. Many of these premature infants are also growth-retarded or small for gestational age and expire during the immediate neonatal period. Many who survive show subsequent abnormal mental and physical development.

Individual twins have mean weights similar to those of singleton fetuses up to 30-32 weeks, after which each twin usually weighs less than a singleton. Slowing of growth occurs earlier with gestations of more than two fetuses. In uncomplicated twin pregnancies the ultrasound biparietal diameters (BPDs) remain similar to those of single fetuses of the same gestational age throughout the third trimester.

Twin birth weights are within 999 gm of each other in 97% of cases. Only 18% of twins vary by between 500 and 999 gm. Weight differences between twins can be constitutional, but may also be due to placental transfusion syndrome, congenital anomalies of one twin, or growth retardation of one twin because of local placental factors.

DIAGNOSIS

Since prematurity contributes significantly to perinatal loss in multiple pregnancy, the prevention of prematurity is of the utmost importance. Unfortunately, many investigators have reported large series in which as many as 20-40% of patients with multiple gestations were not diagnosed until delivery. Any patient who presents with a uterine fundus larger than expected for gestational dates, severe hyperemesis gravidarum, or onset of pregnancy-induced hypertension (PIH) prior to 20 weeks should have an ultrasound examination to determine if there is more than one fetus. In particular, women with a family history of twins or those who have received ovulation-inducing agents such as clomiphene citrate (Clomid, Serophene) and pituitary gonadotropin should be screened for possible multiple pregnancy.

ANTEPARTUM MANAGEMENT

Once the diagnosis of multiple pregnancy is established, the patient should be seen every 2 weeks until 28 weeks of gestation, and weekly thereafter. Any anemia, if present, should be accurately diagnosed and appropriately treated. Bed rest with bathroom privileges can be instituted at 28 weeks and continued until 36 weeks to prevent premature labor, though the efficacy of this therapy remains controversial.

The obstetrician should be acutely aware of the patient's condition at all times. At the first sign or symptom of premature labor or PIH, the patient should be admitted to the hospital. If she is in premature labor with intact membranes and cervical dilation < 4 cm, consideration should be given to suppressing labor with ritodrine hydrochloride (Yutopar). Patients in advanced labor with cervical dilation of 4 cm or more or with evidence of chorioamnionitis should be delivered regardless of gestational age.

Patients with mild PIH before 36 weeks should be placed at bed rest and followed in the hospital with weekly nonstress fetal heart rate testing (NST). Two fetal heart rates can usually be tested simultaneously without difficulty. As long as the NST remains reactive and the patient's condition remains stable or improves, delivery may be delayed until fetal maturity is achieved. Delivery is warranted, however, if the maternal or fetal condition deteriorates.

Urinary estriols are of little value in assessing the well-being of twins. In 89% of twin pregnancies resulting in one stillbirth or growth-retarded infant, 24-hour urine estriol values are within normal limits.

Ultrasound evaluation of BPDs is highly recommended to detect growth problems. With predelivery differences in BPDs between 2 and 6 mm, the incidence of low birth weight in the smaller twin is 40%. When the predelivery difference exceeds 6 mm, the incidence of growth retardation in the smaller twin is 71%.

Patients admitted after 36 weeks with mild PIH may be candidates for delivery. If there is any question regarding fetal maturity, a transabdominal amniocentesis should be performed on one of the fetal amniotic sacs to obtain fluid for a lecithin-sphingomyelin ratio. In general, an L/S ratio of 2.0:1 or more obtained from one fetal sac designates a mature pregnancy. However, when ultrasound evaluation has demonstrated significant developmental differences between twins, the L/S ratio obtained from one sac cannot be assumed valid for the other fetus. If it is technically impossible to tap both sacs, then fluid surrounding the smaller twin should be evaluated.

Any patient with a multiple gestation who presents with severe PIH or eclampsia is a candidate for delivery regardless of gestational age. The patient's condition should be stabilized over a 4- to 6-hour period during which intravenous magnesium sulfate is administered, as necessary, to lower systolic blood pressure below 200 mm Hg and diastolic below 110 mm Hg. Care must be taken, however, to maintain adequate uterine blood flow; hence, maternal blood pressure should not be lowered much below 150/90.

INTRAPARTUM MANAGEMENT

In all cases of twin gestation, both fetal heart rates should be monitored during labor. A fetal ECG electrode should be applied to the scalp of the first fetus, while the second fetus should be monitored by a Doppler ultrasound device placed on the maternal abdomen. A transcervical catheter may also be placed to record intrauterine pressures. These measures ensure that both fetuses will be appropriately followed throughout labor.

As long as no labor or fetal heart abnormalities are detected, vaginal delivery may be anticipated. After delivery of the first twin, the condition of the second twin should continue to be monitored until it is delivered. This is best done by placing a fetal ECG electrode on the second twin's presenting part. As long as the second twin's condition remains satisfactory, labor is allowed to continue and vaginal delivery should be expected.

Occasionally, after delivery of the first twin, the second twin's condition may be jeopardized by sudden umbilical cord prolapse or abruptio placentae. In such cases, a version extraction or total breech extraction should be done.

Cesarean section is recommended in multiple gestations of 27 weeks or greater if more than two fetuses are present or if the first of two fetuses is presenting in transverse or breech position. Cesarean section prevents the birth anoxia and birth trauma that so often accompany breech and premature births in multiple gestation. In patients at term, however, with the first twin in vertex position, vaginal delivery may be anticipated for both twins regardless of the presentation of the second. At the University of Southern California, we have found that a carefully performed total breech extraction or version extraction of the second twin at term is unassociated with significant neonatal injury or mortality.

SUMMARY

Patients with multiple gestation require early diagnosis, early treatment of any medical or obstetric complication during the antepartum period, and bed rest from 28 to 36 weeks of gestation to prevent premature labor. Vigilant prenatal obstetric care, careful intrapartum monitoring, and judicious use of cesarean section in premature twin gestations will ensure the best possible maternal and infant outcome.

SUGGESTED READING

Babson SG, Phillips DS: Growth and development of twins dissimilar in size at birth. *N Engl J Med* 289:937, 1973

Benirschke K, Kim CK: Multiple pregnancy. *N Engl J Med* 288:1276, 1329, 1973

Berkowitz RL: Ultrasound in the antenatal management of multiple gestations. In Hobbins JC, ed: *Diagnostic Ultrasound in Obstetrics, Clinics in Diagnostic Ultrasound Series*, vol 3. New York: Churchill Livingstone, 1979, p 69

Cohen M, Kohl SG, Rosenthal AH: Fetal interlocking complicating twin gestation. *Am J Obstet Gynecol* 91:407, 1965

Farooqui MO, Grossman JH, Shannon RA: A review of twin pregnancy and perinatal mortality. *Obstet Gynecol Surv* (suppl) 28:144, 1973

18

Preterm Labor and Delivery

RICHARD H. PAUL, M.D.

A simplistic definition of preterm delivery is any delivery occurring prior to 37 weeks' gestation or when the newborn weight is less than 2,500 gm. It should be noted that infants of diabetic mothers born prior to 37 weeks often weigh more than 2,500 gm. Likewise, in cases of intrauterine growth retardation, infants born at term often weigh less than 2,500 gm.

Although exceptions are frequent, preterm birth (as defined above), which occurs in 7-10% of all births, accounts for more than 75% of perinatal mortality. Of particular interest is the group of neonates weighing less than 1,500 gm. The incidence is less than 2%; yet this group contributes more than 80% of neonatal mortality, as well as much morbidity.

ETIOLOGY

The etiology of preterm labor may be broadly associated with various factors. One of the more common is spontaneous premature rupture of membranes. The cause of premature rupture and its role in provoking preterm labor remain unknown. This should be no surprise, considering our basic lack of understanding of the onset and control of even normal labor. In the final analysis, about half of preterm births cannot be associated with an identifiable factor such as placental abruption, premature rupture of membranes, uterine anomalies, multiple gestations, etc.

DIAGNOSIS

Another dilemma facing the physician is the difficulty in establishing the diagnosis of preterm labor. Erroneous diagnoses may approach 50%, making judgments regarding therapy difficult. In view of the risk of preterm birth, treatment is usually begun without waiting for clear evidence of labor.

Initial steps in evaluating the patient include observation and bed rest, estimation of gestational age, and ruling out contraindications to inhibition of preterm labor. The most common contraindications include amnionitis, fetal anomalies or death, and severe maternal hemorrhage. Patients with premature rupture of membranes and minimal vaginal bleeding, although classically considered contraindications, may be candidates to receive tocolytic agents on an individualized basis. This approach seems not unreasonable when dealing with the markedly premature fetus (<34 weeks), considering our current techniques for evaluating bleeding, intrauterine infection, and fetal maturity.

MANAGEMENT

Bed rest alone has been associated with successful abeyance of threatened preterm birth in 40-60% of cases. The theoretical basis for such a response involves increased uterine blood flow that should occur with bed rest. Another nonpharmacologic approach that may be instituted during initial evaluation is rapid intravenous infusion of a crystalloid solution such as lactated Ringer's. Should uterine activity subside with this approach over a brief period of observation, no further steps need be taken.

When inhibition of uterine activity is indicated, pharmacologic therapy may be used. Numerous agents have been proposed. Although some advocate antiprostaglandins (aspirin, indomethacin), their side effects are potentially hazardous.

The most widely used tocolytic agents are: (1) ethanol, (2) magnesium sulfate, and (3) β-mimetics.

Ethanol

Ethanol is thought to suppress labor by inhibiting oxytocin release. An initial loading dose of 7.5 ml/kg/hour of a 9.5% ethanol solution is given for 2 hours. This is followed by a maintenance dose for 6-10 hours at an infusion rate of 1.5 ml/kg/hour. Favorable success rates in the range of 70-80% are reported.

Side effects are bothersome and include nausea and vomiting. When overdosage occurs, aspiration, respiratory depression, and death may result. Patient acceptance of this therapy may be a problem; many refuse to submit to a repeat course when indicated.

Magnesium Sulfate

Magnesium sulfate decreases motor end plate sensitivity and acts as an antagonist to calcium, which is intimately involved in uterine contractility. Few studies and only limited clinical data exist regarding the efficacy of this approach. However, the widespread acquaintance with magnesium sulfate therapy for preeclampsia makes it an attractive choice.

An initial 3- to 4-gm intravenous loading dose is given over 5-15 minutes. This is followed by an infusion of 1 to 2 gm/hour. Success of this therapy seems to depend on early administration, with the most benefit occurring at < 2 cm dilation. Side effects relate to overdosage and can be recognized by careful monitoring of deep tendon reflexes and respiratory rate. Calcium gluconate, 10 ml of a 10% solution, is an effective antidote for toxicity.

β-Mimetics

These epinephrine-like substances have an impressive inhibitory effect on uterine smooth muscle. They also provoke varying degrees of cardiovascular responses that must be carefully considered. The ideal agent would be specific for β_2 receptors, inhibiting uterine contractions while causing only minor cardiovascular effects. The only approved substance currently available in the United States (and the most costly) is ritodrine hydrochloride (Yutopar). Isoxsuprine (Vasodilan) and terbutaline (Brethine, Bricanyl) are less costly and have been successfully used in treating preterm labor, but lack specific FDA approval for this indication. Both terbutaline and ritodrine are more β_2-specific and superior to isoxsuprine; they are less likely to provoke maternal side effects such as hypotension and tachycardia.

At times the preterm pregnancy will present in an advanced stage of labor. Most authors advise against prolonged attempts at labor inhibition when the cervix is 4 cm or more dilated. On the other hand, short-term labor suppression may be undertaken to administer corticosteroids, to transfer the patient to a hospital with neonatal intensive-care facilities, or to make preparations for cesarean delivery.

Assuming expert neonatal facilities are available, intrapartum care becomes the focal point, and questions arise about the validity of commonly used surveillance methods. It has been shown that fetal heart rate patterns have the same pathophysiologic significance and acid-base relationship in preterm fetuses as in their term counterparts. However, the preterm fetus appears to lack the usual reserve or tolerance to stress seen in mature fetuses. Thus careful observation and prompt intervention are essential to assure delivery of a non-asphyxiated neonate.

An additional consideration is the effect that the method of delivery has upon outcome. The very-low-birth-weight ($<1,500$ gm) infant is apparently vulnerable to minimal traumatic events, and it appears that atraumatic delivery is extremely important for optimal outcome. From accumulating evidence, cesarean section would appear to be of probable benefit in cases of very-low-birth-weight infants, even with cephalic presentation.

SUGGESTED READING

Bowes WA, Gabbe SG, Bowes C: Fetal heart rate monitoring in premature infants weighing 1500 grams or less. *Am J Obstet Gynecol* 137:791, 1980

Garite TJ, Freeman RK, Linzey EM, et al: The use of amniocentesis in patients with premature rupture of the membranes. *Obstet Gynecol* 54:226, 1979

Hobel CJ, Hyvarinen M, Oh W: Abnormal fetal heart rate patterns and fetal acid-base balance in low birth weight infants in relation to respiratory distress syndrome. *Obstet Gynecol* 39:83, 1972

Martin CB Jr, Siassi B, Hon EH: Fetal heart rate pattern and neonatal death in low birth weight infants. *Obstet Gynecol* 44:503, 1974

Naeye RL, Peters EC: Causes and consequences of premature rupture of fetal membranes. *Lancet* 1:192, 1980

Paul RH, Koh KS, Monfared AH: Obstetric factors influencing outcome in infants weighing from 1001 to 1500 grams. *Am J Obstet Gynecol* 133:503, 1979

Rush RW: Contribution of preterm delivery to perinatal mortality. *Br Med J* 2:965, 1976

Thiaganajah S: The use of magnesium sulfate as the primary tocolytic agent to prevent premature delivery. *Am J Obstet Gynecol* 142:840, 1982

Zanini B, Paul RH, Huey JR: Intrapartum fetal heart rate: the correlation with scalp pH in the pre-term fetus. *Am J Obstet Gynecol* 136:43, 1980 .

19

Premature Labor: Treatment With β-Mimetics

JEFFREY P. PHELAN, M.D.

Sparked by the observations of Rucker in 1925 that epinephrine relaxes uterine musculature, investigators have searched for the ideal tocolytic agent. With the identification of two types of adrenoreceptors, α and β, by Ahlquist in 1948, and of two types of β receptors, β_1 and β_2, by Landsman in 1967, interest in adrenergic stimulation as a method of treating premature labor has grown exponentially. This latter finding has been a catalyst for the development of more specific agents that inhibit uterine activity and produce minimal side effects.

β_1 receptors predominate in the heart, small intestine, and adipose tissue, while β_2 receptors predominate in the smooth muscle of the uterus, bronchioles, blood vessels, and diaphragm. Therefore, a β_1 agent would stimulate the heart and increase the heart rate, while a β_2 agent would primarily cause uterine relaxation. Though the ideal agent does not exist, currently available β_2 amines (isoxsuprine, terbutaline, and ritodrine) have proven to be effective inhibitors of preterm labor while producing minimal side effects.

INDICATIONS FOR TOCOLYSIS

Currently recommended criteria for selecting candidates for treatment of premature labor include: uterine gestation between 20 and 36 weeks, estimated fetal weight less than 2,500 gm, immature fetus (lecithin-sphingomyelin ratio $< 2:1$), and confirmation of diagnosis of premature labor. The minimal criteria for diagnosing premature labor are at least one regular contraction every 10 minutes and/or a change in the effacement or dilation of the cervix.

CONTRAINDICATIONS TO TOCOLYSIS

Maternal contraindications to uterine tocolysis are largely related to uterine factors; for example, amnionitis, uterine hemorrhage, and advanced labor (cervical dilation > 4 cm); or to evidence of eclampsia or severe preeclampsia. In addition, β_2 agents are contraindicated in gravidas with hyperthyroidism, cardiac disease (especially with arrhythmia), pulmonary hypertension, and diabetes mellitus.

Fetal contraindications to tocolysis include fetal demise, fetal distress, or a known fetal malformation incompatible with life.

SIDE EFFECTS

Maternal

Intravenous infusion of β_2 amine agents causes maternal tachycardia, widening of the pulse pressure, and transient hypokalemia, hyperglycemia, and hyperinsulinemia. Additional metabolic side effects, including lactic acidosis, have been reported, although the clinical significance is unknown.

Minor side effects associated with β_2 amines include nausea, headache, sweating, tremor, nervousness, and palpitations. Isoxsuprine may cause an allergic reaction manifesting as pruritic papular rash.

Chest pain has been described with β_2 amine usage and usually resolves with discontinuation of therapy. However, rare instances of angina pectoris with ST-segment depression have been encountered.

Another potentially life-threatening side effect is *pulmonary edema*, which may develop suddenly in patients receiving β_2 amines, often in conjunction with corticosteroids. As this condition is frequently related to fluid overloading, intravenous infusions should be limited and closely monitored. If pulmonary edema develops, β_2 amine therapy should be discontinued and the edema managed by conventional means.

Fetal and Neonatal

Maternal β_2 amine administration may cause fetal tachycardia. Neonatal side effects are infrequently encountered, but include hypoglycemia, hypotension, hypocalcemia, and ileus. Neonatal side effects are more common when the last intravenous dose is given less than 5 hours before delivery, gestational age is less than 32 weeks, or maternal side effects have appeared during drug administration.

Discontinuation of β_2 amine infusion should be considered whenever any of the following major side effects is encountered: maternal heart rate >150 beats per minute, fetal heart rate >200 bpm, maternal systolic blood pressure >180 mm Hg or diastolic pressure <40 mm Hg, more than 6 PVCs (premature ventricular contractions) per minute, chest pain, and signs and symptoms of pulmonary edema.

THERAPEUTIC GUIDELINES

The patient under consideration for uterine tocolysis with a β_2 agent should have, in addition to an admitting history and physical exam, a baseline laboratory evaluation. This should include ECG, serum electrolytes, complete blood count, and serum creatinine.

Before therapy is initiated, the patient should be prehydrated (<500 ml) and placed in the left lateral recumbent position. During tocolysis with a β_2 amine, maternal heart rate and blood pressure, uterine activity, and fetal heart rate should be continuously monitored. Continuous monitoring of maternal heart rhythm would also be prudent. In view of the metabolic alterations associated with β_2 amine usage, serum electrolytes should be measured at intervals of 4-6 hours. Potassium replacement may be necessary during protracted infusions.

DOSAGE AND ADMINISTRATION

Isoxsuprine hydrochloride (Vasodilan), although not approved by the FDA for use as a tocolytic agent, has been used widely since the early 1960s in the treatment of premature labor. The initial intravenous dosage is usually 0.25-0.5 mg/minute and is titrated to suppress uterine activity and to remain within maternal cardiovascular tolerance. The infusion may be required for up to 24 hours. After complete cessation of uterine activity for 12 hours, the infusion should be discontinued and 5-20 mg administered intramuscularly every 3-6 hours for a 24-hour period. Thereafter, the same dose is administered orally until 37 weeks' gestation unless obstetric judgment dictates earlier discontinuation of therapy.

Terbutaline sulfate (Brethine, Bricanyl), one of the newer class of β_2 amines, is currently marketed as a bronchodilator. Since the early 1970s, it has been used increasingly in the treatment of premature labor. However, this agent, like isoxsuprine, is not approved by the FDA for this indication.

Terbutaline is also administered initially by the intravenous route, followed by subcutaneous and, later, oral therapy. The effective intravenous tocolytic dosage ranges from 10-80 μg/minute with an initial loading dose of 25 μg. The dosage is then titrated to achieve the desired tocolytic effect, with adjustments every 10 minutes until uterine activity has abated. After inhibition of uterine contractions, the infusion is continued at a maintenance level for 12 hours. Following intravenous therapy, 0.25-0.5 mg is given subcutaneously every 2-4 hours for a period of 12-24 hours. Thereafter, oral maintenance therapy of 2.5-5 mg every 4-6 hours is continued until 37 weeks' gestation unless obstetric conditions dictate earlier discontinuation.

Ritodrine hydrochloride (Yutopar) has been more extensively studied in prospective, double-blind, controlled investigations than any other such agent. Currently, ritodrine is the first and only drug approved by the FDA for treatment of premature labor.

Ritodrine therapy is begun intravenously with an initial dosage of 50-100 μg/minute. The dosage is increased by 50 μg/minute every 10 minutes until contractions cease or unacceptable side effects develop. The maximum IV dosage is 350 μg/minute. Treatment is considered a failure if labor progresses despite use of the maximum dosage. If therapy is successful, the infusion should be continued for 12-24 hours following cessation of contractions.

Oral maintenance therapy, started approximately 30 minutes before the infusion is stopped, consists of 10 mg every 2 hours or 20 mg every 4 hours for the first 24 hours. The maximum oral dosage is 120 mg/day. Thereafter, in the absence of uterine activity, the maintenance dose is 10-20 mg every 4-6 hours until 37 weeks unless obstetric judgment dictates earlier discontinuation.

SUMMARY

As with any form of therapy employing potent agents in a clinical situation with major implications, careful selection of candidates for β_2 amine treatment is mandatory. Evaluation of both obstetric and medical factors that might contraindicate therapy with this class of drug is essential. Perhaps the most difficult clinical judgment is predicated not on the potential side effects of the tocolytic agents, but on the relative risks versus benefits of preterm delivery or continuation of pregnancy.

SUGGESTED READING

Barden TP, Peter JB, Merkatz IR: Ritodrine hydrochloride: A betamimetic agent for use in preterm labor. I. Pharmacology, clinical history, administration, side effects, and safety. *Obstet Gynecol* 56:1, 1980

Brazy JE, Little V, Gumm J, Pupkin M: Risk: Benefit considerations for the use of isoxsuprine in the treatment of premature labor. *Obstet Gynecol* 58:297, 1981

Caritis SN, Edelstone DI, Mueller-Hueback E: Pharmacologic inhibition of preterm labor. *Am J Obstet Gynecol* 133:557, 1979

Horowitz JJ, Creasy RK: Allergic dermatitis associated with administration of isoxsuprine during premature labor. *Am J Obstet Gynecol* 131:225, 1978

Jacobs MM, Knight AB, Arias F: Maternal pulmonary edema resulting from betamimetic and glucocorticoid therapy. *Obstet Gynecol* 56:56, 1980

Merkatz IR, Peter JB, Barden TP: Ritodrine hydrochloride: A betamimetic agent for use in preterm labor. II. Evidence of efficacy. *Obstet Gynecol* 56:7, 1980

Tye KH, Desser KB, Beuchimol A: Angina pectoris associated with use of terbutaline for premature labor *JAMA* 244:692, 1980

20

Chorioamnionitis: Its Significance and Treatment

KEE SENG KOH, M.D.

Chorioamnionitis is an acute inflammation of the fetal membranes. The likely causative organisms are those that commonly inhabit the vagina and cervical canal. It occurs in 0.5-1.0% of all pregnancies, threatening both maternal and fetal welfare. Despite the potential seriousness of this condition, it presents major diagnostic and therapeutic problems for the physician.

ETIOLOGY

The infecting microorganisms may enter the amniotic cavity by any of three possible routes:
1. Ascending infection, either via intact membranes or, more commonly, after the membranes have ruptured
2. Transplacental infection
3. Descending infection from the abdominal cavity through the fallopian tubes (only remotely possible).

Predisposing factors are: premature rupture of membranes (infection occurs in 3-25% of cases of membrane rupture lasting longer than 24 hours); repetitive vaginal examinations; internal FHR (fetal heart rate) monitoring; and amniocentesis. The incidence of infection is higher in patients of low socioeconomic status.

CLINICAL FEATURES

The clinical signs of chorioamnionitis are often difficult to detect even in the presence of established infection. From the practical point of view, the presumptive diagnosis is usually based on the following factors:
1. A temperature above 100.4°F or 38°C in the absence of any other obvious causes of fever, including dehydration
2. Purulent or malodorous amniotic fluid
3. Presence of bacteria with or without leukocytes in a Gram-stained specimen of the amniotic fluid. The specimen may be obtained by transabdominal amniocentesis or through an intrauterine pressure catheter, provided that the first 10 cc of aspirated fluid are discarded.

Additional clinical features of chorioamnionitis may include:
1. Uterine tenderness
2. Maternal tachycardia
3. Fetal tachycardia
4. Maternal leukocytosis.

It is often difficult to correlate the clinical picture of intrauterine infection with the findings of bacteriologic and histologic studies of the placenta, umbilical cord, and fetal membranes after delivery.

PERINATAL COMPLICATIONS

The presence of chorioamnionitis does not indicate that fetal or neonatal infection is present, but suggests that such infection may occur. Possible consequences of intrauterine bacterial infection include:
1. No clinical effects; only signs such as newborn bacterial colonization
2. Premature birth, with an increased risk of neonatal respiratory distress
3. Intrauterine death
4. Perinatal infection.

Ascending infection enters the fetus through the oral and nasal routes. Thus, the effects are mainly in the lungs and gut, though there may be a spread to the bloodstream. Transplacental infection is characterized by fetal septicemia, with organisms lodging in hematopoietic tissues, the brain, meninges, heart, and adrenals, but with a predilection for the liver and spleen.

The premature and dysmature fetus may be less competent to deal with intrauterine infection. Lanier and co-workers reported a 50% rate of fetal loss when chorioamnionitis was present. Pryles and co-workers earlier reported a 57% incidence of neonatal illness when maternal fever was present.

MATERNAL COMPLICATIONS

Maternal mortality is exceedingly rare. Chorioamnionitis and its attendant complications (particularly septic shock, disseminated intravascular coagulation, and acute renal failure), when promptly recognized, no longer play a major role in maternal deaths.

Chorioamnionitis and postpartum endoparametritis, when untreated, can progress to a more chronic pelvic infection with subsequent risk of infertility, ectopic pregnancy, and menstrual disturbance.

With recent advances in obstetric care, intrapartum biophysical and biochemical monitoring, neonatal intensive-care facilities, potent antibiotics, safer blood transfusions, and better analgesia and anesthesia, the maternal and perinatal outcomes in cases of chorioamnionitis have improved considerably when compared with older published data.

At LAC/USC (Los Angeles County/University of Southern California) Medical Center, a retrospective study was undertaken of 140 patients of low socioeconomic status who developed chorioamnionitis between 1975 and 1977. The results suggested that both perinatal and maternal complications associated with chorioamnionitis (particularly sepsis), when promptly recognized and treated, are not catastrophic. Four neonatal deaths occurred, none related to sepsis; two of these infants weighed less than 2,000 gm. There were no maternal deaths, but 38 patients (27.1%) developed postpartum infections. Cesarean section did not appear to improve either perinatal or maternal outcome.

MANAGEMENT

Early diagnosis and prompt treatment remain the cornerstones of management. Evacuation of the uterus, regardless of fetal maturity, is mandatory. In the face of infection, spontaneous labor usually ensues; if not, oxytocin induction is usually done.

Cesarean section is performed only if there is an obstetric indication, since it carries an increased risk of septic pelvic thrombophlebitis and abdominal wound infection. Extraperitoneal cesarean section is probably not indicated today because of the availability of effective antibiotics and the lack of surgical expertise in this operation. Cesarean hysterectomy for those who have completed their families is probably ill-advised today, since it is a major operative procedure performed in a highly vascular and contaminated field. The complications and morbidity of hysterectomy in patients with chorioamnionitis include bladder injury, cuff cellulitis or abscess, broad-ligament hematomas, anemia, wound infections, pulmonary embolism, and fistulas.

Maternal antibiotic therapy is indicated postpartum following a thorough septic work-up. A Gram stain of the amniotic fluid may guide initial therapy. Full doses of broad-spectrum antibiotics should be given. The combination of ampicillin (1 gm IV q6h) and gentamicin (60 mg IV q8h) is administered until the patient has been afebrile for 48 hours. Despite the paradox of seemingly "inappropriate" antibiotic coverage (anaerobes, especially *Bacteroides fragilis*, play an important role in pelvic infection), excellent clinical results have been achieved with this regimen. Clindamycin (300 mg IV q6h) or chloramphenicol (500 mg IV q6h) are usually reserved for conditions that do not respond to the initial postpartum therapy.

Not all neonates born out of a septic intrauterine environment require antibiotics. Individualized care is advised. Careful examination and investigation of newborns should lead to better means of determining which ones require antibiotics. Aids to early diagnosis of congenital infection are:

1. Gastric aspirate: Gram stain and cell count
2. Blood culture
3. Total and differential white count
4. Urine: cell count, Gram stain, and culture
5. Cerebrospinal fluid: cell count, Gram stain, and culture
6. Chest x-ray.

The presence of more than 5 pus cells/hpf in a gastric aspirate taken at birth suggests the need for antibiotic treatment. The combination of ampicillin (150 mg/kg/24 hours) and gentamicin (5-6 mg/kg/24 hours) is usually adequate. This approach covers a wide range of organisms, yet limits potential toxicity of the initial therapy.

SUGGESTED READING

Clark DM, Anderson GV: Perinatal mortality and amnionitis in a general hospital population. *Obstet Gynecol* 31:714, 1968

Douglas RG, Stromme WB: Management of complications during labor. In *Operative Obstetrics*, ed 3, ch 11. New York: Appleton-Century-Crofts, 1976, p 390

Koh KS, Chun FH, Monfared AH, et al: The changing perinatal and maternal outcome in chorioamnionitis. *Obstet Gynecol* 53:730, 1979

Lanier JR Jr, Scarbrough RE Jr, Fillingim OW, et al: Incidence of maternal and fetal complications with rupture of the membranes before onset of labor. *Am J Obstet Gynecol* 93:398, 1965

Pryles CV, Steg NL, Nair S, et al: A controlled study of the influence on the newborn of prolonged premature rupture of the amniotic membranes and/or infection in the mother. *Pediatrics* 31:608, 1963

21

Post-term Pregnancy

SZE-YA YEH, M.D.

Post-term pregnancy is a confusing and controversial subject. This is partly due to improper use of terminology; for example, the confusion of "post-term pregnancy" with "postmature syndrome." There is also a great deal of controversy in the management of post-term pregnancy. It is generally understood that perinatal morbidity and mortality are higher in post-term pregnancy. The purpose of this chapter is to review the previous reports on this subject, evaluate our experience, and recommend a management scheme.

TERMINOLOGY

"Post-term pregnancy" refers to any pregnancy that lasts beyond 42 weeks or 294 days from the first day of the last menstrual period. Under strict criteria, these numbers should be adjusted according to the length of the menstrual cycle of the pregnant woman. If her menstrual cycle was longer than 28 days, then the gestational period can last longer than 42 weeks before the pregnancy becomes "post-term."

Other terms used synonymously with "post-term pregnancy" include "postdatism" and "postdate" or "prolonged pregnancy." However, under no circumstances should "postmaturity syndrome" be used as a synonym for "post-term pregnancy." "Postmaturity syndrome" refers to fetal dysmaturity, which is present in a small proportion of post-term gestations. In order to avoid confusion, the best term to use in describing the postmaturity syndrome is "dysmaturity."

INCIDENCE

Only 5% of all pregnancies deliver on the expected date of confinement. Approximately 10% of all pregnancies last beyond 42 weeks, and approximately 3% continue beyond 43 weeks. Of these post-term pregnancies, 20% will result in dysmaturity.

It has been suggested that the incidence of post-term pregnancy may be related to maternal age and parity, but convincing evidence is lacking. There is an impression that elderly primigravidas tend to have higher incidences of prolonged pregnancy. A woman who has carried one pregnancy beyond term has a 50% chance for another post-term pregnancy.

ETIOLOGY

The exact etiology of prolonged pregnancy is unknown. However, fetal corticosteroid secretion may play a role, because pregnancies with anencephalic fetuses are often post-term. A study by Nwosu et al suggested that fetal adrenal insufficiency may play a key role in prolonged gestation.

SIGNIFICANCE

The majority of post-term pregnancies result in normal outcomes; however, certain problems are associated with prolonged periods of gestation. It is important to understand these problems so that the proper management can be instituted.

Alterations in Pregnancy Growth Parameters

Classic features in postdate pregnancies with dysmature infants include: decrease in fundal height; decrease in abdominal circumference (Ballantyne-Runge sign); and static or falling maternal weight.

Amniotic fluid volume normally reaches a peak of about 980 ml at 33-34 weeks' gestation and gradually decreases to 540 ml by 41-42 weeks. Beischer et al, using a dilution technique, studied the amniotic fluid volume in 114 patients with post-term pregnancies, and concluded that the average amniotic fluid volume at 42 weeks is 484 ml; at 43 weeks, 332 ml; and at 44 weeks, 162 ml. Increased incidences of umbilical cord accidents and higher concentrations of meconium when there is passage prior to labor are associated with decreased amniotic fluid volume. The latter makes the resuscitation of the newborn more difficult and enhances the possibility of meconium aspiration and pneumonitis.

Macrosomia

In post-term pregnancies, 20% of infants weigh over 4,000 gm (9 lb) at birth, a two-fold increase over the incidence in normal-term pregnancies. About 3% of post-term infants weigh over 4,500 gm (a three-fold increase). Increased incidences of cesarean section, difficult delivery, birth trauma, and shoulder dystocia are associated with increased birth weight.

Meconium-Stained Amniotic Fluid

The reported incidence of meconium-stained amniotic fluid in post-term pregnancies at delivery ranges from 27-43%. Although meconium is associated with increased perinatal morbidity and mortality, its presence in fluid obtained by amniocentesis in post-term pregnancy is not an indication for termination by either elective induction or cesarean section. Green and Paul found that the finding of clear or meconium-stained amniotic fluid in prolonged pregnancies yielded significant increases in both false-positive and false-negative results. In a controlled study, Knox et al found that use of amniocentesis in post-term pregnancy management achieved no better results than use of the contraction stress test. They also found that induction of labor after discovery of meconium through amniocentesis resulted in a higher incidence of failed induction and cesarean delivery. Therefore, amniocentesis is not recommended for routine management of post-term pregnancies.

However, the presence of meconium in the amniotic fluid is a warning sign that some underlying problem, such as dysmaturity, oligohydramnios, or meconium aspiration may exist. In such cases, continuous intrapartum fetal heart rate monitoring, scalp blood pH determinations, and active resuscitation of the newborn are mandatory.

Congenital Anomalies

It is generally reported that the incidence of congenital anomalies increases to 8-10% in prolonged pregnancies. The major anomalies are usually of the nervous system, e.g., anencephaly, hydrocephaly.

Increased Perinatal Mortality

It has been reported that perinatal mortality increases gradually as gestation advances beyond 42 weeks. But most of these data were obtained before techniques for antepartum fetal surveillance and intrapartum fetal monitoring were available. Perinatal mortality rates in cases managed with these new techniques must be determined.

Intrapartum Fetal Distress

Because prolonged gestation is associated with a higher incidence of placental insufficiency, oligohydramnios, and umbilical cord accidents, intrapartum fetal distress is more commonly seen in cases of post-term pregnancy. Recent observations showed no statistically significant increase in the occurrence of late and variable decelerations in prolonged gestation. However, these observations do not negate the need for intrapartum fetal monitoring in all post-term patients.

Fetal Dysmaturity (Postmaturity Syndrome)

Fetal dysmaturity is the most significant problem associated with prolonged pregnancy. It occurs in 2-6% of all pregnancies after 38 weeks' gestation, and in as many as 20% of post-term pregnancies. The cause is thought to be chronic placental insufficiency. Clifford described the syndrome in three clinical stages—stage I: loss of subcutaneous tissue plus desquamation, long nails, abundant hair, alert facies, and loss of vernix in clear amniotic fluid; stage II: all the features of stage I plus greenish meconium-stained amniotic fluid, membranes, and cord; and stage III: all the features of stages I and II plus yellowish meconium staining, indicating prolonged exposure.

Consequences of dysmaturity include: (1) increased perinatal mortality (3-5%), (2) increased incidence of fetal distress due to placental insufficiency and cord accident, and (3) neonatal problems including respiratory distress, meconium aspiration, asphyxial organ damage, hypoglycemia, polycythemia, and hyperviscosity syndrome.

MANAGEMENT

Objectives
Three major objectives in the management of the post-term pregnancy are: (1) to avoid fetal dysmaturity syndrome, (2) to avoid unnecessary induction of labor and unnecessary cesarean section, and (3) to provide safe delivery.

Principles
Early screening and continuous follow-up are necessary to establish reliable obstetric dates. With the following criteria, a good estimate of gestational age can be made: (1) positive pregnancy test by 6 weeks, (2) first examination before 12 weeks to confirm that uterine size agrees with estimated dates, (3) fetal heart tones audible with the DeLee stethoscope at 20 weeks, and (4) B-scan ultrasound examination before 28 weeks.

It is very important for obstetric patients to be seen initially before 12 weeks of gestation, and to be re-evaluated at 20 weeks. At that time, the fundus of the uterus will reach the level of the umbilicus, and fetal heart tones should be audible with the DeLee stethoscope. In cases of discrepancy between uterine size and dates, ultrasound examination can be used to confirm gestational age.

At 42 weeks' gestation, antepartum fetal assessment should begin promptly to minimize perinatal morbidity and mortality. Assessment should include: twice weekly fetal heart rate testing (nonstress test, contraction stress test), and ultrasonic evaluation of amniotic fluid volume and fetal movement. Elective induction of labor is indicated when one of these tests shows abnormal results, obstetric dates are reliable, and the cervix is open and effaced.

Management Protocol at LAC/USC Medical Center
At LAC/USC (Los Angeles County/University of Southern California) Medical Center, the protocol for the management of possible post-term pregnancy (Fig. 21-1) is as follows: Patients with pregnancies lasting longer than 41 weeks are classified into "good obstetric dates" and "poor obstetric dates" groups according to the criteria described above.

In the "good obstetric dates" group, pelvic examination is performed first. If the cervix is found to be inducible (i.e., Bishop's score of 9 or greater), elective induction is performed. If not, nonstress tests (NSTs) are done twice weekly. The contraction stress test (CST) is done when a nonreactive NST is obtained. Pregnancy is terminated only when the CST is abnormal or when ultrasonography shows evidence of oligohydramnios.

For the "poor obstetric dates" group, the NST is performed once a week. If the NST is nonreactive, the CST is done. Pregnancy is terminated when the CST is abnormal or when ultrasonography shows evidence of oligohydramnios.

Our protocol does not recommend termination of pregnancy at any specific gestational age. As long as antepartum fetal surveillance tests indicate good fetal condition and the cervix is not effaced, the pregnancy is allowed to continue until spontaneous labor occurs or abnormal test results indicate termi-

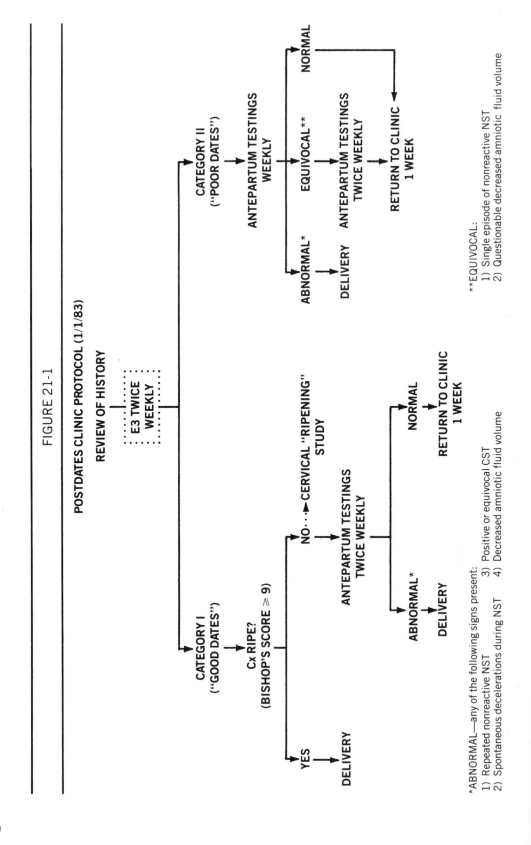

FIGURE 21-1

POSTDATES CLINIC PROTOCOL (1/1/83)

REVIEW OF HISTORY

E3 TWICE WEEKLY

CATEGORY I ("GOOD DATES")

Cx RIPE? (BISHOP'S SCORE ≥ 9)

YES → DELIVERY

NO ⋯► CERVICAL "RIPENING" STUDY

ANTEPARTUM TESTINGS TWICE WEEKLY

ABNORMAL* → DELIVERY

NORMAL → RETURN TO CLINIC 1 WEEK

CATEGORY II ("POOR DATES")

ANTEPARTUM TESTINGS WEEKLY

ABNORMAL* → DELIVERY

EQUIVOCAL**

ANTEPARTUM TESTINGS TWICE WEEKLY

NORMAL

RETURN TO CLINIC 1 WEEK

*ABNORMAL—any of the following signs present:
1) Repeated nonreactive NST   3) Positive or equivocal CST
2) Spontaneous decelerations during NST   4) Decreased amniotic fluid volume

**EQUIVOCAL:
1) Single episode of nonreactive NST
2) Questionable decreased amniotic fluid volume

nation. Under this management protocol, several infants were delivered past 44 weeks' gestation without any apparent complications. However, in private practice, it is not unreasonable to consider termination of pregnancy at 43 weeks or later providing a successful induction of labor and a safe delivery can be anticipated.

CONCLUSION

Post-term pregnancy, a confusing and controversial subject, is one of the more difficult problems encountered in obstetric practice. It has been reported that perinatal morbidity and mortality increase with prolonged gestation. However, careful antepartum and intrapartum fetal evaluation can minimize the risks to the mother and fetus.

SUGGESTED READING

Anderson AB, Lawrence KM, Turnbull AC: The relationship in anencephaly between the size of the adrenal cortex and the length of gestation. *J Obstet Gynaecol Br Commonw* 76:196, 1969

Beischer NA, Brown JB, Smith MA, Townsend L: Studies in prolonged pregnancy. II. Clinical results and urinary estriol excretion in prolonged pregnancy. *Am J Obstet Gynecol* 103:483, 1969

Beischer NA, Brown JB, Townsend L: Studies in prolonged pregnancy. III. Amniocentesis in prolonged pregnancy. *Am J Obstet Gynecol* 103:496, 1969

Beischer NA, Evans JH, Townsend L: Studies in prolonged pregnancy. I. The incidence of prolonged pregnancy. *Am J Obstet Gynecol* 103:476, 1969

Bishop EH: Pelvic scoring for elective induction. *Obstet Gynecol* 24:266, 1964

Browne JCM: Postmaturity. *JAMA* 186:1047, 1963

Clifford SH: Postmaturity—with placental dysfunction. Clinical syndrome and pathologic findings. *J Pediatr* 44:1, 1954

Evans TN, Koeff ST, Morley GW: Fetal effects of prolonged pregnancy. *Am J Obstet Gynecol* 85:701, 1963

Green JN, Paul RH: The value of amniocentesis in prolonged pregnancy. *Obstet Gynecol* 51:293, 1978

Klapholz H, Friedman EA: The incidence of intrapartum fetal distress with advancing gestational age. *Am J Obstet Gynecol* 127:405, 1977

Knox GE, Huddleston JF, Flowers CE: Management of prolonged pregnancy: Results of a prospective randomized trial. *Am J Obstet Gynecol* 134:376, 1979

Lindell A: Prolonged Pregnancy. *Acta Obstet Gynecol Scand* 35:136, 1956

Magram HM, Cavanagh WV: The problem of postmaturity. A statistical analysis. *Am J Obstet Gynecol* 79:216, 1960

Miller FC, Read JA: Intrapartum assessment of the postdate fetus. *Am J Obstet Gynecol* 141:516, 1981

Nwosu U, Wallach EE, Boggs TR, Bongiovanni AM: Possible adrenocortical insufficiency in postmature neonates. *Am J Obstet Gynecol* 122:969, 1975

Pritchard JA, MacDonald PC: *Williams Obstetrics*, ed 16. New York: Appleton-Century-Crofts, 1980, pp 949-952

Queenan JT, Thompson W, Whitfield CR, Shah SI: Amniotic fluid volumes in normal pregnancies. *Am J Obstet Gynecol* 114:34, 1972

Vorherr H: Placental insufficiency in relation to postterm pregnancy and postmaturity. *Am J Obstet Gynecol* 123:67, 1975

Yeh SY, Read JA: Management of postterm pregnancy in a large obstetric population. *Obstet Gynecol* 60:282, 1982

Zwerdling MA: Factors pertaining to prolonged pregnancy and its outcome. *Pediatrics* 40:202, 1967

22

Diagnosis and Management of Intrauterine Growth Retardation

LAWRENCE D. PLATT, M.D.

Intrauterine growth retardation (IUGR) represents an important diagnostic and management problem for the obstetrician. Recent data suggest a significant reduction in both physical and mental development of babies affected by IUGR when compared with normal controls at 12 months of age.

DEFINITION

A satisfactory definition has still not been agreed upon. Some feel IUGR was present whenever a baby weighs less than the *tenth centile* for the normal population at birth. Others feel this is too insensitive an index; thus, the *fifth centile* is often used. In discussing definitions, it is important to realize that each obstetric population studied is unique; and it is not possible to use the same growth charts for different populations.

NORMAL FETAL GROWTH

Fetal growth depends upon a balance between the natural growth potential of the fetus and the fetal environment, the latter being controlled by placental and maternal factors.

What constitutes normal fetal growth is unclear. Much of the data on fetal growth have been derived from animal experiments, and it is by no means clear that extrapolation to the human situation is justifiable. Other data have come from fetuses born as the result of spontaneous premature labor, or fetuses delivered prematurely for an obstetric complication. It seems unlikely that these infants represent a normal population.

The available data suggest that increases in fetal length and weight describe a sigmoid curve when plotted against gestational age. The drive for fetal growth appears to be genetically controlled, but will be influenced by a number of factors. Physiologic control of fetal size appears to operate via a maternal restraining mechanism. The nature of this restraint has not been identified, but it may operate through an immunologic mechanism controlling placental proliferation. It is fundamental, of course, that the fetus must be provided with adequate nutrients and oxygen if growth is to proceed normally.

FACTORS ASSOCIATED WITH ABNORMAL FETAL GROWTH

The factors associated with IUGR may be considered under two categories: (1) maternal, and (2) fetal and placental.

Maternal Factors

The influence of *small maternal stature, poor maternal weight gain and low prepregnancy weight, cigarette smoking,* and *low social class* on fetal growth are well recognized. It has been shown in many studies that all of the above factors, working individually or in combination, will be associated with a reduction in birth size. Often the common denominator is low social class; patients in this group should be considered particularly at risk. Severe maternal malnutrition has been associated with IUGR, but, in most of these cases, caloric intake was less than 500 kilocalories a day. Such poor diets are rare in civilized societies.

Certain maternal diseases are known to be associated with growth retardation. These include moderate to severe hypertension, especially in the presence of proteinuria; renal disease; cyanotic cardiac and pulmonary disease; chronic urinary tract infections (possibly); and chronic debilitating diseases, especially when complicated by vascular problems.

Fetal and Placental Factors

Congenital anomalies may be associated with IUGR. Together with intrauterine infections, they probably represent about 10% of cases.

Placental damage as a result of partial separation may occur at any stage of pregnancy. If it is an early event, the regenerative capability of the placenta will probably enable full function to be restored. However, such damage occurring later in pregnancy may permanently reduce the efficiency of the placenta and give rise to IUGR.

DIAGNOSIS AND ASSESSMENT

Since about 50% of growth-retarded infants show moderate to severe acidosis at birth, it is essential that attempts be made to identify this group antenatally. The diagnosis of IUGR depends upon an obstetric history, clinical examination, and ancillary aids.

The most important aspects of the history involve the factors mentioned above that have been associated with IUGR. Thus, the mother's social history, including her diet, habits (smoking, drinking, drugs), and type of habitation should be considered very important. Elucidation of the previous obstetric history with particular reference to birth weights, gestational ages, and neonatal courses is also essential.

Careful assessment of gestational age is required, since the diagnosis of IUGR will be impossible without these data. Clinical examination of the patient should be performed as early in pregnancy as possible, and, in cases judged to be at risk, should be repeated at regular intervals throughout the pregnancy. It has been shown that IUGR is diagnosed in only 30-40% of cases by clinical assessment alone. However, the obstetrician may improve the diagnostic rate by continually attempting to assess fetal weight in every patient examined. Further, the simple measurement of fundal height may allow identification of 50% of growth-retarded fetuses. Finally, suspicion should be aroused when amniotic fluid volume seems decreased.

The use of ultrasound in obstetrics has brought a new perspective to the diagnosis of IUGR. Several parameters have been measured in an attempt to evaluate fetal growth. The best known has been the biparietal diameter (BPD) of the fetal skull. The BPD has been shown to increase almost linearly until about the 36th week, after which a flattening of the curve is normally noted. Early serial measurements allow for accurate assessment of the gestational age, and also identify cases in which marked flattening of the BPD curve appears prior to the 36th week. But such an approach may identify no more than 50% of growth-retarded fetuses, and does not allow for the "head-sparing" (or "brain-sparing") phenomenon, in which growth-retarded infants have virtually normal head sizes. These infants are said to have suffered asymmetrical growth retardation.

To further evaluate the fetus, a technique was devised to measure fetal girth at the level of the liver. The liver is severely affected by intrauterine starvation, and its diminished size is reflected in a smaller than normal fetal girth. Yet another technique has been devised by Gohari, which assesses total uterine volume.

Recently, we have described a simple ultrasound screening method for IUGR. This technique involves identification of amniotic fluid volume with real-time ultrasound. *If a pocket of amniotic fluid larger than 1 cm can be seen in a vertical depth, the likelihood that the fetus is growth-retarded is less than 5%.* Conversely, *when less than 1 cm of fluid is seen, there is a 40% chance that the fetus will be growth-retarded.*

Finally, a recent report has demonstrated that, by measuring the fetal BPD and crown-rump length (CRL) in the third trimester, an even larger proportion of IUGR fetuses will be identified.

Further assessment of fetal status may be achieved by both biophysical and biochemical techniques. Antepartum fetal heart testing, using either a non-stress or stress technique, is useful. The biophysical profile has also been shown to be helpful. Biochemical evaluation should be performed. Tulchinsky believes urinary estriols may be more reflective of fetal size than plasma estriols. The use of plasma levels of human placental lactogen (hPL) remains controversial, although as many as 70% of pregnancies complicated by IUGR will show low hPL levels.

MANAGEMENT

Since the diagnosis of IUGR is so difficult, it has been almost impossible to devise a management/treatment scheme. It appears that there are two basic types of growth retardation—symmetrical and asymmetrical.

Symmetrical retardation appears early in pregnancy, perhaps around 18-20 weeks. It may be associated with genetic abnormalities or intrauterine infections, and it appears that there is a reduction in total cell number rather than cell size. Certainly, "head-sparing" is not apparent; and after birth, these babies have a higher incidence of mental handicaps and grow into physically smaller children. Treatment of patients in this group, even if identified, is unlikely to be helpful. Early damage to the placenta by abruption or perhaps reduced placental perfusion secondary to vascular disease may be associated with symmetrical growth retardation. Under these circumstances, bed rest in the lateral recumbent position may improve placental blood flow and allow the fetal growth velocity to be normalized.

Asymmetrical growth retardation occurs later in pregnancy and will often be associated with hypertension of any etiology or antepartum hemorrhage. Under these circumstances, total cell number is not affected, and fetal growth potential is inhibited by failure of the placenta to deliver sufficient nutrients and oxygen. Treatment depends on fetal lung maturation, which is often accelerated in IUGR. If examination of the amniotic fluid obtained by amniocentesis suggests full lung maturation, it is best to deliver the baby. Close fetal monitoring is necessary during labor, as fetal distress is likely to occur in one-third of these cases. A positive oxytocin challenge test in the presence of IUGR has been associated with a 75% incidence of severe fetal distress during labor. If lung maturation is not present, the patient should be put at bed rest and fetal status evaluated daily until maturation occurs or some other obstetric factor indicates the need for delivery (i.e., severe preeclampsia or heavy vaginal bleeding).

NEONATAL OUTCOME

The immediate neonatal period is a time of great risk for the growth-retarded infant. For this reason, any fetus diagnosed antenatally as suffering from IUGR should be delivered in a "high-risk" center.

Older studies have demonstrated that the first 72 hours following birth are particularly critical. Because of intrauterine starvation, stores of glycogen and fat are low. This can lead to both hypoglycemic attacks and a failure of temperature control. Blood glucose levels below 40 mg% may cause cerebral damage. Hypocalcemia and hyponatremia may be present, the former often diagnosed after the baby has become "jittery" or convulsed. Polycythemia and increased blood viscosity may cause sludging in the capillaries, possibly resulting in cerebral, pulmonary, and peripheral damage. The enterocolitis sometimes seen in IUGR infants may have a similar etiology.

The long-term prognosis has not been entirely assessed. Many studies have failed to distinguish between symmetrical and asymmetrical patterns of growth retardation. Certainly, the outcome in these two groups is likely to be very different. There is some evidence that *in asymmetrical head-sparing growth retardation, subsequent neurologic development is normal*. Once these infants are delivered from the growth-inhibiting environment in which they existed, they grow rapidly, usually attaining their potential growth centile within 6 months. However, when growth retardation is symmetrical, the babies grow to be small children. These children may have lower IQs and may be more likely to manifest other neurologic deficits later in life.

SUMMARY

IUGR is an important complication of pregnancy. Diagnosis is difficult; once it is made, management depends on the degree of growth retardation and the state of lung maturation. The neonatal course can be precarious in the immediate postdelivery period. The long-term effect on outcome in these children is, at the moment, unclear, but it would appear that, as a group, they are more likely to demonstrate some level of cerebral dysfunction.

SUGGESTED READING

Bergner L, Susser MW: Low birthweight and prenatal nutrition: An interpretative view. *Pediatrics* 46:946, 1970

Bowes WA, Droegemueller W: Management of IUGR. *Contemp Ob/Gyn* 2:10, 1974

Cetrulo CL, Freeman RK: Bioelectric evaluation of IUGR. *Clin Obstet Gynecol* 20:979, 1977

Gohari P, Berkowitz RL, Hobbins JC: Prediction of IUGR by determination of total intrauterine volume. *Am J Obstet Gynecol* 127:255, 1977

Low JA, Galbraith RS, Muir D, Killen H, Karlhmar J, Campbell D: Intrauterine growth retardation: A preliminary report of long-term morbidity. *Am J Obstet Gynecol* 130:534, 1978

Manning FA, Hill LM, Platt LD: Qualitative amniotic fluid volume determination by ultrasound—Antepartum detection of IUGR. *Am J Obstet Gynecol* 139:254, 1980

Manning FA, Platt LD, Sipos L: Antepartum fetal evaluation—Development of a fetal biophysical profile. *Am J Obstet Gynecol* 135:787, 1980

Neilson JP, Whitfield CR, Atchison TC: Screening for the small for dates fetus: A two stage ultrasonic examination schedule. *Br Med J* 280:1230, 1980

Ounsted M, Ounsted C: On fetal growth rate. *Clin in Develop Med* 46, 1973

Tulchinsky D, Ryan KJ: *Maternal-Fetal Endocrinology*. Philadelphia: Saunders, 1980

Usher R, McLean F: Intrauterine growth of live-born Caucasian infants at sea level: Standards obtained from measurements in 7 dimensions of infants born between 25 and 44 weeks of gestation. *J Pediatr* 74:901, 1969

23

Premature Rupture of the Membranes

RAUL ARTAL, M.D.

Premature rupture of the membranes remains one of the major causes of premature labor. In some of the more recent studies, it has been reported that premature labor is preceded by premature rupture of membranes in about 30% of cases.

Premature rupture of the membranes is defined as the spontaneous breaking of the chorioamniotic membranes anytime prior to the onset of labor. It is still generally agreed that etiology is unknown. In experimental studies, membranes that ruptured prematurely as well as normal membranes were found to withstand pressures as high as or higher than those generated by labor, suggesting that uterine contractions do not cause membrane rupture.

We have postulated and partially demonstrated a process of accelerated aging, comprised of different stages, in prematurely ruptured membranes. Due to an inherited defect, membrane integrity may be altered at its formation during the cross-linking of collagen, as a consequence of lower maternal serum copper levels. Later in pregnancy, the membranes may be damaged by enzymatic depolymerization of the collagen fibers. Similar damage may be inflicted by proteolytic enzymes released during an inflammatory process or by collagenase-like enzymes released from seminal fluid.

DIAGNOSIS

Diagnosis is usually made from the typical history: a "sudden gush of water" originating in the vagina. The diagnosis may be confirmed by vaginal examination with a sterile speculum and by two tests: the Nitrazine paper test, whereby the fluid is shown to be alkaline; and the ferning or arborization test, in which the dried fluid is shown to produce a ferning pattern. In cases where there is still doubt, cytologic studies can detect fetal cells resulting from desquamation of fetal skin, which color orange with the Nile blue stain.

In the past, much attention has been paid to a condition called a "high leak." Patients diagnosed as having premature rupture of the membranes would be found to have intact membranes upon arriving for delivery. The speculation was that the membranes had resealed. It is my belief that such a condition does not exist; that the confusion arises because some patients collect excessive amounts of amniotic fluid between the amnion and the chorion during the first half of gestation. On occasion, the chorion ruptures, allowing this fluid to escape, while the amnion remains intact for the rest of gestation. To confirm such a diagnosis, cytologic studies should be done to demonstrate the absence of fetal cells in the fluid. Such a diagnosis could save unnecessary treatment and hospitalization.

MANAGEMENT

The management of patients with premature rupture of the membranes has caused many controversies in the past; even today, there is no generally accepted approach. Management protocols instituted in different hospitals have usually been guided by each hospital's success in providing care for premature infants and in preventing chorioamnionitis. The management problems originate from the delicate balance needed between preventing chorioamnionitis in the mother and avoiding delivery of a premature baby.

Chorioamnionitis

About 90% of patients go into labor within 48 hours of membrane rupture. The incidence of chorioamnionitis increases progressively with time elapsed between rupture and delivery. Different studies have quoted an incidence of chorioamnionitis as high as 10%.

The criteria set for the diagnosis of chorioamnionitis are quite arbitrary: In the absence of any obvious cause for infection, any patient with rupture of membranes who has a temperature greater than 38°C or 100.4°F is considered to have chorioamnionitis until proven otherwise. Purulent or malodorous amniotic fluid is usually indicative of chorioamnionitis. Demonstration of bacteria, with or without white blood cells, in amniotic fluid obtained under sterile conditions is an ominous sign. But chorioamnionitis may be present despite negative cultures. Infections with *Mycoplasma*, anaerobic bacteria, or viruses have an effect similar to those caused by aerobic bacteria.

Once chorioamnionitis is suspected, maternal blood should be obtained for white cell count and cultures. In addition, in some institutions, measuring blood levels of C-reactive protein has proven very helpful in predicting chorioamnionitis. Elevated levels indicate impending infection long before clinical signs have been established. Amniotic fluid should be obtained by amniocentesis, under ultrasonographic guidance, for Gram-staining, white blood cell count, and quantitative cultures. Once the neonate is born, gastric fluid should be aspirated and blood should be drawn for cultures.

The use of prophylactic antibiotics in premature rupture of membranes remains very controversial. Most authorities do not recommend it in the absence of obvious infection.

Once the diagnosis of chorioamnionitis has been made, regardless of gestational age, expeditious evacuation of the uterus becomes desirable because of the high incidence of maternal morbidity and infant morbidity and mortality. In the past, mothers with premature rupture of the membranes who became infected have died of complications such as toxic shock, disseminated intravascular coagulation, and renal failure; such occurrences are very rare today. When neonates of the same birth weight are compared, perinatal mortality is significantly higher when chorioamnionitis is present.

Expectant Observation

In the absence of chorioamnionitis, delivery is indicated when there is evidence of fetal distress or fetal maturity. But with an immature fetus at low risk for developing infection, the course of action should be conservative; in other words, expectant observation. A few studies indicate that prolonged rupture of the membranes can lower the incidence of respiratory distress syndrome; however, other studies have shown no advantage for infants born after prolonged rupture. In the absence of a mature lung profile, administration of betamethasone is warranted.

In our institution, we developed a protocol for the treatment of patients with premature rupture of the membranes prior to 36 weeks' gestation. Amniocentesis is performed; despite reduced amounts of amniotic fluid, the procedure is successful in about 50% of patients. The amniotic fluid is analyzed for fetal lung profile, white blood cells, and bacteria. If the fetal lung profile indicates maturity or a Gram-stained smear indicates the presence of white blood cells and bacteria, the patient will be delivered. If no evidence of infection is found or no fluid is obtained, and gestational age is between 28 and 34 weeks, betamethasone (12 mg IM) is given to accelerate fetal lung maturity, with a second dose 24 hours later. If there is still no evidence of chorioamnionitis, patients are managed expectantly at bed rest in the hospital; theoretically chorioamnionitis may be acquired more readily at home.

During this period, the patient's peripads are collected, and amniotic fluid is squeezed out and used for lung profile determinations. Patients are closely monitored for signs of chorioamnionitis. Temperature is measured every 8 hours; complete blood counts are done initially at 12-hour intervals, then once a day. A significant increase in white blood cells with a 50% increase in bands is considered indicative of infection.

Newborns of patients with premature membrane rupture are at risk of developing group B streptococcal sepsis. At initial evaluation, during the sterile speculum exam, vaginal cultures are obtained. Results can be available within 8 hours. If colonization with group B β-hemolytic streptococci is found, the patient is delivered with intrapartum ampicillin coverage.

SUMMARY

There is a definite correlation between the length of the latent period and chorioamnionitis. Perinatal morbidity and mortality are due to chorioamnionitis or prematurity. The use of prophylactic antibiotics remains controversial. Prolonged premature rupture of the membranes may be associated with a lower incidence of respiratory distress syndrome in the newborn. Maternal steroid therapy appears to be beneficial. Real-time ultrasonography and amniocentesis are significant clinical aids.

SUGGESTED READING

Artal R, Burgeson R, Fernandez FJ, et al: Fetal and maternal copper levels in patients at term with and without premature rupture of membranes. *Obstet Gynecol* 53:608, 1978

Artal R, Burgeson RE, Hobel CJ, et al: An in vitro model for the study of enzymatically mediated biomechanical changes in the chorioamniotic membranes. *Am J Obstet Gynecol* 133:656, 1979

Artal R, Sokol RJ, Newman M, et al: The mechanical properties of prematurely and non-prematurely ruptured membranes. *Am J Obstet Gynecol* 125:655, 1976

Berkowitz RL, Bouta BW, Warshaw JE: The relationship between premature rupture of the membranes and the respiratory distress syndrome. *Am J Obstet Gynecol* 124:712, 1976

Danforth DN, Hull RW: The microscopic anatomy of the fetal membranes with particular reference to the detailed structure of the amnion. *Am J Obstet Gynecol* 75:536, 1958

Evans MI, Hajj SN, DeVoe LD, et al: C-reactive protein as a predictor of infectious morbidity with premature rupture. *Am J Obstet Gynecol* 138:648, 1980

Garite TJ, Freeman RK, Liuzey EM, et al: Prospective randomized study of corticosteroids in the management of premature rupture of membranes and the premature gestation. *Am J Obstet Gynecol* 141:508, 1981

Gibbs RS, Castillo MS, Rodgers PJ: Management of acute chorioamnionitis. *Am J Obstet Gynecol* 136:709, 1980

Golde S: The use of obstetric peripads in the collection of amniotic fluid in patients with rupture of the membranes. *Am J Obstet Gynecol* (in press)

Gunn GC, Mishell DR, Morton DG: Premature rupture of the fetal membranes. A review. *Am J Obstet Gynecol* 106:469, 1970

Johnson JW, Daikeku NH, Niebyl JR, et al: Premature rupture of the membranes and prolonged latency. *Obstet Gynecol* 57:547, 1981

Jones MD Jr, Burd LI, Bowes WA Jr, et al: Failure of association of premature rupture of membranes with respiratory distress syndrome. *N Engl J Med* 292:1253, 1975

Naeye RL: Factors that predispose to premature rupture of the fetal membranes. *Obstet Gynecol* 60:93, 1982

Naeye RL, Peters EC: Causes and consequences of premature rupture of fetal membranes. *Lancet* 1:192, 1981

Niswander KR, Gordon M: *The Women and Their Pregnancies. The collaborative perinatal study of the National Institute of Neurological Diseases and Stroke of the US Department of Health, Education, and Welfare Public Health Service, National Institutes of Health.* Philadelphia: Saunders, 1972, pp 427-434

Schreiber J, Benedetti T: Conservative management of preterm premature rupture of the fetal membranes in a low socioeconomic population. *Am J Obstet Gynecol* 136:92, 1980

Thiebeault DW, Emmanouilides GC: Prolonged rupture of fetal membranes and decreased frequency of respiratory distress syndrome and patent ductus arteriosus in preterm infants. *Am J Obstet Gynecol* 129:43, 1977

24

Management of Breech Presentation

FRANK C. MILLER, M.D.

Probably no other subject in clinical obstetrics arouses such controversy and diversity of opinion as the intrapartum management of breech presentation. The debate, for the most part, concerns what constitutes a safe delivery for both mother and baby. In general, older obstetricians, thoroughly trained and experienced in the mechanical art of breech extraction, and with a healthy concern for maternal complications associated with cesarean section, favor vaginal delivery. Younger obstetricians, mindful of the perinatal risks associated with the vaginal route, prefer cesarean section. Both sides have supporting arguments. This chapter marshals the pertinent published data concerning the arguments for and against cesarean section for all breech deliveries.

CAUSES OF PERINATAL MORTALITY IN BREECH PRESENTATION

There is little doubt that breech delivery presents a potential problem to the practitioner. Although breech presentation comprises only 3% of all deliveries, it is associated with a perinatal mortality rate that is three to five times that associated with cephalic presentation. Significant morbidity rates add to the overall perinatal loss associated with breech presentation. Five principal causes of breech perinatal mortality (listed in approximate order of importance) are: (1) prematurity, (2) congenital malformations, (3) birth injury, (4) birth anoxia, and (5) umbilical cord prolapse.

Prematurity, in and of itself, is recognized as the most significant cause of perinatal mortality in obstetrics today. The overall prematurity rate in any institution approaches 8-10%, but the prematurity rate associated with breech presentation exceeds 25%.

Congenital malformations have been reported to occur two to three times more often in breech than in cephalic presentations. Some studies suggest that up to 20% of premature breech babies have significant congenital anomalies. Fetal disorders associated with breech presentation include congenital hip dislocation, hydrocephaly, anencephaly, meningomyelocele, and familial dysautonomia.

Birth injury occurs significantly more often in vaginal breech than in cephalic deliveries. Birth injuries such as fracture of long bones, soft tissue injury, brachial plexus injury, and intracerebral hemorrhage secondary to tentorial tears often are related to difficult breech extraction or to vaginal delivery of a significantly premature infant. Vaginal delivery of breech infants with de-flexed heads in utero has been associated with fractures of the cervical spine and severe injury to the spinal cord. Although birth trauma is decreased by use of cesarean section, it is not eliminated.

Birth anoxia often results from umbilical cord entrapment during delivery or secondary to difficult delivery of the after-coming head.

Umbilical cord prolapse, a true obstetric emergency, occurs much more often in breech than in cephalic presentations. The incidence of cord prolapse in cephalic presentations is less than 0.5% and is only slightly greater in frank breech presentations (about 0.5-0.9%). The overall incidence in complete and incomplete breech presentations is 5%, and in footling breech presentations the incidence exceeds 10%. The significance of cord prolapse is open to question. The vast majority of cord prolapses (90%) occur in the second stage of labor and during delivery and are not nearly as potentially harmful as early (first stage) prolapse.

MANAGEMENT TECHNIQUES AND ASSOCIATED RISKS

Obstetric attempts to reduce breech perinatal risk at delivery have included external cephalic version, x-ray pelvimetry, Piper forceps, and cesarean section. While all these techniques may improve outcome, only cesarean section has consistently resulted in significantly lowered perinatal mortality rates, approaching zero for term infants. Routine cesarean section for breech presentation prevents the umbilical cord prolapse, birth injury, and birth anoxia associated with vaginal delivery. Cesarean section, however, will not erase the breech perinatal risk associated with prematurity or congenital malformations. In addition, cesarean section is a major operative procedure with its own risks to the mother, including anesthetic complications, hemorrhage, and infection, as well as intraoperative injury to bowel and bladder. Because neither vaginal nor cesarean delivery is entirely safe for both mother and fetus, the controversy continues.

At Women's Hospital, Los Angeles County/University of Southern California Medical Center, we are especially concerned about the risks of vaginal delivery for the premature breech fetus, so we recommend cesarean section for all breech presentations estimated to weigh between 750 and 2,000 gm. Prior to cesarean section, real-time ultrasound or abdominal x-ray must be used to detect any structural abnormalities in the fetus. If an anencephalic or grossly deformed fetus is detected, vaginal delivery is allowed.

At our institution, a randomized prospective study of selected patients with frank breech presentation was conducted. Patients with an estimated fetal weight betweeen 2,500 and 3,800 gm were allowed to labor and deliver vaginally if they had adequate x-ray pelvimetry (Table 24-1) and no evidence of a deflexed fetal head. All candidates for vaginal delivery were monitored for fetal heart rate and uterine activity throughout labor and were compared with a group of matched patients undergoing elective cesarean section.

TABLE 24-1. X-RAY PELVIMETRY, MINIMAL MEASUREMENTS

Pelvic plane	cm
Inlet:	
Transverse	11.5
Anteroposterior	10.5
Midpelvis:	
Transverse	10.0
Anteroposterior	11.5

For breech patients with anticipated vaginal delivery, a continuous epidural anesthetic was preferred for both labor and delivery. When epidural anesthesia was not available, satisfactory results were obtained in most cases with a pudendal anesthetic coupled with halothane general anesthesia for delivery of the after-coming head.

To ensure better control and avoid possible trauma, Piper forceps were applied for delivery of the after-coming head. In the patient group studied, those who met the selection criteria for vaginal delivery suffered no perinatal mortality. There was some perinatal morbidity secondary to delivery trauma. This occurred not with the delivery of the head, but consisted of brachial plexus injury secondary to nuchal arms. (The incidence was 2 in 30 vaginally delivered breech infants.) From this study, we conclude that it seems reasonable to allow vaginal delivery in carefully selected cases of term frank breech presentation.

We are currently studying the applicability of a similar selective protocol in term breech infants with nonfrank presentation. To date, 105 nonfrank breech presentations at term (estimated weight > 2,000 gm) have been studied. The x-ray pelvimetry guidelines in Table 24-1 were also used for this study. Patients who qualified for a trial of labor met the following criteria: estimated fetal weight between 2,000 and 4,000 gm; adequate x-ray pelvimetry measurements; and normal-appearing fetus without deflexed head on ultrasound. Of these patients, 44% were delivered vaginally. There was no difference in neonatal morbidity between those delivered vaginally and those delivered by cesarean section.

Antepartum external cephalic version has now been added to our management choices. We have performed almost 200 of these procedures with only minor problems. Selection is limited to mature fetuses (37-39 weeks) with normal fetal heart rate testing (i.e., reactive nonstress test). A β-mimetic (currently ritodrine hydrochloride given by infusion pump at 100 μg/minute for 10 minutes) is given to relax the uterus and facilitate manipulation. In our pilot study, we were able to significantly lower the need for cesarean section by successful turning in 80% of our cases. The widespread applicability of this method is controversial. Intensive fetal and maternal observation is required in a hospital setting to minimize risks.

SUMMARY

We believe that the use of selective delivery protocols and external cephalic version with tocolysis at term offer two important alternatives to routine cesarean section for the breech-presenting infant.

SUGGESTED READING

Berendes HW, Weiss W, Deutschberger J, et al: Factors associated with breech delivery. *Am J Public Health* 55:708, 1965

Brenner WE, Bruce SR, Hendricks CH: The characteristics and perils of breech presentation. *Am J Obstet Gynecol* 118:700, 1974

Collea JV, Rabin S, Weghorst G, Quilligan EJ: Randomized management of term frank breech presentation. *Am J Obstet Gynecol* 131:186, 1978

Gimovsky ML, Walloa RL, Schifrin BS, Paul RH: Randomized management of the non-frank breech presentation at term—A preliminary study. (work in progress)

Mayer PS, Wingate MC: Obstetric factors in cerebral palsy. *Obstet Gynecol* 51:399, 1978

Morgan HS, Kane SH: An analysis of 16,327 breech births. *JAMA* 187:108, 1964

Rovinsky JJ, Miller JA, Kaplan S: Management of breech presentation at term. *Am J Obstet Gynecol* 115:497, 1973

Saling E, Wolfgang MH: External cephalic version under tocolysis. *J Perinat Med* 3:115, 1975

Van Dorsten JP, Schifrin BS, Wallace RL: Randomized control trial of external cephalic version with tocolysis in late pregnancy. *Am J Obstet Gynecol* 141:417, 1981

25

Postpartum Uterine Atony

LESTER T. HIBBARD, M.D.

Uterine atony is the principal cause of postpartum hemorrhage and is associated with a number of factors, including prolonged labor, oxytocin augmentation of labor, overdistension of the uterus by twins or hydramnios, general anesthesia, chorioamnionitis, malnutrition, grand multiparity, fetal macrosomia, uterine apoplexy, and dystocia. The diagnosis is easily made by palpation of a relaxed uterine fundus, followed by careful vaginal inspection to rule out coexisting cervical or vaginal lacerations, and manual exploration of the uterus to rule out retained placental fragments or membranes and uterine rupture. Whenever the possibility of uterine atony can be anticipated, advance preparations should include establishment of an intravenous line using a large-bore needle or cannula and crossmatching of the patient's blood.

Initial management of atony includes establishment of an infusion of 5% dextrose in lactated Ringer's solution or normal saline containing 20 to 40 units of oxytocin. Crossmatched blood (2 to 4 units) should be available. Then the placenta and membranes are manually removed, and the fundus is both elevated and massaged through the abdominal wall.

If the initial response is unsatisfactory, 0.2 mg of ergonovine (Ergotrate) can be given either intramuscularly or slowly intravenously (to minimize the risk of drug-induced hypertension). As an alternative, 10 units of oxytocin (Pitocin, Syntocinon) can be injected into the cervix. Or, if available, 0.25 mg of 15-methylprostaglandin $F_{2\alpha}$ can be administered intramuscularly, and repeated up to a total of 4 doses if necessary. In abdominal delivery, the same dose may be administered into the myometrium. 15-Methylprostaglandin $F_{2\alpha}$ is contraindicated in patients with a history of asthma or glaucoma.

If atony persists, a gloved fist should immediately be placed in the vagina, pushing the uterus up and out of the pelvis, with the other hand providing counterpressure through the abdominal wall to anteflex the fundus over the vaginal fist. (At this point, the lower uterine segment should be palpated carefully to make certain that a rupture was not overlooked at the initial examination.) If atony can be corrected by this maneuver, the uterus should be held in an elevated position for at least 5 more minutes. If atony recurs, fundal elevation should be maintained by external abdominal pressure for another hour, because uterine prolapse can also cause continuing hemorrhage.

When the above measures fail and the patient is jeopardized by continuing active hemorrhage, the lower abdominal aorta should be occluded by transabdominal compression against the sacral promontory while blood replacement and other measures are being prepared. At this point a uterine pack can be considered. Under light inhalation anesthesia, a gloved hand is inserted into the lower uterine segment while a 5-yard strip of sterile 4-inch gauze is fed into the fundus by packing forceps. Packing is systematic, beginning in one corner and passing from side to side until the entire cavity and lower uterine segment are filled. If successful, the pack is removed in 18 to 24 hours. Infection and continuing hemorrhage behind the pack are the principal complications. Hot intrauterine douches are sometimes recommended, but we have not been impressed with their effectiveness.

For stubborn cases, operative intervention may be necessary. Before considering hysterectomy, bilateral ligation of the ascending uterine arteries should be tried. This is easily and quickly accomplished by passing absorbable sutures through the angles of the lower uterine segment and around the vessels, taking care not to perforate the bladder. (If in doubt, a bladder flap should be mobilized.) Additional hemostasis can be obtained by placing second sutures around the ovarian branches of the ascending uterine arteries in the cornual areas. Experience with this procedure suggests that reproductive function is not seriously jeopardized by arterial ligation.

As an alternative, ligation of the hypogastric arteries can be considered, particularly when the cervical branches of the uterine arteries seem to be contributing to the hemorrhage. In practice, hypogastric ligation does not seem to add much to uterine artery ligation, and certain additional risks are involved, particularly when the operator is unfamiliar with the procedure. Possible complications include inadvertent ligation of the external iliac artery and laceration of the underlying hypogastric vein. Both are potentially lethal.

One other approach for intractable cases involves angiography by way of the right common femoral artery followed by the deposition of a material, such as Gelfoam particles, that induces clot formation in the bleeding vessel.

Hysterectomy may become necessary as a last resort. Total hysterectomy is most often performed, although a subtotal operation would probably be just as effective and a good deal safer for a patient who has become a poor operative risk.

Finally, it should not be forgotten that uterine atony can be associated with a coagulation disorder. In that event, correction of the clotting deficiency becomes a vital step in the patient's management.

SUGGESTED READING

Brown BJ, et al: Uncontrollable postpartum bleeding: New approach to hemostasis through angiographic arterial embolization. *Obstet Gynecol* 54:361, 1979

Hayashi M, et al: Management of severe postpartum hemorrhage due to uterine atony using an analogue of prostaglandin $F_{2\alpha}$. *Obstet Gynecol* 58:426, 1981

Moir DD, Amoa AB: Ergometrine or oxytocin? Blood loss and side-effects at spontaneous vertex delivery. *Br J Anaesth* 51:113, 1979

Toppozada M, et al: Control of intractable atonic postpartum hemorrhage by 15-methyl prostaglandin $F_{2\alpha}$. *Obstet Gynecol* 58:327, 1981

Weekes LR, Gandhi S: Five year study of postpartum hemorrhage: Queen of Angels Hospital, 1973-1977. *J Natl Med Assoc* 71:829, 1979

26

Placenta Previa

JEFFREY P. PHELAN, M.D.

Placenta previa occurs in about 1:200 pregnancies. A higher incidence is found in gravidas with a prior history of abortion, placenta previa, or cesarean section. By definition, placenta previa is the location of the placenta in the area of the lower uterine segment, near or covering the internal os. The various types are classified according to degree of placental encroachment on the os. For example, total covering of the cervical os by the placenta is known as *complete* or *total previa*. In *partial previa*, only a portion of the os is occluded. In *low-lying previa*, the placenta occupies the lower uterine segment, but does not occlude the os.

DIAGNOSIS

Classically, the patient with placenta previa presents with a history of painless, bright red vaginal bleeding. However, pain accompanying vaginal bleeding, while frequently the hallmark of abruptio placentae, may be seen in 10-11% of patients with placenta previa. About 20% will present with uterine activity. In addition, due to the placenta's location in the lower uterine segment, unstable lies and malpresentation are frequently encountered.

When third-trimester vaginal bleeding occurs and the diagnosis of placenta previa is considered, immediate establishment of an intravenous line with a 16-gauge needle is indicated. The line should be kept patent with fluids. Simultaneously, blood should be drawn for type and crossmatch, clotting profile, hemoglobin, and hematocrit.

As part of the diagnostic work-up, real-time or B-scan ultrasound should be performed. Ultrasound is much better at ruling out placenta previa than ruling it in. For example, if the placenta is located in the uterine fundus, or high on the anterior or posterior wall, placenta previa can be ruled out with a high degree of accuracy. However, if the placenta is located in the lower uterine segment, the diagnostic accuracy of ultrasound is related to the type of previa (complete > partial > low-lying).

Even though ultrasonography is useful, the only sure method of accurately diagnosing placenta previa is a vaginal examination. However, *a vaginal exam should not be done unless complete preparations have been made for delivery of the infant.*

Due to the development of the lower uterine segment, a placenta that was infringing on the cervical os in early pregnancy will frequently appear to migrate to a higher position in the uterus with advancing gestation. Therefore, many cases of placenta previa in early pregnancy will be found to have resolved themselves later in gestation.

MANAGEMENT

When placenta previa is suspected sonographically in a hemodynamically stable patient, management is based on the gestational age of the fetus. In the preterm pregnancy (≤36 weeks' gestation or immature phospholipid profile), delivery and expectant management are the available alternatives.

Expectant management should be reserved for cases in which the fetal heart rate pattern and maternal clotting profile are normal; and in which the presenting acute bleeding episode has not persisted. In the occasional patient who presents with previa and premature labor, but without hemorrhage, an attempt at tocolysis should be considered.

Expectant management involves mandatory hospitalization with bed rest. In addition, the following should be considered: (1) ultrasonography every two weeks, (2) weekly antepartum fetal surveillance, (3) assurance of availability of crossmatched blood, (4) maintenance of maternal hematocrit > 30%, and (5) administration of RhoGAM to the Rh-negative gravida. (RhoGAM dosage should be determined by the Kleihauer-Betke technique, which quantitates the volume of fetal red cells in the maternal circulation.)

When bleeding has completely ceased, the patient may be ambulated. If no further bleeding occurs after 2 days of ambulation, the patient may be considered for discharge from the hospital to home care. Discharge of the patient should be contingent upon a home environment that is conducive to a rapid return to the hospital at the first sign of bleeding. Crossmatched blood should remain readily available.

Indications for delivery of the preterm previa patient are as follows: (1) continued moderate bleeding, (2) persistent labor, (3) estimated acute blood loss > 500 ml, (4) evidence of coagulation defect, and (5) evidence of fetal pulmonary maturity.

In the term pregnancy (>36 weeks' gestation or mature phospholipid profile), a double set-up examination should be done in the operating room with the team ready for either vaginal delivery or immediate cesarean section. If complete previa has been noted sonographically, or fetal heart rate abnormality, malpresentation, or heavy vaginal bleeding (>500 ml) is present, a double set-up examination can be avoided.

If placenta previa is confirmed at the double set-up examination, a cesarean section should be performed. The uterine incision should be made so as to avoid the placenta, thereby reducing the likelihood of maternal and fetal blood loss. Fetal blood loss can be significant; anemias occur in about 19% of fetuses. As a result, it is prudent to have (O-negative) blood available in the operating room for transfusion of the fetus if necessary.

After cesarean delivery, patients with placenta previa tend to have an increased incidence of placenta accreta and uterine atony. Therefore, gentle traction of the placenta and close postpartum observation are mandatory. Persistent bleeding or postpartum atony unresponsive to oxytocics may require uterine artery, ovarian artery, or hypogastric artery ligation. If these approaches fail to stop maternal hemorrhage, a hysterectomy is necessary.

SUGGESTED READING

Breen JL, Neubecker R, Gregori CA, Franklin JE: Placenta accreta, increta, and percreta. A survey of 40 cases. *Obstet Gynecol* 49:43, 1977

Cotton DB, Read JA, Paul RH, Quilligan EJ: The conservative aggressive management of placenta previa. *Am J Obstet Gynecol* 137:687, 1980

Hibbard LT: Placenta previa. *Am J Obstet Gynecol* 104:172, 1969

Read JA, Cotton DB, Miller FC: Placenta accreta: Changing clinical aspects and outcome. *Obstet Gynecol* 56:31, 1980

Schmitz HE, O'Dee NJ, Isaacs JH: Placenta previa. A survey at the Lewis Memorial Maternity Hospital. *Obstet Gynecol* 3:3, 1954

27

Premature Separation of the Placenta (Abruptio Placentae)

SAMUEL L. BRUCE, M.D.

Definition. Abruptio placentae is the separation of the normally implanted placenta after the 20th week of gestation and before the birth of the fetus.

Etiology. The basic etiology of abruptio placentae is unknown, but the following have been implicated as possible contributing factors:

1. Short umbilical cord
2. External trauma to the maternal abdomen
3. Sudden decompression of the uterus
4. Uterine anomalies or tumors
5. Inferior vena cava occlusion
6. Maternal folate deficiency
7. Chronic vascular diseases, e.g., chronic hypertension, in the mother
8. High parity
9. Previous placental abruption.

Incidence. The reported incidence varies from 0.2% to 2.4%. The recurrence rate in subsequent pregnancies is 11%. The incidence is also increased in patients of high parity, but not significantly with age. Over 50% of abruptions occur prior to the 36th week of gestation. When the abruption is accompanied by fetal death, there is a 30% chance that the fetus will die in a future pregnancy if abruption occurs.

Types of abruption. Classically, there are three types:

1. *External or revealed bleeding.* This occurs when some blood dissects between the membranes and the uterus and escapes through the cervix. This type accounts for 85% of cases.
2. *Concealed hemorrhage.* In this type of abruption, blood does not escape externally, but is retained between the detached placenta and the uterus or extravasates into the amniotic cavity. This accounts for 15% of cases. Concealed hemorrhage is more often seen in patients with hypertensive vascular disease. It occurs when:
   a. There is effusion of blood behind the placenta, but the margins remain attached

b. The membranes remain attached and the blood gains access into the amniotic cavity

c. The fetal presenting part is so firmly applied to the cervix that the blood cannot escape.

Concealed hemorrhage carries with it more dangerous consequences for the mother. Classically, it presents as maternal shock that is out of proportion to the amount of apparent blood loss.

3. *Marginal placental rupture.* This variant of external bleeding represents placental separation limited to the margin of the organ.

The basic pathologic process in abruptio placentae is initiated by hemorrhage into the decidua basalis. The decidua then splits, leaving a thin layer adherent to the myometrium. As the clot thus formed retroplacentally enlarges, more and more of the placenta separates and the situation worsens.

Diagnosis. The classic history is that of the patient who notices the sudden onset of vaginal bleeding associated with crampy or continuous abdominal pain. The bleeding may be minimal in amount in cases of concealed abruption. There is usually overt vaginal bleeding in external or revealed abruption, as well as in marginal placental rupture. In addition to pain and vaginal bleeding, other signs of abruption include:

1. Increased uterine activity (hypertonic uterus), with an elevation in the resting tone of the uterus. The uterus may also be irritable and contract with slight manipulation. There is usually some tenderness on palpation of the uterus, and this may be either localized or generalized.

2. Hypovolemia secondary to the bleeding, with tachycardia and shock. In concealed abruption, shock will be out of proportion to the amount of blood lost.

3. Absence of fetal heart tones in cases of severe abruption (>50% separation of the placenta).

4. Enlarging uterus due to the accumulation of retroplacental blood.

5. Bloody amniotic fluid on rupture of membranes. In some cases of concealed abruption, the retroplacental hemorrhage ruptures into the amniotic sac.

MANAGEMENT

An intravenous infusion should be started with a large-bore needle or catheter. The intravenous line should be kept patent with lactated Ringer's solution, 5% dextrose in normal saline, or just normal saline. Blood should be drawn for hematocrit, type and crossmatch (for at least 2 units of whole blood), fibrinogen, platelets, fibrin degradation products, and partial thromboplastin time (PTT). A separate tube of blood should be saved for the clot observation test. Coagulation failure is diagnosed if no clot is formed in 6 minutes or the clot formed is lysed within 60 minutes. If no clot is formed in 30 minutes, this may mean the fibrinogen level is less than 100 mg%.

Maternal assessment. Maternal blood pressure, heart rate, respiratory rate, fluid intake, and urine output must be monitored. Height of the uterine fundus is also marked to help diagnose a change in uterine size secondary to enlarging retroplacental clot.

Fetal assessment. Fetal heart tones should be auscultated. If placenta previa has been ruled out, vaginal examination should be performed. Because of the decrease in placental surface area that occurs with abruption, the placenta's respiratory function may be compromised, and the fetus may become hypoxic and acidotic. Fetal distress may, therefore, be seen as tachycardia, decreased fetal heart rate (FHR) variability, late decelerations, terminal bradycardia, and death.

In mild abruption with slight bleeding in a stable mother with a preterm fetus, conservative management may be attempted. The patient must be observed closely for further bleeding or any signs of pain or increasing abruption. However, in most patients, the pregnancy must be terminated.

In mild abruption with a term-size fetus, or in moderate to severe abruption regardless of gestational age, the pregnancy should be terminated. Placenta previa is ruled out by B-scan, when available, or by double set-up. Then, if there is no contraindication to vaginal delivery, amniotomy is performed, a direct monitoring system is put into place, and labor is augmented with oxytocin if necessary (this is usually not necessary). Unmatched O-negative blood may be used until matched blood is available.

Unless the cervix is completely dilated and the vertex is low in the pelvis, cesarean section, under general anesthesia, is done when any of the following is present:

1. Fetal distress
2. Steady bleeding—moderate or heavier
3. Failure of the uterus to relax between contractions
4. Failure of labor to begin within 4 hours
5. Progression of the abruption
6. Progressive fall in fibrinogen levels.

It is recognized that maternal complications and neonatal outcome are directly related to the length of time between onset of abruption and delivery. Some authorities believe this interval should not exceed 6 hours. Therefore, vaginal delivery should be attempted only if the delay is judged safe for both mother and fetus. Maternal and fetal parameters can change rapidly, and careful monitoring is essential. With a dead fetus, a longer interval may be warranted, but a cesarean may still be required for maternal indications.

Complications.

1. *Renal failure* (1.2-3.9%). This could manifest as oliguria or anuria, which may be due to renal tubular or cortical necrosis.
2. *Hemorrhage.* In addition to the severe hemorrhage that can occur acutely, these patients are also susceptible to postpartum hemorrhage due to uterine atony. This is especially true in patients with Couvelaire uteri.
3. *Coagulation failure.* Abruptio placentae is the most common cause of consumption coagulopathy (disseminated intravascular coagulation) in pregnancy. It occurs in about 30% of cases associated with fetal death.

The mechanism is believed to be release of thromboplastin into the circulation, which initiates intravascular coagulation, hypofibrinogenemia, and a decrease in platelets and factors V and VIII. This may trigger the fibrinolytic system and lead to the appearance of fibrin degradation products in the circulation.

4. *Uteroplacental apoplexy* (Couvelaire uterus), which is the extravasation of blood into the uterine musculature and beneath the uterine serosa. It is usually not an indication for hysterectomy. Most cases respond to oxytocics, but uterine atony may be a problem. If there is no response to oxytocics, ergonovine, or intramyometrial prostaglandins, then surgical treatment (including ligation of uterine or hypogastric arteries, or hysterectomy) may be considered. Further management depends on the severity of the abruption, the amount of blood loss, the presence of shock, and coagulation competency.

Management of coagulation failure. As mentioned above, one of the possible complications of abruptio placentae is the development of maternal hypofibrinogenemia (<100 mg/100 ml of plasma). Below this level, blood will usually fail to clot. If disseminated intravascular coagulation (DIC) should develop in association with abruptio placentae, prompt removal of the products of conception is the best treatment method. Replacement of clotting factors may sometimes be of use. In actively bleeding patients with severely depleted clotting factors, replacement using fresh, whole blood or frozen plasma is the treatment of choice.

There is controversy regarding the use of fibrinogen in these cases. In general, both fibrinogen and cryoprecipitate are less useful, because fibrinogen lacks factors V and VIII and cryoprecipitate lacks factor V. In addition, both may cause hepatitis. Many patients with fibrinogen levels below 100 mg/100 ml do not bleed from hypofibrinogenemia. Therefore, if active hemorrhage has ceased, fibrinogen need not be given despite low levels. Also, since hypofibrinogenemia rapidly corrects itself postpartum, in the absence of hemorrhage fibrinogen need not be given despite low postpartum levels.

When fresh, whole blood or frozen plasma is not available for a DIC patient with persistent bleeding and low fibrinogen levels, or for a patient with low fibrinogen levels being considered for abdominal delivery, then fibrinogen should be given. The recommended dose is 4-8 gm. A 4-gm dose of fibrinogen raises the blood level 100 mg/100 ml.

Heparin. The purpose of using heparin is to inhibit further coagulation, allowing restitution of blood coagulation factors. Some authors have reported favorable results, but very few institutions use this as a routine mode of treatment. In cases of persistent postpartum hemorrhage with low fibrinogen and high fibrinolysin levels, a heparin trial may be undertaken. But in general, experience with this treatment is limited.

When anticoagulation is used, it should always be by intravenous heparin. The usual anticoagulant doses should be used, with the aim of maintaining the

PTT at twice the normal value. This is done best with a constant rate of infusion, although intermittent boluses of heparin (e.g., 5,000 units q4h) may be adequate.

Anticoagulation is rarely needed in DIC associated with abruption. Clotting factor replacement is usually the treatment of choice. The use of antifibrinolytic agents, such as ϵ-aminocaproic acid, to prevent clot lysis and the development of fibrin degradation products is generally not recommended because: (1) clot lysis may be beneficial, and (2) these agents cross the placenta and may be harmful to the fetus.

Mortality. The maternal mortality associated with abruptio placentae varies from 0% to 1% depending on the series. The reported perinatal mortality is about 50%.

SUGGESTED READING

Beller FK, Uszynski M: Disseminated intravascular coagulation in pregnancy. *Clin Obstet Gynecol* 17:250, 1974

Bonnar J, McNicol GP, Douglas AS: The behavior of the coagulation and fibrinolytic mechanism in abruptio placentae. *J Obstet Gynaecol Br Commonw* 76:799, 1969

Gilditch IM, Boyce NE Jr: Management of abruptio placentae. *JAMA* 212:228, 1970

Hibbard CM: Abruptio placentae, preeclampsia and essential hypertension. *J Obstet Gynaecol Br Commonw* 69:282, 1962

Hibbard CM, Jeffcoate NA Jr: Abruptio placentae. *Obstet Gynecol* 27:155, 1966

Knab DR: Abruptio placentae. *Obstet Gynecol* 52:625, 1978

Lunan CB: The management of abruptio placentae. *J Obstet Gynaecol Br Commonw* 80:120, 1973

Pritchard JA, Brekken AL: Clinical and laboratory studies on severe abruptio placentae. *Am J Obstet Gynecol* 97:681, 1963

Pritchard JA, Mason R, Corley M, Pritchard S: Genesis of severe placental abruption. *Am J Obstet Gynecol* 108:22, 1970

Sher G: A rational basis for the management of abruptio placentae. *J Reprod Med* 21:123, 1978

28

Placenta Accreta

JEFFREY P. PHELAN, M.D.

Since the classic report on placenta accreta by Irving and Hertig in 1937, revolutionary changes have occurred in obstetrics. Based on a retrospective review and their own experience, these authors described a clinical entity characterized by placental adherence and an associated maternal mortality rate of 37.2%. With the advent of antibiotics and blood banking facilities, Fox reviewed 622 cases from 1945 to 1969 and found that maternal mortality had declined to 9.5%. Because of further changes in maternal, fetal, and neonatal intensive care and monitoring during the 1970s, the experience at LAC/USC (Los Angeles County/University of Southern California) Medical Center was recently reviewed to assess their impact on the outcome of patients with placenta accreta.

Placenta accreta is defined both clinically and pathologically. Clinically, it is the abnormal adherence, complete or partial, of the placenta to the underlying uterine wall. The histopathologic diagnosis is subclassified into three entities depending on depth of penetration of the placental villi. In *placenta accreta vera*, the placental villi adhere directly to the myometrium due to partial or complete absence of the decidua basalis. In *placenta increta*, there is deep invasion of villi into the myometrium. Penetration of placental villi through the entire thickness of the uterine wall is considered *placenta percreta*. Cases are also classified as *complete:* the entire placenta is abnormally adherent; *partial:* more than one cotyledon is abnormally adherent; or *focal:* a single cotyledon is adherent.

In a recent review of the histopathology of placenta accreta by Breen et al, the frequency by type was as follows: accreta 77.5%, increta 17.5%, and percreta 5.0%; and by degree of adherence: focal 20.0%, partial 17.5%, and complete 62.5%.

ETIOLOGY

Possible predisposing factors that have been associated with placenta accreta include: advanced maternal age, grand multiparity, multiparity alone, prior cesarean section, prior uterine surgery, infection or malformation, prior D&C, prior postpartum hemorrhage or manual removal of the placenta, and placenta previa. Currently, the more dominant etiologies are placenta previa, prior cesarean section, or both. In the LAC/USC Medical Center review, an associated placenta previa was found in 14 of 22 cases (63.6%). Of these, six had had one or more prior cesareans.

INCIDENCE

Prior to 1950, the reported incidence of placenta accreta was 1:30,000 deliveries. Since that time, the mean reported incidence has increased in each decade as follows: 1:19,000 in the 50s, 1:15,000 in the 60s, and 1:7,000 or less in the 70s. At the LAC/USC Medical Center from 1975 to 1979, the incidence was 1:2,562 deliveries. While enhanced awareness and better reporting may be responsible for the reported increase, a true increase may have occurred. This increase, despite decreasing average family size, may be related to the increased use of cesarean section or uterine instrumentation (D&C) for spontaneous and induced abortions.

DIAGNOSIS

While bleeding with placenta previa and severe, crampy, abdominal pain during pregnancy have been associated with placenta accreta, the diagnosis can be made only at the time of delivery. In the classical clinical situation, there is an inability to remove all or part of the placenta, associated with varying degrees of hemorrhage. The amount of hemorrhage (estimated to average 3,826 ml in the LAC/USC series) will vary from a little, as in cases of untraumatized complete placenta accreta, to profuse with partial accreta.

MANAGEMENT

Over the years, the clinical management of the patient with placenta accreta has changed dramatically due to advances in technology, blood banking, and antibiotics. Prior to 1950, immediate hysterectomy was advocated because of high maternal mortality associated with conservative approaches. Since 1950, several authors have reported successful outcomes in patients managed conservatively, i.e., without hysterectomy. At LAC/USC, a conservative approach (curettage, suturing of the bleeding site, and/or uterine or hypogastric artery ligation) was attempted in 12 of 22 cases. It was successful in eight.

Once the diagnosis of placenta accreta has been made, treatment must proceed rapidly. The choice between conservative management and immediate hysterectomy will depend on degree of hemorrhage and type of placenta accreta. In the patient with minimal bleeding and a small, partial or focal placenta accreta, conservative management appears justified. On rare occasions, success has been reported with the placenta left in situ. Because these patients are at greater risk of infection, delayed hemorrhage, re-operation, and mortality, this approach should be limited to patients with complete or partial accreta without bleeding. In patients with extensive hemorrhage, immediate hysterectomy is the preferred approach. In any case of massive bleeding, component blood replacement is essential to prevent or correct any coagulation difficulty—still the leading cause of maternal death in these cases.

During this century, maternal mortality from placenta accreta has declined from 37.2% (Irving and Hertig, 1937), to 9.5% (Fox, 1945-1969), to 3.1% during the 70s.

There has been a similar improvement in fetal and neonatal survival. In the LAC/USC series, there were no losses among 24 infants delivered in 22 cases of placenta accreta. This is in contrast to the 9.6% stillborn rate cited by Fox, and the overall loss rates of 35%, reported by McKeogh and D'Errico in 1951, and 25%, reported by Breen et al in 1977. Since, historically, most perinatal deaths were associated with maternal bleeding, ruptured uterus, ante- and intrapartum distress, and prematurity, a strong argument can be made that this improvement is due to better obstetric care in general and better antepartum and intrapartum surveillance (i.e., monitoring) in particular. Improved neonatal care and universal cesarean section for an atraumatic delivery in placenta previa with accreta seem to have improved the outcome for premature infants.

SUMMARY

There seems to be an increase in the incidence of placenta accreta, with placenta previa and prior cesarean section being the dominant associations. Management may be individualized in certain cases, but rapid recognition and treatment are essential, as a large blood loss with associated coagulation problems remains the lethal factor in this disease. With better maternal-fetal surveillance and general obstetric-surgical care, maternal and fetal mortality and morbidity have declined greatly.

SUGGESTED READING

Breen JL, Neubecker R, Gregoni CA, Franklin JE: Placenta accreta, increta, and percreta. A survey of 40 cases. *Obstet Gynecol* 49:43, 1977

Fox H: Placenta accreta, 1945-1969. *Obstet Gynecol Surv* 27:475, 1972

Irving FC, Hertig AT: A study of placenta accreta. *Surg Gynecol Obst* 64:178, 1937

McKeogh RP, D'Errico E: Placenta accreta: Clinical manifestations and conservative management. *N Engl J Med* 245:159, 1951

Read JA, Cotton DB, Miller FC: Placenta accreta: Changing clinical aspects and outcome. *Obstet Gynecol* 56:31, 1980

Weekes LR, Greig LB: Placenta accreta. A twenty year review. *Am J Obstet Gynecol* 113:76, 1972

29

The Significance of Meconium During Labor

FRANK C. MILLER, M.D.

The classic signs of "fetal distress" have been described as alterations in fetal heart rate (FHR) and passage of meconium. There is disagreement, however, about the precise significance of these signs, alone or together.

The presence of meconium with no other sign of fetal distress is reported to be associated with a perinatal mortality rate ranging from 1% to 13.5%. In 1955, Resnick reported a perinatal mortality rate of 8% with an abnormal FHR and thin meconium, and 32% with an abnormal FHR and thick meconium. In cases in which the FHR was below 110 beats per minute, Fenton and Steer found a perinatal mortality rate of 3.5% in the presence of thin meconium, and 21.4% with thick meconium. Recent studies have confirmed that thick meconium is associated with higher rates of fetal morbidity and mortality than is thin meconium.

It is apparent that there is no agreement about perinatal morbidity and mortality rates associated with meconium and various other clinical signs of fetal distress. Indeed, in recent years the significance of meconium as a reliable sign of fetal distress has been questioned. Clinical experience confirms that in many instances of fetal asphyxia and distress no meconium is passed. Conversely, meconium is often found without signs of fetal distress.

CAUSES OF MECONIUM PASSAGE

A review of the mechanism proposed for meconium passage may prove helpful in attempting to evaluate its significance in the amniotic fluid. Passage of meconium in utero may result from various stimuli. Walker found that fetuses passing meconium had lower umbilical vein oxygen saturation than did normal fetuses. Saling postulated that fetal hypoxia produces vasoconstriction in the fetal gut resulting in hyperperistalsis and sphincter relaxation, with passage of meconium. Hon suggested that meconium passage may be related not to hypoxia but to vagal activation from cord compression, especially in a mature fetus. Fenton and Steer considered the passage of meconium to be a normal physiologic function, perhaps a sign of increasing fetal maturity. Certainly the incidence of finding meconium in the amniotic fluid increases with gestational age. Passage of meconium is probably due to one, or a combination, of these causes.

EVALUATING FETAL RISK

Fetal biochemical and biophysical monitoring should provide a means by which the fetus with meconium passage may be more accurately evaluated.

Hobel found a good correlation between a fetal scalp blood pH below 7.25 and a 1-minute Apgar score under 7 if signs of fetal distress (meconium and/or abnormal FHR) were present. In his study, 40 of the 76 high-risk fetuses evaluated were associated with meconium in the amniotic fluid. A significant degree of fetal acidosis was found in early labor in the meconium group, whereas fetuses with no meconium, but with abnormal FHR patterns, developed acidosis later in labor. Infants with slight meconium, with or without abnormal FHR patterns, did as well as controls, judged by the 1- and 5-minute Apgar scores. The heavy-meconium group, with or without moderate or severe FHR abnormalities, had the lowest 1- and 5-minute Apgar scores in the study group.

In a study by our group, 366 high-risk patients with singleton pregnancies and vertex presentation were monitored during labor in the perinatal intensive-care delivery room. In all cases, maternal and fetal heart rate and intrauterine pressure were continuously monitored. Fetal scalp blood was sampled routinely during early labor, at 5-cm dilation, and at delivery. Umbilical cord arterial and venous blood samples were obtained at delivery. Newborn arterial blood samples were taken 4, 8, 16, 32, and 64 minutes after birth. All specimens were analyzed for pH, pO_2, pCO_2, and base deficit. Of the 366 patients, 106 (29%) had meconium in the amniotic fluid at some time during labor. This high incidence may be characteristic of high-risk populations and should not be considered the expected incidence.

Mean 1- and 5-minute Apgar scores were significantly lower for the infants with meconium passage than for the non-meconium group. The lowest scores were in the group with initially clear fluid but subsequent meconium passage during labor. The infants with meconium present at rupture of membranes also had slightly lower scores than did the controls. When meconium was found only at delivery, there was no reduction in Apgar score compared with the control group.

Infants with thick meconium had the lowest mean 1-minute Apgar score. The thin-meconium group also had scores that were lower, but not significantly, than the control scores. Therefore, it appeared that infants with thick-meconium passage during labor were at highest risk of having depressed Apgar scores.

There was no apparent difference in incidence of FHR deceleration patterns between the meconium and non-meconium groups when compared as groups or as any of the subgroups. When evaluating late decelerations in the meconium and non-meconium groups using χ^2 analysis, there was no statistical difference in incidence of low Apgar scores between meconium and non-meconium patients when there were late decelerations with fewer than 10% of the uterine contractions. However, with more than 10%, there was a marked and highly significant increase ($p < 0.01$) in the incidence of low Apgar scores in the meconium group. If the fetus was acidotic (pH < 7.25) and had more than 10% late decelerations, the Apgar score was found to be low in both meconium and non-meconium groups, as one would expect.

These data indicate that without signs of fetal distress (late decelerations), meconium in the amniotic fluid does not jeopardize outcome. However, when distress occurs in the presence of meconium, the likelihood of neonatal depression is greater than when meconium is absent.

MECONIUM ASPIRATION

In cases of fetal distress in the presence of meconium, the following series of events may occur and result in meconium aspiration: Fetal asphyxia may cause pulmonary vasoconstriction and reduced blood flow; fetal gasping would then occur secondary to asphyxial insult, with aspiration of meconium into the trachea. With the reduction of pulmonary fluids, the self-cleansing action of the tracheobronchial tree is lost, and meconium in the pharynx confers the potential for aspiration.

Meconium aspiration syndrome can be eliminated almost entirely by immediate deep suction of the nasopharynx after delivery of the fetal head but before delivery of the thorax. If meconium is present in the hypopharynx, tracheal suction under direct vision becomes necessary.

SUMMARY

It seems clear that meconium passage per se does not indicate fetal distress. But fetal asphyxia associated with meconium enhances the potential for aspiration and a poor neonatal outcome. In all cases when meconium is present in the amniotic fluid, the FHR should be monitored continuously during labor. If any abnormal FHR changes are noted, fetal blood sampling for acid-base analysis is indicated.

Special care must be taken to avoid factors that can cause fetal asphyxia, such as uterine hyperstimulation and maternal hypotension, either positional or secondary to conduction anesthesia and/or other medication. Every attempt should be made to avoid a difficult or traumatic delivery with inherent increase in fetal compromise and asphyxia. At delivery, trachea and pharynx should be suctioned carefully in an attempt to prevent aspiration. Positive pressure respiration should be avoided until adequate tracheal cleansing, under direct vision, has been accomplished, to prevent the forcing of meconium deeper into the respiratory tract.

SUGGESTED READING

Carson BS, Losey RW, Bower WA, Simmons MA: Combined obstetric and pediatric approach to prevent meconium aspiration syndrome. *Am J Obstet Gynecol* 126:712, 1976

Fenton AN, Steer CM: Fetal distress. *Am J Obstet Gynecol* 83:354, 1962

Hobel CJ: Intrapartum clinical assessment of fetal distress. *Am J Obstet Gynecol* 110:336, 1971

Hon EH: The fetal heart rate. In Carey HM, ed: *Modern Trends in Human Reproductive Physiology*, ch 16. London: Butterworth, 1963, p 245

Meis PJ, Hall M, Marshall JR, Hobel CJ: Meconium passage: A new classification for risk during labor. *Am J Obstet Gynecol* 131:509, 1978

Miller FC, Sacks DA, Yeh SY, Paul RH, Schifrin BS, Martin CB, Hon EH: Significance of meconium during labor. *Am J Obstet Gynecol* 122:573, 1975

Resnick L: Fetal distress: A comparison of fetal mortality in relation to meconium staining of the liquor amnii postmaturity. *S Afr Med J* 29:857, 1955

Saling EW: *Foetal and Neonatal Hypoxia in Relation to Clinical Obstetric Practice*. London: Edward Arnold, 1968, p 117

Walker J: Meconium staining and lower umbilical vein oxygen saturation. *J Obstet Gynaecol Br Emp* 61:162, 1954

30

Abnormal Labor

FRANK C. MILLER, M.D.

Normal labor is the process by which uterine contractions cause progressive effacement and dilation of the cervix with descent and expulsion of the products of conception. Abnormal labor (dystocia) is characterized by unusually slow progress of cervical dilation. It may be secondary to a variety of maternal and/or fetal conditions. Subnormal or hypotonic uterine contraction is the most frequently cited cause of abnormal progress in labor. Maternal factors such as age, parity, and pelvic size and configuration frequently contribute to dystocia. Fetal factors include size, presentation, position, number of fetuses present, and hydramnios.

EVALUATION OF UTERINE ACTIVITY

Although it is generally agreed that uterine activity is directly related to progress in labor, until relatively recently, the only method of assessing uterine activity was by palpation of the maternal abdomen. The frequency and duration of uterine contractions may be evaluated with this technique, but intensity cannot be accurately assessed. Because uterine activity is difficult to measure directly, it has traditionally been evaluated indirectly by measuring progressive cervical dilation.

The graphic portrayal of cervical dilation plotted against time was introduced in 1954 by Friedman. Prior to that time, abnormalities of labor were generally described in terms of duration of aberrant uterine activity. Abnormal labors were described as dysfunctional, desultory, or as uterine inertia, terms that conveyed little real information. Accurate measurement of cervical dilation, however, could be performed on all patients, and this information was reproducible and universally available.

The use of the labor curve documented the similarity in the rate of cervical dilation in multiparous and nulliparous women, especially during the active phase of labor. Once the expected pattern of cervical dilation during normal labor was established, individual patients could be compared against the "normal labor curve," and abnormal patterns could serve to alert the physician to potential problems.

The labor curve is divided into two major parts, the latent phase and the active phase (see Fig. 30-1). The latent phase begins with the onset of labor

FIGURE 30-1

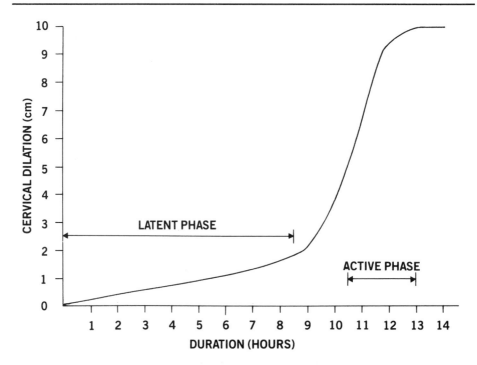

Two major components of the labor curve are the latent phase and the active phase. The active phase of labor is generally predictable and will follow the standard curve very closely. The latent phase is less predictable and may vary several hours within a normal range.

and ends with the active (acceleration) phase. The active phase begins with the upswing of the cervical dilation curve, leading into the linear phase of maximum slope with rapid dilation. The mean duration of the latent phase is approximately 5 hours for multiparas and 9 hours for nulliparas.

MANAGEMENT OF THE LATENT PHASE

Management of the prolonged latent phase is a somewhat controversial subject. Friedman reports that a prolonged latent phase is not associated with increased perinatal mortality. However, the likelihood of cesarean delivery is increased.

If the diagnosis of labor is in question and the membranes are intact, the best method of treatment is sedation and analgesia. If the patient is in false labor, the contractions will usually cease, and only observation is necessary. If labor persists, there is frequently improvement in the quality of the uterine contractions, and the patient will enter active progressive labor.

Advocates of active labor management state that the important decisions are made in the first 2 hours of labor and that many labor complications are the products of passive management. Active management consists of stimulating labor to shorten the latent phase, so that active labor begins sooner and the total duration of labor is shortened. In theory, a reduction in the duration of labor should benefit the patient by reducing the chances of infection, hemorrhage, and exhaustion.

During the latent phase, much of the uterine activity is expended to accomplish effacement of the cervix. Therefore, cervical dilation is much slower than during the active phase. A good guideline for management is to allow 6-8 hours of good uterine activity during the latent phase before considering the diagnosis of failure to progress in labor.

When possible, the patient should labor in the lateral position. This prevents supine hypotension and improves uterine blood flow, as well as frequently improving the quality of uterine contractions. There is no good evidence that amniotomy will reduce the duration of the latent phase, and it increases the risk of amnionitis.

Following rupture of membranes, direct measurement of uterine activity by the intrauterine pressure catheter technique should be used whenever possible to help assess the quality of the contractions.

MANAGEMENT OF THE ACTIVE PHASE

During the active phase of labor, the lowest normal rate of cervical dilation in nulliparas is 1.2 cm/hour, and in multiparas, 1.5 cm/hour. In contrast, the *average* rate of dilation in normal labor is 3+ cm/hour for nulliparas and 5+ cm/hour for multiparas. A protracted active phase is frequently associated with relative cephalopelvic disproportion, excessive sedation or analgesia, and conduction anesthesia.

Arrest of labor is the cessation of progress of cervical dilation during the active phase. If cephalopelvic disproportion can be ruled out and uterine activity is less than optimal (contractions less frequent than every $2\frac{1}{2}$ to 3 minutes and intensity less than 50 mm Hg), uterine activity may be augmented by oxytocin (Pitocin, Syntocinon). Adequate uterine activity generally corresponds to approximately 150-250 Montevideo units.

X-ray pelvimetry is not required before oxytocin is given, provided clinical assessment indicates normal pelvic configuration. The policy of the American College of Obstetricians and Gynecologists concerning pelvimetry is as follows: "X-ray pelvimetry provides limited additional information to physicians involved in the management of labor and delivery. It should not be a prerequisite to clinical decisions concerning obstetrical management. Reasons for requesting x-ray pelvimetry should be individually established."

Oxytocin is the most commonly used drug during labor. There is little doubt that it is also the most frequently abused. Because there is no way to predict precisely how sensitive the uterus will be to a given dosage, extreme caution must be used during administration. Ideally and practically, oxytocin should be given intravenously in a dilute solution by controlled, continuous infusion.

The two most popular systems for intravenous administration are the peristaltic-type pump mechanisms (IVAC or similar units) and the syringe injection system, such as the Harvard infusion pump. The advantage of the IVAC system is that small increases and decreases in rate can be made easily without changing the concentration of the oxytocin or the size of the syringe.

The most commonly used concentration of oxytocin is 10 units (1-ml ampule) in 1,000 ml of intravenous solution (usually 5% dextrose in water). This provides a concentration of oxytocin of 1 mU for each 0.1 ml of intravenous solution.

The amount of oxytocin required to initiate or augment labor is much less than is commonly employed in clinical practice. At term, required dosage is frequently as low as 2 mU/minute and seldom exceeds 16 mU/minute. Utilizing an oxytocin concentration of 1 mU/0.1 ml will require an infusion rate of only 0.1-1.0 ml/minute. Such low infusion rates require careful regulation to prevent hyperstimulation. Prior to term, when the uterus is less responsive to oxytocin, larger doses may be required to stimulate uterine contractions.

The oxytocin should be given using a two-bottle (piggyback) technique. The oxytocin infusion is attached to the primary infusion near the point of administration to the patient. This allows more careful regulation of the oxytocin without restricting the amount of fluids the patient may receive from the primary infusion. It is important to remember that oxytocin is present in the IV tubing below the level of connection with the primary infusion, and injections into the tubing will result in a bolus of oxytocin.

The half-life for oxytocin in the blood is quite short (about 4 minutes) but the half-life of its effect on uterine activity is between 20 and 30 minutes. Therefore, at least 15-20 minutes should elapse between each increase in oxytocin infusion rate to prevent a cumulative effect and hyperstimulation.

There is no place in modern obstetrics for intramuscular injections of oxytocin. Although buccal oxytocin is approved by the FDA, indications for its use are very limited. Its only stated advantage is that it does not require an IV for administration. However, no oxytocic drug should be administered without the precautions of an IV and very close observation.

If a tetanic uterine contraction occurs, the infusion of oxytocin should immediately be discontinued. Administration of oxygen to the mother is initiated, and she is placed in the lateral position to relieve any pressure on the inferior vena cava. The tetanic contraction usually abates within minutes. If it does not, the patient should be delivered as expeditiously as possible. Recently, β-mimetic agents have been recommended for the treatment of tetanic uterine contractions. When the patient has no medical contraindications to the use of these drugs, 125 μg of terbutaline sulfate (Brethine, Bricanyl) or 50 μg of ritodrine hydrochloride (Yutopar) may be administered slowly by a single intravenous injection.

SUGGESTED READING

Caldeyro-Barcia R, Pose SV, Alvarez H: A quantitative study of the actions of synthetic oxytocin on the pregnant human uterus. *J Pharmacol Exp Ther* 121:18, 1957

Friedman EA: Indications and techniques of inducing labor. In *Oxytocin Induced Labor*. Greenwich, Ct: CPC Communications, 1976

Friedman EA: *Labor: Clinical Evaluation and Management*, ed 2. New York: Appleton-Century-Crofts, 1978

Friedman EA: The graphic analysis of labor: *Am J Obstet Gynecol* 68:1568, 1954

Miller FC: Uterine activity, labor management and perinatal outcome. *Semin Perinatol* 2:181, 1978

O'Brien WF, Cefalo RC: Evaluation of x-ray pelvimetry in abnormal labor. *Clin Obstet Gynecol* 25:57, 1982

O'Driscoll K, Jackson RJ, Gallagher JT: Active management of labour and cephalopelvic disproportion. *J Obstet Gynaecol Br Commonw* 77:385, 1970

Quality Assurance in Obstetrics and Gynecology. Washington, DC: The American College of Obstetricians and Gynecologists, 1981

31

Use of the Vacuum Extractor in Obstetrics

RICHARD H. PAUL, M.D.

The vacuum extractor as an aid to delivery has been more widely used in Europe than in the United States. Its use in this country has been limited, for the most part, to a few medical centers and teaching institutions. In general, the vacuum extractor may be used in lieu of forceps when delivering a fetus with a vertex presentation.

There are presently two types of vacuum extractors available for clinical use. The Malmström extractor uses metal cups 40-60 mm in diameter. The newer Kobayashi extractor is made of silicone rubber with a diameter of 65-75 mm. Both are attached to the scalp by negative pressure.

ADVANTAGES AND CONTRAINDICATIONS

The advantages of using the vacuum extractor rather than forceps for assisting delivery include: (1) decreased maternal soft-tissue trauma, (2) elimination of the need for conduction or general anesthesia, (3) a lesser diameter presented to the maternal soft tissues during extraction, (4) a maximum traction force limited to 40 pounds before disengagement of the cup, and (5) the pathway of least resistance will be followed by the head.

Contraindications to the use of the vacuum extractor, where forceps might be used instead, are: (1) fetal prematurity, (2) face presentation, and (3) breech delivery requiring application to the after-coming head. Although recommended by some, the use of the vacuum extractor with an undilated cervix or with a completely dilated cervix but the vertex at 0 station or above is also contraindicated. Such use is associated with a high rate of complications.

The use of the vacuum extractor in cases of fetal distress with a completely dilated cervix often results in a successful outcome. However, when the fetus is known to be compromised, the least traumatic and most prompt method of delivery should be chosen. Thus, when the compromised fetus is in the high midpelvis, an expeditious cesarean section is probably best, despite its association with increased maternal morbidity. When the compromised fetus is in the lower pelvis, a skilled forceps delivery is usually faster and safer for the fetus than vacuum extraction.

The vacuum extractor may be indicated when a second twin presents in the vertex position. However, with proper monitoring, spontaneous delivery generally occurs and is preferable to operative intervention.

COMPLICATIONS

Maternal

Maternal complications associated with the use of the vacuum extractor are mainly related to lacerations and improper applications. Applications inadvertently including the cervix may cause cervical avulsion. In nearly all comparative series, the vacuum extractor is associated with less maternal morbidity than forceps, when used in similar clinical situations. In general, third- or fourth-degree laceration occurs in about 1-4%, and vaginal laceration in about 5-10% of patients delivered by vacuum extraction.

Fetal

Fetal complications associated with the use of the Malmström extractor are frequent, but fortunately not of major clinical consequence. The most common complication is scalp ecchymoses, found in about half of the infants. Cephalhematoma occurs in about 10% of cases, but is usually self-limited and only rarely results in significant cerebral irritability or hyperbilirubinemia. Scalp lacerations occur in 5-10% and are more frequent with cup detachment or leakage of the seal with the scalp. The most serious complication, intracranial hemorrhage, has never been conclusively linked to the vacuum extractor, although sporadic reports exist in the literature. Many observers feel this complication is related to the coexistent clinical complications rather than the vacuum extraction procedure.

TECHNIQUE

Technique differs slightly between the Malmström and Kobayashi extractors. With the former, a 50- or 60-mm cup is usually used. If possible, the cup is applied over the occiput, with the anterior fontanelle preferably being avoided. If monitoring is necessary, the fetal scalp electrode may need to be removed and reapplied after the cup is in place. The cup is usually considered safe to apply following fetal scalp blood sampling, but there is no large body of evidence to support this opinion.

Negative pressure should be increased gradually from 0 to 0.7 kg/sq cm in 2-minute increments over 8-10 minutes. It is initially necessary to spend this time establishing a seal with the fetal scalp to ensure optimum results with traction. More rapid establishment of negative pressure is acceptable with reapplication or in an expeditious delivery attempt for fetal distress.

Traction on the handle attached to the vacuum cup should be exerted along the axis of the vagina and at a right angle to the cup. Torque or oblique torsion will result in disengagement during traction. Reapplication is acceptable when detachment occurs, but should not be reattempted multiple times. Some operators place one hand on the cup to prevent slippage or loss of vacuum during traction. Traction is usually applied only during uterine contractions, concomitant with maternal expulsive effort. The total time for use of the vacuum extractor from initial application to delivery should not exceed 30 minutes. If no significant descent is accomplished within this time, it is safer to deliver the fetus abdominally.

Used as described above, the vacuum extractor fails to effect delivery in about 5% of attempted cases. When failure occurs, cesarean section should be done unless the fetus is crowning and can be delivered by Ritgen maneuver or an easy low forceps procedure. Failed vacuum extraction followed by a midforceps procedure has been associated with serious fetal and maternal injury and is to be condemned.

The Kobayashi extractor appears to offer a number of advantages over the Malmström extractor. However, it has not yet received large-scale clinical trials in this country. The silicone-rubber Kobayashi cup is folded, inserted into the vagina, and applied to the fetal scalp. A blue line indicates where the posterior fontanelle should lie. Vacuum suction is established, and traction can then be applied.

Many American physicians have been reluctant to use the Malmström extractor because of the risk of fetal scalp trauma. Clinical trials with the Kobayashi extractor report a decreased incidence of scalp trauma. The reluctance to use the vacuum extraction method may be overcome if these results are confirmed in the United States.

SUGGESTED READING

Chalmers JA: *The Ventouse: The Obstetric Vacuum Extractor*. Chicago: Year Book, 1971

Gries JB, Bieniarz J, Scommegna A: Comparison of maternal and fetal effects of vacuum extraction with forceps or cesarean deliveries. *Obstet Gynecol* 57:571, 1981

Mishell D, Kelly JV: The obstetrical forceps and the vacuum extractor: An assessment of their compressive force. *Obstet Gynecol* 19:204, 1962

Plauché WC: Fetal cranial injuries related to delivery with the Malmström vacuum extractor. *Obstet Gynecol* 53:750, 1979

Plauché WC: Vacuum extraction: Use in a community hospital setting. *Obstet Gynecol* 52:289, 1978

32

Vaginal Delivery Following Cesarean Birth

RICHARD H. PAUL, M.D.

Currently, 15-20% of all deliveries in the United States are by cesarean section. The rate of cesareans increased approximately three-fold during the 1970s. The trend toward frequent cesarean delivery has caused concern, since it imposes a significantly higher maternal risk than vaginal delivery. It is also associated with increased cost and longer hospitalization. An additional concern involves later pregnancies in patients with a history of cesarean section: Repeat cesareans are usually done, exposing patients to further risk. Thus, the dictum "once a section, always a section" mandates growing numbers of cesarean births.

Obstetric patients are increasingly concerned with this issue. Physicians these days are more frequently hearing the question: "Is it possible for me to deliver vaginally having had a cesarean section?" The first responsibility of the physician is to assess the facts as they relate to the medical feasibility of such an approach. Second, the physician must know how to decide whether a trial of labor is practical in a given case.

INDICATIONS FOR CESAREAN DELIVERY

A good place to start assessing this issue is a review of the indications for the first cesarean section. The most commonly encountered indication is the diagnosis of dystocia or cephalopelvic disproportion. However, 30-40% of primary cesarean sections result from causes that are unlikely to recur in later pregnancies, such as breech presentation, fetal distress, and a series of other miscellaneous obstetric complications, including third-trimester bleeding and prolapsed cord.

INITIAL CONSIDERATIONS

The management of a patient with a previous section begins with the constructive development of rapport and a frank discussion of the facts relating to possible vaginal delivery. The patient's wishes should be considered in choosing the mode of delivery. It would seem unwise to attempt labor in a patient who did not want to try it. Likewise, a trial of labor should be considered only for patients fulfilling certain specific criteria. Finally, it is extremely important to have the physical facilities, medical support, and services that can permit maximum safety in such an approach.

EXCLUSION FACTORS

In general, our approach has been to avoid trials of labor in patients with more than one previous cesarean section. When there has been only one prior section, we make a concerted effort to obtain the operative report of the procedure. We exclude patients with a history of a section by vertical uterine incision. The history of a morbid postoperative course following the previous cesarean section is a relative contraindication to vaginal delivery. Additional contraindications include fetal malpresentation or macrosomia, antepartum complications such as diabetes or preeclampsia, placenta previa, and evidence of severe pelvic contracture.

PREREQUISITES

Prerequisites for consideration of vaginal delivery are as follows: (1) absence of the exclusion factors noted above, (2) availability of maternal and fetal intensive-care capabilities, (3) blood bank services with immediate access to blood, (4) facilities for beginning emergency cesarean section within 5 to 10 minutes, and (5) patient acceptance of the approach. A previous vaginal delivery is not a prerequisite.

INTRAPARTUM AND POSTPARTUM MANAGEMENT

During the trial of labor, electronic fetal heart rate monitoring is essential to provide a constant evaluation of fetal status. Following amniotomy, direct or internal methods are used, since they provide the most accurate information on which to base clinical decisions. An indwelling urinary catheter should be inserted to detect hematuria, which may herald uterine rupture. Heavy sedation and conduction anesthesia are used only with caution, since they may inhibit the patient's perception of pain associated with scar dehiscence.

When labor progresses poorly and is associated with inadequate uterine activity, we permit the cautious administration of oxytocin, but only with an infusion pump and direct intrauterine pressure measurement.

If scar separation is suspected at any time during labor, prompt intervention is indicated. Tipoffs to uterine rupture include: (1) onset of lower abdominal pain, (2) onset of hematuria or vaginal bleeding, (3) maternal shock, or (4) fetal distress.

Following vaginal delivery, the uterine cavity is palpated to make sure that the previous scar has not separated. When a small window defect is felt, but no bleeding is present, we have followed a conservative approach. Immediate outcome in this group has been good, but management of subsequent pregnancies remains to be defined. When hemorrhage is present or the defect is large, operative intervention is necessary. Repair is usually accomplished; occasionally, hysterectomy is indicated.

IMPLICATIONS

About 50-75% of patients who have had a previous cesarean section may be candidates for attempted vaginal delivery in a subsequent pregnancy. Of the patients undertaking a trial of labor, one-half to two-thirds will be successfully delivered vaginally.

Based on our experience and the cases reported in the literature, it appears that labor following a previous cesarean birth is an acceptable medical approach for selected patients. However, practical realities make it very difficult for many hospitals to provide such a service. The necessary time commitment and immediate availability of the physician and surgical support staff, possibly extending over many hours, would create enormous problems for many community hospitals. But the practicality issues should not be confused with the medical issues involved. Obviously, the physician must consider both these factors and offer a trial of labor only after fully informing the patient.

In summary, current trends in obstetrics indicate that patients are increasingly asking about vaginal delivery following cesarean birth. It is not unreasonable to undertake a trial of labor in properly selected patients. In general, the patients' enthusiasm for this process makes it a positive and fulfilling experience. It would appear that patients requesting this approach can often be safely managed, and that facilities offering such services will increasingly be in demand.

SUGGESTED READING

Cesarean Childbirth, Pub 82-2067. Washington, DC: National Institutes of Health, Dept of Health and Human Services, 1981

Gibbs C: Planned vaginal delivery following cesarean section. *Obstet Gynecol* 23:507, 1980

Lavin JP, Stephens RJ, Miodovnik M, Barden TP: Vaginal delivery in patients with a prior cesarean section. *Obstet Gynecol* 59:135, 1982

Meier PR, Porreco RP: Trial of labor following cesarean section: A two year experience. *Am J Obstet Gynecol* 144:671, 1982

Merrill B, Gibbs C: Planned vaginal delivery following cesarean section. *Obstet Gynecol* 52:50, 1977

Rosen M: Cesarean section rates: What the Task Force found. *Contemp Ob/Gyn* 18:27, 1981

Saldana L, Schulman H, Reuss L: Management of pregnancy after cesarean section. *Am J Obstet Gynecol* 135:555, 1975

33

Suppression of Postpartum Lactation

DANIEL R. MISHELL JR., M.D.

The suppression of puerperal breast engorgement and lactation is a controversial issue. Inhibition of lactation is usually accomplished by (1) hormonal inhibition with estrogens alone or in combination with androgens, (2) mechanical compression of the breasts, with or without fluid restriction, and (3) use of bromocriptine mesylate (Parlodel), a peptide ergot alkaloid.

The administration of intramuscular long-acting estrogen preparations, often with androgens, is widely used in the United States to inhibit postpartum lactation. The benefits derived from the use of these steroids have to be weighed against their potential risks and compared with the benefits and risks of bromocriptine and mechanical compression alone.

HORMONE THERAPY VERSUS PLACEBO

Postpartum breast engorgement and lactation normally begin 40-72 hours after delivery and persist for at least 1 week in the absence of nursing. During this period, the symptoms may be treated by such measures as breast binders, ice packs, and analgesics. The degree to which hormonal preparations are superior to these means, and to placebos, varies in different studies, depending on the study population, experimental design, and the specific drugs being evaluated.

The conclusion of most prospective studies has been that long-acting intramuscular estrogen preparations effectively prevent symptoms, without rebound engorgement, in about 80% of patients. This rate is significantly better than that obtained with placebos.

For example, Morris and associates, in a randomized, double-blind study, compared a testosterone enanthate-estradiol valerate combination (Deladumone) with a placebo. When evaluated on the third, fourth, and fifth postpartum days, the hormonal preparation was significantly more effective than the placebo in preventing lactation, engorgement, and discomfort. Similar results were obtained by questionnaire at 14 days postpartum. At the 6-week examination, the placebo- and drug-treated groups were indistinguishable in regard to breast and uterine involution, lochia, and resumption of menses. In another randomized, double-blind study, Varga et al found that oral stilbestrol suppressed postpartum lactation to a significantly greater extent than placebo.

A problem with nearly all randomized drug-placebo studies dealing with inhibition of lactation is the lack of use of breast binders in the placebo group. But in a double-blind, placebo-controlled study performed by Schwartz and associates, all patients were fitted with tight bras soon after delivery. On the third and fourth postpartum days, patients treated with any of the three estrogens used in the trial—chlorotrianisene (TACE), diethylstilbestrol, and Deladumone—had significantly less breast tenderness and lactation than the placebo group. However, about half of all patients had continued or rebound breast engorgement after leaving the hospital, and the differences between the four groups were not significant 5 weeks postpartum.

The results of this study indicate that estrogen therapy is superior to the use of breast binding alone in suppressing postpartum breast tenderness and lactation during the first few postpartum days. But this improvement is not sustained during the next few weeks.

The benefits of estrogenic drugs must be weighed against their risks and side effects. The most important of these is their reported association with venous thrombosis and thromboembolism. Retrospective studies have suggested such a relationship, but the actual incidence of thrombosis in estrogen-treated puerperas is unknown. Although the incidence may be presumed to be low, estrogens should not be administered to patients with a history of thrombosis or thromboembolism. Breast carcinoma and active hepatic disease are also contraindications. Uterine subinvolution and endometrial hyperstimulation have been reported to occur more frequently with estrogen therapy, but the addition of an androgen to the estrogenic agent appears to prevent these effects.

In summary, long-acting estrogen-androgen preparations are effective in preventing puerperal breast engorgement, lactation, and discomfort in about 80% of patients. Their use carries very low risk in most cases. Nevertheless, their use is not mandatory, and in most patients the symptoms of breast engorgement may be relieved by nonhormonal methods.

ALTERNATIVE DRUG THERAPY

In an attempt to avoid the potential risks (mainly thromboembolism) of estrogens, other drugs, such as clomiphene citrate (Clomid, Serophene) and bromocriptine (bromoergocryptine), have been used to suppress lactation.

Unlike estrogens, which inhibit the action of prolactin in the breast tissue, bromocriptine directly suppresses pituitary secretion of prolactin. In recommended doses of 2.5 mg bid with meals for 14 days, bromocriptine is very effective in preventing breast secretion, engorgement, and congestion.

Several randomized studies have compared bromocriptine with estrogen (either diethylstilbestrol or chlorotrianisene). In these studies, bromocriptine was found to be as or slightly more effective in inhibiting lactation and breast engorgement. No comparison with Deladumone or breast binders and ice packs has been reported, and there are no prolonged studies to determine the incidence of symptoms several weeks after therapy is stopped.

About one-fourth of women receiving bromocriptine report adverse symptoms. The most common are headache, dizziness, nausea, vomiting, and skin rash. Bromocriptine also produces hypotension in about one-third of patients; therefore, treatment should not be initiated until at least 4 hours after delivery and after vital signs have stabilized. Since bromocriptine does not affect clotting factors, it would appear to be the preferred choice for use in the first 2 weeks postpartum in patients at increased risk for thromboembolism. These include women over 35, those with a past history of thrombophlebitis or thromboembolism, and those who were delivered by cesarean section.

Steroids are as effective as bromocriptine in preventing symptoms in women without these risk factors. But in comparison with breast binders and ice packs, symptomatic relief with medication is superior only during the first few weeks postpartum.

After lactation has been initiated, bromocriptine is still useful in lactation suppression, because of the low prolactin levels it produces. The estrogenic agents are not equally effective at this stage. Thus, bromocriptine is the agent of choice for the inhibition of lactation in women who must discontinue nursing for any reason.

SUGGESTED READING

Jeffcoate TNA, et al: Puerperal thromboembolism in relation to the inhibition of lactation by oestrogen therapy. *Br Med J* 4:19, 1968

Morris JA, Creasy RK, Hohe PT: Inhibition of puerperal lactation. Double-blind comparison of chlorotrianisene, testosterone enanthate with estradiol valerate and placebo. *Obstet Gynecol* 36:107, 1970

Schwartz DJ, et al: A clinical study of lactation suppression. *Obstet Gynecol* 42:599, 1973

Turnbull AC: Puerperal thromboembolism and the suppression of lactation. *J Obstet Gynaecol Br Commonw* 75:1321, 1968

Varga L, et al: Suppression of puerperal lactation with an ergot alkaloid: A double-blind study. *Br Med J* 2:743, 1972

TWO

PERINATAL MEDICINE

34

Pregnancy Monitoring With α-Fetoprotein

LAWRENCE D. PLATT, M.D., and MAURICE DRUZIN, M.D.

α-Fetoprotein (AFP) is the major circulating protein of the early fetus. It is an α-globulin with unknown physiologic function. Synthesis occurs mainly in the fetal liver, yolk sac, and gastrointestinal tract, but a small placental contribution has also been demonstrated.

NORMAL CONCENTRATIONS OF AFP

The concentration of AFP in fetal tissue varies. In fetal blood it peaks at 2-3 mg/ml between the 12th and 14th weeks of gestation, after which the level decreases as pregnancy progresses. In amniotic fluid, AFP is present at microgram, not milligram, levels. Like fetal serum levels, amniotic fluid levels of AFP reach a peak in early pregnancy and decline sharply during the second trimester. The major source of AFP in amniotic fluid may be fetal urine.

In other fetal tissues, the concentration of AFP reaches a peak between the 22nd and 32nd weeks of gestation and parallels circulating maternal levels. Maternal serum levels occur in nanogram amounts. In the mother, circulating AFP normally rises progressively beginning at the seventh week, reaches a peak around 32 weeks (27-36 weeks), and then declines toward term. The range of values around the mean is very wide, particularly in the last weeks of pregnancy. In normal, nonpregnant adults, the basal level of AFP is approximately 25 ng/ml, with a half-life of 1-6 days. Levels of AFP are not affected by oral contraceptives.

MEASUREMENT OF AFP

Since AFP has no biologic activity, measurement depends on immunologic methods. Numerous techniques are used, including immunodiffusion, immunoelectrophoresis, hemagglutination inhibition, and radioimmunoassay (RIA). A sensitive technique is required for detecting nanogram amounts of AFP in pregnancy, and RIA is the only assay with this degree of sensitivity. Because of limited availability of highly purified protein for iodination and standardization, there may be different ranges of normal in different laboratories, and this must be borne in mind when interpreting results.

ABNORMAL LEVELS OF AFP

Nonpregnant Adults

Primary carcinoma of the liver (hepatoma) and some cancers of germinal tissues lead to elevation of blood AFP levels. These increases presumably reflect the tendency of dedifferentiated cells to return biochemically to the embryonic state. Elevation of AFP levels may also be found in some non-neoplastic conditions of the liver, and the possibility of an extrauterine source of AFP production should always be remembered in the differential diagnosis of abnormally increased levels of AFP during pregnancy.

Early and Midpregnancy

Early abortion. It has been shown that after the 13th week of gestation, abortion is more frequent in women with abnormal levels of serum AFP and symptoms of threatened abortion. The abnormal levels are of two types. Low levels occur in blighted ovum with absent fetus. High levels are found in intrauterine demise. A possible mechanism for the elevated levels in this case might be disturbance of the placental site, but this theory is controversial.

Abnormal elevations of AFP do not correlate as well with poor outcome if clinical symptoms are absent.

Trophoblastic disease. Maternal AFP levels are in the nonpregnant range in many cases of hydatidiform mole and in all cases of choriocarcinoma, presumably because of the absence of fetal tissue.

Neural tube defects. The detection of these defects (NTDs) is perhaps the most important application of AFP testing in maternal serum and amniotic fluid. Elevated amniotic fluid levels of AFP in the second trimester can detect anencephaly with 95% accuracy, and open spina bifida with 85% accuracy. Elevated maternal serum AFP levels in the second trimester lead to detection of more than 80% of cases of anencephaly and 40% of cases of open spina bifida. In closed spina bifida (about 10% of cases), AFP levels are normal or only slightly increased.

The source of the increased amniotic fluid AFP is presumably leakage of fetal cerebrospinal fluid or transudation from fetal capillaries directly exposed to the amniotic fluid. The source of elevated maternal levels of AFP is presumably amniotic fluid absorbed through the membranes.

Amniotic fluid analysis for AFP levels is important in cases where NTDs are strongly suspected, such as patients who themselves have an NTD or who have had a previous pregnancy with NTD. The risk of NTD is two to five times higher in this group than among normal women.

The risks of amniocentesis make amniotic fluid AFP determination impractical as a screening procedure. Routine maternal serum AFP screening is performed in Britain, but the general-population risk in the United Kingdom is greater than in the United States, with an overall frequency of 5-7:1,000 compared with 1-2:1,000. Nevertheless, ongoing studies suggest that routine screening may soon be recommended in the United States.

To minimize the incidence of results that are either false-positive (high levels, normal fetus) or false-negative (normal levels, affected fetus) in determination of maternal serum levels of AFP, selection of the normal range is critical. Setting a high level reduces false-positive rates, but also reduces the number of cases detected. Setting a lower level improves the detection rate, but at the expense of an increase in false-positives.

False-negative results arise from the fact that the range of values in affected cases overlaps the normal range. Technical errors can also occur. Up to 20% of all mothers whose fetuses have open NTDs may have normal serum AFP values. Failure of detection will not lead to termination of a normal pregnancy, but false-positive results may. Therefore, the reasons for false-positive results should be kept in mind:

- Overlap of the upper end of the normal range with the lower end of the abnormal range
- Technical errors in estimation
- Multiple pregnancy
- Concurrent maternal liver disease
- Collection of blood samples after amniocentesis, which increases fetomaternal bleeding and consequently elevates maternal serum AFP.

To eliminate these errors, all high levels should be checked by repeated measurement on the same sample, and another sample should be collected and analyzed within a few days. Careful attention to history, physical examination, and use of ultrasound should eliminate most of the other reasons for false-positive results.

Another extremely important point is accurate dating of the gestation, because abnormal levels at a certain gestational age may be normal for a different gestational age. Therefore, careful history-taking combined with physical exam and ultrasonic scanning should be utilized to obtain as accurate an estimation of gestational age as possible. The optimal time for sampling is 16-18 weeks' gestation.

Amniocentesis for the measurement of amniotic fluid AFP and stage II ultrasound examination by an experienced ultrasonographer should always be performed as the final confirmatory steps in the detection of an NTD. These should always precede consideration of pregnancy termination.

Other congenital abnormalities. Elevated levels of amniotic fluid AFP have been observed in encephalocele, hydrocephalus, esophageal atresia, tetralogy of Fallot, congenital nephrosis, 45,X monosomy, exomphalos, gastroschisis, pilonidal cyst, and cystic hygroma.

The cause of the raised AFP in these conditions is obscure. In esophageal atresia, it is suggested that the mechanism is reduced clearance of amniotic protein due to failure of swallowing. In congenital nephrosis, the source is likely to be fetal urine. Whenever a raised AFP level is found and no NTD or anomaly is identified by a single ultrasound scan, the patient should be referred for a second exam to a center recognized as having special ultrasound competence.

In most hands, the identification of a small NTD is difficult. Other tests to identify false-positive elevations have been described. These tests, which are currently under investigation and available in only a few centers in the United States, include tests for rapidly adhering cells, acetylcholinesterase, and neural proteins. Samples can be sent to these labs for evaluation. Currently, the gel electrophoresis technique for measurement of acetylcholinesterase seems to be of most assistance. In this test, a band is identified only when an NTD is present.

Late Pregnancy

In late pregnancy there is an extremely wide normal range of maternal serum AFP levels, and deviation from normal is likely to be found only with the most severe pathologic conditions.

Relationship to weight and gestational age. No consistent relationship between amniotic fluid AFP levels and fetal weight and gestational age has been found. Some studies have suggested that low levels of AFP are associated with either low birth weight or an increase in perinatal mortality. Others have shown that elevated levels of AFP are associated with low birth weight.

Multiple pregnancy. Maternal serum AFP levels are elevated in patients with multiple pregnancies.

Fetal demise. Maternal serum AFP levels may be increased in association with fetal death between 20 and 36 weeks' gestation. It has not been determined whether there is a consistent rise just prior to fetal death. The cause is probably disturbance of the placental site.

Hypertensive disorders and diabetes mellitus. Overall maternal levels of AFP in chronic hypertension and diabetes have been shown to be lower than in normal or other high-risk groups. An adequate explanation for this observation is unknown.

Rh-immunization. In mild or moderate disease or in severe cases in which the baby survived, AFP levels in amniotic fluid were normal in a study by Whyley et al on 60 patients. However, in severe cases with an unfavorable fetal outcome, 42% of patients showed elevated levels.

Antepartum hemorrhage. High AFP levels have been found in blood lost per vaginam in some cases of abruptio placentae. Mennuti et al reported that AFP levels in maternal serum increased significantly following genetic amniocentesis in 8.4% of patients. They attributed this finding to fetal-maternal bleeding. In the same study, they showed that there was a significantly higher frequency of spontaneous abortion in those patients in whom the AFP rose following amniocentesis. We have recently reported this observation and have shown that up to 14% of patients will show a rise in AFP levels 15 minutes postamniocentesis.

SUMMARY

The use of maternal serum AFP as a screen for open NTDs is gaining wide acceptance. The importance of this surveillance is not only to establish the incidence of NTDs, but also to detect variations in incidence among population groups. When maternal serum AFP is elevated, ultrasound examination must be performed to rule out erroneous dating, fetal demise, tubal pregnancy, or congenital anomalies associated with these elevations. If these cannot be detected, amniocentesis should be carried out under ultrasound guidance to measure levels of amniotic fluid AFP. When findings are normal, reasonable assurance can be given the patient with regard to the chance that her baby will not have an anomaly. When the level is greater than 5 standard deviations above the mean, the chance the fetus will be abnormal is high. Both ultrasound and ancillary biochemical testing, such as acetylcholinesterase measurement, should be completed to confirm the diagnosis. If the results are still inconclusive, invasive testing methods such as fetoscopy should be considered. When the level of amniotic fluid AFP is between 3 and 5 SD above the mean, both ultrasound and repeat amniocentesis should be completed prior to ancillary biochemical testing; if these are still inconclusive, the invasive method can then be applied. In the United States, most authorities would agree that the chance of having an NTD with an amniotic fluid AFP less than 3 SD above the mean is remote. Nevertheless, a careful second ultrasound exam should be carried out at a special center. This is especially true for patients with a high risk, such as those with previous affected children. With the combined use of AFP and ultrasound, the rate of detection of open spina bifida between 10 and 26 weeks' gestation approaches 100%.

SUGGESTED READING

Ferguson-Smith MA, Gibson AM, Whitfield CR, et al: Amniocentesis and the alpha fetoprotein screening programme. *Lancet* 1:39, 1979

Kjessler B, Johansson SGO, Liobjork G, et al: Alpha fetoprotein levels in maternal serum in relation to pregnancy outcome in 7158 pregnant women prospectively investigated during their 14th-20th week post last menstrual period. *Acta Obstet Gynecol Scand* 69:25, 1977

Macri JN, Weiss RR: Prenatal serum alpha fetoprotein screening for neural tube defects. *Obstet Gynecol* 59:633, 1982

Menutti MT, Brummond W, Crombleholme WR, et al: Fetal maternal bleeding associated with genetic amniocentesis. *Obstet Gynecol* 55:48, 1980

Milunsky A, Alpert E, Weff RK, Frigoletto F: Prenatal diagnosis of neural tube defects. IV. Maternal serum alpha fetoprotein screening. *Obstet Gynecol* 55:60, 1980

Seppala M: Immunologic detection of alpha fetoprotein as a marker for fetal-pathology. *Clin Obstet Gynecol* 20:737, 1977

Whyley GA, Ward H, Hardy NR: Alpha-fetoprotein levels in amniotic fluid in pregnancies complicated by Rhesus iso-immunization. *J Obstet Gynaecol Br Commonw* 81:459, 1974

35

Antepartum Fetal Evaluation

RICHARD H. PAUL, M.D.

One of the long-term goals of those caring for pregnant patients has been to identify every compromised fetus. Historically, physical examination and observation of fetal heart tones formed the basis of fetal care. The inadequacies of this approach became more evident as maternal mortality fell in the 1940s and 1950s and attention was directed toward decreasing perinatal mortality.

EARLY DEVELOPMENTS IN FHR MONITORING

During the late 1950s, continuous recording of the fetal heart rate (FHR) began to emerge as a means of basic evaluation of the human fetus. Hon, Quilligan, Caldeyro-Barcia, and others led in the search for the meaning of FHR patterns, and this form of fetal assessment was first introduced into clinical care during the late 1960s. The area of initial intensive study was the intrapartum period, which is time-limited, is known to stress the fetus, and permits direct access to the fetus following rupture of the membranes. One of the most significant findings that emerged from these investigations was that FHR patterns could be associated with specific pathophysiologic causes.

Observations of antepartum FHR had been carried out in the 1950s by Hon and Wohlgemuth, with the specific intent of fetal assessment. They explored the possibility that maternal exercise (stress) might alter the FHR in the compromised fetus. The abdominal wall fetal electrocardiogram (FECG) served as the counting signal, and the FHR had to be laboriously calculated and retrospectively plotted. Minimal antepartum study was undertaken during the 1960s, when the primary focus of fetal evaluation continued to be the intrapartum period.

Interest in antepartum FHR testing (AFHRT) in the United States was renewed in the early 1970s. Although there had been sporadic reports on the potential of AFHRT from Hammacher, Posé, Kubli, and others, few substantive data were produced. The approach taken by Freeman, Schifrin, and others evolved from concepts gained through intrapartum studies, which had established that the FHR pattern of late decelerations was often associated with a compromised outcome. These investigators reasoned that if late decelerations often denoted a pathologic fetal state during labor, they might well form the basis for AFHRT.

The obvious obstacle to this approach was that the stress factor during labor (uterine activity) was usually minimal or absent during the antepartum period. Thus, in order to mimic labor, it was usually necessary to administer oxytocin to produce uterine contractions, or stress, which formed the basis for the contraction stress test. The term "oxytocin challenge test" (OCT) thus came into usage—but in fact it is a misnomer.

Accumulating experience with the contraction stress test (CST), still acclaimed by some, has led to disenchantment because of its inherent drawbacks and the emergence of a simple alternative approach in the form of the nonstress test (NST). The major problems with the CST approach are the length of time required, the need for an intravenous infusion, confusion and variation in interpretation of results, relative contraindications, and a high false-positive rate, which at times has exceeded 50%. In addition, the fact that such testing must be carried out in a hospital setting is a distinct drawback.

European experience with the NST approach proposed by Hammacher in the late 1960s showed it to have many advantages, and this approach was studied and documented by Rochard, Schifrin, and their colleagues. Schifrin developed study protocols that integrated both the NST and CST into a scheme that forms the basis for much of our current approach. At present, AFHRT relies primarily on an initial NST with selective use of the CST—required in fewer than 2% of patients. Several studies have shown that this testing approach can be used successfully in an outpatient setting.

TEST METHOD

Current testing utilizes standard, commercially available monitors, such as the Corometrics or Hewlett-Packard. The most practical technique uses an ultrasonic transducer to obtain the FHR and a tocodynamometer for recording uterine contractions (UC).

Careful attention must be paid to the patient's position, to avoid supine hypotension. This requires frequent checks (every 5-10 minutes) of the maternal blood pressure. It is highly desirable to have this done by a skilled person who can interpret the results consistently.

INDICATIONS

Although some recent reports by Schifrin and others suggest routine antenatal testing is beneficial, the most common indications for testing are postdates pregnancy, diabetes mellitus, hypertensive disorders, suspected growth retardation, and miscellaneous factors known to be associated with increased fetal risk. Testing is usually begun at 30-32 weeks, when intervention on the basis of fetal condition might be considered.

TESTING PROTOCOL

All patients undergo an NST as the primary test. This involves recording FHR in relation to UC and looking for accelerations of the FHR that are specifically related to fetal movements. When two or more qualifying accelerations occur within a 10-minute "window," the pattern is called reactive. Such tests are considered normal and have been associated with good outcome. A nonreactive NST fails to achieve the required FHR accelerations over a 40-minute observation period, and is considered abnormal. To qualify as reactive, FHR accelerations must reach or exceed 15 bpm and the overall duration of the rise and return to baseline must exceed 15 seconds. This observation is most often associated with fetal movement, which is evident to the mother and a trained observer.

The usual testing interval following a reactive test is weekly; this arbitrary approach probably grew out of the practice of seeing patients weekly in late pregnancy. More frequent testing has been suggested, particularly in high-risk situations, and would seem to be reasonable. Unfortunately, minimal data are available to support such an approach, and any interval would currently have to be chosen on an empiric basis.

Our current approach utilizes the NST for screening all high-risk patients. If there is a reactive pattern, the patient is retested in 1 week. (If the patient is diabetic or the pregnancy is postdates, retesting is done twice weekly.) A nonreactive pattern may be due merely to fetal sleeping or nonactivity; when nonreactivity is observed, the fetus is therefore stimulated by manipulation for 1 minute and an additional 20-minute observation period is begun. If a reactive pattern then occurs, the patient is retested in 1 week.

If the NST persistently remains nonreactive, the patient is usually retested later the same day. An acceptable alternative would be to perform a CST. On retesting, most patients will demonstrate a reactive pattern and will thus be retested in 1 week. When a CST is undertaken following persistent nonreactive NSTs, fetal movements and concomitant FHR accelerations will often be evident; in fact, few such completed CSTs have been found to be abnormal. Thus, when a reactive pattern occurs during the CST, the CST is stopped, the test is called reactive, and a repeat NST is done in 1 week. Using this approach, fewer than 2% of patients tested will require completion of a CST.

CSTs are handled as follows: A positive result (persistent late decelerations) usually prompts delivery unless the fetus is immature or the fetal condition may benefit from correction of a maternal disorder. Negative and suspicious, or equivocal, CSTs are repeated within 24 hours. The persistence of a nonreactive NST followed by a negative CST is associated with a higher incidence of fetal loss than a normal reactive test group.

RESULT

This approach, with minor modifications, used over the past 7 years has shown that reactive NSTs appear to be equivalent to negative CSTs in predicting good outcome. Although the CST continues to play a role in the overall scheme, it is utilized in very few patients. A major advantage of using the NST as the primary approach is that the length of AFHRT is dramatically shorter than required for the CST. Additionally, the NST can be easily done in an outpatient or office setting.

AFHRT provides useful clinical information in the individualized care of high-risk patients. The incidence of unanticipated death is less than 0.5% among tested high-risk groups. Preliminary results of testing a large group of normal patients in office settings by Schifrin and collaborators also suggest its benefit as a routine screening approach. This individualized assessment is more predictive than classically used high-risk scoring systems. Refinement and simplification of the testing scheme are being evaluated. Additional biophysical indicators, such as observation of fetal chest wall movements and ultrasonically determined amniotic fluid volume, will provide useful supplementary information in cases of abnormal tests. Thus, it is likely that a more comprehensive biophysical profile will assist in antepartum fetal evaluation.

SUGGESTED READING

Druzin ML, Gratacos J, Paul RH: Antepartum fetal heart rate testing: VI. Predictive reliability of "normal" tests in the prevention of antepartum death. *Am J Obstet Gynecol* 137:746, 1980

Evertson LR, Gauthier RJ, Schifrin BS, Paul RH: Antepartum fetal heart rate testing: I. Evolution of the nonstress test. *Am J Obstet Gynecol* 133:29, 1979

Gauthier RJ, Evertson LR, Paul RH: Antepartum fetal heart rate testing: II. Intrapartum fetal heart rate observation and newborn outcome following a positive contraction stress test. *Am J Obstet Gynecol* 133:34, 1979

Keegan KA Jr, Paul RH: Antepartum fetal heart rate testing. IV. The nonstress test as a primary approach. *Am J Obstet Gynecol* 136:75, 1980

Keegan KA Jr, Paul RH, Broussard PM, McCart D, Smith MA: Antepartum fetal heart rate testing. V. The nonstress test—an outpatient approach. *Am J Obstet Gynecol* 136:81, 1980

Rochard F, Schifrin BS, Goupil F, et al: Nonstressed fetal heart rate monitoring in the antepartum period. *Am J Obstet Gynecol* 126:699, 1976

Schifrin BS, Foye G, Arato J, Kates R, MacKenna J: Routine fetal heart rate monitoring in the antepartum period. *Obstet Gynecol* 54:21, 1979

36

Fetal Lung Maturity

STEVEN H. GOLDE, M.D.

Hyaline membrane disease is the largest contributor to the neonatal mortality rate, accounting for 12,000 deaths annually in the United States. In terms of morbidity, it is the leading cause of admission to the neonatal intensive-care unit. The proven reliability of amniotic fluid analysis in the determination of fetal lung maturity places responsibility on the obstetrician to fully understand and evaluate this function before embarking on the elective termination of pregnancy.

Avery and Mead discovered that the lung fluid of newborns contains substances that produce stable foams and are present only in lung specimens from mature fetuses. Soon after, Clements determined that phospholipids were the active compounds responsible for this vital function. Based on these findings, Gluck and others developed methodology that permitted semiquantification of the phospholipid components. These tests evolved into the present lecithin-sphingomyelin (L/S) ratio and shake tests. Further refinements and greater understanding of phospholipid function have expanded these methods to include the phospholipid lung profile, which is the most comprehensive amniotic fluid analysis of lung maturity to date.

PULMONARY SURFACTANT

Pulmonary surfactant is composed of 80-90% lipid, 10-20% protein, and 1-2% carbohydrate. It is secreted by the type II pneumocyte directly into the alveolar space in the form of lamellar packets. It spreads over the alveolar surface and provides an air-surfactant interface that lowers the alveolar surface tension. Lowering the surface tension stabilizes the alveoli as their volume decreases with expiration. This follows from the law of Laplace:

$$P = \frac{2T}{r}$$

where P = outer pressure, T = surface tension, and r = radius of the alveolus. With high surface tension, greater pressure is required to maintain a fixed radius. This radius must not decrease below the size required for the maintenance of functional residual capacity (the reserve air in the lungs at the conclusion of a forced expiration), or atelectasis will occur. The initial expansion of the neonate's lungs requires opening pressures of 60-80 cm H_2O while pressures of only 2-8 cm H_2O are necessary for each breath thereafter. The marked reduction in force required is due to the decrease in surface tension provided by surfactant. Without adequate surfactant, the neonate is condemned to repeat its first breath over and over again, dying of hypoxia and exhaustion.

The major surfactant phospholipids are lecithin (80%), phosphatidylglycerol (10-15%), and phosphatidylinositol (5-10%). Lecithin is really a family of phospholipids having two fatty acid chains attached to a glycerol backbone along with a phosphocholine molecule. The most active of the lecithins is dipalmitoyl-lecithin (DPPC), with two fatty acid chains of palmitic acid (16 carbon atoms in a straight chain without a double bond). Phosphatidylglycerol (PG) has essentially the same structure except that glycerol replaces choline. Phosphatidylinositol (PI) contains the 6-carbon polyalcohol myoinositol in place of the choline molecule.

METHODS OF DETERMINING FETAL MATURITY

Biophysical Tests

Over the past decade, several methods for the determination of fetal maturity have been described. They can be classified into three main groups. Group I includes biophysical determinants of fetal age: distal and proximal femoral epiphyses, cephalometry for biparietal diameter (BPD) measurement, and the presence of fetal squamous cells in amniotic fluid stained with Nile blue sulfate. The first two represent attempts to approach the problem through low-risk, noninvasive techniques.

Because of wide variation in the physical variables measured, all these methods have large false-positive and false-negative rates and should be used with caution. Cephalometry may serve as a useful screening approach in certain circumstances. Hobbins and co-workers have described unacceptably high false-positive and false-negative rates in BPDs between 8.7 and 9.0 cm. The false-positive rate of 6% (i.e., immature fetus) using the larger value is particularly disturbing.

We have prospectively collected data using a larger minimum BPD of 9.2 cm (or the presence of a grade III placenta) as determined with real-time equipment. We have not encountered a single case of respiratory distress syndrome in over 200 nondiabetic patients. It must be emphasized that all patients were rigorously screened for the presence of diabetes using a 2-hour post-Glucola blood glucose value of <140 μg/dl as indicative of absence of diabetes. Using this technique, we have reduced our amniocentesis rate by more than 50%.

Amniotic Fluid Analysis

Group II tests involve amniocentesis but measure parameters other than surfactant concentration: creatinine, cortisol, protein, prolactin, and bilirubin. Correlation with fetal maturity is high with these tests, but they still have unacceptable false-positive and false-negative rates. Maturity in high-risk situations such as diabetes, Rh-isoimmunization, growth retardation, and premature labor is poorly determined by these methods, greatly limiting their utility.

Pulmonary Surfactant Determinations

Group III can be subdivided into screening tests and semiquantitative methods of surfactant detection (Table 36-1).

Screening tests. Shake (foam stability) tests are relatively easy to do and are reproducible as long as strict attention is paid to the details of the method. Only a trained laboratory technologist should do the test, because false-positive results occur if the protocol is varied. While the test has a high false-negative rate of 30-60%, it has a very low false-positive rate. Thus, positive tests predict the presence of lung maturity with good accuracy. The test requires only 15 minutes and minimal laboratory equipment and thus can serve as an adequate screening test.

Change in absorbance at 650 nm (ΔOD_{650}) relies on the fact that surfactant phospholipids increase the turbidity of amniotic fluid. The technique is reproducible and rapid and requires only a spectrophotometer capable of reading in the near infrared at 650 nm, which is available in most hospital laboratories. The false-positive rate is very low, but the false-negative rate is high (30-60%).

Microviscosimetry relies on a biophysical principle of quantum state changes in dye dispersed in lipid membranes and is technically simple and rapid to perform, although it requires expensive equipment. Preliminary testing of this method suggests that intermediate values obtained may reflect intermediate risks of respiratory distress syndrome, so that this method may be of potential benefit in grading risks.

Semiquantitative tests. There are several modifications of the L/S ratio test that yield differing end points for maturity. The clinician needs to know what

TABLE 36-1. MATURITY VALUES FOR SURFACTANT SCREENING TESTS

Test	Maturity value	Comment
Shake (foam stability)	Stable ring of foam in third tube ($+1+1+$ reaction)	Must be run on uncontaminated samples only
FSI (foam stability index)	Stable ring of foam in $\geq 47\%$ tube	Must be run on uncontaminated samples only
ΔOD_{650}	≥ 0.150	Must be run on uncontaminated samples only
FELMA (microviscosimetry)	<0.320	Must be run on uncontaminated samples only

TABLE 36-2. MATURITY VALUES FOR SURFACTANT TESTS

Test	Maturity value	Comment
L/S ratio	≥2.0:1	Must be run on uncontaminated samples only
Lung profile		
L/S ratio	≥2.0:1	Any sample with PG ≥2% is mature
DPPC	>50%	
PI	Variable	In absence of PG, the L/S ratio, % DPPC, and % PI will yield a graded probability of lung maturity. The higher the L/S, % DPPC, and % PI, the greater the likelihood of mature surfactant
PG	≥2.0%	

the maturity values are for his own laboratory. The advantage is a low false-positive rate of 1-3% in very large reported series (over 2,100 cases available from the literature), with a false-negative rate of 30-60% in most series. A risk gradient can be assigned to intermediate values, providing more information to the clinician.

FIGURE 36-1

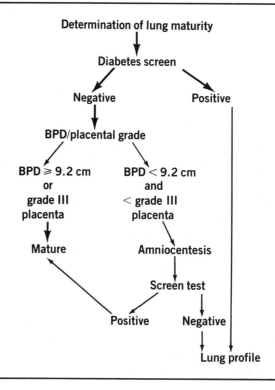

TABLE 36-3. LUNG PROFILE EVALUATION

Parameter	Critical value	Comment
L/S ratio	≥2.0:1	This has the same interpretation as the standard L/S ratio, but should be used with caution in the diabetic, isoimmunized, or parabiotic twin pregnancy
% precipitable lecithin (% DPPC)	≥50%	DPPC is the active lecithin fraction, and its concentration rises in parallel with L/S ratio. It ensures high-quality lecithin
% PI	No absolute value	PI concentration increases until about 36 weeks' gestation, then decreases until term. It can be estimated when PG is likely to appear by knowledge of PI content
% PG	≥2.0%	PG represents final maturation of surfactant. It ensures that hyaline membrane disease will not occur, even in diabetic pregnancy

Modifications of the L/S ratio measure total lecithin concentration or lecithin palmitate/stearate ratios. The drawback of these methods is that they require sophisticated technology and highly trained personnel, and take several hours to perform.

The lung profile (phospholipid profile) is really a modification of the L/S ratio but provides more data, since levels of DPPC, PI, and PG are obtained. It requires two-dimensional chromatography or complex solvent systems. Table 36-2 summarizes the L/S ratio and lung profile.

From the above, the following approach can be taken to maximize the risk/benefit ratio (see Fig. 36-1). Patients who are likely to undergo elective termination or indicated induction before the onset of labor at term should be screened for diabetes and Rh-isoimmunization. If the fetal BPD is 9.2 cm or greater (or there is a grade III placenta) and the patient is not diabetic, delivery can be undertaken without prior amniocentesis. If there is diabetes or Rh disease, fetal BPD less than 9.2 cm, and less than a grade III placenta, amniocentesis should be performed. A screening test should be employed and delivery permitted if this shows maturity. One exception is in the diabetic pregnancy, where knowledge of the PG content is important.

If intermediate or negative screening results are obtained, a full lung profile should be done for maximum data retrieval (Table 36-3). The lung profile should also be performed in all cases of diabetes because of the possibility of delayed lung development. The presence of blood or meconium precludes the use of amniotic fluid screening tests but not the lung profile, since PG is present in significant quantity only in lung effluent and can be detected in the presence of contaminants. The screening tests all yield false-positive results in the presence of these substances, and the L/S may be falsely high or low. This approach will help to decrease the need for amniocentesis while providing maximum utility of the laboratory. It also provides a means of conserving valuable laboratory time and personnel. Most hospitals should be able to establish screening tests with currently available equipment and personnel. More sophisticated testing can be handled at regional centers established to maintain proper quality controls and expertise.

SUGGESTED READING

Clements JA, Platzger ACG, Tierney DF, et al: Assessment of the risk of the respiratory-distress syndrome by a rapid test for surfactant in amniotic fluid. *N Engl J Med* 286:1077, 1972

Golde SH, et al: Fetal lung maturity—The adjunctive use of ultrasound. *Obstet Gynecol* 142:445, 1982

Golde SH, Mosley GH: A blinded comparison study of the lung phospholipid profile, fluorescence microviscosimetry, and the L/S ratio. *Am J Obstet Gynecol* (in press)

Golde SH, Vogt JF, Gabbe SG, et al: The clinical evaluation of the FELMA microviscosimeter in the prediction of fetal pulmonary maturity *Obstet Gynecol* 54:639, 1979

Goldstein P, Gershenson D, Hobbins JC: Fetal biparietal diameter as a predictor of a mature lecithin/sphingomyelin ratio. *Obstet Gynecol* 48:667, 1976

Hallman M, Kulovich M, Kirkpatrick E, et al: Phosphatidylinositol and phosphatidylglycerol in amniotic fluid: Indices of lung maturity. *Am J Obstet Gynecol* 125:613, 1976

Kulovich MV, Hallman MB, Gluck L: The lung profile: I. Normal Pregnancy. *Am J Obstet Gynecol* 135:57, 1979

37

Use of Glucocorticoids to Induce Fetal Pulmonary Maturity

STEVEN H. GOLDE, M.D.

At LAC/USC (Los Angeles County/University of Southern California) Medical Center, perinatal care is provided for a large volume of high-risk indigent patients. Approximately 8% of the neonates we deliver weigh less than 2,500 gm. This low-birth-weight group accounts for 80% of our perinatal mortality. More significantly, while only 1.5% of our newborns weigh less than 1,500 gm, this small group accounts for 67% of our perinatal mortality. Prematurity and the accompanying hazard of respiratory distress syndrome (RDS) remain a significant cause of perinatal mortality.

The clinical and laboratory investigations of the past decade produced increasing interest in the pharmacologic induction of pulmonary maturity in premature fetuses. Although many pharmacologic agents, such as β-sympathomimetics, thyroxine, and prolactin, have been studied for this purpose, the majority of clinical studies have used glucocorticoids. Both the naturally occurring steroid cortisol (or hydrocortisone) and the synthetic steroids betamethasone, dexamethasone, and methylprednisolone have been used for the induction of pulmonary maturity.

MECHANISM OF GLUCOCORTICOID ACTION

The exact mechanism by which glucocorticoids are thought to reduce the incidence of RDS is not known. However, several theories have been proposed. Ballard and his co-workers have shown there are specific glucocorticoid receptors in the cytoplasm of fetal pulmonary epithelial cells. They proposed that the protein receptors combine with the glucocorticoid; this complex changes configuration and migrates to the nucleus, where it attaches to acceptor sites on the chromatin. Messenger RNA is thought then to transcribe an encoded enzyme produced in the cytoplasm. There is no agreement as to which enzyme is primarily induced—or, indeed, which enzyme is primary in effecting surfactant synthesis.

Hallman demonstrated that surfactant could be synthesized and released by the addition of cyclic AMP analogs to rabbit lung slices. This suggests another mechanism using cyclic AMP as a second messenger to promote surfactant production. Finally, Johnson and colleagues demonstrated an increase in maximum lung volumes in rhesus monkey fetuses after betamethasone administration, but could not show increased phospholipid concentrations or lower surface tensions. They speculated that the major effect of antenatal betamethasone is on connective tissue elements, with a minimal effect on alveolar surfactant.

CLINICAL STUDIES

Many clinical trials have evaluated the efficacy of antenatal corticosteroids in inducing fetal pulmonary maturity. The first and, until relatively recently, the only well-designed double-blind study was that of Liggins and Howie in New Zealand. This study employed 12 mg of betamethasone against a cortisone "placebo" group in a randomized, double-blind trial of 853 patients admitted for premature labor before 36 weeks' gestation. Two injections of drug, given 24 hours apart, were administered. Liggins and Howie found that betamethasone was effective in reducing the incidence of RDS by 63% compared with placebo if treatment occurred within 24 hours to 7 days before delivery.

Betamethasone was not effective if given less than 24 hours before delivery, suggesting that this interval may be necessary for surfactant production. The finding that betamethasone was not more effective than placebo if given more than 7 days before delivery might have been due to normal gestational maturation, as the incidence of RDS did substantially fall (from 23.7% to 2.2%) in the "control" group. Similarly, Liggins and Howie found no benefit of betamethasone in fetuses more mature than 34 weeks' gestation. This lack of effect may also be explained by the expected degree of endogenous surfactant production in fetuses beyond 34 weeks.

The Ballards showed similar effects of betamethasone at the same dosage in a smaller study done in the United States. The drug was ineffective in neonates weighing under 750 or over 1,250 gm. Babies under 750 gm are not likely to have reached development of functional alveoli; those above 1,250 gm are likely to have attained more mature surfactant levels spontaneously.

Finally, a recent collaborative study done under the auspices of the National Institutes of Health, using dexamethasone (4 mg qid) in a 48-hour treatment course, substantiated the findings discussed above. The investigative group further noted that if L/S ratios were not obtained (this test was not required unless the pregnancy was beyond 34 weeks' gestation), there was no difference in the rate of RDS between treated and control groups. If the L/S ratio was <2.0:1 (those infants actually at risk for RDS), maternal steroid treatment decreased the incidence of RDS by 50%. The study also demonstrated no improvement if the fetus was male, in cases of preeclampsia, or in premature rupture of the membranes.

LONG-TERM EFFECTS OF TREATMENT

Many questions still remain. One of great concern is: Will the fetus, infant, child, or adult who has been treated in utero pay a price for this treatment?

We do not have the answer in human subjects. However, a somewhat reassuring study by Ballard suggests that the levels of betamethasone in cord serum, when expressed as cortisol equivalents, were similar to cortisol levels reached in response to stress—such as RDS. Though the follow-up is short, no adverse effects have yet been attributed to steroid therapy directed at accelerating human pulmonary maturity. On the other hand, animal studies report the following adverse effects of steroids in developing organisms: (1) decreased body weight, (2) decreased total cell number, (3) decreased DNA synthesis in the brain, (4) impaired myelination, (5) small lungs, (6) behavioral changes, (7) thymic weight decreases, (8) inhibition of phagocytosis, and (9) gliosis in brains of rhesus monkeys. All of these studies used doses that were proportionately much larger than those employed clinically. However, the principle that glucocorticoids accelerate cellular differentiation at the expense of cellular division may still operate even at the lower doses used in humans.

PRECAUTIONS

Because of the undefined potential for long-term effects on growth, brain development, immunologic competence, social functions, and so on in humans who were treated in utero, we strictly control the use of glucocorticoids. Only those patients between 28 and 32 weeks (900-1,500 gm) are candidates unless surfactant levels are shown to be below mature values after 32 weeks. Whenever possible, we attempt to document the absence of lung maturity by amniocentesis. We use the regimen described by Liggins and Howie, i.e., 12 mg of betamethasone IM stat and 12 mg in 24 hours. Attempts are made to postpone delivery as long as possible. Intravenous magnesium sulfate or a β-mimetic agent, such as terbutaline (Brethine, Bricanyl), is utilized when needed for suppression of premature labor in order to obtain at least a full 48-hour course of therapy.

An ultrasound examination is performed on each patient for fetal biparietal diameter, placental localization, amniotic fluid volume assessment, and selection of a site for amniocentesis. If a site for amniocentesis is found, amniocentesis is performed before betamethasone is given, in order to document fetal pulmonary immaturity by amniotic fluid screening tests or lung profile and to rule out occult amnionitis, based on bacteria in the amniotic fluid, whether or not membranes are intact. The drug is not administered if the screening tests are positive or the L/S ratio is greater than 2.0:1, if phosphatidylglycerol is present, if bacteria are found in the amniotic fluid, or when in our clinical judgment delivery cannot safely be delayed for at least 24 hours or premature delivery is not likely to occur within 7 days. Continuous external fetal heart rate monitoring and tocodynamometry are utilized with all patients in premature labor to rule out fetal distress and to aid in the assessment of uterine activity.

The safety of betamethasone in the patient with ruptured membranes remains a subject of concern. Some data indict its use in these patients. The NIH collaborative study was unable to show any benefit in this group of patients, and the experience of Garite and Freeman suggests that these women face the additional hazard of infection. We avoid vaginal examinations, and we hospitalize these patients until either fluid stops leaking or delivery occurs. The presence of amnionitis is a clear indication to undertake delivery. Evidence suggests that prolonged rupture of the membranes in and of itself may accelerate fetal pulmonary maturation. Corticosteroids are given only if there is a demonstrable need on the basis of surfactant studies.

Finally, one must remember that the prevention of RDS, even in the most optimistic of these glucocorticoid studies, was never 100%. The prevention of RDS still must include certain standard principles of modern obstetric care:

1. Inhibition of premature labor
2. Intensive intrapartum monitoring to allow rapid detection and prompt assessment and treatment of subtle signs of distress in very small premature fetuses
3. Along with prevention of stressful labor, avoidance of traumatic delivery of these fragile babies—a precaution of critical importance.

SUGGESTED READING

Ballard RA, Ballard PL, Granberg JP, Sniderman S: Prenatal administration of betamethasone for prevention of respiratory distress syndrome. *Pediatrics* 94:97, 1979

Brehier A, Benson BJ, Williams MC, Mason RJ, Ballard PL: Corticosteroid induction of phosphatidic acid phosphatase in fetal rabbit lung. *Biochem Biophys Res Commun* 77:883, 1977

Collaborative Group on Antenatal Steroid Therapy: Effect of antenatal dexamethasone administration on the prevention of respiratory distress syndrome. *Am J Obstet Gynecol* 141:276, 1981

Epstein MF, Farrell PM, Sparles JW, Pepe G, Driscoll S, Chez RA: Maternal betamethasone and fetal growth and development in the monkey. *Am J Obstet Gynecol* 127:261, 1977

Garite TJ, Freeman RK, Linzey EM, et al: Prospective randomized study of corticosteroids in the management of premature rupture of membranes and the premature gestation. *Am J Obstet Gynecol* 141:508, 1981

Hallman M: Induction of surfactant phosphatidylglycerol in the lung of fetal and newborn rabbits by dibutyryl adenosine 3':5'-monophosphate. *Biochem Biophys Res Commun* 77:1094, 1977

Johnson JWC, Mitzner W, London WT, Palmer AE, Scott R: Betamethasone and the rhesus fetus: Multisystemic effects. *Am J Obstet Gynecol* 133:677, 1979

Liggins GC, Howie RN: A controlled trial of antepartum glucocorticoid treatment for prevention of the respiratory distress syndrome in premature infants. *Pediatrics* 50:515, 1972

Zuspan FP, Cordero L, Semchyslyn S: Effects of hydrocortisone on lecithin-sphingomyelin ratio. *Am J Obstet Gynecol* 128:571, 1977

38

Electronic FHR Monitoring: What Every Practitioner Must Know About the Equipment

FRANK C. MILLER, M.D.

The pioneer work of Hon and associates in the development of reliable methods for continuous intrapartum plotting of instantaneous fetal heart rate has profoundly influenced modern obstetrics. When used properly, intrapartum FHR monitoring has resulted in the virtual disappearance of intrapartum death and a significant decline in the incidence of intrapartum fetal asphyxia and its consequences. When used improperly, FHR monitoring may lead to dramatic and often unnecessary increases in the incidence of cesarean section. The effect of direct FHR monitoring on maternal febrile morbidity has not been clearly established. Isolated instances of fetal trauma or sepsis associated with placement of the scalp electrode have been reported. However, the advantages of FHR monitoring far outweigh the disadvantages.

THE CARDIOTACHOMETER

The instantaneous rate of each of a sequence of cardiac cycles is inversely proportional to the interval between cycles; that is, rate is equal to 60,000 divided by the interval in milliseconds. Thus, if there is an interval of 600 msec between the beginning of one cycle and the beginning of the next, the instantaneous rate is 100 beats per minute (bpm); with an interval of 400 msec the instantaneous rate is 150 bpm; and with a 300-msec interval the rate is 200 bpm. The FHR monitor calculates intervals between fetal heart cycles and converts them to proportional voltage outputs, which in turn are used to drive a pen on the strip chart recorder. (In simple terms, then, the FHR monitor is a cardiotachometer.) The electrical and mechanical activities of the heart provide several markers that can be used to calculate cycle intervals, and these form the basis for different methods of monitoring FHR.

THE DIRECT (INTERNAL) SYSTEM

The direct (internal) system involves placement of a stainless steel spiral electrode a short depth (2-3 mm) into the subcutaneous tissue of the presenting fetal part after the membranes have ruptured. The second pole of the bipolar electrode is in contact with the maternal vaginal fluid, and thus with the mother. The two leads from the spiral electrode are then connected to a maternal ground plate, usually on the patient's thigh. The resulting electrical signal is a mixture of maternal and fetal ECG complexes (as the fetus is a conductor and in contact with the mother).

The fetal signal far exceeds the mother's, and an automatic gain control amplifier increases the amplitude of the fetal signal. The peak of the fetal R wave triggers the cardiotachometer. The direct system allows for precise measurement of instantaneous heart rate variability, short- and long-term.

Troubleshooting the Direct System

Evaluation of the noisy or uninterpretable record. The monitor works by measuring the interval between two triggers and converting it to an instantaneous rate. When the system is attached properly, the triggers are fetal R waves. An improperly attached spiral electrode or ground plate results in a low signal-to-noise ratio, making a portion of the triggers noise instead of fetal R waves. This results in random wide, rapid fluctuation in the recorded rate. To eliminate this problem, auscultate fetal heart tones to rule out an arrhythmia, then check the electrode placement and ground plate and reposition them if necessary. A defective electrode or monitor is rarely responsible; the problem is nearly always a result of poor contact. Rapid, intermittent changes in heart rate every three to five beats may represent a true fetal arrhythmia—most commonly premature ventricular contractions. This can be confirmed by direct analysis of the fetal ECG signal on the oscilloscope or by auscultation of a fetal heart rate irregularity.

Evaluation of persistent bradycardia. The monitor can measure only the time interval between successive triggers (R waves) and cannot discriminate between maternal and fetal sources of R waves. Thus, if the spiral electrode is connected to the cervix or vagina, the monitor will record maternal heart rate. A dead fetus will conduct the maternal ECG complexes, which may be transmitted by the spiral electrode on the fetal scalp to the monitor and be converted to a rate, giving an erroneous diagnosis of fetal bradycardia. Finally, the fetus may have a true bradycardia as a result of distress or, rarely, congenital heart block.

It is a wise policy to determine that a bradycardia recorded on the monitor is indeed fetal, not maternal, in origin. This is accomplished by simultaneous recording or auscultation of the maternal heart rate or palpation of the pulse along with auscultation or real-time ultrasound evaluation of the fetal heart. These simple maneuvers can avoid the tragic mistake of cesarean section for apparent fetal distress that in reality represents a normal maternal heart rate!

THE INDIRECT (EXTERNAL) SYSTEM

There are three common methods for indirect, or external, recording of the fetal heart rate. Two of these systems, Doppler ultrasound and phonocardiogram, derive the heart rate signal from the mechanical activity of the heart. The Doppler system sends out continuous ultrasound energy and then detects frequency shifts of the sound as it is reflected from moving heart structures such as the ventricular walls, septum, or valves. The Doppler system is a very reliable means of obtaining an FHR signal. In order to conduct and receive the ultrasound signal, a coupling gel must be applied to the maternal abdomen for proper interface.

The phonocardiogram detects the sounds produced by the fetal heart and converts them to a rate. This system is purely passive and does not require any preparation of the maternal abdomen. With either system, the mechanical motion that provides the signal may vary from cycle to cycle. For example, a valve motion may provide one trigger and a septum motion the next. Thus, neither system provides meaningful information about beat-to-beat variability or short-term variability.

A change in the relationship of either the Doppler or phonocardiogram transducer to the fetal heart caused by movement of either the mother or the fetus can result in a loss of the fetal heart rate signal. Because these shifts occur frequently, most external systems that rely on mechanical movement of the heart contain an editing capability. The essential function of the editing is to improve the cosmetic appearance of the fetal heart rate record. The specific characteristics of the editing logic vary from one manufacturer to another, and the user is advised to become familiar with the specific system in the machine that is being used.

With external systems there is a refractory period of a few milliseconds after each first heart sound. This is to prevent counting the second heart sound as a separate beat. Editing may result in doubling the heart rate when the actual rate falls below 80-90 bpm, or halving a rapid rate (more than 180 bpm). Doubling of the FHR occurs when the true heart rate is so slow that the first and second heart sounds are counted as separate heartbeats. Halving of a rapid heart rate may occur when the second heartbeat falls within the refractory period immediately following a recorded heartbeat.

The third method of external recording of fetal heart rate relies on the fetal ECG signal conducted to the surface of the maternal abdomen. The magnitude of this signal at a given point on the abdomen varies with fetal position, and so the electrodes are moved systematically until the largest fetal ECG complex is detected. The signal obtained is a mixture of both fetal and maternal ECG complexes and is processed so that the heart rate is derived from the fetal signal. Most abdominal wall fetal ECG systems contain editing logic that injects an artificial signal when fetal and maternal ECG complexes coincide (based on the assumption that there was a fetal signal hidden by the longer maternal signal). Some contain more extensive logic to average the heart rate and produce a better cosmetic result. When used with minimal or no editing, this system can provide a reasonably accurate estimate of both beat-to-beat and long-term variability. Most monitors have a switch that allows or defeats editing.

Troubleshooting the Indirect System

The most frequent cause of an unsatisfactory external record of fetal heart rate is improper positioning of the transducer. This problem is readily corrected by moving the transducer until a clear, distinct fetal heart rate is obtained, then fixing the transducer in this position. Frequently all that is required is a small adjustment in the angle of the transducer. Occasionally, in very obese patients, it is impossible to monitor the FHR with external systems. In a very thin patient, the maternal abdominal aorta can be the source of a signal, leading to an erroneous diagnosis of fetal bradycardia.

METHODS OF RECORDING UTERINE ACTIVITY

The Direct System

The direct, or internal, system involves placement of a fluid-filled plastic catheter through the vagina and cervix into the uterine cavity and then connecting the other end to a pressure-sensitive transducer. The transducer converts the hydrostatic pressure of the fluid column and intrauterine pressure to a proportional voltage. It is essential that the transducer be placed over the estimated position of the catheter tip—that is, at a point that intersects with a horizontal plane midway through the abdomen—and then opened to air and calibrated. When properly calibrated, the direct system can precisely measure intrauterine resting tone and the amplitude of uterine contractions. The resting tone is helpful in evaluating states of altered uterine contractility—either endogenous, as in abruption, or exogenous, as in overstimulation with oxytocin. A falsely elevated resting tone occurs when the pressure transducer is placed below the tip of the intrauterine catheter. Similarly, true resting tone may be falsely low when the transducer is above the catheter tip.

Perforation of the lower uterine segment by the ridged catheter guide has been reported. Care must be taken not to allow the guide past the tips of the examining fingers during catheter insertion. The flexible catheter is very unlikely to cause a perforation. Although there has been much concern regarding intrauterine infection with the use of the catheter, there is no evidence of an increased incidence of infection when the length of labor and duration of ruptured membranes are controlled.

The Indirect System

The indirect system of recording uterine activity involves placement of a pressure-sensitive device, a tocodynamometer, on the maternal abdomen, usually in the region of the uterine fundus. The tocodynamometer detects the forward rotation of the uterus with a contraction and produces an electrical sign reflecting uterine activity. This system provides accurate information on the frequency and duration of contractions, but does not indicate their intensity; nor does it provide information about uterine resting tone. Thus the use of an external system to gauge the rate of oxytocin infusion may be hazardous. The external systems for measuring uterine activity are purely passive and are not associated with any known maternal or fetal complication.

SUGGESTED READING

Hon EH: Instrumentation of fetal heart rate and fetal electrocardiography. III. Fetal ECG electrodes: Further observations. *Obstet Gynecol* 30:281, 1967

Hon EH: *An Atlas of Fetal Heart Rate Patterns*. New Haven, Ct: Harty Press, 1968

Hon EH: Intrapartum fetal electrocardiography. In Crosigani PG, Pardi G, eds: *Fetal Evaluation During Pregnancy and Labor*. New York: Academic Press, 1971, p 240

Paul RH, Hon EH: A clinical fetal monitor. *Obstet Gynecol* 35:161, 1970

Paul RH, Petrie RH: *Fetal Intensive Care*. North Haven, Ct: William Mack Co, 1979

39

Interpretation of FHR Records: Baseline Heart Rate and Variability

BARRY S. SCHIFRIN, M.D.

Proper control of the fetal heart rate requires a well-oxygenated myocardium capable of responding to impulses arising from a responsive, well-oxygenated central nervous system.

CONTROL OF FETAL HEART RATE

Regulation of the heartbeat is a complex function involving both intrinsic and extrinsic factors. Any area of the heart may serve as pacemaker. Because the spontaneous discharge frequency of the sinoatrial node is faster than any other focus, it predominates. At term the fetal heart responds predictably to a host of neural and humoral influences that modify the regular pacing action of the SA node. Thus atropine, epinephrine, and stimulation of the fetus cause tachycardia, while drugs such as acetylcholine and propranolol, and maneuvers such as cord compression and stimulation of the trigeminal nerve area, slow the FHR. The effects of these drugs and maneuvers increase with advancing gestation.

The fetus undergoes sleep/wake (rest/activity) cycles akin to those in the normal newborn. During activity, accelerations and decelerations are quite common and variability (to be discussed below) is increased. When neural and humoral influences that affect pacemaker function are diminished in the fetus as a result of prematurity, drug effects, asphyxia, or sleep, the rate of discharge is quite regular. These responses highlight the limited value of auscultation of heart rate for assessment of fetal condition. No longer is it reasonable to believe that every bradycardia or tachycardia represents either fetal distress or a step on the road to fetal death. Aberrations in FHR pattern provide early information about developing fetal hypoxemia and acidemia as well as a number of other neurologic and cardiac events.

EFFECTS OF UTERINE CONTRACTIONS

The evaluation of electronic fetal monitoring patterns consists of the assessment of FHR changes in relation to uterine contractions (UC). Contractions represent a repetitive stimulus and stress to the fetus. UC are frequently accompanied by fetal cardiac accelerations (these are most prominent before labor or in a nonvertex presentation). Other possible effects of UC include pressure on the fetal presenting part, with the potential of increased intracranial pressure and trauma, and trapping of the umbilical cord between the fetal body and extremities or between the fetus and the uterine wall.

The most consistent effect of UC, however, is impairment of uterine blood flow in direct proportion to the duration and amplitude of contractions. During contractions the fetus is functionally isolated from exchange of oxygen with the mother. This decrease in oxygen availability is usually well tolerated, and there is little evidence that these effects of contractions are cumulative. If contractions are excessive or the fetal blood is anemic, they will cause a fall in oxygen content of the blood and late decelerations will appear.

In the considerations of FHR patterns presented below, fetal distress is defined only in relationship to UC. In the absence of UC, the patterns of distress (baseline tachycardia, decreased variability) are far more insidious and less amenable to early detection.

TERMINOLOGY OF FHR MONITORING

As understanding of the significance of FHR patterns improved, a new terminology became necessary. *Baseline features* refer to those occurring between contractions, while *periodic changes* are those related to UC. Thus bradycardia, tachycardia, and variability refer to baseline changes while accelerations and decelerations describe FHR changes associated with UC.

Baseline Heart Rate

The baseline heart rate is the rate observed between contractions. The average baseline FHR at term is about 140 beats per minute (bpm) with the range of normal from 120 to 160 bpm. Maturation of vagal function produces a small, progressive decrease in heart rate with advancing gestational age. By definition, a new baseline heart rate requires a change in baseline of at least 10 minutes' duration.

A baseline fetal heart rate of less than 120 bpm is bradycardia. In most instances, a fetal bradycardia of 100-120 bpm is a normal variant and consistent with a normal outcome, especially if associated with normal variability. However, bradycardia may also signal fetal problems, such as sustained umbilical cord compression, severe fetal hypoxia, or a cardiac arrhythmia. It must be emphasized that sustained bradycardia with absent variability, as distinguished from a sudden deceleration, is a late sign of fetal asphyxia.

Fetal heart block, another cause of sustained bradycardia, may be best diagnosed by auscultation of an irregularity of the fetal heart or by direct analysis of the fetal ECG, available from a scalp electrode. Rarely, an apparent fetal bradycardia may represent the maternal heart rate. In the direct (internal) mode, a dead fetus may nevertheless transmit the maternal ECG complex. This problem is readily solved by simultaneous monitoring of the maternal and presumed fetal pulses or by noting the absence of fetal heart motion with

Doppler or real-time B-scan ultrasound. In the external mode, the ultrasound transducer may inadvertently detect pulsation in maternal vessels, irrespective of the viability of the fetus.

Fetal tachycardia is defined as a baseline fetal heart rate in excess of 160 bpm. The most commonly identified cause of fetal tachycardia is maternal fever. On occasion, though, tachycardia may represent fetal sepsis long before it has been manifested as maternal fever. When combined with late or variable decelerations, it carries an ominous connotation. Tachycardia alone may be an early sign of hypoxemia and acidemia if contractions are infrequent or absent. During labor, tachycardia unassociated with decelerations is usually related to a cause other than hypoxia. β-Mimetic drugs such as isoxsuprine (Vasodilan) and ritodrine (Yutopar) and anticholinergic drugs such as atropine and scopolamine may cross the placenta and cause fetal tachycardia. Maternal catecholamines do not cross the placenta readily and so do not affect FHR directly. Other causes of fetal tachycardia include cardiac arrhythmias, such as paroxysmal atrial tachycardia.

Fetal Heart Rate Variability

Beat-to-beat variability appears to represent the continuous and subtle interaction of the sympathetic and parasympathetic nervous systems as they determine the appropriate heart rate (and cardiac output) for the fetus. Reflex neural inputs such as those related to fetal chest wall movement (respirations) or local cardiac factors may influence variability, as well as those impulses originating in higher cortical centers of the fetal brain.

Under normal circumstances FHR is continuously modulated by parasympathetic (vagal) and sympathetic input. These countervailing influences, one to slow the heart, the other to increase the rate, contribute to the irregular undulations in the heart rate pattern termed variability. Variability has been divided, in turn, into long- and short-term components. Abrupt, short-lived, unpredictable changes in beat-to-beat interval are referred to as short-term variability. More gentle, predictable oscillations of 2 to 5 cycles per minute with an amplitude varying from 5 to 15 bpm are referred to as long-term variability. While short-term variability is difficult to quantitate, its presence reflects an intact, well-oxygenated autonomic nervous system and is the single most reliable indicator that the fetus is not hypoxic.

Adequate short-term variability (beat-to-beat changes), even if other signs suggest hypoxia, usually presages a good outcome. Generally, long- and short-term variability rise and fall in unison. Thus most classifications of variability in fact represent an evaluation of long-term variability.

Variability is best assessed in a period of stable baseline heart rate between or just before contractions. Decreased variability (<5 bpm) may reflect fetal hypoxemia and acidemia. Severely compromised infants invariably show decreased to absent variability along with decelerations. More commonly, decreased variability without decelerations reflects drugs administered during labor. Narcotics, tranquilizers, and local and general anesthetics all diminish both long- and short-term variability. This effect on variability should not be regarded as asphyxia, but as a pharmacologic property.

Decreased variability may also reflect fetal sleep or inactivity. Sleep/wake cycles in the fetus are reflected in the variability patterns of the heart rate. During the rest phase, movements, accelerations, and variability are minimal. During activity, accelerations are accompanied by normal variability. These alternating episodes are easily seen during antepartum FHR testing, and may also be seen during labor.

The clinical significance of increased variability (>15 bpm) is not completely understood. In most instances, increased variability is associated with a normal outcome; in other instances, it has been associated with a short umbilical cord or mild fetal asphyxia.

A heart rate composed only of long-term variability in which the oscillations are regular is termed sinusoidal heart rate. Initially it was associated with a grave prognosis in the anemic, Rh-isoimmunized fetus. Subsequently it was found in anemic fetuses irrespective of etiology, as well as in fetuses with CNS or cardiac anomalies. However, in many instances a "sinusoidal" pattern may be found in otherwise normal fetuses. In fact, the pattern is found in about 50% of fetuses following administration of narcotics to the mother during labor. When a persistent sinusoidal pattern is encountered during labor, scalp sampling and ultrasound examination are indicated.

40

Periodic Changes in FHR

BARRY S. SCHIFRIN, M.D.

Periodic changes in fetal heart rate related to uterine contractions (UC) are referred to as accelerations and decelerations. Acceleration of the FHR in association with movements or uterine contractions is a common observation. In the antepartum period, the appearance of FHR accelerations of at least 15 beats per minute (bpm) with fetal movement or UC forms the basis for the reactive nonstress test, a reliable indication of fetal well-being. Similar benign correlations have been made when FHR accelerations appear during labor. Such accelerations are common occurrences early in labor or in nonvertex presentations.

In some instances, periodic accelerations may result from selective umbilical vein occlusion while the arteries remain open. In this circumstance, the venous return to the right heart is decreased and the fetus develops a reflex acceleration. Such periodic accelerations may anticipate later development of variable decelerations. One often sees a periodic acceleration immediately before and after a variable deceleration (so-called "shoulders"). These brief, erratic accelerations accompanying variable decelerations are probably of little consequence, especially with good variability.

Rebound accelerations, on the other hand, refer to accelerations following variable decelerations. They carry an ominous prognosis. In this instance, variability is absent and there are no preceding accelerations. The presence of this combination of features strongly suggests fetal compromise with autonomic imbalance.

Three kinds of periodic FHR decelerations—early, variable, and late—have been defined. They are identified by their relationship to the onset of UC and by their waveform, or shape.

EARLY DECELERATIONS

Early decelerations are benign and rarely associated with fetal acidosis. An early deceleration begins simultaneously with the onset of the contraction, reaches its nadir at or near the peak of the contraction, and returns to the baseline before or at the end of the uterine contraction. The waveform mimics the waveform of the underlying UC. In a given sequence, the amplitude and duration of the deceleration are proportional to the amplitude and duration of the UC. Early decelerations usually drop 10-15 bpm below baseline at their nadir. They rarely fall more than 30 bpm or below 100 bpm.

Early decelerations are reflex (vagal) in origin and appear to be due to compression of the fetal head. They can be reproduced in the fetus or newborn by manual compression and can be blocked with atropine. Early decelerations may occur throughout labor but are seen most frequently in advanced labor, as the vertex begins its descent into the pelvis, and throughout the second stage of labor. Early decelerations are rarely observed in the breech presentation. No specific therapy is indicated for early decelerations.

VARIABLE DECELERATIONS

Variable decelerations are the most common patterns observed. They frequently develop without warning late in the first stage of labor and are believed to be related to cord compression. They can be produced in experimental animals or humans by occlusion of the umbilical cord, and can be precipitated or relieved by maneuvers that alter the relationships among the cord, fetus, and uterine wall.

Occlusion of the umbilical vein and arteries causes a sudden rise in fetal blood pressure, which in turn produces a vagal reflex slowing of the fetal heart. Variable decelerations are so named because they vary in duration and in relationship to the onset of UC. Helpful features in distinguishing a variable deceleration include the presence of periodic acceleration immediately before and after ("shoulders"). In addition, the initial fall in rate may be very abrupt, producing a change of 30 bpm or greater over 1-2 seconds. Recovery is usually rapid. Variable decelerations may mimic early or late decelerations, but the recurrence of intermittent decelerations of varying timing and waveform with variable relationship to UC usually enables one to identify the pattern correctly.

Variable decelerations can frequently be eliminated by changing the position of the patient and giving her oxygen by face mask. An estimate of the cumulative effect of repeated variable decelerations on fetal condition can be made by examining the responses of the baseline heart rate and variability to the deceleration. If variability and baseline rate remain normal, babies are usually born in good condition irrespective of the frequency or character of the decelerations. Decreasing variability and rising baseline rate are indications that the decelerations, no matter what their amplitude, are distressing the fetus.

Severe variable decelerations may occasionally be accompanied by brief episodes of cardiac asystole (heart block). These episodes seem to represent an exuberant vagal response, usually in healthy fetuses. They are invariably associated with average or increased baseline variability after the deceleration and the outcome has uniformly been good. Commonly, such severe variable decelerations contain a brief episode of bradycardia at about 60 bpm with absent variability. This represents nodal rhythm and, like the occasional episode of asystole, should be treated like any other severe variable deceleration.

LATE DECELERATIONS

Late decelerations result from a fall in fetal pO_2 produced by the interruption of intervillous blood flow. The degree of fall in fetal pO_2 depends on the size and duration of the UC and the amount of fetal reserve. If uterine activity is excessive, it may embarrass even the most resilient fetus. However, in the compromised fetus with uteroplacental insufficiency, even small, short UC may cause a fall in pO_2 and a late deceleration.

The mechanism by which fetal hypoxia causes late decelerations is not fully known, but at least two pathways may be involved. The more common is the vagal response initiated by hypoxia. Here aortic body chemoreceptors in the fetus detect the falling pO_2 and induce a vagal discharge to slow the heart. The reflex late deceleration is characterized by an increase in variability during and usually after it. Reflex late decelerations imply that the fetal central nervous system is intact, and therefore the fetus is not likely to be severely depressed. Nevertheless, even with good variability, late decelerations warrant immediate evaluation. The second, and much more sinister, mechanism producing late deceleration is direct hypoxic depression of the fetal myocardium. Direct late decelerations are characterized by a lack of heart rate variability. Recurrent late decelerations with absent variability require immediate fetal evaluation and usually delivery.

A late deceleration of the FHR is so named because the onset of the deceleration occurs late in relation to the onset of UC. The nadir is reached after the peak of the contraction and returns to baseline beyond the end of the contraction. The amplitude of fall in heart rate with a late deceleration may be as small as 5-10 bpm or as much as 60 bpm. As with early decelerations, the amplitude and duration of late decelerations are proportional to the intensity and duration of UC. While true late decelerations may be subtle, they are nevertheless repetitive. Isolated late decelerations, no matter how typical, should not be considered a sign of hypoxia. Late decelerations of the fetal heart rate are a potentially ominous periodic pattern that requires prompt attention.

41

Fetal Blood Sampling

FRANK C. MILLER, M.D.

The two most commonly used techniques for intrapartum assessment of the "high-risk" fetus are continuous FHR monitoring and intermittent fetal capillary blood acid-base evaluation.

The investigation of fetal acid-base balance was pioneered by Ylppo, who reported in 1916 that by adult standards, human fetal cord blood was acidotic. The current technique of fetal scalp blood sampling was introduced by Saling in 1963. Fetal capillary blood pH is of clinical interest because it is directly related to tissue oxygenation. With inadequate oxygenation, the fetus will suffer brain damage and ultimately death.

pO_2 reflects fetal status only at the time of sampling, without any memory of the preceding levels. Blood pH is influenced by both respiratory and metabolic factors and therefore may reflect both rapid (respiratory) and/or prolonged (metabolic) changes. pH is used more often than pO_2 for evaluating fetal acid-base status because pO_2 measurement is subject to more technical error, and pO_2 is subject to more rapid fluctuation.

In a simplified way, changes in carbon dioxide (respiratory) will inversely affect pH. Retention of carbon dioxide will cause a reduction in pH (respiratory acidosis) while a decrease in carbon dioxide will result in an elevated pH (respiratory alkalosis). The effect on respiratory pH is rapid; the metabolic pH is slower to respond and return to normal.

The fetus is subject to both respiratory and metabolic acidosis. A major function of the placenta is to serve as the fetal lung. Conditions that intermittently interrupt the normal blood flow to and from the placenta, such as umbilical cord compression, will cause an increase in fetal pCO_2 and a fall in pH. More prolonged or chronic conditions that reduce the oxygen supply to the fetus interfere with normal aerobic metabolism, with subsequent increased production of metabolic acids.

TECHNIQUES OF FETAL SCALP BLOOD SAMPLING

The patient may be in the lithotomy or the Sims position. The cervix must be dilated at least 3 cm to allow the endoscope to be well applied to the presenting part. The necessary equipment may be obtained in a disposable kit or made up individually.

The Monoject kit (Sherwood Medical Industries, St. Louis) contains:

1 endoscope	10 Critocaps
6 swabs	1 pellet Critoseal
1 lancet (2 × 2 mm)	5 "fleas"
3 capillary tubes (heparinized)	1 magnet
1 sample carrier	1 packet of silicone gel

The only additional requirement is a light source.

The fetal head must be well down into the pelvis; if not, an assistant may be required to maintain pressure to prevent displacing the head during the procedure. The scalp is wiped dry, and silicone gel is applied to the proposed puncture site. The silicone will cause the blood to bead up after the scalp puncture for easy collection in a capillary tube. The fetal hair may need to be parted to get good exposure to the scalp. The scalp puncture is done with a 2 × 2 mm blade on a long handle with firm pressure held for a count of 4-5. Care must be taken not to perform the puncture over the fontanelles. Usually one puncture is sufficient, although there is no danger in more than one puncture as long as the site can be observed afterward to assure hemostasis. To reduce the likelihood of breakage, special care must be taken not to bend or twist the blade.

The capillary tube is held with the tip just in contact with the blood as it beads from the puncture. The blood will collect in the tube by capillary action. In theory, the blood should be collected between contractions to reflect fetal baseline status, but in practice the capillary flow is frequently better during a uterine contraction. The pH values are not significantly different as long as there are no profound FHR changes with contractions. Following collection, pressure is held over the puncture site through at least two contractions to assure hemostasis.

pH and blood gas analysis may be done with as little as 75 to 100 μl of blood (each capillary tube will hold 255 μl). pH alone may be determined with less than 50 μl of blood. The time required for analysis is only minutes if the blood gas analyzer is ready for use. A delay of more than 15-20 minutes from sample to analysis is unacceptable for clinical management.

The Corometrics pH analyzer utilizes a self-standardizing cassette and needs only 30 μl of blood in a capillary tube. Results are printed in 2-3 minutes and are immediately available if the equipment is located on the labor floor. No technician is needed.

NORMAL ACID-BASE RANGE

There is a considerable range of so-called normal blood gas values (Table 41-1). Modanlou and others have clearly shown that the fetal pH normally decreases as labor progresses. There is also a correlation between fetal acidosis and progressive severe FHR patterns. Apgar scores correlate in a general way with fetal pH values in late labor, although there is considerable overlap. Bowe and co-workers reported a false-normal pH 10.4% of the time and a false-abnormal pH in 7.5% of cases.

TABLE 41-1. NORMAL RANGE OF BLOOD GAS VALUES

pH	7.25-7.35
pCO_2 (mm Hg)	35-45
pO_2 (mm Hg)	18-28
Base excess	-5-0

TABLE 41-2. CONDITIONS THAT MAY RESULT IN A FALSE-NORMAL pH

Maternal hyperventilation
Drugs
Airway obstruction (newborn)
Prematurity
Infection
Congenital anomalies
Asphyxia between sampling and delivery

TABLE 41-3. CONDITIONS THAT MAY RESULT IN A FALSE-ABNORMAL pH

Timing of blood sampling in relation to uterine contractions
Stage of labor when sampling is done
Maternal acidosis
Anesthesia and/or analgesia
Small amount of bleeding from scalp, with slow collection
Delay in analyzing sample
Caput (this is controversial)

Table 41-2 lists conditions that may result in a false-normal pH, as revealed by low Apgar scores. Table 41-3 summarizes some causes of false-abnormal pH, as revealed by good Apgar scores.

There is evidence from several sources that fetal scalp blood is a reliable index of the fetal central circulation. Bowe et al reported a positive correlation between the pH of the scalp blood just prior to delivery and the pH of the umbilical artery and vein.

Adamsons et al compared the pH of blood taken simultaneously from the scalp of a rhesus monkey fetus and from the carotid artery and jugular vein. They reported that capillary blood remained representative even under conditions of extreme asphyxia. The capillary blood more closely resembled the jugular venous blood.

In practice, fetal scalp blood pH is used primarily to supplement FHR monitoring. FHR monitoring has the advantage of providing a record that immediately reflects changes in the fetal condition, and it can be performed almost universally. When there is a question about the FHR pattern, a pH determination may help clarify it. When the two tests agree—whether normal or abnormal—confidence in diagnosis is increased.

It is difficult to establish exact limits of pH that require intervention, but a decreasing pH that reaches the 7.20 range, or a pH less than 7.20 that persists despite changing the maternal position, turning off oxytocin, and giving oxygen by mask would mandate prompt intervention.

Currently there is considerable interest in clinical evaluation of continuous pH electrodes. The advantages of continuous pH determination during labor are obvious. To date, however, the results have been less than encouraging. The electrodes are functional and accurate. However, their application is technically cumbersome and their reliability has still to be proven.

SUGGESTED READING

Adamsons K, Beard RW, Cosmi EV, Myers RE: The validity of capillary blood in the assessment of the acid-base state of the fetus. In Adamsons K, ed: *Diagnosis and Treatment of Fetal Disorders*. New York: Springer-Verlag, 1968, p 175

Bowe ET, Beard RW, Rinster M, Poppers PJ, Adamsons K, James LS: Reliability of fetal blood sampling. *Am J Obstet Gynecol* 107:279, 1970

Kubli FW, Hon EH, Khazin AF, Takemura H: Observations on heart rate and pH in the human fetus during labor. *Am J Obstet Gynecol* 104:1190, 1969

Modanlou H, Yeh SY, Hon EH, Forsythe A: Fetal and neonatal biochemistry and Apgar score. *Am J Obstet Gynecol* 117:942, 1973

Tejani N, Mann L, Bhakthauathsalan A: Correlation of fetal heart rate patterns and fetal pH with neonatal outcome. *Obstet Gynecol* 48:460, 1976

Young DC, Gray JH, Luther ER, Paddle LJ: Fetal scalp blood pH sampling: Its value in an active unit. *Am J Obstet Gynecol* 136:276, 1980

42

Effects of Drugs on FHR

RICHARD H. PAUL, M.D.

The fetal heart rate forms the primary basis of objectively evaluating fetal well-being. The clinical use of FHR monitoring has emerged largely in the last 10 years, and monitoring is now done in the majority of births in the United States. Widespread experience has shown that many procedures and drugs affect the fetus, as revealed by changes in FHR. At best, the FHR is merely an indirect reflection of fetal status. However, careful observation of changes in FHR, coupled with our present understanding of the pathophysiology of FHR response, permits us to draw some conclusions regarding the effects of various drugs used in clinical care of the pregnant patient.

FHR responses to drugs may be evoked by multiple mechanisms. Three primary factors must be considered individually and collectively with drug administration: direct effects on the fetus, effects on response to uterine activity, and effects on the maternal cardiovascular system. Each of these factors can significantly affect the FHR response; at times, a combined effect involving all factors is seen. In general, most drugs cross the placenta—a notable exception is heparin. Succinylcholine crosses the placenta, but only slowly.

ANTEPARTUM PERIOD

Except for propranolol (Inderal) and phenobarbital, we know little about the FHR effects of most drugs used during the antepartum period. Propranolol, a sympathetic blocking agent, may cause fetal bradycardia, which, if unrecognized as drug-induced, may lead to unnecessary intervention. Phenobarbital as used in the treatment of "mild hypertension" or preeclampsia has been shown roughly to double the incidence of abnormal patterns during antepartum FHR testing.

There is little doubt that many other drugs affect FHR characteristics. Our identification and understanding of these agents are grossly deficient at this time. Furthermore, even though an unusual or suspect observation is made, interpretation of its clinical significance is difficult.

INTRAPARTUM PERIOD

One should assume that drugs commonly administered to the mother, except as noted above, will rapidly cross the placenta to the fetus. Agents such as antibiotics, vitamins, and anesthetic gases clearly enter the fetal compartment, but scanty information exists regarding their effects on FHR.

Compared with the antepartum period, intrapartum observations regarding effects of various drugs on FHR form a larger area of understanding, including the following major categories:

- Narcotic analgesics
- Local anesthetic agents
- Labor-inhibiting agents
- Anticonvulsant sedatives
- Oxytocics
- Agents affecting the autonomic system.

It must be re-emphasized that many of these agents may evoke their effects through various mechanisms. For instance, a local anesthetic agent may directly affect the fetus, the uterus, and the maternal vascular system.

The principal observed effect of narcotic analgesics is their propensity to decrease FHR variability. This is thought to reflect a depressant effect on the fetal central nervous system after rapid transplacental passage. Quantitative data regarding such effects are minimal but worthy of investigation. The clinical significance of such observations is also unknown, but conscious recognition of this effect is important since FHR variability is significant in FHR interpretation. More subtle FHR effects that may emerge as narcotic agents are evaluated relate to their apparent effects on uterine activity. Narcotic-induced increases in uterine activity may be due to direct myometrial stimulation or indirectly related to pain relief and changes in maternal catecholamine release. Narcotic-provoked respiratory arrest and maternal hypoxia will be dramatically reflected in the FHR. This complication can be largely avoided by careful patient observation and appropriate drug dosage.

Local anesthetic agents can produce FHR changes by two principal mechanisms: First, their oxytocic capability can interfere with uteroplacental exchange or cause umbilical cord compression. More commonly, FHR changes are due to alterations in the maternal cardiovascular system. The primary problem involved with techniques such as saddle block or epidural anesthesia is their blocking effect on sympathetic tone, and the secondary hypotension. The fetus often responds to such insults with typical late deceleration patterns. Less commonly, as with paracervical block, the agent's local vasoconstrictive effect on the uterine arteries reduces uterine blood flow and produces fetal stress, as reflected in FHR changes.

Studies on labor-inhibiting agents have mostly involved attempts to inhibit premature labor. FHR measurements during these studies have usually been limited to external modes, which impose severe limitations on FHR evaluation. Thus, little information exists regarding the effects of the most widely used of these drugs: ritodrine (Yutopar), ethanol, and isoxsuprine (Vasodilan). Intrapartum experience with administration of the β-sympathomimetics is limited, although it is known that when these drugs are given over a period of hours, the FHR tends to rise and variability diminishes. The chronic oral administration of such drugs is probably associated with similar FHR changes, but some of these effects may be counterbalanced by the usual tendency of the FHR to fall as the fetus matures.

Anticonvulsant sedative agents are often used intrapartum to treat pregnancy-induced hypertension. Chronic administration of magnesium sulfate, the drug most commonly used, is often associated with diminished FHR variability over 12-24 hours, in contrast to the increased variability seen within minutes of IV administration. Other anticonvulsant sedative agents, such as diazepam (Valium), barbiturates, and hydroxyzine (Vistaril), all appear to diminish FHR variability.

The ability of oxytocin to induce uterine tetany and dramatic FHR decelerations or bradycardia needs little explanation. The resultant cessation of intervillous blood flow and fetal hypoxemia cause profound FHR changes. Carefully controlled oxytocin administration produces little apparent FHR effect as a result of direct transfer of the agent. As mentioned, local anesthetics may exert oxytocic effects. Dimenhydrinate (Dramamine) and narcotics may also be associated with excessive uterine activity.

Drugs that affect the autonomic nervous system pass to the fetus and evoke FHR responses. Propranolol may cause fetal bradycardia, whereas atropine or scopolamine will modify or eliminate most vagally mediated deceleration responses. Atropine may also produce fetal tachycardia and loss of FHR variability when used in therapeutic dosages. Use of these vagolytic agents to alter abnormal FHR patterns is contraindicated.

Numerous additional agents no doubt have effects that could be reflected in the FHR. Their basic mechanisms must be individually considered. For example, an antihypertensive agent such as hydralazine (Apresoline) would probably cause FHR changes by reducing maternal blood pressure. The physiologic effect of antepartum and intrapartum administration of drugs—and no less their associated FHR changes—must be a critical area of extensive future research.

SUGGESTED READING

Keegan KA, Paul RH, Broussard PM, McCart D, Smith MA: Antepartum fetal heart rate testing. III. The effect of phenobarbital on the nonstress test. *Am J Obstet Gynecol* 133:579, 1979

Miller FC, Quesnel G, Petrie RH, Paul RH, Hon EH: The effects of paracervical block on uterine activity and beat-to-beat variability of fetal heart rate. *Am J Obstet Gynecol* 130:284, 1978

Nochimson DJ, Riffel HD, Yeh SY, Kreitzer MS, Paul RH, Hon EH: The effects of ritodrine hydrochloride on uterine activity and the cardiovascular system. *Am J Obstet Gynecol* 118:523, 1974

Petrie RH, Yeh SY, Murata Y, Paul RH, Hon EH, Barron BA, Johnson RJ: The effect of drugs on fetal heart rate variability. *Am J Obstet Gynecol* 130:294, 1978

Wong R, Paul RH: Methergine induced uterine tetany treated with epinephrine: A case report. *Am J Obstet Gynecol* 134:602, 1979

Yeh SY, Paul RH, Cordero L, Hon EH: A study of diazepam during labor. *Obstet Gynecol* 43:363, 1974

43

Diagnosis and Treatment of Fetal Distress

BARRY S. SCHIFRIN, M.D.

The term "fetal distress" is universally used to connote fetal hypoxia. It must be emphasized, however, that no technique now available reliably predicts hypoxia except in the terminally ill fetus. The value of newer techniques of electronic fetal monitoring and fetal blood sampling lies in the accuracy with which they predict that fetuses will not be asphyxiated.

FHR RESPONSES TO HYPOXIA

Hypoxia is but one of several factors with a potential for fetal/neonatal compromise. Drugs, infection, trauma, and congenital anomalies may contribute to low Apgar scores, disordered neonatal adaptation, or subsequent disability or death without materially influencing FHR patterns or blood pH. In general, low Apgar scores due to these causes cannot be reliably predicted.

The FHR responses to hypoxia are varied. They depend not only on the rapidity of onset and the intensity of the asphyxial episode, but also on the frequency and intensity of uterine contractions. In the absence of significant uterine activity, the fetus will respond to slowly developing asphyxia with tachycardia—a response presumably mediated through discharge of sympathomimetic amines from the adrenal medulla. Under these conditions of minimal stress, tachycardia represents an early compensatory response to asphyxia. As the insult is prolonged, variability decreases. When compensation is no longer possible, the heart rate becomes unstable and slows, and death ensues. During labor, the earliest signs of distress are late or variable decelerations, which are followed by the changes in baseline rate and variability to be described. If the asphyxial insult is acute and/or profound, the fetus will respond with bradycardia irrespective of the presence or absence of contractions.

DIAGNOSIS AND TREATMENT OF FETAL DISTRESS
USING FHR PATTERNS

The clinical signs of fetal evaluation during labor are usually divided into four categories: reassuring, suspicious, threatening, and ominous. Each category consists of an evaluation of both baseline and periodic changes.

Reassuring Patterns

Baseline features of reassuring patterns include average variability and stable FHR. Periodic features include absent decelerations, early decelerations, mild variable decelerations, and uniform accelerations.

Early decelerations are not caused by hypoxia and do not appear to be associated with poor outcome. Mild variable decelerations (often indistinguishable from early decelerations) appear totally innocuous, especially if associated with mild variable accelerations ("shoulders") before and after. Uniform accelerations invariably signify a healthy, reactive fetus. But most important, the presence of normal variability strongly suggests that there is no fetal indication for intervention.

Suspicious Patterns

Baseline features of suspicious patterns include tachycardia (>160 bpm), bradycardia (<120 bpm), and decreased variability. In the suspicious group, periodic decelerations are absent.

Each of the baseline changes in the suspicious category may be associated with fetal hypoxia. But when such changes are not accompanied by decelerations, the mechanism is usually other than hypoxia. Clinically, maternal fever secondary to amnionitis is the most common discoverable etiology of fetal tachycardia. The fetal and maternal heart rates rise in direct proportion to the fever. Frequently a normal rate can be restored by prompt treatment of the underlying cause or by cooling the mother when the fever is excessive. Drugs, especially atropine and β-sympathomimetics, may increase fetal heart rate. Fetal tachyarrhythmias may also be responsible for heart rates in excess of 160 bpm.

Baseline bradycardia, as opposed to a prolonged deceleration, is a late sign of fetal asphyxia. While moribund fetuses will invariably have bradycardia along with absent variability, the majority with persistent heart rates below 120 bpm are not asphyxiated. Many fetuses with heart rates in the range of 90-120 bpm exhibit no objective compromise. They usually display average baseline variability. Baseline bradycardia in the range of 50-80 bpm may signal complete heart block, which can be diagnosed easily by fetal ECG analysis. Severely asphyxiated fetuses with bradycardia usually have sinus rhythm.

Decreased variability may signify loss of fine autonomic control of the heart rate from many causes. Decreased variability during labor may be seen with adequate oxygenation in premature fetuses, or when drugs are given to the mother during labor. All barbiturates, tranquilizers, and anesthetics, local or general, have the capacity for reducing variability. It is for these reasons that we recommend that monitoring be started before the mother is given any medication with the potential for altering FHR patterns. It must be emphasized that decreased variability in the absence of decelerations during labor is almost invariably related to an etiology other than asphyxia—usually medication. If an asphyxial insult is superimposed on a fetus whose heart rate variability is diminished by medications, decelerations will appear.

Suspicious patterns usually require no therapy. A search for the underlying cause should be made. If hypoxia cannot reasonably be excluded, a fetal blood sample should be obtained. With a suspicious pattern, potentially compromising drugs or anesthetic techniques should be avoided until it is certain that an explanation other than hypoxia exists for this pattern.

Threatening Patterns

Baseline features of threatening patterns include stable rate and average variability. Periodic features include periodic late decelerations as well as variable decelerations.

Threatening patterns represent unequivocal fetal insult related to impaired uterine blood flow (late decelerations) or impaired umbilical blood flow (variable decelerations). Although other mechanisms have been proposed for these decelerations, their relationship to compromised blood flow is well established by clinical observation. Late decelerations associated with good variability are usually found during episodes of compromise in a fetus with a previously normal pattern. This combination is found when the mother develops supine hypotension with or without conduction anesthesia, and excessive uterine activity secondary to oxytocin. More important, these episodes are usually correctable with conservative measures.

The management of late decelerations includes (1) turning the patient on her side to eliminate supine hypotension and improve uterine blood flow, (2) administering oxygen by mask (5 l/minute), (3) correction of hypotension, if present, and (4) stopping oxytocin infusion. The patient should be examined vaginally. If delivery is not imminent, a fetal scalp blood sample should be analyzed for pH. If this is not possible and late decelerations persist despite conservative therapy, delivery by cesarean section is indicated. Repetitive late decelerations with a normal fetal scalp blood pH (>7.25) may be observed provided the fetal blood is sampled every 30-60 minutes, the pH remains normal, and a falling trend in pH is absent. A scalp pH of less than 7.20 is an indication for immediate delivery.

In the majority of instances, no obvious explanation for variable decelerations will be found. However, as the frequency of decelerations increases and the ability to correct the pattern diminishes, the likelihood of some obvious cord problem increases. Factors that increase the likelihood of variable decelerations include ruptured membranes, oligohydramnios, vasa previa, nuchal cord, and short or prolapsed cord. As with late decelerations, we give little attention to the amplitude or, within reason, the duration of the deceleration, but rather judge the impact of the deceleration on the basis of the changes in baseline variability and rate associated with it. If baseline variability and rate remain stable, conservative maneuvers are implemented and cesarean section is not performed.

Threatening patterns warrant measures directed at correcting the underlying disturbance in fetal or placental blood flow. In the majority of instances these patterns are correctable by eliminating oxytocin, turning the mother on her side, and administering oxygen by mask. Recovery can usually be anticipated. It is axiomatic that prevention is more important than therapy. Elimination of the supine position and judicious use of oxytocin infusion are appropriate safeguards in all patients. Bicarbonate and glucose infusions are not of demonstrable value.

The response of variable decelerations to corrective measures is less predictable than the response of late decelerations. Often these patterns can be corrected or their severity reduced by maneuvers designed to alter the relationship among fetus, cord, and uterine wall. Thus, altering the mother's position—lateral, supine, or Trendelenburg—will frequently improve the pattern. If such maneuvers provide no relief, placing the patient in the knee-chest position will occasionally correct the pattern. If that fails, and if rising heart rate and loss of variability have been superimposed on the variable decelerations and intervention is considered, gentle elevation of the vertex may ameliorate the pattern. Elevation of the vertex, however, should be undertaken only in the delivery room lest it cause prolapse of the cord.

While variable decelerations are more common in the second stage of labor, their interpretation and therapy are the same in both the first and second stages. Except when the head is crowning and delivery is imminent, therapy should be governed by the conservative principles elaborated above—that is, by attempts at intrauterine resuscitation.

Ominous Patterns
Baseline features of ominous patterns include absent baseline variability, unstable rate, and bradycardia or tachycardia. Periodic features include late decelerations, variable decelerations, and rebound accelerations.

Ominous patterns combine periodic features of the threatening category with the baseline patterns of the suspicious category. These patterns strongly suggest severe fetal compromise. The mechanisms behind these individual changes have already been discussed. Rebound accelerations ("overshoot") are uniform accelerations following variable decelerations of any amplitude. Absent baseline variability is a constant feature of this pattern, but baseline tachycardia need not be present. More than any other pattern, the combination of decreased variability and variable decelerations with overshoot strongly suggests autonomic imbalance. It may be seen following atropine administration or in premature fetuses as well as in those who are severely asphyxiated.

An unstable rate with absent short-term variability that is occasionally sinusoidal is an added clue that fetal compensatory mechanisms have been exhausted. Such patterns have been reported in dying fetuses and in those severely affected with Rh-isoimmunization. Cardiac denervation in the experimental animal produces a similar combination of unstable heart rate and absent short-term variability.

Before fetal death, only the ominous baseline changes may be present; late or variable decelerations may be absent. Bradycardia is common at this time, but the rate may occasionally be in the normal range. Heart rate changes in the terminally ill fetus are rarely dramatic. Cardiac arrest may occur, but unlike the abrupt, unpredictable episodes of asystole and nodal rhythm seen at the nadir of variable decelerations, these are predictable, associated with sinus rhythm, and invariably fatal.

While the same conservative measures advocated for threatening patterns should be applied to the patient with ominous patterns, preparations should be made for expeditious delivery, as recovery is unlikely.

INDICATION FOR INTERVENTION

While many fetal monitoring records would demonstrate unequivocal fetal distress, intervention by operative delivery is only rarely necessary. The indication for intervention on behalf of the fetus is nonremediable fetal distress. This philosophy represents an attempt to use the monitoring pattern to determine whether or not the maternal-placental unit is capable of sustaining the fetus. With intact placental function and fetal blood flow, operative delivery does not appear warranted. The intact placenta is a faster, safer, and more efficient apparatus for resuscitating the fetus than any man-made device.

If patterns of distress are not remediable, intervention should be undertaken as quickly as is consistent with maternal and fetal safety. Under this concept, no arbitrary time between onset of distress and optimal delivery is definable, nor can we safely state how much hypoxia is tolerable without compromise. Rather, it seems appropriate to aspire to the minimum amount of exposure to hypoxia. To this end, avoidance of the supine position during labor and restricting potentially compromising techniques to demonstrably normal fetuses become reasonable objectives.

44

Abnormal FHR Patterns:
A Management Approach

RICHARD H. PAUL, M.D.

Fetal heart rate (FHR) monitoring forms the primary basis of assessing fetal well-being during labor. Likewise, antepartum FHR testing is proving useful in the identification and therapy of the distressed, or jeopardized, fetus during the last months of pregnancy. With the widespread availability of continuous FHR-monitoring equipment, clinicians are faced with the challenge of interpreting data and acting in the best interests of the mother and fetus.

Basing patient management on a single observation or "test" is unusual in medicine. In this case, one biological variable—FHR—is used in an attempt to deduce total condition.

Before the advent of FHR monitoring, fetal viability was assessed by auscultating fetal heart tones (FHT). The efficacy of this approach has never been scientifically documented. In fact, the ability to define fetal status on the basis of FHT has significant limitations: They are heard intermittently, they must be averaged, and counting errors can occur. The widespread clinical adoption of continuous FHR recording in the 1970s has eliminated these disadvantages. Continued clinical experience will further elucidate the value of FHR monitoring. Essential to proper interpretation of FHR data is detailed knowledge of the instrumentation used and a full understanding of its limitations.

The fundamental observations of FHR were derived in the 1960s, using direct techniques. These investigations laid the foundations for determining normal and abnormal FHR. A normal FHR falls in the range of 120-160 beats per minute (bpm), demonstrates variability, and shows no appreciable deviations from a constant level (e.g., 140 bpm) during uterine contractions. An abnormal FHR might fall outside the 120-160-bpm range, lack variability, and change significantly in response to uterine contractions. Contractions impede uterine blood flow and thus periodically stress the fetus, often causing changes in both FHT and FHR.

BASIC FHR PATTERNS

The early focus of FHR monitoring was on falls in rate, since these had been clinically associated with compromised outcome. Observations led to the recognition of three basic deceleration patterns whose time of onset was related to the onset of uterine contraction (UC): early decelerations, late decelerations, and variable decelerations. Early and late decelerations exhibit a constant waveform, while the waveform of variable decelerations is inconsistent.

Numerous investigators slowly elucidated the pathophysiology of these observations and their potential clinical significance. Early decelerations result from pressure applied to the vertex, or head compression; late decelerations are caused by decreased uteroplacental oxygen exchange; and variable patterns are due to compression of the umbilical cord. The operational terms that evolved were thus head compression (HC), uteroplacental insufficiency (UPI), and cord compression (CC). Both UPI and CC are capable of provoking hypoxia, brain damage, and death, depending on the duration and severity of their occurrence.

The major reason for identification of the various FHR patterns is to take corrective steps to remove the threat to the fetus. For example, the basic problem of CC is easy to understand and therapy is aimed at relieving the mechanical factors that provoke it. Therapy of CC consists simply of the following steps:

1. Rule out a prolapsed cord
2. Alter the maternal position in an attempt to relieve the mechanical pressure on the cord.

The factors causing UPI are more complex, but may be broadly classed as excessive uterine activity, decreased intervillous blood flow secondary to low perfusion pressure, and separation of exchange surfaces, as in placental abruption. Abruption cannot be remedied, but correction of hypotension and decreasing oxytocin-induced excessive activity are possible.

MAJOR PROBLEMS OF MANAGEMENT

The major problems of management occur when FHR patterns are difficult to interpret or when recognizable pathologic patterns are uncorrectable. Simplistic therapy has faded with continuing clinical observations. Additional FHR characteristics, such as variability and acceleration, are now commonly evaluated in an attempt to judge the significance of so-called ominous deceleration patterns. FHR variability has been uniformly associated with improved outcome. Likewise, the occurrence of accelerations, particularly during antepartum FHR testing, has a positive prognostic meaning. Both variability and acceleration apparently reflect intact CNS responses, thus indicating fetal well-being at the time of observation.

The clinical approach to managing abnormal FHR patterns rests on what one defines as abnormal. Corrective steps to normalize the FHR may be undertaken empirically; when they are successful, no further therapy is necessary. The problem arises when a suspect FHR pattern persists and the danger to the fetus must be quantitatively assessed. The fact that uterine contractions are a fetal stress is readily accepted. The clinical dilemma is clearly the differentiation of stress from distress. A human experimental approach to this question is clearly impossible, so one must accept end points other than death and permanent damage in defining a management approach.

Once an abnormal FHR pattern type has been identified and persists despite attempts at correction, questions of pathologic significance arise and must be individually evaluated. Clearly an abnormal pattern in early labor would call for a different response than in the closing minutes of labor. The quantitative significance of FHR abnormalities may be derived from two observations: baseline FHR characteristics and fetal acid-base determinations. With persistent stress, the FHR usually rises gradually to more than 160 bpm and variability diminishes. These findings are commonly seen after an identifiable acute stress, such as a tetanic contraction due to overstimulation with oxytocin. These same FHR findings may emerge more slowly when the stress factors are intermittent, such as repetitive uterine contractions. Although tachycardia may reflect a stress response secondary to fetal asphyxia, it often may also merely reflect maternal pyrexia. Likewise, decreased variability may be due to maternal analgesia, fetal sleep states, immaturity, or congenital anomalies. Thus the limitations of a quantitative interpretation of FHR are apparent and an additional parameter is needed in order to devise proper management.

OTHER TESTS

The Apgar score is beneficial in retrospectively judging the significance of FHR patterns, but is of no prospective use. However, measurements of fetal scalp blood gases and pH during labor have greatly increased understanding of the pathophysiology of FHR patterns. The major deficiencies of fetal scalp blood sampling are its intermittency and circumstances that preclude its use.

Fetal scalp blood analysis is useful if one accepts that stress in the absence of acidosis is tolerable. Labor in the presence of abnormal FHR patterns that are not associated with acidosis can be managed expectantly, depending on the mother's clinical status and availability of repeat pH sampling. The practicality of such an approach must be assessed case by case.

MANAGEMENT OF ACUTE PROBLEMS

On occasion an acutely abnormal FHR pattern, such as a profound fall to 60 bpm, cannot be associated with an identifiable, remediable cause. When empirical measures fail, such as ruling out prolapse of the cord and altering the maternal position, and the pattern persists for 60-90 seconds, one must assume that fetal asphyxia is occurring. Movement to an operative facility is indicated and monitoring should be reinstituted. If the fetal bradycardia is not corrected, delivery is best accomplished expeditiously. The general aim should be to deliver such a fetus within 10 minutes, since times beyond this have been associated with brain damage in experimental animals.

Expedited delivery often results in an infant who obviously was not subjected to total asphyxia as judged from cord acid-base values and Apgar scores. In retrospect, the fall in FHR was probably mediated through reflex mechanisms rather than provoked by hypoxic myocardial depression. One must acknowledge the protective adaptability of the fetus as reflected in the FHR and realize the limitations of quantitative FHR interpretation.

CONCLUSION

A normal FHR is uniformly associated with a nonacidotic fetus and an infant born in good condition. The definition of abnormal is limited by what we are willing to accept as end points that would justify such a diagnosis. Clearly, many currently diagnosed "abnormal" patterns fall within the tolerance of a given fetus to stress factors. The main goals of therapy are to restore blood flow through the umbilical cord or to the intervillous space. Obviously, both CC and UPI can coexist, and the resultant FHR pattern cannot be clearly defined.

Whenever FHR patterns are difficult to interpret or confusing, the additional information provided by fetal acid-base evaluation is most useful. In the final analysis, one is faced with the dilemma of attempting to define the degree of abnormality while avoiding the very clear end point of brain damage or death that would confirm the diagnosis. Techniques such as continuous fetal pH evaluation are currently being tested and will no doubt soon assist us in our attempts to define and manage abnormal FHR patterns.

SUGGESTED READING

Greiss FC Jr: Concepts of uterine blood flow. In Wynn RM, ed: *Obstetrics and Gynecology Annual*. New York: Appleton-Century-Crofts, 1973, pp 55-83

Hon EH: Electronic evaluation of the fetal heart rate. VI. Fetal distress—A working hypothesis. *Am J Obstet Gynecol* 83:333, 1962

Hon EH: *An Atlas of Fetal Heart Rate Patterns*. New Haven, Ct: Harty Press, 1968

Lauersen NH, Miller FC, Paul RH: Continuous intrapartum monitoring of fetal scalp pH. *Am J Obstet Gynecol* 133:44, 1979

Martin CB: Regulation of the fetal heart rate and genesis of FHR patterns. *Sem Perinatol* 2:131, 1978

Parer JT, Krueger TR, Harris JL: Fetal oxygen consumption and mechanisms of heart rate response during artificially produced late decelerations of the fetal heart rate in sheep. *Am J Obstet Gynecol* 136:478, 1980

Paul RH: Fetal distress. In Quilligan EJ, Kretchmer N, eds: *Perinatal Medicine*. New York: Wiley, 1980, pp 317-332

Paul RH, Khazin Suidan A, Yeh SY, Schifrin BS, Hon EH: Clinical fetal monitoring. VII. The evaluation and significance of intrapartum baseline FHR variability. *Am J Obstet Gynecol* 123:206, 1975

Zanini B, Paul RH, Huey JR: Intrapartum fetal heart rate: The correlation with scalp pH in the pre-term fetus. *Am J Obstet Gynecol* 136:43, 1980

THREE

GYNECOLOGY

45

Prepubertal Vulvovaginitis

PAUL F. BRENNER, M.D.

ETIOLOGY

The most common gynecologic complaint of premenarchal patients is vaginal discharge. The risk of vaginal infections in young girls is increased by an exposed introitus, a thin vaginal mucosa, and poor perineal hygiene. Failure of the labia minora to develop prior to puberty leaves the vaginal introitus relatively unprotected. The unestrogenized vaginal mucosa is very thin and easily susceptible to infection should bacteria gain access to the vagina. Most significant is failure to instruct and observe girls in proper perineal hygiene. Girls who wipe the perineum from the rectum toward the vagina after defecation carry bacteria toward the exposed introitus and thin vaginal mucosa.

A vaginal discharge in a premenarchal patient may be physiologic. The vaginal mucosa and cervix are quite sensitive to estrogen. Small elevations of estrogen in the peripheral circulation increase the amount of cervical mucus present and the number of cells desquamated from the vaginal mucosa. These changes produce a clear mucous discharge. Some estrogen of maternal origin remains in the infantile circulation for the first 2 or 3 weeks of life, and an increase in endogenous estrogen in the early months of puberty just before menarche produces a physiologic leukorrhea.

A pathologic vaginal discharge in premenarchal patients may be specific in origin or due to mixed infection with enteric organisms. There are several specific causes of vulvovaginitis in children. A streptococcal or staphylococcal infection may be associated with a recent infection involving these bacteria elsewhere in the body, most commonly the upper respiratory tract. *Candida* vaginitis is an uncommon cause of leukorrhea in a young girl, but whenever it is present, the child should be tested for diabetes mellitus. The thin, unestrogenized vaginal mucosa of a prepubertal patient does not contain glycogen and will not sustain the *Candida albicans* microbe. Trichomonas vaginitis is also an uncommon cause of leukorrhea in a prepubertal child.

Gonococcal vaginitis occurs in prepubertal girls of all ages. Whether this infection is most commonly the result of contact with inanimate objects, such as bed linen, or is due to sexual contact is not resolved. When a young girl has a culture positive for gonorrhea, the immediate members of the family should be screened to detect the individual harboring the gonococcus.

Complaints by the patient of perianal irritation and pruritus, and/or a history of parasites in other family members, suggests that pinworms (*Enterobius vermicularis*) are the cause of the vulvovaginitis. The "Scotch Tape test" is used to identify the pinworm eggs.

Congenital anomalies in which a communication exists between the vagina and the rectum or bladder can be the cause of a vaginal discharge that has been present since birth. A foreign body in the vagina can also produce vulvovaginitis. The vaginal discharge associated with a foreign body is characteristically purulent and bloody. A foreign body may be a solid object, like a button or small part of a toy, but most commonly it is tissue paper. A bloody, purulent vaginal discharge may rarely be the result of a tumor.

The pertinent points in the history include the character of the discharge, the length of time the discharge has been present, the presence of blood, the method of perineal hygiene, recent infections that might be streptococcal or staphylococcal in origin, recent venereal disease or parasites among immediate members of the family, perianal pruritus, and a foreign body in the vagina.

EXAMINATION

The external genitalia and perineum are inspected with the child in the supine position, her knees apart and the soles of her feet approximated. The inspection and subsequent vaginoscopy cannot be rushed. Attempts to hasten the procedure only result in an inadequate examination and a frightened patient. The success of the examination depends on the physician's willingness to take the time necessary to gain the confidence of the young patient, the patient's cooperation, and previous attempts at inspection and examination. Attempts to examine the patient in the knee-chest position are less successful, as she cannot see or assist in the examination. The more the patient is involved in assisting with the examination, the more likely it is to be successful.

The patient is instructed to use each index finger to separate the labia. This gives the physician the opportunity to inspect the external genitalia and perineum and allows the patient to retain control of the exam. If discharge is present at the introitus, wet mounts, one using saline and another using potassium hydroxide, are prepared and examined for *Trichomonas* and *Candida*. The discharge is cultured for *Neisseria gonorrhoeae* on chocolate agar and placed on Stuart's medium and on a slide for a Gram stain. If the history and/or inspection of the perineum are consistent with pinworms, a "Scotch Tape test" is performed. With a cooperative child, discharge can be collected from the vagina with a plastic eyedropper, which is less irritating to the patient than a cotton swab. A glass instrument should not be placed in a young girl's vagina, as it may break if the child moves.

An attempt should be made to examine the vagina of every child with prepubertal vulvovaginitis with the child awake. A variety of instruments are available for vaginoscopy of young patients, including specially designed vaginoscopes, the Killian nasal speculum, veterinary otoscopes, and urethroscopes. An air urethroscope is an excellent instrument for examination of the prepubertal vagina. An otoscope with veterinarian attachments is both practical and inexpensive. Again, it is important for the patient to assist in the vaginoscopy. She should be given the opportunity to become familiar with the instruments and should be permitted to guide the examiner's hand as the vaginoscope is inserted into her vagina.

Anytime the discharge is mixed with blood or the patient or her parents indicate that a foreign body has been placed in the vagina, adequate inspection of the vagina must be carried out. In such cases, if vaginoscopy cannot be completed successfully with the patient awake, she should be anesthetized. If the discharge does not contain blood, there is no history of a foreign body, and vaginoscopy is unsuccessful with the patient awake, vaginoscopy under anesthesia need not be performed; a gentle rectal exam should be substituted.

TREATMENT

Specific treatment is available for pinworms (mebendazole, or Vermox; one 100-mg chewable tablet), *Candida* vaginitis (nystatin oral suspension, or Mycostatin or Nilstat; 100,000 units/ml, 1-2 million units/day in 4 divided doses), *Trichomonas* vaginitis (metronidazole, or Flagyl; 15 mg/day in 3 divided doses for 7 days), and streptococcal, staphylococcal, or gonococcal vaginitis (ampicillin 50 mg/day in 3 or 4 divided doses for 10 days). Foreign bodies require removal from the vagina.

The treatment of children with mixed bacterial vaginal infection includes instructions on proper perineal hygiene, systemic antibiotics, and topical corticosteroid therapy. The importance of wiping the perineum from front to back, away from the vagina, following defecation must be stressed. Cotton underpants, which absorb discharge, are preferred to those made of synthetic fibers such as nylon, which hold discharge against vulvar tissue. Vulvar irritation may also be reduced by changing underpants frequently during the day and by using white underpants and toilet paper (free of colored dyes), and loosely fitting clothing. Skirts are better than tight slacks.

Sitz baths 2-4 times a day in warm water bring temporary relief of vulvar symptoms, but soap should be avoided. If vulvitis is present, hydrocortisone cream 1% or Mycolog cream should be applied after each sitz bath.

Systemic antibiotics are used to treat mixed bacterial vulvovaginitis. Oral liquid preparations are selected and administered in divided doses, the total dose corresponding to the patient's weight. This three-fold regimen of improved perineal hygiene, topical corticosteroids, and systemic antibiotics resolves 95% of all mixed bacterial vaginal infections in premenarchal patients.

In addition to the presence of blood in the discharge and history of a foreign body in the vagina, persistent leukorrhea that fails to respond to therapy is an indication for vaginoscopy even if it requires anesthesia. Even if the vaginitis fails to respond completely, the vulvitis is generally markedly improved, enhancing the possibility of vaginoscopy without anesthesia. If a specific etiology is not found by vaginoscopy, persistent vulvovaginitis is treated with estrogen cream (Premarin) 0.5 gm applied locally for 10 consecutive nights.

SUGGESTED READING

Altchek A: Pediatric vulvovaginitis. *Pediatr Clin North Am* 19:559, 1972

Capraro VJ: Vulvovaginitis and other local lesions of the vulva. *Clin Obstet Gynecol* 1:533, 1974

Capraro VJ, Capraro EJ: Vaginal aspirate studies in children. *Obstet Gynecol* 37:462, 1971

Capraro VJ, Gallego MB: Vulvovaginitis in children. *Pediatr Ann* 3:74, 1974

Davis TC: Chronic vulvovaginitis in children due to Shigella flexneri. *Pediatrics* 56:41, 1975

Felman YM, William DC, Corsaro MC: Gonococcal infections in children 14 years or younger. *Clin Pediatr* 17:252, 1978

46

Vulvovaginitis

SUBIR ROY, M.D.

ETIOLOGY

Vulvovaginitis, the most common problem in gynecologic office practice, has many causes and is often transmitted by sexual contact. The cardinal symptom of vaginitis is an abnormal vaginal discharge. If the vulva is involved, the patient may also complain of pruritus, burning pain, dysuria, and dyspareunia. The cause of the symptoms is usually one or more microorganisms. A vaginal discharge can also be physiologic when due to mucus secretion from the endocervix at midcycle or to desquamation of epithelial cells premenstrually. Sometimes chemical irritation, an allergen, or a foreign body will produce an inflammatory reaction. Other factors that contribute to vulvovaginitis are poorly cornified vaginal epithelium, as seen in prepubertal girls and postmenopausal women, fecal contamination from the anus, sexual intercourse, chronic cervicitis, pregnancy, excessive local heat and moisture, broad-spectrum antibiotic therapy sufficient to destroy the normal bacterial flora, and coexisting systemic disease, particularly diabetes.

The vagina is normally acidic (pH 3.5-4.5) because of the lactic acid produced by Döderlein's bacillus (*Lactobacillus acidophilus*). Cervical mucus, menstrual blood, overgrowth of other organisms of the vaginal flora, and progesterone all raise the vaginal pH and favor the growth of trichomonads and *Gardnerella vaginalis* (previously known as *Corynebacterium vaginale* or *Haemophilus vaginalis*).

The history should include accounts of any previous vaginal infections and their treatment, as well as hygienic, contraceptive, and sexual practices. Microscopic examination of a wet smear will help to differentiate among infections due to fungi, trichomonads, and bacteria.

TRICHOMONAS

Trichomoniasis of the urogenital tract is caused by the flagellated protozoan *Trichomonas vaginalis*, a sexually transmitted microorganism found in adults of either sex. A moderate rise in vaginal pH favors its growth. Another factor encouraging trichomonal infection is local erosion resulting from chemical or mechanical trauma, neoplasms, or other forms of vaginal infection. Presumably there is no significant host immunity to *Trichomonas*.

Clinical Picture

Asymptomatic carrier. Approximately 15% of women in the reproductive years of life harbor *T. vaginalis*, but only one-third of these women have symptoms and signs of local inflammation, probably because the organism is more virulent. Asymptomatic carriers are identified by wet mount preparations at the time of routine gynecologic examination. These women should be treated to prevent transmission of the disease and to minimize the possibility that an acute infection will eventually be established.

Active infection. Trichomoniasis usually produces a malodorous discharge that may be frothy, profuse, thick or thin, and green, yellow, gray, or white. If the vulva is involved, there may be local pain, itching, dyspareunia, dysuria, or urinary frequency. Erythema and edema of the vulva and vagina and punctate subepithelial hemorrhages or strawberry marks on the vagina and cervix are sometimes observed.

Diagnosis

In 80% or more of cases, a wet smear prepared with warm saline and examined immediately will contain motile trichomonads. They are easily identified by their size, shape, and flagellate motion. Other cases may be identified by cytologic smear, although there is a considerable incidence of both false-positive and false-negative reports. Staining methods add little to diagnosis, and cultures are seldom needed.

Systemic Treatment

The drug of choice is metronidazole (Flagyl), and an adequate dose for most patients is 500 mg every 12 hours for 5 days (a smaller amount than recommended by the manufacturer) or 250 mg tid for 7 days. Since the teratogenic potential of metronidazole is unknown, it seems prudent to withhold this drug during pregnancy. The short-term cure rate with this regimen approaches 98% and the complication rate is 10%, consisting chiefly of gastrointestinal complaints. Long-term cure rates depend on whether trichomoniasis is also eradicated from patients' sexual partners.

Topical Treatment

A number of topical preparations are available, including suppositories, creams, and douches. They are not particularly effective, but may be useful in controlling symptoms in patients with multiple sexual partners when the partners cannot be treated.

Therapy for Sexual Partners

Ideally, male sexual partners should be examined and treated *if indicated*. The diagnosis of trichomonads in the male is made on a wet mount of a urethral discharge obtained spontaneously or after prostatic massage. As a compromise, a couple can be treated concurrently. The male should use a condom during therapy to reduce the risk of reinfection. An alternative for the male partner is to abstain from intercourse for a month (or use a condom) in hopes that the infection will clear spontaneously.

Resistant Disease

Continuing or recurring symptoms may be due to a coexisting pathogen such as *Candida*, to recurrent infection from an untreated sexual partner, to drug resistance or poor drug absorption, or to local inactivation of the drug by vaginal bacteria. In the last case, oral metronidazole should be repeated at a dose of 500 mg tid for 10 days.

CANDIDA

Vulvovaginitis due to *Candida* is usually caused by the species *C. albicans*, a dimorphic fungus that forms yeastlike buds, pseudohyphae, and hyphae. This ubiquitous organism is frequently found as a saprophyte on the skin and in the bowel, oropharynx, and vagina. When host defenses are impaired, it becomes a pathogen. *C. albicans* is currently the most common cause of vaginitis during the reproductive years.

Factors that presumably predispose to candidal vulvovaginitis include an excess of vaginal glucose, as occurs in pregnancy or diabetes; a reduction in vaginal bacterial flora, as occurs with the use of broad-spectrum antibiotics; and an excess of local moisture, as occurs during hot, moist weather or with tightly fitting clothing.

Clinical Picture

Vulvitis. A candidal infection usually involves both the vulva and the vagina. The major vulvar symptom is pruritus, which may be associated with dysuria, dyspareunia, and local pain. The skin is erythematous, slightly edematous, and often excoriated.

Vaginitis. A typical vaginal discharge is thick, whitish, and resembles cottage cheese. The vagina may be erythematous but often appears normal.

Diagnosis

Candidiasis that produces a typical cheesy discharge can be diagnosed on sight. Other cases can be diagnosed by microscopic examination of a wet smear prepared by mixing a sample of the discharge with a few milliliters of normal saline to which several drops of 10% potassium hydroxide have been added. *Candida* cells are oval or round and approximately the size of a red blood cell. Elongated buds and pseudomycelia may also be present. Still other cases will require a culture for confirmation. Either Sabouraud's or Nickerson's medium inoculated with cells from a cotton swab will show evidence of growth in 2 or 3 days.

Treatment

1. The vagina is first cleansed as thoroughly as possible to remove excess discharge before the start of treatment.

2. A topical antifungal agent is prescribed. These are the most effective:
   - Nystatin (Mycostatin, Nilstat) vaginal tablets, 1 in the morning and 1 at night for 14 days
   - Miconazole nitrate (Monistat 7) cream, 1 applicatorful intravaginally nightly for 7 days
   - Clotrimazole (Gyne-Lotrimin, Mycelex-G), 1 applicatorful intravaginally nightly for 7-14 days, or 1 tablet intravaginally nightly for 7 days, or 2 tablets intravaginally nightly for 3 days.
3. Although messy and somewhat irritating, gentian violet solution (1% aqueous) is an effective adjuvant that can be applied at an office visit.
4. Coexisting vulvitis is best treated by local application of a corticosteroid cream plus an antifungal agent—for example, Mycolog ointment, which has a higher pH than the vagina and therefore does not burn when applied to the vulva.
5. Clothing that increases local heat and moisture, such as nylon underwear and tightly fitting garments, should be avoided.
6. Intercourse should be avoided during the first few days of treatment or until it is no longer painful.
7. Broad-spectrum antibiotics (such as tetracycline for the treatment of acne) should be discontinued until the vulvovaginitis is eradicated.

Treatment Failure
1. Re-examine the patient carefully to be certain that symptoms are not due to the emergence of a coexisting pathogen such as *Trichomonas*.
2. Evaluate the possibility of reinfection from a candidal infection of the patient's sexual partner's penile skin.
3. Re-treat the patient with combined topical and oral medication (1 nystatin tablet 4 times a day) or alternate vaginal preparations with 1% aqueous gentian violet painted on the vagina on 5 consecutive days.
4. Evaluate the possibility that the patient may have undiagnosed diabetes.

BACTERIA

When vulvovaginitis is due to neither *Trichomonas* nor *Candida*, the diagnosis is usually labeled "nonspecific vaginitis." In the majority of these cases, however, the infection is due to a specific, though unidentified, bacterium.

Gardnerella Vaginalis
The most common form of bacterial vaginitis is caused by *Gardnerella vaginalis*, a small, gram-negative rod and facultative anaerobe, in association with other anaerobic organisms. A superficial infection produces erythema, small, punctate hemorrhages, and a homogeneous gray, malodorous discharge. The diagnosis can be confirmed by finding "clue cells"—stratified squamous cells with a granular appearance due to a coating of organisms.

Local treatment with triple sulfa or nitrofurazone (Furacin) cream for 10-14 days is sometimes ameliorative but usually not successful. Ampicillin 500 mg

4 times a day for 5 days may eradicate *Gardnerella*, but since it also kills *Lactobacillus* it raises the vaginal pH, leading to reinfection. Metronidazole 500 mg twice daily for 7 days is the treatment of choice. It eradicates *G. vaginalis* and other anaerobes while sparing the lactobacilli. If reinfection occurs, the patient's sexual partner should also be treated with metronidazole on the supposition that he is harboring the organism.

Neisseria Gonorrhoeae
Gonococcal infection is discussed in Chapter 49.

Colon Bacilli
A persisting vaginitis, particularly in children, can result from repeated contamination of the vulvar area by feces. Although any of the usual inhabitants of the lower bowel can be involved, *Escherichia coli* is most likely to be the offending organism. Teaching proper hygiene usually cures the infection. Acute vaginitis usually responds to a 4-5-day course of oral ampicillin.

Bacteroides species are often found in the vagina and may on occasion cause vaginitis that produces a malodorous discharge. A symptomatic infection from which *B. fragilis* has been cultured can be treated with oral metronidazole 250 mg tid or clindamycin (Cleocin) 300 mg qid for 10 days.

Miscellaneous Bacteria
Many other bacteria are capable of causing vaginitis. Examples are streptococci, which produce a thin, watery discharge, and staphylococci, which can occur in hospital personnel.

VIRUSES

Herpes Simplex Virus
The most common venereal disease in women in many parts of the country is herpetic infection of the vagina and vulva. This topic is covered in Chapter 48.

Condyloma Acuminatum
Condyloma acuminatum is thought to be a viral venereal infection that produces multiple small warts. These lesions are found most often on the vestibule but may also involve the labia, perianal skin, vagina, and cervix. Large lesions tend to coalesce and become secondarily infected.

Treatment is tedious and protracted. For small lesions, the best drug is podophyllin (20% in tincture of benzoin or a 25% ointment) applied directly to individual lesions. The surrounding skin should be protected against the irritating effects of this drug by a coating of petrolatum, and the residual podophyllin should be washed away with soap and water 1 to 2 hours later.

Therapy should be repeated at weekly intervals until all lesions are cleared. Any other coexisting infections, such as trichomoniasis or candidiasis, should be treated concurrently. Extensive lesions may require electrocautery, cryosurgery, laser therapy, or surgical excision under anesthesia.

CHEMICALS AND ALLERGENS

Almost any agent that comes into contact with the vulva or vagina can cause erythema, irritation, ulceration, and/or discharge. The list includes soaps, douche materials, bubble bath, contraceptive preparations, powder, cloth, dyes, perfumed or colored toilet paper, and local medications. Treatment begins with elimination of as many of these items as possible, including a change from nylon to cotton underwear.

ATROPHIC VAGINITIS

This topic is covered in Chapter 107 on hormone replacement therapy for menopausal symptoms.

CERVICITIS

If the primary source of a vaginal discharge is extensive cervicitis, cautery, cryosurgery, or laser therapy may be necessary once neoplastic disease has been ruled out.

PEDICULOSIS

An infestation with *Phthirus pubis* will cause chronic vulvar irritation but can easily be missed unless a careful examination is made for this tiny louse. Lindane (Kwell) lotion or shampoo is the treatment of choice. Clothing and linen should be changed frequently. Repeat treatment in 1 week is commonly required, as is treatment of sexual partners.

PEDIATRIC VULVOVAGINITIS

Infections in children are covered in Chapter 45.

SCABIES

Scabies is due to the mite *Sarcoptes scabiei*, which produces small, itchy subcutaneous burrows, papules, and vesicles along the wrists, finger webs, and torso. Treatment is the same as for pediculosis.

SUGGESTED READING

Chen KCS, Forsyth PS, Buchanan TM, et al: Amine content of vaginal fluid from untreated and treated patients with nonspecific vaginitis. *J Clin Invest* 63:828, 1979

Gardner HL: *Haemophilus vaginalis* vaginitis after twenty-five years. *Am J Obstet Gynecol* 137:385, 1980

Kaufman RH: The origin and diagnosis of "nonspecific vaginitis." *N Engl J Med* 303:637, 1980

McCormack WM, Evard JR, Laughlin CF, et al: Sexually transmitted conditions among women college students. *Am J Obstet Gynecol* 139:130, 1980

Pheifer TA, Forsyth PS, Durfee MA, et al: Nonspecific vaginitis: Role of *Haemophilus vaginalis* and treatment with metronidazole. *N Engl J Med* 298:1429, 1978

Spiegel CA, Amsel R, Eschenbach D, et al: Anaerobic bacteria in nonspecific vaginitis. *N Engl J Med* 303:601, 1980

47

Sexually Transmitted Diseases

SUBIR ROY, M.D.

Venereal diseases may be caused by a variety of agents. Bacterial diseases include syphilis, gonorrhea, chancroid, and granuloma inguinale. Lympho-granuloma venereum is caused by *Chlamydia*. Venereally transmitted *Myco-plasma* species include *M. hominis* and the T strain. Infections with herpes simplex type 1 and 2 and condyloma acuminatum are caused by viruses. Trichomonal vaginitis is caused by a protozoan while pediculosis pubis is caused by a louse.

SYPHILIS

The primary lesion of syphilis appears after 10-90 days of incubation (average, 21 days) and consists of single or multiple chancres on the anus, vulva, vagina, cervix, nipples, or mouth. Regional lymph nodes will probably be enlarged. If a chancre is discovered, syphilis is best diagnosed by a dark-field examination to demonstrate the spirochete, *Treponema pallidum*. To obtain a good speci-men, the lesion is cleansed, abraded, and blotted free of blood, and a sample of oozing serum is placed on a slide and covered with a coverslip.

Serologic tests for syphilis become positive 4 or 5 weeks following an initial infection, or 1-2 weeks after a chancre appears. The nonspecific *Treponema* tests, such as flocculation tests (VDRL, Kline, Mazzini, Hinton, etc.) or com-plement fixation tests (Wassermann, Kolmer), are diagnostic if the titer is 1:32 or higher. Tests showing titers lower than 1:32 should be repeated and a spe-cific test for treponemal antibodies (TPI, FTA-ABS) should be performed be-cause of the likelihood of obtaining a false-positive result with the comple-ment fixation tests.

Secondary syphilis is manifested by cutaneous and mucous membrane le-sions or by condylomas (condyloma latum) of the anogenital region. Because these lesions are teeming with spirochetes, either a dark-field examination or a biopsy can be used for diagnosis. Latent syphilis has no clinical manifesta-tions and is diagnosed on the basis of positive serology after neurologic (nega-tive cerebrospinal fluid) and cardiovascular involvement has been ruled out. It is also necessary to rule out other diseases that can produce a positive blood test: acute fevers, collagen disease, mononucleosis, malaria, leprosy, yaws, and lymphogranuloma.

Penicillin is the drug of choice. Primary or secondary syphilis is treated with intramuscular procaine penicillin G 600,000 units daily for 8-10 days or intramuscular procaine penicillin G in 2% aluminum monostearate 2.4 million units followed by 1.2 million units on the third and sixth days. Patients who are allergic to penicillin can be treated with tetracycline or erythromycin 30 gm over a 10-day period. In latent syphilis with negative cerebrospinal fluid, the patient can be given either benzathine penicillin G 3 million units weekly for 3 weeks or procaine penicillin G 600,000 units daily for 10-15 days. Follow-up serologic and cerebrospinal fluid tests are necessary to evaluate the effectiveness of the treatment; they should be done every 3 months for the first year following treatment and every 6 months in the second year. In the case of primary syphilis, 98% of adequately treated patients will become seronegative within the first year.

During pregnancy, the recommended treatment for primary syphilis in the first and second trimesters is IM benzathine penicillin G 2.4 million units, repeated in 7 days. In the third trimester, use IM procaine penicillin G with 2% aluminum monostearate 2.4 million units followed by 1.2 million units on the 4th, 8th, and 12th days. Latent syphilis with a negative cerebrospinal fluid requires IM benzathine penicillin G 2.4 million units, repeated in 14 days.

GONORRHEA

Gonorrhea is covered in Chapter 49.

GRANULOMA INGUINALE

Granuloma inguinale is due to a gram-negative bacterium, *Calymmatobacterium granulomatis*, that may be sexually transmitted, possibly by anal intercourse. The initial papular lesion ulcerates and spreads via the lymphatics to regional lymph nodes, with pseudobubo formation in the inguinal areas. Suppuration and sinus formation are rare in female patients; when they do occur, the lesions may mimic carcinoma. The diagnosis is made by the observation of Donovan bodies (intracellular bacteria) in a biopsy specimen.

The treatment of choice is tetracycline 2 gm daily for 14-21 days. Other antibiotics, such as erythromycin, kanamycin (Kantrex), and ampicillin, are also effective. If the response is poor, treatment may be extended. Treatment of relapses is often necessary.

CHANCROID (SOFT CHANCRE)

Chancroid is a superficial infection caused by a small gram-negative rod, *Haemophilus ducreyi*. The typical lesion is a painful, shallow, circular vulvar ulcer with a necrotic, erythematous base. Regional lymph nodes are often enlarged. Dark-field examination eliminates the diagnosis of a syphilitic chancre, and a Gram stain of a smear usually demonstrates the bacilli arranged in a characteristic cluster.

Sulfisoxazole (Gantrisin) 4 gm daily for 10-14 days or tetracycline 2 gm daily for 7-10 days is usually effective. A follow-up test for syphilis is advisable.

LYMPHOGRANULOMA VENEREUM

Lymphogranuloma venereum is produced by a bacterium, *Chlamydia trachomatis*. The initial small erosion or ulcer may progress by lymphatic spread to the femoral and inguinal lymph nodes. Lymphatic buboes with ulceration and drainage are relatively uncommon in women. Lymphatic spread to the perirectal and pelvic nodes produces proctitis, followed by strictures and fistula formation. The urethra can also be involved. About 80% of patients will have a positive Frei test if injected intradermally with 0.1 ml of the antigen. A complement fixation test is more accurate in the earlier stages of the disease. Biopsies may be obscured by necrosis and infection and are not always diagnostic. Serologic tests for syphilis are apt to give a false-positive result.

Triple sulfa 4 gm daily for 2 weeks or tetracycline 2 gm daily for 10-15 days is effective in treating the earlier stages of this disease. A rectal stricture will require a colostomy.

MYCOPLASMAS

Mycoplasma hominis and T strains of this genus (unique bacteria that have no cell wall) frequently inhabit the vagina, are commonly associated with pelvic infections, and can be transmitted sexually.

While *Mycoplasma* has been implicated as a possible cause of abortion, chorioamnionitis, low-birth-weight infants, bartholinitis, salpingitis, tubo-ovarian abscess, urinary tract infection, and infertility, it appears to have a low rate of virulence. The antibiotic of choice is tetracycline 1 gm daily for 7 days following a loading dose of 1-2 gm.

OTHER DISEASES

Herpes simplex is discussed in Chapter 48, and condyloma acuminatum, trichomoniasis, pediculosis, and scabies are discussed in Chapter 46.

SUGGESTED READING

Abrams AJ: Lymphogranuloma venereum. *JAMA* 205:59, 1968

Alergant CB: Chancroid. *Practitioner* 209:624, 1972

Ribiero J: Granuloma inguinale. *Practitioner* 209:628, 1972

Sparling PF: Diagnosis and treatment of syphilis. *N Engl J Med* 284:642, 1971

Taylor-Robinson D, McCormack WM: The genital mycoplasmas. *N Engl J Med* 302:1003, 1980

48

Genital Herpes

LESTER T. HIBBARD, M.D.

The herpesvirus hominis (or herpes simplex virus) type 2 is a DNA virus that replicates in nuclei of host cells, is not destroyed despite the development of special antibodies, and is responsible for most viral infections of the lower genital tract. The type 2 virus almost always involves the genital tract and is usually transmitted by sexual contact. A few cases of genital herpes are also caused by the type 1 virus, which usually involves the oropharynx or the eye, and are the result of oral-genital contact. Like gonorrhea, genital herpes occurring in women is frequently asymptomatic and is detected only by a Papanicolaou smear.

Symptomatic primary genital herpes infections are usually more severe than recurrent infections and are accompanied by varying degrees of fever, anorexia, malaise, and inguinal adenopathy. The vulva, vagina, cervix, urethra, perineum, and buttocks can be involved by vesicular, ulcerating lesions that may persist for 3 to 6 weeks. There is some vaginal discharge accompanied by local tenderness, pain, and dyspareunia when the vulva is involved. The initial lesions are vesicles that rupture and progress to shallow ulcers covered by a whitish membrane.

Recurrent infections are common despite the presence of specific viral antibodies, but the symptoms are less severe than in primary infections, and of shorter duration. As a rule, both primary and recurrent infections are self-limiting and heal without scar formation.

DIAGNOSIS

Multiple vesicles or intensely painful vulvar and perineal ulcerations often make the diagnosis obvious. Vaginal and cervical lesions tend to be macerated. The differential diagnosis between herpes and other lesions causing vulvovaginal ulcerations can best be made by cultures, but is more easily and practically made by the demonstration of multinucleated giant cells, nuclear degeneration, and intranuclear inclusions using a Papanicolaou stain on a smear from a vesicle or ulceration. Antibody testing is not useful because the results are usually confused by pre-existing antibodies to a type 1 infection. Because herpes is often associated with other venereal infections, gonorrheal cultures and a serology test should be performed.

TREATMENT

In the past, the treatment of genital herpes has been largely unsatisfactory despite a multitude of suggested remedies. Acute inflammatory reactions should be cleansed with a povidone-iodine solution. Cold compresses of 1:4,000 benzalkonium chloride or 1:6,000 potassium permanganate solutions 4 times daily, local and systemic analgesics, and broad-spectrum antibiotics for secondary bacterial infections are helpful. Steroids are contraindicated because they enhance replication of the virus. Freezing, photodynamic inactivation, iodine, alcohol, ether, antimetabolites, idoxuridine, lecithin, and 2-deoxy-D-glucose have been disappointing. The newest recommendation for a primary infection is an antiviral ointment containing acyclovir (Zovirax) applied locally 6 times daily for 6 or 7 days. This preparation apparently alleviates symptoms and hastens healing, but is not effective in the treatment of recurrent attacks. The value of immunotherapeutic agents (such as BCG vaccine) for recurrent herpes has not been established.

COMPLICATIONS

The major complication of genital herpes is a secondary bacterial infection, which increases the patient's discomfort and interferes with treatment. Other complications, such as meningoencephalitis, urethral strictures, and lymphatic suppuration, are rare. But it should be kept in mind that herpes often coexists with other venereal infections such as gonorrhea or trichomoniasis, and that a herpetic infection during pregnancy can be responsible for abortion, premature labor, and lethal infection of the newborn infant. Congenital herpetic infection is also possible, although the fetus will probably be protected by antibodies formed in response to a previous maternal herpes type 1 infection of the oropharynx or eye. In addition, there is reason to suspect that the type 2 virus is carcinogenic to the cervix.

An active herpetic infection during the third trimester of pregnancy poses additional problems. As long as the lesions remain infectious, vaginal birth is associated with a high rate of neonatal herpes and neonatal death. If birth is even a possibility before the lesions are healed, one or more viral cultures should be obtained. A positive culture is an indication for cesarean section and a negative culture justifies a vaginal delivery. If there is insufficient time to obtain a culture report before the anticipated date of delivery, an elective section should be considered. Most laboratories require a week or longer to complete a culture. When labor begins before the evaluation of herpetic lesions has been completed, a section is indicated unless the membranes have been ruptured long enough to guarantee that the fetus has become infected. One study suggests that intrauterine infection is highly likely if the membranes have been ruptured for 4 hours. Since neonatal herpes is highly lethal, using 7 or 8 hours (instead of 4) as the threshold for allowing vaginal delivery will probably save a few more infants. A herpetic infection in the first trimester is occasionally the cause of spontaneous abortion, but rarely the cause of a fetal infection that would justify a therapeutic abortion.

SUGGESTED READING

Goodheart CR: Herpes virus and cancer. *JAMA* 211:91, 1970

Grossman JJ, Wallen WC: Management of genital herpes simplex virus infection during pregnancy. *Obstet Gynecol* 58:1, 1981

Guinan ME, et al: The course of untreated recurrent genital herpes simplex infection in 27 women. *N Engl J Med* 304:576, 1981

Whiteley RJ, et al: The natural history of herpes simplex virus infection of mother and newborn. *Pediatrics* 66:489, 1980

Zervoudakis IA, et al: Herpes simplex in amniotic fluid of unaffected fetus. *Obstet Gynecol* 55(suppl):168, 1980

49

Pelvic Infection

SUBIR ROY, M.D.

The vaginal flora contains both aerobic and anaerobic organisms, at average concentrations of 10^8 and 10^9/gm of vaginal fluid, respectively. A study of cultures obtained sequentially throughout the menstrual cycle showed that the concentration of anaerobic organisms was relatively constant but that the concentration of aerobes was almost 100-fold less during the last premenstrual week than in the first week after menstruation. When the portal for entry to the upper genital tract is violated, as during cervical instrumentation or hysterectomy, an inoculum of potentially pathogenic organisms may be introduced, leading to infection.

BIPHASIC INFECTIONS

Studies by Bartlett and colleagues have shown that when an inoculum of mixed aerobic and anaerobic organisms is introduced into an abdominal operative site, the initial stage of peritonitis—predominantly due to the aerobe *Escherichia coli*—is produced. In these studies, done in mice, animals that survived the initial stage of infection later developed abscesses that were found to be due to the pathogenic effects of anaerobic bacteria, mainly *Bacteroides fragilis*. It was postulated that the aerobic bacteria died after using up all the available oxygen, but in the course of tissue destruction provided a more fertile field for the proliferation of anaerobes, resulting in abscess formation.

EVIDENCE OF ANAEROBIC INFECTION

An infection due to anaerobic organisms should be suspected if an abscess with a fecal odor is encountered, if gas is observed in purulent material, especially on an x-ray of the pelvic organs, if septic pelvic thrombophlebitis develops in a seriously ill patient, if nongonococcal intracellular organisms (e.g., *Veillonella*) are seen on a Gram stain of abscess material, or if a culture report of "no growth" is received although the patient is obviously septic; in this last case, poor sampling or culture technique is probably responsible for the lack of results.

Proper technique is to obtain the culture sample from the margin of the abscess. The center of an abscess contains desquamated cells and nonviable materials; it is at the margins where rapid bacterial proliferation occurs. Material from the margin of an abscess may be aspirated into a glass syringe, which is then stoppered and taken to the microbiology laboratory for direct plating. Another technique is to do anaerobic culturing directly into a gas pack, although this is somewhat cumbersome and impractical unless appropriately trained personnel are in the operating theatre to handle the cultured material. Perhaps the easiest way to obtain cultures for both anaerobic and aerobic organisms is to use a Port-A-Cul transport medium, which can maintain a culture for 24-48 hours.

SALPINGITIS

Salpingitis, or "febrile menses," usually occurs immediately following the onset of menstruation. It is accompanied by fever of 100-102°F associated with vaginal discharge and diffuse, usually bilateral, pain or appreciation of a mass on bimanual examination. The salpingitis is usually due to more than one organism and is sexually transmitted: *Neisseria gonorrhoeae* accounts for 30-80% of cases in the United States. *Chlamydia trachomatis* has been implicated in fewer than 20% of salpingitis cases, usually by immunologic screening rather than by culture in the United States, while it is cultured in more than 50% of cases in Sweden. Anaerobic bacteria occur in approximately 50% of cases, particularly in repetitive infections. *Mycoplasma hominis* has been associated with 10-15% of salpingitis cases in Sweden. *Ureaplasma urealyticum*, viruses, and other organisms may also be implicated in salpingitis.

Incidence
Salpingitis occurs in about 12:1,000 of the 36 million women under 35 years of age (based on 1970-1974 data); during 1981, approximately 1 million cases of salpingitis were reported. Incidence is highest among women 15-24 years old.

Prevalence
Salpingitis tends to occur in proportion to the number of sexual partners a woman has. Approximately 10-15% of women of reproductive age have had salpingitis. Among sexually active women, those using no contraceptive method have 3.42 cases per 100 woman years, IUD users have 5.21 cases, oral contraceptive users have 0.91 cases, and barrier users have 1.39 cases. Thus IUD users are at slightly increased risk for salpingitis compared with women who use no contraceptive method, whereas women who use a barrier method or oral contraceptive would appear to be significantly protected.

Sequelae
Twenty-five per cent of women with salpingitis will eventually suffer chronic abdominal pain, infertility, and/or ectopic pregnancy. Chronic abdominal pain was the major complaint in 17% of salpingitis patients studied by Falk. A 1980 study by Westrom showed that 18% of women who had had salpingitis complained of chronic abdominal pain, compared with only 5% of women who had no history of salpingitis.

Studies in Scandinavia showed that the incidence of complaints of infertility could be correlated with the number of episodes of salpingitis. Tubal occlusion was found in 11% of women who had had one episode of salpingitis, in 23% of those who had had two episodes, and in 54% of those with a history of three or four episodes. Tubal occlusion may also be related to the severity of a given episode of salpingitis. Based on 1970-1974 statistics, the rate of infertility as a result of salpingitis was approximately 15%. Brought forward to the 1980s, this figure means that approximately 100,000 American women are rendered infertile each year because of salpingitis.

The rate of ectopic pregnancy was 1:300 pregnancies in 1979 among women who had never had salpingitis. In women with a history of this condition, the incidence of ectopic pregnancies increased to 1:16 in 1980. It is currently estimated that 25,000 ectopic pregnancies are attributable to salpingitis in the United States each year.

Diagnosis

Salpingitis is frequently overdiagnosed clinically. In recent studies in which laparoscopy was utilized to confirm or refute the clinical diagnosis of salpingitis, it was confirmed in only 62% of patients. Among the rest, 22% of patients had normal findings, 5% had ovarian cysts, 4% had ectopic pregnancies, 3% had appendicitis, 1% had endometriosis, and 3% had other conditions. The important differential diagnoses to keep in mind are the two critical ones—ectopic pregnancy and appendicitis. Unless the clinical picture and pelvic findings are entirely consistent with salpingitis, and in the absence of pelvic peritonitis, where surgery may be imprudent, a diagnostic laparoscopy is recommended in order to make the correct diagnosis.

Both gonococcal and nongonococcal salpingitis may cause mild, severe, or rebound abdominal tenderness, purulent vaginal discharge, cervical tenderness, unilateral or bilateral adnexal tenderness, or an adnexal mass greater than 6 cm in diameter. However, liver tenderness and a purulent cervical exudate are found twice as often in gonococcal as in nongonococcal disease.

Principles of Therapy

For suspected gonococcal salpingitis, since there is no clinical way to distinguish between non-penicillinase-producing and penicillinase-producing gonococci, the routine therapy has been probenecid (Benemid) given before the administration of procaine penicillin or doxycycline (Vibramycin). If there is reason to suspect a penicillinase-producing gonococcus, the usual therapy is spectinomycin (Trobicin), cefoxitin (Mefoxin), or one of the third-generation cephalosporins such as cefotaxime (Claforan) or moxalactam (Moxam).

If the patient has a clinical salpingitis presentation but a Gram stain of the endocervical swab reveals no gram-negative intracellular diplococci and no pelvic mass can be palpated, one should suspect *Chlamydia*. The appropriate therapy for a chlamydial infection is tetracycline, doxycycline, or erythromycin. If a pelvic mass is present, suspect *Bacteroides fragilis*. The encapsulated species of *B. fragilis* is most often associated with abscess formation; indeed, the capsule alone may produce an abscess. Various combinations of antibiotics are usually effective in the therapy of salpingitis with a mass, including clindamycin (Cleocin) with gentamicin (Garamycin) with or without penicillin. Clindamycin and gentamicin are not effective against enterococci; however, these organisms may not be pathogenic in gynecologic infections.

Other therapies are chloramphenicol with gentamicin, cefoxitin with or without gentamicin, cefotaxime alone, or a cephalosporin with a specific anaerobic agent, such as cefotaxime with clindamycin or any cephalosporin with clindamycin or metronidazole (Flagyl). If the patient with salpingitis has an IUD that has been in place for some time, suspect *Actinomyces israelii*; penicillin is the treatment of choice for this organism. If the patient develops a bulging cul-de-sac abscess extending beyond the cervical os, colpotomy drainage should be performed. A ruptured tubo-ovarian abscess is a surgical emergency requiring a total abdominal hysterectomy and bilateral salpingo-oophorectomy.

Among the hospital-acquired infections are those of operative wounds. Infections that occur less than 48 hours postoperatively, particularly if they are associated with erysipelas, may be due to group A β-hemolytic streptococci, which produce a hyaluronidase. The treatment of choice is penicillin or ampicillin. If, however, there is early abscess development, suspect a group B β-hemolytic streptococcus; here the treatment of choice is ampicillin with or without gentamicin. If postoperative infection occurs more than 48 hours postoperatively, suspect *B. fragilis* and use the same combination of therapies employed for salpingitis with a mass.

Dosage Regimens
Four regimens may be employed for outpatient treatment of salpingitis:
1. Aqueous procaine penicillin 4.8 million units IM in two divided doses, with probenecid 1 gm PO approximately 30 minutes prior to the penicillin injections. This therapy is usually followed by ampicillin or amoxicillin 500 mg PO qid for 10 days.
2. Ampicillin 3.5 gm PO or amoxicillin 3 gm PO followed by ampicillin 500 mg PO qid for 10 days.
3. Tetracycline 500 mg PO qid for 10 days if the patient is not pregnant, or doxycycline 200 mg PO to start, then 100 mg bid for 10 days.
4. Cefoxitin 2 gm IM followed by cephradine (Anspor, Velosef) 500 mg PO qid for 10 days.

The most complete inpatient treatment of salpingitis is triple antibiotic therapy. Aqueous crystalline penicillin 5 million units IVPB q6h should be administered with gentamicin at a rate of 5 mg/kg/day IM or IV in three divided doses, which averages about 80 mg q8h. With aminoglycoside therapy, serum creatinine and aminoglycoside levels must be monitored to prevent the development of nephrotoxicity by appropriately adjusting the dose. Vigilance for the development of ototoxicity must also be maintained. Anaerobic coverage for *B. fragilis* may be provided by one of the following agents: clindamycin 600 mg IVPB q6h—also has good activity against *Chlamydia* and is effective against one-third of the gonococcal strains at LAC/USC; chloramphenicol 500 mg IV q6h—not widely used because of the risk of aplastic anemia (1:50,000, the majority of cases occurring after oral therapy) and the advent of newer anaerobic agents; and metronidazole 15 mg/kg (usually 1 gm) as a loading dose, then 7.5 mg/kg (usually 500 mg) IVPB q6h—a bactericidal agent with wide tissue distribution, effective only against obligate anaerobes, and packaged at physiologic pH. Alternative regimens are clindamycin with gentamicin at the dosages above or moxalactam or cefotaxime 1 or 2 gm IVPB q8h.

If the patient exhibits obvious symptomatic improvement, as evidenced by reduction of fever and tenderness, over the first 24 to 48 hours, it is recommended that parenteral therapy be continued until she has been afebrile for 48 hours. At that time, she should undergo a pelvic examination and be observed for an additional 24 hours, still on parenteral therapy. If the fever does not return, she can be discharged home on oral medication. The duration of oral and parenteral antibiotic therapy combined should equal 10 days.

If the patient again develops a fever, parenteral therapy should be continued with adjustments as necessary. If no residual masses are present at the pelvic exam, a broad-spectrum cephalosporin such as cephradine or ampicillin at a dose of 500 mg qid may be used for a total of 10 days of therapy. If a residual mass is present, either clindamycin 300 mg qid or metronidazole 250 mg qid might be added if it was the anaerobic agent used during parenteral therapy. If a cephalosporin available only parenterally was used, then cephradine 500 mg qid may be used for the oral phase of therapy.

For patients who have responded more gradually, parenteral therapy can be continued for a week or more, particularly if preservation of fertility is desirable. If a third-generation cephalosporin was used and response was slow, an anaerobic agent (e.g., clindamycin or metronidazole) could be added after 48-72 hours.

About 10% of serious pelvic infections fail to respond to antibiotic therapy within 72 hours. If an abscess is enlarging rather than regressing, surgical intervention may be necessary, with appropriate drainage or resection of involved structures. A unilateral adnexectomy may be indicated in a woman with an unresponsive unilateral tubo-ovarian abscess who desires to keep her fertility. If the patient has no demonstrable site of infection but has a spiking fever suggestive of septic pelvic thrombophlebitis, a trial of heparin in addition to the antibiotic therapy is recommended at a dose of 5,000 units IV q4h or a loading dose of 5,000 units followed by continuous infusion of 1,000 units/hour while maintaining the partial thromboplastin time at 1.5-2.5 times the normal value.

UPDATE ON TREATMENT OF ACUTE SALPINGITIS

The Centers for Disease Control recently released new recommendations for the treatment of acute salpingitis. The CDC guidelines recommend combination therapy for all patients and hospitalization and parenteral therapy in all but mild cases without an adnexal mass or IUD.

Inpatient parenteral antibiotic regimens recommended are: (1) cefoxitin (Mefoxin) plus doxycycline (Vibramycin) for patients with gonococcal salpingitis without pelvic mass or IUD; and either (2) clindamycin (Cleocin) plus an aminoglycoside, or (3) metronidazole (Flagyl) plus doxycycline for nongonococcal salpingitis, recurrent salpingitis, or salpingitis associated with a mass or an IUD.

All these regimens are to be given IV for at least 4 days or until the patient has been afebrile for at least 48 hours, whichever is longer. Following discharge from the hospital, the antimicrobial effective against *Chlamydia trachomatis* is continued orally to complete 10-14 days of treatment.

For outpatient treatment, it is recommended that *one* of the following be given *along with* probenecid (Benemid) 1 gm PO and *followed by* doxycycline 100 mg PO bid × 10-14 days: (1) cefoxitin 2 gm IM, (2) amoxicillin 3 gm PO, (3) ampicillin 3.5 gm PO, or (4) aqueous procaine penicillin 4.8 million units IM at two sites.

Outpatients so treated should be re-evaluated 48-72 hours after initiation of antibiotic therapy. Those not responding favorably should be hospitalized. Sexual partners of patients with acute salpingitis should be similarly treated.

SUGGESTED READING

Centers for Disease Control: Sexually transmitted diseases—Treatment guidelines, 1982. *MMWR* 31(suppl), 1982.

Falk HC: Interpretation of the pathogenesis of pelvic infections as determined by cornual resection. *Am J Obstet Gynecol* 52:66, 1946

Ginsburg DS, Stern JL, Hamod KA, Genadry R, Spence MR: Tubo-ovarian abscess: A retrospective review. *Am J Obstet Gynecol* 138:1055, 1980

Holmes KK, Eschenbach DA, Knapp JS: Salpingitis: Overview of etiology and epidemiology. *Am J Obstet Gynecol* 138:893, 1980

Onderdonk AB, Weinstein WM, Sullivan NM, Bartlett JG, Gorbach SL: Experimental intraabdominal abscesses in rats: II. Quantitative bacteriology of infected animals. *Infect Immun* 10:1256, 1974

Rees E: The treatment of pelvic inflammatory disease. *Am J Obstet Gynecol* 138:1042, 1980

Senanayake P, Kramer DG: Contraception and the etiology of pelvic inflammatory disease: New perspectives. *Am J Obstet Gynecol* 138:852, 1980

Weinstein WM, Onderdonk AB, Bartlett JB, Gorbach SL: Experimental intraabdominal abscesses in rats: I. Development of an experimental model. *Infect Immun* 10:1250, 1974

Westrom L: Incidence, prevalence and trends of acute pelvic inflammatory disease and its consequences in industrialized countries. *Am J Obstet Gynecol* 138:880, 1980

50

Prevention of Postoperative Gynecologic Infection

SUBIR ROY, M.D.

Contamination by endogenous bacteria may occur at the time of gynecologic operations despite vigorous preoperative vaginal cleansing. The combination of hemostatic sutures around crushed tissue, blood products, and bacterial contaminants from the vagina may lead to postoperative abdominal wound infections, pelvic (cuff) cellulitis, or pelvic abscesses. Prolonged hospitalization with therapeutic antibiotic administration and a second operation may be necessary before the patient recovers.

PROPHYLACTIC ANTIBIOTICS

A variety of techniques may be used to reduce infection following gynecologic surgery. Foremost is the use of prophylactic antibiotics. Following are guidelines for the use of prophylactic antibiotics in gynecologic surgery:

1. The operation should carry a significant risk of developing postoperative wound infection.
2. The operation should be expected to cause a significant degree of bacterial contamination.
3. The antibiotic used for prophylaxis should have demonstrable laboratory and clinical evidence of effectiveness against some of the contaminating microorganisms.
4. A short-term, low-toxicity regimen of antibiotics should be used.
5. The benefits of prophylactic antibiotics must outweigh the dangers of their use.

Effectiveness

In general, the use of prophylactic antibiotics at the time of vaginal hysterectomy, regardless of menopausal status, has been shown to reduce the incidence of operative site infection. Data for abdominal hysterectomy suggest that antibiotic prophylaxis reduces the incidence of postoperative urinary tract infections as well as wound infections if the rate of wound infections in the control group is high. Only 2 of 12 abdominal hysterectomy studies demonstrated a reduction in postoperative pelvic cellulitis.

These discrepancies are largely due to the varied drug regimens and definitions of outcome in reported studies. Some authors have lumped together standard febrile morbidity or all infection-related complications while others have carefully defined and categorized outcome in terms of fever index, pelvic (vaginal cuff) cellulitis, vaginal cuff abscess, urinary tract infection, wound infection, need for therapeutic antibiotics (a sum of the four previous diagnoses), and duration of postoperative hospitalization. Only when randomized groups are actually similar in terms of entry characteristics can the outcome of prophylaxis be meaningfully compared.

Timing of Administration

In suitably chosen subjects, prophylactic antibiotics have reduced operative site infection from 40-70% to 5-20% following vaginal hysterectomy, and from 20-30% to 5-10% following abdominal hysterectomy. A study by Burke demonstrated that prophylactic antibiotics had no benefit if administered more than 3 hours after bacterial contamination occurred. To be effective, these agents should be administered before any elective procedure requiring antibiotic prophylaxis. A short-term course not to exceed about 24 hours postoperatively is currently recommended.

Choice of Agents

A variety of agents have been successfully utilized: ampicillin, doxycycline (Vibramycin), metronidazole (Flagyl), and several cephalosporins, which because of their broad antibacterial spectrum and low toxicity have become popular prophylactic agents. These include cephalothin (Keflin), cephradine (Anspor, Velosef), cefazolin (Ancef, Kefzol), cefoxitin (Mefoxin), cefotaxime (Claforan), and moxalactam (Moxam). Although metronidazole is considered effective only against obligate anaerobes, it is also successful when administered prophylactically.

The newer agents, such as cefoxitin, cefotaxime, and moxalactam, provide a broader spectrum of antibacterial coverage than the earlier agents and can be administered over a shorter period. A shorter treatment course is thought to make it less likely that resistant organisms will emerge—always a concern when antibiotics are administered prophylactically. However, these newer agents should not be utilized for prophylaxis unless associated with a significant reduction of operative site infection following gynecologic surgery relative to older, less potent agents. Studies to test this hypothesis are under way.

Prophylactic Regimens

Table 50-1 summarizes various prophylactic regimens. The first dose of antibiotic should be administered while the patient is awake in order to observe her for adverse reactions. Two patients receiving cephalothin for the first time while under anesthesia apparently died from anaphylaxis. The initial dose of antibiotic is usually administered 30-60 minutes prior to incision in order to achieve satisfactory serum and tissue levels. Cefoxitin must be diluted with

TABLE 50-1. PROPHYLACTIC ANTIBIOTIC REGIMENS

Drug	Preoperative dose	Intraoperative dose	Postoperative dose
Ampicillin	—	500 mg IV	500 mg IV q6h × 4
Cefazolin	1 gm IV	500 mg-1 gm IV	500 mg-1 gm IV q6h × 4
Cefotaxime	1 gm IM*	1 gm IV q90-120m × 3-4	
Cefoxitin	2 gm IM*	—	2 gm IVPB q6h × 2
Cephalothin	1 gm IV	1 gm IV	1 gm IV q6h × 4
Cephradine	2 gm IV	—	—
	1 gm IV	—	500 mg IV q6h × 4
Doxycycline	200 mg IV over 1 hour 2-4 hours preop	—	200 mg IV or PO qd × 2
Metronidazole	1 gm IV	—	0.5-1 gm IV 6 hours after first dose
Moxalactam	2 gm IM*	—	—

*Currently under investigation.

lidocaine prior to intramuscular injection to reduce pain at the injection site. A normal prothrombin time or 10 mg of vitamin K is required prior to moxalactam administration, since this drug (like other broad-spectrum agents with significant biliary excretion) may lead to hypothrombinemia with or without bleeding.

Other factors, such as operative time, estimated blood loss, regrowth of vaginal flora, and associated procedures performed at the time of hysterectomy, have been studied. The subjects at highest risk of postoperative infection seem to be those with the greatest amount of surgery—e.g., vaginal hysterectomy with the Pereyra procedure or abdominal hysterectomy with the Burch procedure. These infections usually begin more than 72 hours after surgery.

OTHER MEASURES

For individuals who are allergic to antibiotics, Swartz and Tanaree have reduced infections following vaginal or abdominal hysterectomy by using closed T-tube suction drainage in the space between the peritoneum and vaginal cuff for 36 hours postoperatively. A vaginal pack coated with a sterile gel rather than an antibiotic cream can also reduce the amount of blood and blood products that accumulate between the peritoneum and vaginal cuff. Osborne et al have reported that hot conization of the cervix, an area that harbors bacteria despite vaginal cleansing prior to hysterectomy, has also reduced postoperative infections. However, this requires additional surgery and may not be cost effective in reducing infections.

It is best not to alter the normal flora of the vagina or abdominal skin prior to surgery. For vaginal hysterectomy patients, an iodophor douche the night before surgery reduces the total number of organisms from about 10^8 to 10^6-

10^7. However, a very thorough preoperative cleansing of the vagina renders it essentially organism-free during the time required to perform a hysterectomy with associated anterior and posterior colporrhaphies. Therefore, douching the night before surgery is not recommended. Patients undergoing exploratory laparotomy or abdominal hysterectomy need simply bathe or shower as usual the night before surgery. Use of an agent such as an iodophor for many days prior to surgery could alter the skin flora and lead to a predominance of gram-negative organisms, resulting in an increased risk of wound infection. It is preferable to have the patient simply remove debris from the skin surface. Skin preparation immediately prior to surgery will reduce the bacterial count sufficiently during the operative period.

Cruse and Foord have shown a reduced postoperative infection rate if patients are shaved just prior to operation, no electrocautery knives or adhesive plastic drapes are used, and no drains are brought through the abdominal incision.

There is no substitute for good operative technique, with attention to hemostasis, in reducing postoperative infections. No antibiotic or other aids will overcome poor operative technique.

SUGGESTED READING

Burke JF: The effective period of preventive antibiotic action in experimental incisions and dermal lesions. *Surgery* 50:161, 1961

Cruse PJE, Foord R: Some factors determining wound infection. A prospective study of 30,000 wounds. In Polle HC Jr, Stone HH, eds: *Hospital-Acquired Infections in Surgery*. Baltimore: University Park Press, 1977, pp 77-85

Duff P: Antibiotic prophylaxis for abdominal hysterectomy. *Obstet Gynecol* 60:25, 1982

Duff P, Park RC: Antibiotic prophylaxis in vaginal hysterectomy. *Obstet Gynecol* 55:1935, 1980

Ledger WJ: Prevention, diagnosis and a treatment of postoperative infections. *Obstet Gynecol* 55:2035, 1980

Osborne NG, Wright RC, Dubay M: Preoperative hot conization of the cervix. *Am J Obstet Gynecol* 133:374, 1979

Roy S, Wilkins J: Comparison of cefotaxime to cefoxitin for prophylaxis of vaginal or abdominal hysterectomy. *Clin Ther* 5(supp A):74, 1982

Swartz WH, Tanaree P: Suction drainage as an alternative to prophylactic antibiotics for hysterectomy. *Obstet Gynecol* 43:305, 1975

51

Chronic Pelvic Pain

LESTER T. HIBBARD, M.D.

Pelvic pain is a diagnostic challenge for several reasons. First, most of the painful stimuli are mediated by the autonomic nervous system, which tends to produce inconsistent patterns of pain that are difficult both to describe and to recognize. Only the parietal peritoneum is innervated by the somatic nervous system. Second, multiple organ systems are involved. Third, a significant amount of pain is psychosexual in origin. Fourth, there are multiple pathogenic mechanisms for the production of pain, including ischemia, inflammation, muscular contractions, capsular distension, disruption, and chemical contamination.

The majority of painful stimuli are mediated either by way of the parasympathetic fibers of the pelvic nerves serving the cervix, urethra, and bladder base, by sympathetic fibers accompanying the ovarian blood vessels, or by sympathetic fibers spreading through the posterior retroperitoneal space in the plexus of Frankenhäuser and then passing over the pelvic brim to form the so-called presacral nerve. Although these nerve pathways can be surgically interrupted, the inconsistent results seldom justify a primary operation.

DIFFERENTIAL DIAGNOSIS

Chronic pain can be defined as pain that has persisted for 2 months or more without relief. Chronic pain is particularly difficult to diagnose because a substantial proportion will be due either to functional causes or to organic causes involving the bowel, the urinary tract, or the musculoskeletal system, instead of to gynecologic pathology.

Functional Pain

Although the percentage of patients with functional pain is difficult to estimate, some appreciation of the extent of the problem is gained from observations that almost 10% of gynecology patients are psychiatrically disturbed and that one-third of patients complaining of pelvic pain give evidence that their pain is a bodily reaction to stress. The diagnosis in such patients can be suspected from the lack of objective pelvic findings of organic disease. The pain is usually dull, persistent, and nonradiating. It tends to be either generalized or variable and shifting.

Other clues pointing toward a functional etiology are a pain that is not present on awakening and is aggravated by stress but is not reproduced by pelvic manipulation. Multiple complaints involving several organ systems and a history of multiple operations also suggest psychogenic pain. Patients with this disorder are often hypersensitive and have minimal pelvic findings in proportion to their complaints.

Diseases of Nonreproductive Structures

Approximately 20% of organic pelvic pain is due to urinary tract disease, and another 20% is due to diseases of the bowel or musculoskeletal system. By far the most common urinary tract lesion causing chronic pain is chronic posterior urethritis. This insidious problem is frequently overlooked because the pain is dull and poorly described and because there are no urinary symptoms, with the possible exception of nocturia, and no significant findings on a routine urinalysis. Since the infection involves the periurethral glands, the diagnosis can be suspected if the wall of the urethra seems thickened, and is confirmed by sounding the urethra with a No. 24 sound to demonstrate a mild to moderate amount of posterior urethral stenosis.

Treatment consists of serial urethral dilations to size 28 or more, followed by a short course of a prophylactic urinary antibiotic such as sulfisoxazole (Gantrisin) 1 gm 4 times daily for 3 or 4 days. Failure of this therapy would suggest an overlooked urethral diverticulum, which can be demonstrated by urethroscopy, a voiding cystourethrogram, or a Davis catheter study. If the bowel or musculoskeletal system is responsible for pelvic pain, the majority of patients will have either colitis or a postural disorder.

Reproductive Tract Disorders

The most common organic lesion of the reproductive tract associated with chronic pelvic pain is endometriosis. The diagnostic evaluation and treatment of endometriosis are covered in Chapters 98 and 99.

Chronic pelvic pain among older parous women suggests several etiologies. Sometimes the clinical picture supports a diagnosis: for example, clear-cut evidence of pelvic relaxation in a patient with pelvic pain and pressure or the finding of a symmetrically enlarged uterus containing adenomyosis in a patient with a history of acquired dysmenorrhea and metrorrhagia.

Other patients, with a lesser amount of relaxation or a seemingly slight enlargement of the uterus, may well have pelvic vascular congestion associated with broad ligament varicosities. There are no clear-cut criteria for the diagnosis of this syndrome, although an attempt to palpate the broad ligament varicosities with the patient in a standing position has been recommended. Observation of large veins on histologic examination of tissue obtained by endometrial biopsy has also been described in patients with this syndrome. Disruption of the cardinal ligaments (the Allen-Masters syndrome) as a cause of pain can be diagnosed by palpating a uterus that can be freely rotated on its long axis.

Adhesions

Another troublesome diagnosis is the presence of pelvic adhesions following infection or an operation. If there are unmistakable findings of pelvic masses or fixation of the adnexal structures, the diagnosis is fairly secure. But lesser adhesions responsible for pain can be diagnosed only by direct observation through a laparoscope.

DIAGNOSTIC AIDS

A number of diagnostic aids can help determine the etiology of puzzling cases of chronic pelvic pain. Relief of pain following inhibition of ovulation with oral contraceptives has been used as a method to diagnose suspected endometriosis, although laparoscopic examination has much greater accuracy. Use of a pessary to relieve symptoms thought to be caused by pelvic relaxation or the rather unlikely possibility of uterine retroversion helps to establish these disorders as the etiology of the pain. When available, pneumogynography may be helpful in the evaluation of vague or confusing pelvic findings such as suspected adhesions. Ultrasound studies are useful to detect an occasional deep-seated cyst or abscess that cannot be adequately palpated because the patient is obese or uncooperative. A hysterosalpingogram may demonstrate tubal disease or a uterine anomaly. Hysteroscopy may reveal an unsuspected polyp.

Visualization of the pelvic structures for diagnosis is more certain but also entails additional risk and expense. Colpotomy, culdoscopy, or minilaparotomy can be used in addition to laparoscopy, which is still the most popular and preferred method for diagnostic evaluation of pelvic pain. Satisfactory visualization of the pelvis can be obtained with the laparoscope in 90% to 95% of patients with a diagnosis of pelvic pain of unknown etiology. In the large majority of cases, no significant lesion will be found. However, a substantial number of these patients with presumably functional pain will be relieved of their symptoms when assured that no organic disease is present. Other patients, with minimal endometriosis or adhesions, may have their symptoms relieved without a major operation if the lesions can be fulgurated or cut with the aid of the laparoscope.

SURGERY

Operations for nonorganic pelvic pain are frequently unsuccessful, particularly if the patient has previously exhibited depression, anxiety, or hysteria. It should be remembered that a hysterectomy is followed by a two- to three-fold greater incidence of postoperative depression than other elective abdominal operations. Although either a presacral neurectomy or resection of the pelvic nerves can effectively relieve such problems as primary dysmenorrhea, the results are sufficiently unpredictable that neither procedure is well accepted as a primary indication for an operation. Suspension of the uterus is probably justified only as part of the conservative surgical management of endometriosis or as an aid in the suspension of prolapsed ovaries that are thought to be contributing to dyspareunia.

SUGGESTED READING

Beard RW, et al: Pelvic pain in women. *Am J Obstet Gynecol* 128:566, 1977

Benson RC, et al: Atypical pelvic pain in women: Gynecologic and psychiatric considerations. *Am J Obstet Gynecol* 77:806, 1959

Lundberg WJ, et al: Laparoscopy in evaluation of pelvic pain. *Obstet Gynecol* 42:872, 1973

Renaer M, et al: Psychological aspects of chronic pelvic pain in women. *Am J Obstet Gynecol* 134:75, 1979

Taylor HC Jr: Pelvic pain based on vascular and autonomic system disorders. *Am J Obstet Gynecol* 67:1177, 1954

52

Dysmenorrhea

JOYCE M. VARGYAS, M.D.

To patients and physicians alike, dysmenorrhea (literally, "difficult monthly flow") refers to cramping pelvic pain that occurs before and during menstruation. Dysmenorrhea falls into two categories: secondary and primary. Secondary, or acquired, dysmenorrhea is defined as painful menstruation related to organic pelvic disease. Primary, or intrinsic, dysmenorrhea is defined as painful menstruation without evidence of an organic defect.

It has been estimated that approximately 50-60% of women suffer from dysmenorrhea; 10% of those women are incapacitated for 1-3 days each month, resulting in a significant loss of working hours. Fortunately, in recent years, extensive research efforts have been made with regard to both the etiology and treatment of the disorder.

SECONDARY DYSMENORRHEA

Diagnosis

Secondary dysmenorrhea is caused by underlying pelvic pathology. Although the patient may have had menstrual cramps since menarche, with secondary dysmenorrhea she is likely to describe a change in the character or location of the pain. Occasionally patients notice an increase in the severity or duration of cramping.

Beyond the history, which may be only suggestive of secondary dysmenorrhea, the pelvic examination can be helpful in establishing the diagnosis of conditions such as endometriosis and myomas. Most helpful in the diagnosis of secondary dysmenorrhea are laparoscopy, hysteroscopy, ultrasound, hysterosalpingography, and/or D&C to confirm or eliminate the finding of pelvic pathology.

Etiology and Treatment

The most frequent cause of secondary dysmenorrhea is endometriosis. Although the exact incidence of endometriosis is unknown, it may be present in nearly half of patients complaining of dysmenorrhea. The severity of pain is frequently unrelated to the extent of the disease. Some patients with severe disease have minimal symptomatology, while others, with only a few endometriotic lesions, have debilitating dysmenorrhea and may have pain at other times in their cycle. The choice of medical and/or surgical treatment depends on the severity of the disease and the needs of the individual patient in terms of reproductive function.

Adenomyosis, another leading cause of dysmenorrhea, is similar to endometriosis in both pathophysiology and type of pain. It is found more often in older women. The mainstay of treatment is hysterectomy. However, because ectopic glandular material may be secreting prostaglandins, which result in increased uterine contractions, a trial of prostaglandin inhibitors in both adenomyosis and endometriosis is worthwhile.

Pelvic congestion syndrome was an entity described in the older literature. There is no scientific evidence for the existence of this syndrome as a cause of pelvic pain. Most women with retroverted uteri and "dilated pelvic veins" are not symptomatically distinguishable from other groups of women, and therefore this diagnosis should not be entertained.

The spasmodic type of dysmenorrhea has been found to be associated with IUD use. The rate of removal of IUDs because of pain and bleeding ranges from 4% to 14% per year of use. Prostaglandin inhibitors have been used successfully to treat this type of pain and may prevent an unnecessary change in type of contraception.

Some authors believe that fibroids and endometrial polyps can increase uterine contractility and lead to a spasmodic type of dysmenorrhea. Prostaglandin levels have been shown to be higher only when menorrhagia was also present in these women, and this finding may explain the former supposition that these processes by themselves caused dysmenorrhea. Again, the treatment is either prostaglandin inhibitors, D&C, myomectomy, or hysterectomy, depending on the diagnosis and the patient's desires.

The obstructive type of dysmenorrhea is found with cervical stenosis and congenital disorders of the müllerian tract, such as rudimentary uterine horn, vaginal atresia, or imperforate hymen. The pain begins with menarche and the only treatment is surgical.

PRIMARY DYSMENORRHEA

Diagnosis

Once the recognizable causes of secondary dysmenorrhea have been excluded, the diagnosis of primary dysmenorrhea may be entertained. The diagnosis is made on the basis of the history and physical exam. Usually patients with primary dysmenorrhea have regular cycles and have experienced pain with menstruation ever since the teen-age years. The dysmenorrhea most likely began approximately 1 year after menarche, since this is a common interval between menarche and the beginning of ovulatory cycles. The patient will frequently complain of associated symptoms such as nausea, vomiting, diarrhea, dizziness, and/or headaches, all resulting from prostaglandin release. These symptoms—including pelvic and low back pain—often begin before the onset of menstrual flow. The patient may have been symptom-free while on oral contraceptives. Finally, the pelvic exam is normal.

Etiology

The prostaglandins are synthesized from phospholipids in the plasma membrane of endometrial cells. It is well known that primary dysmenorrhea occurs only in ovulatory cycles and, therefore, only in the presence of progesterone. It is believed that regression of the corpus luteum and a decrease in progesterone cause disruption of the lysosomes containing enzymes such as phospholipase, thus triggering the onset of menstruation and the conversion of phospholipids in the endometrial cell membranes into prostaglandins.

Prostaglandins have been identified and measured in endometrial tissue, and both PGE_2 and $PGF_{2\alpha}$ have been found in higher levels in the endometrium during the luteal phase than in the follicular phase of the ovulatory cycle. Moreover, it has been shown that patients with dysmenorrhea have higher endometrial levels of prostaglandins than women with no complaints of dysmenorrhea. The metabolites of prostaglandins, which may be measured in peripheral plasma samples, are also found to be elevated in women with dysmenorrhea as compared with normal subjects.

It is known that intravenous $PGF_{2\alpha}$ will produce menstrual-like cramps and intense uterine contractions increased in amplitude and frequency, plus an increased resting tone. It is believed that the resulting pain is essentially ischemic, with the release of prostaglandins causing contractions and a reduction in blood flow. It has also been postulated that the pain may be simply secondary to increased uterine activity or, more specifically, secondary to an increased sensitization of nerve terminals to pain by the prostaglandins.

Treatment

Former treatment modalities for dysmenorrhea resulted in only occasional success and certainly lacked a sound scientific basis. Narcotic medications decreased the cramping sensations, but frequently at the expense of the patient's ability to function. Cervical dilation seems to provide some relief by permitting a more rapid efflux of blood and endometrium containing prostaglandins, but the relief is only temporary. Presacral neurectomy was utilized when more conservative measures failed, but this appears to be a rather radical form of treatment.

The greatest degree of past success was achieved by the use of oral contraceptives. The inhibition of ovulation suppresses the levels of prostaglandins, thereby decreasing uterine contractions. Oral contraceptives still remain a very useful mode of therapy for the young woman who desires contraception as well as relief of dysmenorrhea.

Once the prostaglandin synthetase inhibitors were tested in well-controlled studies, the treatment of menstrual cramps was revolutionized and the missing link between prostaglandins and dysmenorrhea was discovered. Chan, Dawood, and Fuchs in 1979 gave credence to what was formerly only speculation. In a double-blind crossover study, they not only demonstrated symptomatic relief from dysmenorrhea in treatment versus control cycles, but also showed a decline in menstrual fluid levels of prostaglandins during treatment.

To date, many studies on the treatment of dysmenorrhea with prostaglandin inhibitors have been done; they have been reviewed by Dingfelder. Several prostaglandin inhibitors have now been approved for use in the treatment of dysmenorrhea: aspirin, ibuprofen (Motrin), naproxen (Naprosyn), naproxen sodium (Anaprox), and mefenamic acid (Ponstel).

Indomethacin (Indocin), phenylbutazone (Butazolidin), and oxyphenbutazone (Tandearil) are effective nonsteroidal prostaglandin inhibitors but are not approved for use in dysmenorrhea because of serious side effects. Tolmetin (Tolectin), fenoprofen (Nalfon), and sulindac (Clinoril) are also very potent but approved only for severe arthritis because of their known toxicity.

Aspirin, although approved, is the weakest of the drugs. In the usual dosages, it was not found to be any more effective than placebo.

Ibuprofen, naproxen, and naproxen sodium are classified as arylpropionic acids, a group of prostaglandin synthetase inhibitors developed in the 1970s. Ibuprofen has been shown to be more effective than indomethacin. Chan compared ibuprofen and placebo. Treatment was begun 2-3 days prior to the expected menstrual cycle at doses of 400 mg PO qid. Ibuprofen afforded good to excellent relief of pain in 100% of cycles, compared with placebo, which appeared to relieve pain in only 20% of cycles. When this "prophylactic" regimen was compared with administration of the drug on day 1 of menses, no difference was seen. It is therefore advisable to start treatment with the onset of menses to avoid administration of the medication in cases of unknown early pregnancy.

Naproxen was given at doses of 250 mg q6h and compared with placebo. In all studies pain relief was good, 61-88%. Naproxen sodium was given at doses of 275 mg q6h after an initial dose of 550 mg and was found to be far superior to placebo, with a quoted 90% success rate. It appears, then, that naproxen has a longer duration of effect than other drugs. Naproxen sodium appears to have a more rapid onset of action than other prostaglandin inhibitors. Comparative studies may indicate that their unique pharmacologic actions may make these drugs advantageous over others.

Most prostaglandin inhibitors act by blocking the enzyme cyclo-oxygenase, thereby preventing the synthesis of prostaglandins, but do not affect the prostaglandins already in the circulation. Fenamates interfere with the synthesis of prostaglandins but also act as prostaglandin antagonists by blocking the action of the prostaglandins at the target organs. The only fenamate approved for use in the United States is mefenamic acid (Ponstel). Budoff originally compared it with placebo, using 250 mg qid, and found an 84% success rate. Subsequent studies using dosages of 250 mg qid and 500 mg tid all demonstrated excellent relief of pain.

All the prostaglandin synthetase inhibitors are effective in the treatment of primary dysmenorrhea and may prove to be beneficial in some cases of secondary dysmenorrhea. The side effects of the approved drugs at the recommended dosages are minimal. Many studies have compared these drugs with placebo, but few have compared the effectiveness of one drug against another. However, such studies are probably unnecessary because in clinical practice what is effective for one patient may not be effective for another. If a trial of one prostaglandin inhibitor in two consecutive cycles fails to relieve dysmenorrhea, a different agent may be prescribed for the next cycle. In this fashion, most women with primary dysmenorrhea are able to use one of the prostaglandin inhibitors with great success.

SUGGESTED READING

Budoff PW: Use of mefenamic acid in the treatment of primary dysmenorrhea. *JAMA* 241:2713, 1979

Chan WY, Dawood MY, Fuchs F: Relief of dysmenorrhea with the prostaglandin synthetase inhibitor ibuprofen: Effect on prostaglandin levels in the menstrual fluid. *Am J Obstet Gynecol* 135:102, 1979

Dawood MY: *Dysmenorrhea.* Baltimore: Williams & Wilkins, 1981

Dingfelder R: Primary dysmenorrhea treatment with prostaglandin inhibitors: A review. *Am J Obstet Gynecol* 140:874, 1981

Halbert DR, Demurs LM: A clinical trial of indomethacin and ibuprofen in dysmenorrhea. *J Reprod Med* 21:219, 1978

Henzl MR, Massey S, Hanson FW, et al: Primary dysmenorrhea: The therapeutic challenge. *J Reprod Med* (suppl) 25:226, 1980

Lundstrom V, Green K: Endogenous levels of prostaglandin $F_{2\alpha}$ and its main metabolites in plasma and endometrium of normal and dysmenorrheic women. *Am J Obstet Gynecol* 130:640, 1978

Pickles VR: Prostaglandins in the human endometrium. *Int J Fertil* 12:335, 1967

Pickles VR, Hall WJ, Best FA, Smith GW: Prostaglandins in the endometrium and menstrual fluid from normal and dysmenorrheic subjects. *Br J Obstet Gynaecol* 12:185, 1965

Roth-Brandel V, Bygdeman M, Wiqvist N: Effect of intravenous administration of prostaglandin E_2 and $F_{2\alpha}$ on the contractility of non-pregnant human uterus in vivo. *Acta Obstet Gynecol Scand*, suppl 5, 49:19, 1970

Williams EA, Collins WP, Clayton SG: Studies in the involvement of prostaglandins in uterine symptomatology and pathology. *Br J Obstet Gynecol* 83:337, 1976

53

The Premenstrual Syndrome

JOYCE M. VARGYAS, M.D.

INTRODUCTION

Premenstrual syndrome (PMS) has received considerable attention in recent years. The astounding lack of knowledge surrounding this problem seems to be due to a combination of apathy, frustration, and the somewhat ill-defined nature of the problem itself. However, with increasing knowledge in the areas of endocrinology, psychiatry, and nutrition, an old problem is being addressed with renewed interest and different attitudes.

PMS encompasses a wide variety of symptoms, ranging in severity from very mild to debilitating. Symptoms include physical discomfort, emotional distress, or both. The syndrome is defined as a cyclical symptom complex that begins anytime from 5 to 11 days prior to the onset of menses, is unique to each patient in type and degree of symptomatology, and disappears with the onset of menses or shortly after. The syndrome appears to worsen with age and parity.

As many as 70% of women experience symptoms, with 20% of these women reporting some degree of incapacitation. Because PMS is so prevalent, the quality of life for many women is impaired and optimal working hours are needlessly sacrificed. It is therefore apparent that the problem warrants serious investigation. Although the gynecologic literature is filled with proposed theories on the etiology and the treatment of the disorder, none of the hypotheses or remedies under consideration has been conclusively tested in well-controlled studies.

DIAGNOSIS

The diagnosis is made by questioning the patient about the type and timing of her symptomatology. Symptoms may include nervous tension, anxiety, hostility, fatigue, food cravings, depression, lethargy, mood swings, decreased self-esteem, breast tenderness, abdominal bloating, and edema. The important factor in making the diagnosis is to be certain these symptoms are present only in the luteal phase. If the patient complains of these problems throughout her cycle, the diagnosis of endogenous depression or anxiety neurosis must be considered.

ETIOLOGY AND TREATMENT

The etiology of PMS has been attributed to elevated serum estrogen levels, decreased progesterone, elevated estrogen-progesterone ratio, and increased progesterone and androgens, depending on the study. Other proposed etiologies have included decreased vitamin B_6 levels, decreased magnesium levels, and vitamin A deficiency. Fluid retention and edema were felt to be secondary to elevated aldosterone in the luteal phase of premenstrual subjects. Hypoglycemia, secondary to a change in insulin receptors, a flattened glucose tolerance curve, hyperinsulinism, and increased carbohydrate tolerance, was also proposed as a possible cause of some symptoms. These findings were obtained only during the subjects' luteal phase.

Other theories pertaining to the etiology of premenstrual syndrome include elevated prolactin and vasopressin levels and, most recently, elevated levels of melanocyte-stimulating hormone and endorphin. Hormone allergy and psychosomatic problems are theories that have been discarded.

At the present time, approximately 300 different treatments for PMS may be found in the gynecologic literature—persuasive evidence for the concept that the number of theories and treatments connected with a disease process is inversely proportional to the amount of scientific knowledge surrounding the entity.

A review of the past and present literature suggests that the etiology and treatment of PMS can be divided into three schools of thought: ovarian steroid abnormalities, nutritional aberrations, and the effects of opioids on the central nervous system and hypothalamic-pituitary axis.

Peripheral steroid levels were one of the first parameters tested. Studies in this area are contradictory. Some researchers have found that progesterone levels in the luteal phase of premenstrual subjects were decreased compared with controls and stated that progesterone treatment was successful. Other investigators have found no decrease in endogenous progesterone levels, and no clinical improvement after trials of progesterone. Despite this conflict, progesterone therapy still appears to be the most popular. The recommended dose is 200-400 mg/day by suppository.

A second major approach to the problem is Abraham's elaborate hypothesis attributing all of the symptomatology and hormonal changes of PMS to dietary habits and nutritional deficiencies. Therapy depends on the individual patient's type of symptoms. High-protein diets low in salt and refined sugar are recommended. In this therapeutic regimen, magnesium is given to decrease extracellular fluid; vitamin A for acne; and vitamin E for breast tenderness.

Vitamin B_6 plays a most important role in this scheme because it is a coenzyme in the conversion of L-dopa to dopamine and an aid in the liver's conjugation of estrogen. Decreased dopamine is thought to cause depression, while increased estrogen is thought to result in anxiety. Vitamin B_6 is prescribed at a dosage of 200-800 mg/day, especially for patients with symptoms of anxiety and nervousness. More conveniently, a combined vitamin therapy for PMS is marketed as an over-the-counter medication known as Optivite.

This therapeutic approach is relatively new, and definitive conclusions concerning its efficacy await more clinical trials. Nevertheless, the benign nature of this treatment, which has no known toxicities or side effects, may warrant a trial for your patients.

A more recent approach, proposed by Reid and Yen, addresses the effect of opioids. Endorphin levels appear to be greater in the luteal phase. Midluteal elevation may be responsible for a decrease in norepinephrine and dopamine, and resulting depression. The subsequent decrease in opioids may then be responsible for the common symptoms of anxiety. Endorphins have also been shown to affect vasopressin, prostaglandins, and pancreatic cells, thereby explaining other physiologic changes during the premenstrual period. Various research groups are currently investigating the effects of narcotic antagonists on PMS.

Modes of therapy that have been found ineffective are danazol and/or bromocriptine, although these agents have been used successfully in the treatment of the isolated symptoms of breast tenderness and engorgement. Antiprostaglandin agents are of no benefit in the treatment of PMS but remain the mainstay of therapy for dysmenorrhea, and therefore may help women who complain of the physical discomforts associated with menstruation itself.

Diuretics were the most frequently prescribed drugs in the past. However, adjustments in nutritional habits seem to be far safer and more advantageous. Trials of spironolactone at dosages of 25 mg bid 7 days before the menses have been reported to be effective by one author. However, the success of aldosterone inhibition as therapy for PMS has not yet been confirmed by others.

Lithium carbonate, major and minor tranquilizers, and sedatives have been used in the past in the treatment of PMS, but the high incidence of toxicity and/or inability to function associated with these agents makes this type of therapy undesirable.

Low-dose oral contraceptives have been used with some success in a few patients and may be tried in young women who also desire contraception. However, studies have shown this therapy to be no more effective than placebo in relieving PMS symptoms.

CONCLUSION

The premenstrual syndrome remains a therapeutic problem for both physician and patient. At the present time, with so little sound scientific data available, it seems that a nutritional approach with vitamin supplementation may be the most beneficial and, at the very least, harmless. If this approach does not appear to be successful in a particular patient, one of the other modes of therapy mentioned here may be tried with great caution. It must be realized that the basis and efficacy of these therapies are not yet established. Fortunately, many investigators are making efforts to perform well-controlled studies on both the etiology and treatment of the premenstrual syndrome. It's to be hoped that the results of these studies will shed some light on this very prevalent disease entity.

SUGGESTED READING

Abraham GE: Premenstrual tension. *Curr Prob Obstet Gynecol* 3(12), August 1980

Backstrom T, Carsteusen H: Estrogen and progesterone in plasma in relation to premenstrual tension. *J Steroid Biochem* 5:257, 1974

Biskind MS: Nutritional deficiency in the etiology of menorrhagia, metrorrhagia, cystic mastitis and premenstrual tension: Treatment with vitamin B_6 complex. *J Clin Endocrinol Metab* 3:227, 1943

Greene R, Dalton K: The premenstrual syndrome. *Br Med J* 1:1007, 1953

Hargrove ST, Abraham GE: Effect of vitamin B_6 on infertility in women with the premenstrual syndrome. *Infertility* 2:315, 1979

Hendler NH: Clinical drug trial spironolactone for premenstrual syndrome. *Female Patient* 5:17, June 1980

Reid RL, Yen SSC: Premenstrual syndrome. *Am J Obstet Gynecol* 139:85, 1981

Reid RL: The premenstrual syndrome: A therapeutic enigma. *Drug Ther* 12:65, 1982

54

Diagnosis of Abnormal
Uterine Bleeding

PAUL F. BRENNER, M.D.

The differential diagnosis of diseases that can cause abnormal uterine bleeding covers almost the entire field of gynecology and some diseases that originate outside the reproductive system. When abnormal uterine bleeding is not due to an organic cause, then, by exclusion, the diagnosis of dysfunctional uterine bleeding is assumed.

Excessive uterine bleeding has been defined in quantitative terms, including menses persisting for more than 7 days, menstrual cycles less than 21 days, and total menstrual blood loss exceeding 80 ml. Rather than these specific figures, however, abnormal uterine bleeding should be defined in terms of deviation from an individual patient's established menstrual pattern: an increase of two or more sanitary pads per day or menses that last 3 or more days longer than usual.

The term abnormal uterine bleeding suggests that the source of the blood is the pelvic organs. However, blood seen in the toilet bowl or on a sanitary napkin can originate from the urinary or the gastrointestinal tract. A urinalysis and stool guaiac test should be performed if the anatomic origin of the bleeding is in doubt.

The differential diagnosis of abnormal uterine bleeding includes organic gynecologic disease, systemic disease, blood dyscrasias, iatrogenic causes, and trauma. The diagnosis of dysfunctional uterine bleeding can be established only by excluding these five categories.

ORGANIC GYNECOLOGIC DISEASE

This category includes tumors, infection of the pelvic organs, and complications of pregnancy.

Tumors

Tumors of the pelvic organs, benign or malignant, can result in abnormal uterine bleeding. The incidence of endometrial carcinoma increases with age. A guideline is that all perimenopausal and postmenopausal bleeding should be considered due to malignancy until proven otherwise. Cancer is not the most common cause of abnormal uterine bleeding in women of this age, but it is the most important. Approximately 10% of all abnormal uterine bleeding in perimenopausal women is due to cancer, and about 25% of all women with postmenopausal bleeding will have cancer.

The Papanicolaou test's value in detecting cervical cancer is well known, but it is considerably less reliable in diagnosing endometrial cancer. The incidence of endometrial carcinoma in women over the age of 35 is sufficiently high to recommend that all women in this age group with abnormal uterine bleeding undergo endometrial biopsy. If examination of an adequate sample of endometrium fails to establish the cause of the bleeding, a D&C should be performed. Women with a long history of oligo-ovulatory or anovulatory menstrual cycles have a higher incidence of endometrial carcinoma. Eighty per cent of women who develop endometrial carcinoma prior to the age of 40 years have polycystic ovarian disease. When abnormal uterine bleeding occurs in these women, their endometrial histology must be determined if they are 30 years of age or older.

Occasionally, a very young patient, who has not yet had her desired number of children, has recurrent episodes of heavy uterine bleeding at the time of menses. This bleeding can be so copious that the patient's hematocrit falls dramatically. Surgical curettage is necessary to stop the bleeding. This history suggests the presence of a submucous fibroid. If the leiomyoma is not detected during curettage, a hysterosalpingogram or hysteroscopy should be performed several days after the bleeding has ceased.

Infections

Vaginitis, cervicitis, endometritis, and salpingitis may cause abnormal uterine bleeding. Uterine and/or adnexal pain on palpation and movement of the pelvic organs, a sensation of increased warmth of the uterus and adnexal structures, and purulent material exuding from the cervical os during bimanual examination should strongly suggest the presence of infection. An elevated temperature, white blood cell count and differential, and erythrocyte sedimentation rate usually indicate infection but do not localize the organs involved in the inflammatory process. A cervical culture for gonorrhea should be taken. When the possibility of pelvic inflammatory disease is high, a Gram stain of the cervical mucus should be prepared to detect gram-negative intracellular diplococci.

Pregnancy Complications

Complications of early pregnancy are an important cause of abnormal uterine bleeding in women of reproductive age. These complications include abortions, ectopic gestations, and trophoblastic disease. A guideline to follow here is that abnormal uterine bleeding in a woman of childbearing age should be considered the result of a complication of pregnancy until proven otherwise. The history and examination must specifically look for symptoms and findings of pregnancy. Whenever appropriate, a pregnancy test is ordered.

When the clinical signs and symptoms suggest the possibility of an ectopic pregnancy, a culdocentesis should be performed to detect hemoperitoneum—nonclotting blood in the peritoneal cavity. A hematocrit should be performed on sanguinous fluid obtained by culdocentesis. A specimen that comes from lysed blood clots usually has a hematocrit of 15% or greater. A culdocentesis specimen with a hematocrit less than 15% when the peripheral hematocrit is considerably higher usually means that the specimen consists of blood-tinged fluid, possibly from a ruptured ovarian cyst. Ultrasonography is an important diagnostic modality when ectopic pregnancy is considered as part of the differential diagnosis. The presence of an intrauterine gestational sac makes the diagnosis of extrauterine gestation unlikely, although the possibility of combined intra- and extrauterine pregnancies does exist. After 5 weeks of gestation, the absence of an intrauterine gestational sac suggests the diagnosis of an ectopic pregnancy.

SYSTEMIC DISEASES

Two systemic diseases should be considered in the diagnosis of abnormal uterine bleeding: hypothyroidism and advanced liver disease. The woman with myxedema usually has amenorrhea, but lesser degrees of thyroid hypofunction are associated with increased uterine bleeding. Weight gain, marked fatigue, cold hands and feet, and failure to perspire in warm weather are symptoms and signs of hypothyroidism. An elevated serum thyroid-stimulating hormone concentration is the most reliable laboratory parameter in confirming this diagnosis.

Estrogens are conjugated in the liver. Advanced hepatic disease may cause abnormal estrogen metabolism, which results in abnormal uterine bleeding. A history of liver disease or excessive ingestion of alcohol and the physical findings of jaundice, hepatomegaly, spider hemangiomas, palmar erythema, and ascites indicate the need to order liver function tests.

BLOOD DYSCRASIAS

Idiopathic thrombocytopenic purpura, leukemia, aplastic anemias, and Minot-von Willebrand syndrome are blood dyscrasias that rarely may first present clinically as abnormal uterine bleeding. Women with a blood dyscrasia can usually be identified by a history of easy bleeding or bruising, a family history of a bleeding disorder, bleeding from other orifices, and excessive bleeding associated with minor trauma, minor surgery, or dental surgery. In addition, they may have ecchymoses or petechiae. A platelet count, examination of the stained blood smear, bleeding time, and partial thromboplastin time are ordered when the history indicates a blood dyscrasia may be likely or when therapy for dysfunctional uterine bleeding fails.

IATROGENIC CAUSES

Iatrogenic causes of abnormal uterine bleeding include estrogens, oral contraceptives, intrauterine devices, corticosteroids, androgens, anabolic agents, hypothalamic depressants, anticholinergic drugs, digitalis, and anticoagulants. There is no specific laboratory test that can determine an iatrogenic cause of abnormal uterine bleeding. A careful history is required to make the correct diagnosis.

TRAUMA

Trauma to the pelvic organs rarely results in abnormal uterine bleeding.

DIFFERENTIAL DIAGNOSIS

It is important in every patient with abnormal uterine bleeding to consider the entire differential diagnosis. Failure to make the correct diagnosis usually is the result of a hasty evaluation that did not include all of the diagnostic possibilities. All women of childbearing age with abnormal uterine bleeding should have a careful history and physical examination, Papanicolaou smear (if not done in the previous 12 months), complete blood count, pregnancy test, and a single-sample endometrial biopsy from the anterior wall of the uterine fundus. Thyroid function tests, liver function tests, studies of the clotting mechanism, Gram stain of the cervical mucus, culdocentesis, and D&C are performed only when indicated by the history and physical examination.

Menorrhagia is excessive and/or prolonged uterine bleeding that occurs at regular intervals. Metrorrhagia is uterine bleeding that occurs at irregular and frequent intervals. Heavy cyclic menstruation referred to as menorrhagia is more likely to be indicative of organic gynecologic disease than the irregular bleeding episodes described as metrorrhagia.

If a diagnosis of dysfunctional uterine bleeding is entertained, the presence or absence of ovulation should be documented by use of a basal body temperature record, serum progesterone concentration, or endometrial biopsy. A biopsy interpreted as secretory endometrium, a serum progesterone level above 3 ng/ml, or a biphasic basal body temperature curve indicates that the patient is ovulatory, that the cause of bleeding is probably organic, and that the endometrial cavity must be investigated by a D&C, hysterosalpingogram, or hysteroscopy. Besides evidence of ovulation, anemia and long-standing complaints of abnormal bleeding are indications for a study of the endometrial cavity. Submucous leiomyomas and endometrial polyps may be found to be the cause of the bleeding in as many as half of these patients. If the patient is anovulatory, or if she is ovulatory and the endometrial cavity is found to be normal, dysfunctional uterine bleeding may be diagnosed.

SUGGESTED READING

Grimes DA: Diagnostic dilatation and curettage: A reappraisal. *Am J Obstet Gynecol* 142:1, 1982

Kadar N, DeVore G, Romero R: Discriminating hCG zone: Its use in the sonographic evaluation for ectopic pregnancy. *Obstet Gynecol* 58:156, 1981

55

Treatment of Dysfunctional Uterine Bleeding

CHARLES M. MARCH, M.D.

Dysfunctional uterine bleeding (DUB) can be defined as entirely abnormal bleeding with no demonstrable organic cause. Therefore, DUB is a diagnosis of exclusion; that is, it can be made only after a complete investigation has ruled out a wide variety of organic lesions.

This diagnosis should be applied only to functional derangements of the hypothalamic-pituitary-ovarian-endometrial axis. Dysfunctional bleeding occurs most often at the extremes of the reproductive years—ages when anovulatory cycles are common. Approximately half of patients are over 40 years old and another 20% are adolescents. In some reported series, DUB has been responsible for up to 10% of all hospital admissions and may be the indication for 25% of all gynecologic surgery. The full impact of dysfunctional bleeding in young women may not be noted until later in life, because a high percentage of these patients are infertile secondary to anovulation. The availability of safe medications for the induction of ovulation has lessened the significance of this feature of DUB.

ETIOLOGY

The predominant cause of DUB is prolonged stimulation of the endometrium by estrogen. This stimulation needs to be prolonged, but not necessarily excessive. It occurs following periods of chronic anovulation secondary to faulty hypothalamic-pituitary-ovarian interactions. Unopposed estrogen stimulation leads to a continuously proliferating endometrium. The endometrium may outgrow its blood supply, or endometrial nutrition may be deficient because of the persistence of a dense acid mucopolysaccharide ground substance. Other explanations include asynchronous development of the stroma, glands, and blood vessels, or overdevelopment of the Golgi-lysosomal complex with the release of excessive amounts of hydrolytic enzymes. Excessive amounts of prostaglandins cause irregular contraction and relaxation of spiral arterioles and thus contribute to endometrial breakdown. All of these conditions can lead to the irregular endometrial shedding characteristic of DUB.

In a small percentage of patients, DUB occurs during ovulatory cycles. In these instances, abnormal bleeding is due to persistence of the corpus luteum (Halban's syndrome). Other causes of ovulatory DUB are defects in the corpus luteum due to either a shortened life span or to inadequate progesterone production, and an overactive fibrinolytic system, which would initiate abnormal bleeding. However, the effect of fibrinolysis on normal uterine bleeding is unknown. Finally, DUB may be caused by a deficiency of endometrial receptors (for either estrogen or progesterone), which would cause an abnormal endometrial response to a normal hormonal milieu.

DIAGNOSIS

A careful history will usually permit a diagnosis of DUB. The site of bleeding must be established with certainty. Differentiation of cyclic from acyclic bleeding is critical. It may be presumed that cyclic bleeding is associated with ovulation, but tests will be necessary to prove that association. The history should include at least the dates of the last three episodes of bleeding, the presence of pain or clots, and the occurrence of premenstrual molimina. The use of medications, as well as a complete contraceptive history and symptoms of pregnancy, should be noted. The extent of bleeding should be assessed from the number of pads used per day as well as the degree of saturation. A history of any extragenital sources of bleeding or easy bruising should be obtained as well.

The extensiveness of the laboratory investigation must be individualized. Following a complete physical examination, studies of the patient's cervical cytology are indicated. Because a complication of an intrauterine or ectopic pregnancy must always be considered, a rapid serum pregnancy test should be done. A complete blood count is also mandatory. In all patients, except perhaps the very young, an endometrial biopsy should be obtained. A single sample taken with a small Rock-Garcia curette, beginning at the top of the fundus, where the response to hormone stimulation is maximal, is usually sufficient. In order to interpret the biopsy properly, the histologic pattern must be correlated with the bleeding pattern.

A treatment guideline for those with DUB is this: A patient who has had only one episode of minimal or moderate bleeding and whose hemoglobin is unchanged may be merely observed. With repeated episodes, despite an unchanged hemoglobin concentration, hormonal therapy should be instituted. For those who have repeated episodes and/or those who have evidence of anemia, a combination of hormonal and iron therapy should be employed. If hypovolemia occurs, regardless of the number of bleeding episodes, curettage and transfusions are mandatory. Curettage should be performed in all cases involving patients over 35 years of age, patients who have failed to respond to hormonal therapy, and patients exhibiting profuse bleeding. Patients who fail to respond to hormonal therapy frequently have a submucosal myoma or endometrial polyps, and therefore hysteroscopy is a valuable adjunct at the time of curettage.

HORMONE THERAPY

Although a variety of medications have been used, including estrogens, progestins, androgens, ergot derivatives, oral contraceptives, and thyroid preparations, therapy should be restricted to estrogens and progestins. For treatment of the acute episode of bleeding, three regimens have been recommended: oral contraceptives alone, progestins alone, and sequential estrogen-progestin therapy. Studies at the University of Southern California have indicated that the most effective regimen for controlling the acute episode, as well as for reducing the frequency of recurrences, is oral administration of conjugated estrogens 2.5 mg 4 times a day. If this regimen is successful, the bleeding will stop, or be markedly reduced, within 2 or 3 days. If so, treatment should be continued for 21 days and medroxyprogesterone acetate (Provera) 10 mg/day should be added for the last 5 days. If the bleeding persists beyond the first 2 or 3 days of therapy, the dose of conjugated estrogens should be doubled for another 2 days. If the bleeding then stops, this higher dose should be continued for the full 21 days with medroxyprogesterone acetate added for the last 5 days. If the bleeding persists despite the higher dose, a D&C should be performed. Intravenous estrogens are more expensive than the oral forms and offer no advantage over oral administration with respect to either speed or efficacy.

Oral contraceptives, at 3 or 4 times the usual dose, are as effective as estrogen alone in arresting the initial bleeding episode. However, the rate of recurrent abnormal bleeding after the medication has been stopped is high. Although pharmacologic doses of estrogen are used to control the bleeding, the sequential estrogen-progestin regimen mimics the hormonal events of the normal cycle. First the estrogen stimulates endometrial growth by causing cellular proliferation, DNA synthesis, mitotic activity, growth of glands, stroma, and vessels, and protein synthesis. Estrogen increases its own endometrial receptors and causes increased synthesis of progesterone receptors. Then the progesterone inhibits endometrial growth by reducing estrogen receptors and mitosis and increasing glycogen storage. The duplication of normal hormonal events may induce more complete sloughing of the endometrium than is seen with the dyssynchronous endometrial response to combined estrogen-progestin preparations.

If the original endometrial biopsy revealed proliferative endometrium, the patient should receive 5 mg of medroxyprogesterone acetate daily for the first 10 days of every month to prevent unopposed estrogen stimulation. This will differentiate the endometrium into a secretory phase and avoid recurrences. If the biopsy revealed secretory endometrium and if the abnormal bleeding recurs, a mechanical defect should be suspected and investigated by either hysterosalpingography or hysteroscopy. After the acute episode, patients who have had normal cyclic bleeding in the past and who desire contraception may use oral contraceptives at the usual dose. However, the continued use of oral contraceptives for anovulatory patients is controversial because many of these women develop a more pronounced endocrinopathy (amenorrhea and/or galactorrhea) as time passes. These symptoms would be masked by pill use, which would produce regular bleeding and inhibit lactation. Therefore a pretreatment prolactin determination and repeat measurements at yearly intervals during pill use are advised. Following the arrest of anovulatory bleeding, the patient who wishes to conceive may have ovulation induced with clomiphene citrate (Clomid, Serophene).

OTHER TREATMENTS

Other drugs, such as ergot derivatives and inhibitors of plasminogen activators, are not very effective for the treatment of DUB and have a high incidence of side effects. Thyroid replacement obviously is indicated only for those with documented hypothyroidism. Androgens may be used to arrest abnormal bleeding, but offer no advantages over estrogens and may cause masculinization. Recently prostaglandin synthetase inhibitors have been shown to be helpful in reducing blood loss in women with menorrhagia. Full evaluation of the use of these agents for the treatment of DUB is currently being undertaken.

CONCLUSION

The prognosis for the patient with DUB depends upon the presence of other gynecologic or systemic disorders as well as the desire for fertility. As with all disorders, a thorough investigation and aggressive management are likely to resolve the acute episode quickly and to reduce the frequency of recurrences.

SUGGESTED READING

Aksel S, Jones GS: Etiology and treatment of dysfunctional uterine bleeding. *Obstet Gynecol* 44:1, 1974

Bromberg YM, Bercovici B: Occult intermenstrual bleeding about the time of ovulation. *Fertil Steril* 7:71, 1956

DeVore GR, Owens O, Kase N: Use of intravenous Premarin® in the treatment of dysfunctional uterine bleeding—A double-blind randomized control study. *Obstet Gynecol* 59:285, 1982

Fraser IS, Baird DT: Blood production and ovarian secretion rates of estradiol-17β and estrone in ovaries with dysfunctional uterine bleeding. *J Clin Endocrinol Metab* 39:564, 1964

Fraser IS, Michie EA, Wide L: Pituitary gonadotropins and ovarian function in adolescent dysfunctional uterine bleeding. *J Clin Endocrinol Metab* 37:407, 1973

Hallberg L, Hogdahl AM, Nilsson L: Menstrual blood loss—A population study. *Acta Obstet Gynecol Scand* 45:320, 1966

March CM: Dysfunctional uterine bleeding. In Mishell DR Jr, Davajan V, eds: *Reproductive Endocrinology, Infertility and Contraception*. Philadelphia: FA Davis, 1979, pp 299-309

Winter JSD, Faiman C: The development of cyclic pituitary-gonadal function in adolescent females. *J Clin Endocrinol Metab* 37:714, 1973

56

Evaluation and Management of Adnexal Masses

JOHN B. SCHLAERTH, M.D.

EVALUATION

In evaluating an adnexal mass, physiologic enlargement of the normal pelvic viscera must be borne in mind. Stool in the rectum, a full urinary bladder, and a pregnant uterus can all masquerade as a pelvic or adnexal mass. A pelvic examination is not adequate unless these possibilities are considered.

Another important point is the technique of examination. An adnexal mass usually occupies the posterior pelvis behind the uterus. Bimanual abdominal-vaginal examination will detect only those masses large enough to fill the posterior pelvis and extend out of the cul-de-sac. The only proper means of clinically evaluating the adnexa is the bimanual abdominal-*recto*vaginal examination. The diagnostic work-up and therapy for adnexal masses depend on the stage of reproductive life in which they occur: the premenarchal, reproductive, or postmenopausal years.

Premenarchal Years

Adnexal masses are rarely detected on pelvic examination in premenarchal girls. Most commonly, a pelvic-abdominal mass gives rise to symptoms of abdominal enlargement, pain, and perception of a mass. Physiologic causes of ovarian enlargement are rare prior to menarche. Consequently, all pelvic-abdominal masses must be presumed to be neoplastic and require a laparotomy without delay. The most common ovarian tumors in this age group are dermoid cysts and malignant germ-cell tumors, which occur with approximately equal frequency.

Reproductive Years

Physiologic cystic enlargement of the ovaries is common in women who ovulate regularly. These are either follicle or corpus luteum cysts. They may achieve a size as large as 10 cm on pelvic examination and are invariably unilateral. At times they cause pain secondary to rupture, hemorrhage, or torsion. Because these physiologic cysts are self-limiting, a conservative course is advisable. Thus, a unilateral cystic adnexal mass less than 10 cm in size can be followed for regression over 4-8 weeks.

It is best to inhibit the pituitary gonadotropins with oral contraceptives during this observation period. If the mass has not appreciably diminished in size or disappeared at the end of this observation period, it must be considered to be a neoplasm and laparotomy is advisable. A cystic adnexal mass may also be detected during pregnancy. In general, the same rules of management apply as for ovulating women, except that oral contraceptives are not used. If the mass is detected very early in gestation, ectopic pregnancy must be ruled out as soon as possible.

If a woman develops a unilateral, cystic adnexal mass while taking oral contraceptives, the mass must be assumed to be neoplastic and an observation time of 4-8 weeks before laparotomy is not warranted. A solid ovarian tumor, bilateral cystic ovarian tumors, and adnexal cysts greater than 10 cm are all presumed to be pelvic neoplasms and laparotomy is advised.

Postmenopausal Years
With cessation of ovarian function, the ovaries gradually grow smaller over a period of several months. Since physiologic cysts cannot develop in these atrophic ovaries, an adnexal mass in a postmenopausal woman is presumed to be neoplastic. Furthermore, since women in this age range have the highest incidence of ovarian carcinoma, immediate laparotomy and surgical treatment are indicated.

The concept of a postmenopausal palpable ovary (PMPO) has become popular. The basis for this concept is that a completely involuted ovary should not be palpable on pelvic examination, and therefore any palpable mass in the adnexa must be viewed with suspicion. While there are few data on operative findings in women in this category, the advanced stage and high mortality of most cases of ovarian cancer at the time of diagnosis emphasize the need for early diagnosis. We therefore prefer to perform a laparoscopy or laparotomy when a PMPO is found, as it could represent an early, curable ovarian carcinoma. How to proceed becomes more difficult when a small mass appears in a woman of advanced age who has other medical problems, such as heart, lung, or kidney disease or diabetes, that make anesthesia risky. In this setting, culdocentesis or paracentesis, with peritoneal lavage to obtain samples for cytology, and serial pelvic examinations to detect enlargement of the mass may be more appropriate.

PREOPERATIVE WORK-UP

Once a patient is found to have an adnexal mass that requires surgery, a number of diagnostic tests bear mention. A chest x-ray and ECG are routine preanesthetic tests. The chest x-ray may reveal a hydrothorax, which can be present with benign or malignant ovarian neoplasms. Pregnancy testing should be done in women of childbearing age. An intravenous pyelogram will delineate the number and position of the kidneys as well as ureter and bladder anatomy. Because adnexal pathology can require retroperitoneal surgery near a ureter, it is wise to obtain this study in most patients. Those with relatively small, freely mobile masses may be exceptions.

Abdominal X-rays

The most common ovarian neoplasm is the dermoid cyst. The majority of dermoid cysts can be diagnosed on abdominal x-ray. The findings include a halo surrounding the neoplasm, calcium specks scattered throughout the mass, or teeth. Preoperative diagnosis of a dermoid cyst is important, as it may have a bearing on the choice of incision and timing of the operation.

Ultrasound

Sonography of the pelvis in patients with an adnexal mass has not proven to be a useful clinical adjunct to abdominal x-rays. It is hoped that refinement of this technique will make it possible to determine whether a neoplasm is malignant or benign and to distinguish functional from neoplastic cysts.

Barium Enema

We do not routinely perform a barium enema in all patients who have adnexal masses. The primary purpose of a barium enema would be to determine whether an adnexal mass is caused by colonic disease. Candidates include patients over the age of 35 who have a history suggestive of diverticulitis, patients who have occult blood in the stool, patients with a history suggestive of appendiceal abscess, and patients in whom the irregularity, fixation, or location of the mass makes one consider a colonic cause.

Sigmoidoscopy is considered an adjunct to the barium enema in evaluating the patient with an adnexal mass that could be colonic in origin.

Upper Gastrointestinal Series

An upper gastrointestinal series is done only if symptoms suggest upper abdominal disease, if there is occult blood in the stool, if there is evidence of metastatic ovarian cancer, or if there are bilateral and/or solid pelvic masses.

Laparoscopy

The place of laparoscopy in the management of an adnexal mass is unclear. Non-neoplastic adnexal masses that can be diagnosed and managed completely by laparoscopy are few. In our experience, endometriosis, asymptomatic hydrosalpinx, and perhaps polycystic ovaries are the only entities that fit into this category. The patient's history usually suggests the diagnosis. There has been some mention of aspiration of benign-appearing ovarian cysts discovered at laparoscopy. From a risk/benefit standpoint, this appears difficult to justify.

Metastatic Neoplasms

Not uncommonly, the ovary is a site of metastatic cancer. The site of the primary cancer is usually the breast, colon, endometrium, or stomach. Most of the time the primary malignancy is obvious, but occasionally the ovarian metastasis is the initial finding while the primary cancer remains clinically occult. Solid ovarian masses, especially if they are bilateral, strongly suggest primary disease elsewhere. Mammography, barium enema, upper gastrointestinal series, and endometrial biopsy should be done in this situation.

SUGGESTED READING

Barber HRK, Graber EA: The PMPO syndrome (postmenopausal palpable ovary syndrome). *Obstet Gynecol* 38:921, 1971

Spanos WJ: Preoperative hormonal therapy of cystic adnexal masses. *Am J Obstet Gynecol* 116:551, 1973

57

Ectopic Pregnancy

PAUL F. BRENNER, M.D.

An ectopic pregnancy is the implantation of the blastocyst outside the endometrial cavity, most frequently in a fallopian tube (95%), but occasionally in the abdominal cavity, an ovary, or the cervix. Tubal gestations most commonly occur in the ampulla, but also may occur in the isthmus, infundibulum, or interstitial portion—in that order of frequency. Ectopic pregnancy is the cause of approximately 12% of all maternal deaths in the United States and accounts for the majority of maternal deaths in the first trimester. The ratio of maternal deaths to ectopic pregnancies varies between 1:250 and 1:800. The most common cause of death is sudden hemorrhage.

Ectopic pregnancy can occur in either parous or nonparous women at any time during the reproductive years. The incidence varies greatly throughout the world, ranging from 1:28 to 1:200 pregnancies.

Approximately three-quarters of patients with extrauterine pregnancies report having abnormal uterine bleeding. A similar proportion indicate a delay in menses of at least 2 weeks. Abdominal pain is a very frequent symptom. It is most often generalized, but can be unilateral; 20% of patients describe the pain as radiating to the shoulder or back. Syncopal symptoms are reported by one-third of women with ectopic pregnancies.

On the initial pelvic examination, the uterus is rarely estimated to exceed 8 weeks' gestational size unless there is coexisting pathology (leiomyomata uteri) associated with the extrauterine gestation. A unilateral adnexal mass is felt on bimanual examination in approximately one-half the cases, and 5-10% of women with an ectopic gestation pass a uterine cast.

DIAGNOSIS

The most important concept relating to ectopic pregnancy is that failure to think of it means failure to diagnose it.

Levels of human chorionic gonadotropin (hCG) are lower in an ectopic pregnancy than in an intrauterine pregnancy of a corresponding gestational age. Therefore, the frequency with which the pregnancy test is positive in ectopic gestations depends on the sensitivity of the test. The agglutination inhibition pregnancy tests have a sensitivity between 200 and 700 mIU/ml hCG and are positive in 80-85% of ectopic pregnancies. Radioimmunoassays of hCG and its β-subunit (β-hCG) have sensitivities varying from 3 to 10 mIU/ml hCG and are almost always positive. The latter tests have two limitations: First, the length of time necessary to complete the assay may be too long to be practical in an emergency. Second, the sensitivity of the hCG assay is so great that midcycle luteinizing hormone (LH) peaks and menopausal LH can cross-react with hCG and cause false-positive results. The β-subunit assay is specific for hCG and will not cross-react with LH. The radioreceptor assay (RRA) has a sensitivity of 100-200 mIU/ml hCG and can be performed in 1-2 hours. The RRA is positive in 89% of ectopic pregnancies. Serial RRAs performed 48-72 hours apart may improve the diagnosis of unruptured ectopic pregnancy, but hCG assays cannot differentiate ectopic pregnancy from other problems of early gestation, such as threatened or missed abortion.

Culdocentesis (performed with a 20-gauge, 3.5-inch spinal needle) is a useful diagnostic procedure in determining the presence of a ruptured ectopic pregnancy. Nonclotting blood obtained by culdocentesis indicates the presence of blood in the peritoneal cavity but does not locate the site of the bleeding. A hematocrit should be performed on all samples of blood collected by culdocentesis. When the hematocrit of the specimen is less than 15% and the peripheral hematocrit is considerably greater, the sample obtained from the peritoneal cavity is most likely, but not necessarily, blood-tinged fluid from an ovarian cyst. Conversely, if the hematocrit of the specimen is greater than 15%, intraperitoneal bleeding has occurred. The accuracy of culdocentesis in the diagnosis of ectopic pregnancy is approximately 95%.

The preoperative hematocrit obtained from patients with ectopic pregnancies has little relation to the amount of the hemoperitoneum found at the time of surgery. Rapid blood loss can occur in patients with ruptured extrauterine gestations before this loss is reflected in the peripheral blood count. The preoperative white blood cell count is elevated in approximately one-half of these patients and may even exceed 20,000/cu mm. Unless an inflammatory process coexists with the ectopic pregnancy, the preoperative temperature usually does not rise above 99.6°F.

The use of ultrasound has been applied to the diagnosis of ectopic pregnancy. If an intrauterine gestational sac is visualized by ultrasonography, the likelihood of an extrauterine gestation is extremely small, although combined intrauterine and extrauterine gestations are possible. After 5 weeks' gestation, if an intrauterine sac is not demonstrated by ultrasonography, the possibility of an ectopic pregnancy must be strongly considered. As the resolution of the equipment and experience of the ultrasonographer improve, the reliability of this diagnostic procedure increases.

For unknown reasons, an ectopic gestation is found more commonly in the right fallopian tube (57%) than the left (43%). In order not to overlook the possibility of an ectopic pregnancy, a physician is obligated to confirm the presence of fetal tissue following a therapeutic abortion. The absence of fetal tissue suggests either that the attempt to evacuate the pregnancy failed or that an ectopic pregnancy is present.

ETIOLOGY

Any process that impedes the passage of the fertilized ovum into the uterine cavity may result in ectopic pregnancy. A history of pelvic inflammatory disease (salpingitis) is associated with a subsequent increased risk of ectopic gestation. Abdominal pelvic surgery, particularly in the area involving or immediately adjacent to the reproductive organs, is another etiologic factor. A history of infertility surgery, particularly salpingostomy, has been shown to be associated with a higher incidence of ectopic pregnancy. About 15-25% of pregnancies following tubal sterilization surgery, including fulguration as well as bilateral tubal ligation, are ectopic. A history of tubal sterilization surgery does not exclude ectopic pregnancy from the differential diagnosis in a woman of reproductive age who has abnormal uterine bleeding and/or lower abdominal-pelvic pain. Pelvic tumors or anomalous development of the salpinx may also hinder transport of the fertilized egg through the fallopian tube.

An increased incidence of ectopic pregnancy is related to certain contraceptive modalities. Women conceiving with an IUD in situ have about a 10-fold higher proportion of ectopic pregnancies (5%) than women who conceive not using an IUD (0.5%). This finding does not indicate that the IUD causes ectopic pregnancies, but that the IUD is 98% effective in preventing intrauterine pregnancies and less effective (90%) in preventing pregnancy in the fallopian tubes. Therefore, the ratio of extrauterine to intrauterine gestations is increased in IUD acceptors who become pregnant with the IUD in situ.

Women who conceive while using gestagen-only oral contraceptives also have a higher incidence of ectopic pregnancy. Women using either an IUD or a gestagen-only oral contraceptive may present with abnormal uterine bleeding and/or abdominal-pelvic pain. The etiology of the bleeding and/or pain should not automatically be attributed to the method of contraception. The possibility of ectopic pregnancy, as well as other organic causes of these complaints, must be considered.

TREATMENT

The treatment of ectopic pregnancy is surgical. The surgical procedure depends on the patient's desire for future fertility, the presence or absence of the contralateral tube, the appearance of the contralateral tube, the presence of a ruptured or unruptured tubal gestation, and the amount of salpinx involved in the ectopic gestation. For women not desiring future fertility, a salpingectomy is performed and should include a resection of approximately one-half of the interstitial portion of the involved fallopian tube.

The abdominal approach is preferred over the vaginal one. Attempts to treat ectopic pregnancies via the vaginal route have required a laparotomy in more than half the cases and are therefore to be discouraged. Elective ipsilateral oophorectomy is not advocated. If the remaining ovary following ipsilateral oophorectomy requires extirpation at a later date, the patient will be left without any functional ovarian tissue. At the present time there is no evidence that fertility is improved or the incidence of ectopic pregnancy is reduced by performing an ipsilateral oophorectomy in the treatment of ectopic pregnancy. Only when the ipsilateral ovary is involved in the ectopic pregnancy, or is diseased, should it be removed.

Conservative surgery for unruptured tubal pregnancy should be preferred for young patients when the involved tube has normal fimbriae and the contralateral fallopian tube is absent or diseased. In achieving the highest term pregnancy rate and the lowest repeat ectopic pregnancy rate, linear salpingostomy appears to be superior to either tubal resection or manual expression of the ovisac, although the procedure to be performed depends upon the findings at the time of laparotomy. When the contralateral tube is found to be diseased, tuboplastic surgery should be delayed until an optimal time.

A unilateral salpingectomy and hysterectomy may be performed if the patient has no desire for future fertility, the contralateral tube has already been removed, and her medical and surgical condition permits this more extensive surgery without undue risk. With in vitro fertilization now a reality, patients desiring further children should not have a hysterectomy even if both tubes have been removed. A hysterectomy may be the procedure of choice if the patient has sustained a ruptured cornual pregnancy.

The informed consent for women taken to the operating room with the preoperative diagnosis of ectopic pregnancy should cover a wide variety of diagnostic and therapeutic procedures: laparoscopy, exploratory laparotomy, unilateral salpingectomy, the conservative tubal surgical options of linear salpingostomy and segmental tubal resection, hysterectomy, bilateral salpingo-oophorectomy, and appendectomy.

The decision to perform ancillary surgical procedures, particularly appendectomy, at the time of treatment of ectopic pregnancy is also controversial, but the literature suggests that operative morbidity and mortality are not increased when appendectomy is performed along with salpingectomy.

About half the women who have had an ectopic pregnancy fail to conceive afterward. Failure to conceive is as high as 70% when the ectopic pregnancy occurs in a previously nonparous woman. The incidence of repeat ectopic pregnancy is 10-20%.

SUGGESTED READING

Brenner PF, Benedetti T, Mishell DR Jr: Ectopic pregnancy following tubal sterilization surgery. *Obstet Gynecol* 49:323, 1977

Brenner PF, Roy S, Mishell DR Jr: Ectopic pregnancy: A study of 300 consecutive surgically treated cases. *JAMA* 243:673, 1980

Cole T, Corlett RC: Chronic ectopic pregnancy. *Obstet Gynecol* 58:63, 1982

Kadar N, DeCherney AH, Romero R: Receiver operating characteristic (ROC) curve analysis of the relative efficacy of a single and serial chorionic gonadotropin determinations in the early diagnosis of ectopic pregnancy. *Fertil Steril* 37:542, 1982

Sherman D, Langer R, Sadovsky G, Bukovsky I, Caspi E: Improved fertility following ectopic pregnancy. *Fertil Steril* 37:497, 1982

58

Uterine Myomas

LESTER T. HIBBARD, M.D.

Myomas of the uterus are a familiar problem to gynecologists as they are the most common kind of uterine tumor. Myomas occur in 20% of women past the age of 35. The majority of patients with myomas are asymptomatic when first encountered and have multiple firm tumors of varying size that are easily palpated by bimanual pelvic examination. While there is no good explanation for their frequency, estrogen appears to be an etiologic factor, since myomas are of clinical importance only during reproductive life and tend to enlarge during pregnancy or when combination oral contraceptives are prescribed.

Myomas range in size from microscopic lesions to huge tumor masses filling the entire abdomen. They are classified according to location as submucous, intramural, or subserous and can be found extending between the leaves of the broad ligament or on the cervix and round ligaments. They are surrounded by a pseudocapsule of areolar tissue from which they derive a somewhat meager blood supply consisting of one or two major vessels and multiple small arteries arranged in random fashion.

DIAGNOSIS

The diagnosis of myomas can usually be made by a pelvic examination, but other causes of uterine enlargement and asymmetry, such as pregnancy, adenomyosis, and congenital anomalies, must be considered. In addition, other kinds of pelvic masses, including ovarian cysts, hydrosalpinx, and endometriosis, can be confused with myomas. Calcified myomas can be diagnosed by x-ray, and submucous tumors can be detected by hysterography, hysteroscopy, or curettage. In puzzling cases, ultrasonography and pelvic pneumography have been helpful.

TREATMENT

Conservative Management

The majority of women with myomas require no treatment and can be followed with periodic pelvic examinations every 6 or 12 months to detect evidence of tumor growth. The indications for surgery depend on symptoms, complications, and the patient's age and desire for pregnancy as well as the size, location, and growth pattern of the tumor.

Hysterectomy

Submucous myomas frequently require hysterectomy because of associated hypermenorrhea, which is probably due to a combination of increased endometrial surface, interference with uterine contractility, increased venular ectasia, and incomplete regeneration of the endometrium. But in planning therapy it should be kept in mind that the bleeding of a myomatous uterus can also be due to other organic causes, such as endometrial polyps, an undetected cancer, or pregnancy as well as hormonal dysfunction, and these possibilities should first be ruled out by appropriate diagnostic procedures. The medical management of bleeding associated with submucous myomas is unrewarding. Hormonal therapy is unsatisfactory, and irradiation produces menopausal symptoms and causes an increase in the risk of subsequent uterine cancer in these patients.

A second indication for hysterectomy is pain produced by infarction, torsion, infection, or impaction of the myomas within the bony pelvis. A third indication is obstruction producing urinary retention, ureteral dilation, or excessive constipation.

Size of itself is an important consideration because an enlarged uterus can mask significant coexisting pelvic disease, such as ovarian neoplasms, particularly if the uterus is larger than the size of a 12-14-week pregnancy.

Rapid growth is another indication for hysterectomy both because additional delay increases the likelihood of operative complications and because of the possibility of uterine sarcoma. The risk of sarcoma associated with myomas is quite small, probably a fraction of 1%, and there is no conclusive evidence that sarcomatous degeneration of pre-existing myomas occurs.

In preparing the patient for surgery, the need for special diagnostic procedures, such as an intravenous pyelogram or barium enema, must be evaluated, particularly if the diagnosis is uncertain. Intravenous pyelography (including a lateral view) is of particular value in demonstrating ureteral displacement by an intraligamentous myoma or even a rare pelvic kidney. But the surgeon must remember that most ureteral injuries are due to failure to expose and identify the ureter in complicated cases rather than to failure to order an intravenous pyelogram.

When surgical exposure is adequate, there are few operative complications. On occasion it is useful to gain better exposure by enucleating one or more large myomas prior to hysterectomy or to perform a subtotal hysterectomy before removing the cervical stump. Because many patients having a hysterectomy for any reason will be in their 40s, a decision regarding ovarian preservation will be necessary. The appropriate age for prophylactic oophorectomy is still a matter of opinion, although age 45 seems to be the national consensus. The risk of dying from ovarian cancer must be balanced against the risk of dying from a complication of estrogen deprivation, such as a fractured hip secondary to osteoporosis. If the decision is to preserve the ovaries, the uterine cavity should be inspected before the abdomen is closed to rule out an undetected malignancy.

Myomectomy

Infertility is an occasional indication for an operation if no other cause for infertility can be demonstrated and if one or more myomas appear to be in a location that might interfere with fertilization or nidation.

Myomectomy in the treatment of infertility or as an alternative to hysterectomy is a relatively simple procedure that gives good results if a few precautions are followed. First, it is important to minimize blood loss by the use of a Bonney clamp or a tourniquet at the uterocervical junction or by local injection of a solution containing 5-10 units of vasopressin (Pitressin) in 10-20 ml of saline. Vasopressin is more effective than a clamp or tourniquet but has the theoretical disadvantage of masking the fact that hemostasis is inadequate. Second, whenever possible, the uterine incisions should be made on the anterior uterine surface to minimize postoperative adhesions. Third, an attempt should be made to remove multiple myomas through one incision. Fourth, a uterine suspension will reduce the risk of adhesions.

Following myomectomy, about 40% of patients will achieve a successful pregnancy and 20% will have a recurrence of myomas necessitating subsequent hysterectomy. It is also possible to remove small submucous myomas by fulguration under hysteroscopic observation. At present this method is probably best left to those physicians who are expert hysteroscopists.

Some submucous myomas become pedunculated and extend through the cervical canal. If the pedicle is elongated, as is usually the case, the myoma can be removed per vaginam by means of a snare or by twisting until the pedicle breaks. The risk of hemorrhage from the base is small, and additional surgery, such as hysterectomy, should be deferred for 6-8 weeks to minimize the risk of operative infection. Often the myomectomy is curative.

Myomas in Pregnancy

A pregnant patient with myomas is at risk of hemorrhage and infarction. If the tumor is submucous or intramural, the patient should be treated medically with a reasonable expectation that the process will subside without having produced premature labor. Only pedunculated subserous myomas that have become infarcted should be surgically removed from a pregnant uterus. But if myomectomy becomes necessary at the time of an abdominal delivery, hemostasis is usually better than anticipated because of myometrial contraction.

SUGGESTED READING

Babaknia A, Rack JA, Jones HW: Pregnancy success following myomectomy for infertility. *Fertil Steril* 30:644, 1978

Brooks GG, Stage HM: The surgical management of prolapsed pedunculated submucous leiomyomas. *Surg Gynecol Obstet* 141:397, 1975

Kobayashi M: *Illustrated Manual of Ultrasonography in Obstetrics and Gynecology*, ed 2. New York: Igaku Shoin, 1980, pp 30-42

Neuwirth RS, Amin HK: Excision of submucous fibroids with hysteroscopic control. *Am J Obstet Gynecol* 126:95, 1976

Ramsey B, Frederick I: The occasional need for myomectomy. *Obstet Gynecol* 53:437, 1979

59

Rectovaginal Injuries

LESTER T. HIBBARD, M.D.

The great majority of rectal injuries encountered in gynecologic practice are due to previous obstetric trauma and consist of either complete perineal tears extending into the rectal wall or rectovaginal fistulas. The successful surgical correction of rectovaginal injuries depends on healthy tissues at the site of injury and good surgical technique, as well as the avoidance of postoperative infection. Under adverse circumstances, even the simplest of operative repairs can fail.

If the fistula or tear is the result of recent trauma or the breakdown of a surgical repair, the operation must be delayed until the injured tissues are free of edema and induration or other evidence of residual infection. This process takes at least 8 weeks, and often longer. On the average, the appropriate waiting period appears to be 12 weeks. Steroids to hasten the disappearance of the inflammatory reaction are not recommended because they interfere with wound healing.

PREOPERATIVE PREPARATION

Preoperative preparation of patients with either perineal tears or rectovaginal fistulas is an important part of the total management of these injuries. Preoperative preparation includes evacuation of the bowel, preferably by at least two cleansing saline enemas. The use of castor oil is often disappointing because it may cause leakage of liquid feces during the operation. In addition, the patient should receive either an antibiotic bowel preparation or a regimen of antibiotic prophylaxis. One antibiotic bowel preparation begins 24 hours before surgery with three oral doses of 1 gm of neomycin and 1 gm of erythromycin every 8 hours. In most situations antibiotic prophylaxis is preferable not only because it is simpler and requires less preoperative hospitalization, but also because the perfect method of antibiotic bowel preparation has yet to be devised.

One effective regimen of antibiotic prophylaxis is cefoxitin (Mefoxin) 1 gm IV on call to surgery and then 1 gm IV every 6 hours for 3-5 days. Other antibiotic regimens give similar results. The use of antibiotics is extremely important because of the considerable risk of postoperative infection, leading to operative failure.

COMPLETE PERINEAL TEAR

A complete perineal tear can be effectively repaired by a layer closure or the Warren flap procedure. Nonabsorbable sutures should be avoided because they can form a nidus of infection and secondary fistula formation. Either chromic catgut or polyglycolic sutures are satisfactory. It does not matter whether a submucosal or through-and-through stitch is used to close the rectal mucosa. What is important is that the muscular coat of the rectum and its fascia be reapproximated with a second layer of sutures. Repair of the rectal sphincter usually requires that some time be devoted to recovering the well-retracted torn ends. The use of a paradoxical incision in the reapproximated sphincter is seldom necessary, but pubococcygeal muscles should be reapproximated because they contribute to fecal continence. In addition, the perineal body and vaginal sphincter should be repaired to restore normal vaginal function.

RECTOVAGINAL FISTULA

A rectovaginal fistula can be repaired either by excision with a three-layer closure of vagina, rectal muscular coat, and rectal mucosa or by laying open the fistulous tract by means of an episioproctotomy, followed by excision of the tract and a three-layer closure. The latter technique is usually to be preferred whenever the fistula involves the perineal body or multiple fistulous tracts are suspected. But with either procedure—as with the repair of a complete perineal tear—careful approximation of the muscular coat of the rectum is the single most important step. Irrespective of the location of the rectovaginal fistula, the use of a diverting colostomy is not indicated as a primary procedure.

REOPERATION

When the first operation for correction of a rectovaginal injury has failed, the success of a second or third operation can be greatly enhanced by the use of a Martius graft to reinforce the area of closure. A Martius graft consists of a flap of bulbocavernosus muscle and its surrounding fat that has been isolated through a longitudinal incision in the labia majora, detached at its anterior pole, brought through a tunnel under the lateral vaginal wall, and fixed in place between the rectum and posterior vagina. The Martius graft should always be used whenever healing is uncertain because of previous scarring or multiple operative failures. The use of a diverting colostomy is never indicated as a primary procedure and is rarely needed following operative failures. Before resorting to colostomy, a repair incorporating a Martius graft should first be tried.

POSTOPERATIVE CARE

The postoperative care of these patients requires no special measures other than the prescription of stool softeners to be used until normal bowel function has been restored.

SUGGESTED READING

Hibbard LT: Surgical management of rectovaginal fistulas and complete perineal tears. *Am J Obstet Gynecol* 130:139, 1978

Martius M: *Martius' Gynecologic Operations*. Boston: Little, Brown, 1956, p 328

Miller NF, Brown W: The surgical treatment of complete perineal tears in the female. *Am J Obstet Gynecol* 34:196, 1937

Russell TR, Gallagher DM: Low rectovaginal fistulas. *Am J Surg* 134:13, 1977

Warren JC: A new method of operation for the relief of rupture of the perineum through the sphincter and rectum. *Trans Am Gynecol Soc* 72:322, 1982

60

Prepubertal Vulvar Lacerations, Hematomas, Sexual Assault, and Labial Adhesions

PAUL F. BRENNER, M.D.

VULVAR LACERATIONS

Frequently, when a physician attends a young child who has recently sustained a vulvar laceration, a single vessel is identified as the source of the bleeding. It is very tempting to secure hemostasis and repair the vulvar laceration with the child under local anesthesia. However, repair can seldom be accomplished under these conditions. Most children do not remain sufficiently still for the sutures to be properly placed and the operative field kept sterile. Instead of achieving hemostasis, attempts to repair vulvar lacerations in children under local anesthesia may create more bleeding. The best advice is to repair all vulvar lacerations under general anesthesia even when the laceration is small and a single pumping vessel is identified as the source of the bleeding. If the location of the laceration suggests that the vagina, urethra, or bladder might be involved in the injury, these structures are examined while the patient is anesthetized.

VULVAR HEMATOMAS

The most common cause of vulvar hematomas in children are "straddle" injuries. While riding a bicycle or climbing on a jungle gym, the child falls with the cross bar between her legs and sustains blunt trauma to the vulva. The single most important feature in the care of vulvar hematomas is to identify the lesion's full extent. Inspection and palpation of the vulva and perineum are not sufficient to define the borders of the collection of blood. A rectal examination must be performed, as there is a large space for the collection of concealed blood, which might be interpreted as a small hematoma if only the perineum is examined. Very rarely, the amount of bleeding is so great that the child goes into shock. If the hematoma has not expanded after 4 hours of observation, the patient has spontaneously voided clear urine, and the hematoma is not large enough to cause her undue distress, a nonsurgical approach may be used: Application of ice packs to the hematoma is all the treatment necessary.

A hematoma that enlarges, causes considerable pain, and/or obstructs the urethra must be treated surgically to evacuate the clots and identify and ligate the actively bleeding vessels.

ALLEGED SEXUAL ASSAULT

Sexual assault evokes so much physical and emotional trauma that most victims of any age endure the sequelae for many years, if not the rest of their lives. The care of the victim of an alleged sexual assault requires a team of specialists that includes a physician, nurse, social worker, and security officer who are specially trained and concerned for persons who have been sexually assaulted. Optimal care should include immediate medical attention, privacy, confidentiality, and adequate medical and social service follow-up.

In the past, physicians have been reluctant to become involved in treating victims of alleged sexual assault, and as a result these patients have been kept waiting. They must be given immediate emergency care so that the extent of their physical and psychological trauma can be evaluated. This trauma may be life-threatening. All of these victims suffer from some degree of psychological shock, which is often very difficult to assess. Privacy and confidentiality are an important part of their total treatment plan.

Not all of the sequelae of a sexual assault can be detected at the initial examination. Follow-up visits with the physician and the social worker are an integral part of the care of a person who has been sexually violated. This team of specialists has many responsibilities in the treatment of alleged sexual assault patients, but the one responsibility it does not have—and should not assume—is to prove or disprove that rape occurred. This decision should be made by the judicial system, not by the medical profession.

The sexual assault of a child is even more devastating than the same crime committed against an adult. The extent of both the physical and the psychological injuries tends to be greater in the prepubertal girl than the adult. The child may never completely recover from the physical and especially the emotional trauma resulting from the attack.

The first priority in the management of an alleged sexual assault patient of any age is to determine whether she has sustained any life-threatening injuries. Attention to these problems takes precedence over all other aspects. If the patient's life is not in immediate jeopardy, the physician then proceeds to define and document carefully the extent of her injuries and collect the specimens and evidence required by the judicial system. Vaginoscopy for the collection of evidence, with the child awake, is attempted for prepubertal girls who do not show evidence of vulvar trauma and vaginal penetration. The collection of evidence includes a dry mount preparation to be examined for the presence of sperm, a dry swab and saline swab taken from the vagina for determination of the presence of acid phosphatase and ABO typing, respectively, and a culture for gonorrhea. If vaginoscopy cannot be adequately performed with the child awake and there is no evidence that she has sustained vaginal penetration, further endeavors to complete the procedure are not advised. When the child has clearly sustained vaginal penetration, she should be placed under general anesthesia for the collection of evidence and repair of the traumatized tissue.

Because of the size of the vaginal canal and the lack of development of the pelvic tissues and support of the reproductive organs, penetration into the peritoneal cavity and total avulsion of the upper vaginal vault are more likely to occur in prepubertal patients who have been sexually violated than in adults. If the peritoneal cavity has been entered, there will be evidence of crepitus and intraperitoneal gas. Avulsion of the upper vaginal vault causes the child to have marked discomfort when walking or talking, and she will develop an ileus. Penetration of the peritoneal cavity and avulsion of the upper vaginal vault must be considered in every child who has evidence of vaginal penetration before she is taken to surgery.

LABIAL ADHESIONS

In young girls at any age prior to puberty, the labia can become fused as the result of adhesions. Fusion may be partial or it may completely occlude the vaginal orifice. The need for treatment is based on the patient's ability to void spontaneously. As long as she can urinate without discomfort, there is no need to initiate therapy. In most cases the labia separate spontaneously as the concentration of endogenous estrogen in the peripheral circulation increases in early puberty. Attempts to separate the labia manually are never indicated, as they are guaranteed to cause both physical and emotional trauma. Almost always these attempts fail, and even more scarring occurs as the labia fuse once again.

If labial adhesions do cause problems in voiding or recurrent urinary tract infections, active treatment must be started. Topical application of 0.5 gm of estrogen cream (Premarin) to the labia for 10-14 consecutive nights is successful in bringing about separation of the labia in almost all cases.

SUGGESTED READING

Breen JL, Greenwald E, Gregori CA: The molested young female: Evaluation and therapy of alleged rape. *Pediatr Clin North Am* 19:717, 1972

Burgess AW, Holmstrom LL: Rape trauma syndrome. *Am J Psychiatr* 131:981, 1974

Caparo VJ: Sexual assault of female children. *Ann NY Acad Sci* 142:817, 1967

Hogan WL: The raped child. *Med Aspects Hum Sexual* 8:129, 1974

Robinson HA, Sherrod DB, Malcarney CN: Review of child molestation and alleged rape cases. *Am J Obstet Gynecol* 110:405, 1971

Soules MR, Pollard AA, Brown KM, Verma M: The forensic laboratory evaluation of evidence in alleged rape. *Am J Obstet Gynecol* 130:142, 1978

Woodling BA, Evans JR, Bradbury MD: Sexual assault: Rape and molestation. *Clin Obstet Gynecol* 20:509, 1977

FOUR

GYNECOLOGIC

UROLOGY

61

Urinary Tract Infection

ROBERT C. CORLETT JR., M.D.

Urinary tract infection is a common problem among women. The magnitude of this problem is suggested by studies among diverse populations in South Wales, Jamaica, and Japan, which have demonstrated a very similar incidence of bacteriuria. It occurs in 4% of women between 16 and 65, compared with 0.5% of men. The prevalence rises with age and parity, with age being the more important factor. In pregnancy, bacteriuria is no more common than in the general population, but it seldom remits spontaneously, whereas in non-pregnant women spontaneous remission is very common. The incidence in young schoolgirls is 1%; in nonpregnant young women, 4%; in pregnant women, 4-7%, depending on the socioeconomic status of the patient population; and in postmenopausal women, approximately 7-10%.

ACUTE CYSTITIS

"Honeymoon cystitis" is a common problem. Although easily treated, its symptoms may be extremely disconcerting. It is most often caused by *Escherichia coli*, and nearly always by one or another species of the Enterobacteriaceae; the pathogenesis will be discussed in greater detail below. Diagnosis is generally simple, with urinalysis and culture confirming suspicions based on the history of dysuria, frequency, urgency, nocturia, and hesitancy. Treatment is somewhat more controversial, but generally one of the many urinary antiseptics—sulfisoxazole (Gantrisin), nitrofurantoin (Furadantin, Macrodantin), methenamine hippurate (Hiprex, Urex) or mandelate (Mandelamine), nalidixic acid (NegGram), trimethoprim-sulfamethoxazole (Bactrim, Septra)—is preferable to a broad-spectrum antibiotic. The duration of treatment need not exceed 7 days for an initial episode. My personal choice is Macrodantin 100 mg qid for 1 week.

The advantages of a highly concentrated urine, with its increased osmolarity and concentration of antiseptic, are probably outweighed by the dilution and washout effect of a very well-hydrated patient, although this hypothesis has not been tested in clinical practice. Similarly, although many antibiotics seem more effective in an alkaline milieu, it is generally recommended that the urine be acidified to inhibit bacterial growth. Acidification can usually be accomplished with oral ascorbic acid, starting with 500 mg bid and increasing the dosage in 500-mg increments until the urinary pH is less than 6.

The exception to these principles would be patients with *Pseudomonas* or other gram-negative organisms resistant to the standard oral agents as tested by disc sensitivity. In instances where the only apparent effective antibiotics are parenteral agents such as colistimethate (Coly-Mycin M) or aminoglycosides, we have found that treatment with oral erythromycin with urinary alkalinization is often effective. Urinary alkalinization can usually be accomplished by having the patient check her own urine with litmus paper while titrating herself with sodium bicarbonate tablets qid, just as she would with ascorbic acid tablets, the difference being that she is attempting to maintain a pH of 8 or greater.

Unfortunately, fewer than half of women with the complaints of frequency, dysuria, urgency, and nocturia have culture-proven bacterial cystitis. The remaining women have sterile urine cultures and are frequently diagnosed as having "the urethral syndrome," "cystourethritis," or some other equally vague malady. This is undoubtedly a heterogeneous group with a number of possible etiologies for their complaints. Atopy may become manifest as irritative urinary tract symptoms that resolve after desensitization or withdrawal of the offending antigen. The loss of estrogen support to the urethra secondary to menopause may result in marked irritative phenomena that respond dramatically to estrogen therapy. Vulvovaginitis or cervicitis may be associated with symptoms of urinary tract infection. Treatment of the underlying disorders will cure the "cystourethritis." There is some support for the hypothesis that a lymphatic connection between bladder and cervix exists and forms a route for organisms to reach the bladder.

RECURRENT URINARY TRACT INFECTION

There has been considerable research in the area of recurrent urinary tract infection in both males and females. Localization studies have shown the primary reservoir in the male to be the prostate gland, and in the female, the vaginal vestibule.

Stamey and colleagues have reported interesting investigations to corroborate this theory. By studying a number of women with a history of recurrent urinary tract infection—but currently without bacteriuria—and comparing them with normal controls, they have demonstrated that patients with recurrent infection tend to have a significantly greater degree of colonization of the vestibule with Enterobacteriaceae. In the same two groups of women, patients with recurrent urinary tract infection had a much greater propensity for alkaline pH of the vaginal introitus. Then, studying scrapings of the vaginal mucosa in vitro, Stamey et al demonstrated that bacterial adherence to the vaginal mucosa was significantly greater in women with a history of recurrent urinary tract infections than in normal controls. Microbial adherence is important in the organism's ability to colonize the surface. Stamey and colleagues concluded that biologic susceptibility to recurrent infections of the urinary tract in women is related to a defect at the cellular level that favors bacterial adherence.

By this type of innovative investigation it has been demonstrated that over 95% of all recurrent infections in women or girls are caused by reinfection by spread of bacteria from the rectum to the vaginal vestibule and then to the urethra and bladder, often with coitus as the precipitating episode. Moore and Hira inquired into the toilet habits of a large number of women with symptoms of cystourethritis and found that in every case wiping was performed from behind forward. Thus, in addition to the trauma and milking action induced by coitus, improper hygiene may play a significant role in the process of recurrent infection.

Several different regimens have proven effective for the treatment of recurrent cystourethritis. If the recurrent episodes can clearly be related to sexual activity, preventive measures should include instructing the patient to void as soon as possible following coitus and to increase fluid intake for 24 hours afterward.

Additionally, if vaginal secretions are scanty, the use of a water-soluble lubricant should reduce the degree of trauma and thus introduce a smaller inoculum into the bladder. These measures may be adequate alone or in combination with one dose of a urinary antiseptic such as nitrofurantoin or trimethoprim-sulfamethoxazole taken around the time of coitus (usually shortly after). While this technique is not consistent with usual methods of appropriate antibiotic therapy, its efficacy has been proven. We usually start by prescribing Macrodantin 50 or 100 mg and maintain that regimen for at least 6 months, at which time the medication may be stopped and recurrences awaited. If recurrences then develop, this regimen should be resumed for an indefinite period.

If recurrent cystitis is not clearly related to coitus, two other methods have been shown to be beneficial. Ingesting one dose of an appropriate antiseptic each night for an indeterminate period is very effective in reducing the number of recurrences. Because the washout phenomenon is not utilized at night, antimicrobial therapy is needed to lengthen the doubling time of bacteria in the bladder urine. Landes et al have shown that application of Betadine gel to the external meatus twice daily produced a significant decrease in the number of recurrent urinary tract infections.

Appropriate management, including a urologic investigation that except for intravenous pyelography can easily be performed in the office, can provide symptomatic relief for the patient, prevent recurrence along with possible deleterious effects to the upper tract, and ameliorate underlying disorders such as urethral diverticula, urethral stenosis, neuropathic bladder, or chronic cervicitis. The minimal urologic work-up for these patients would include urinalysis, culture and sensitivity, IVP, cystourethroscopy, and cystometry. Additional measures, such as David catheter urethrography, uroflowmetry, and urethral pressure profiles, may be indicated for the patient who fails to respond to therapy. If the physician is not trained to perform endoscopic investigation of the lower urinary tract for cases of persistence or recurrence, a urologic consultation should be obtained.

SUGGESTED READING

Fair W, Timothy M, Millar M, Stamey T: Bacteriologic and hormonal observation of the urethra and vaginal vestibule in normal premenopausal women. *J Urol* 104:426, 1970

Landes R, Melnick I, Hoffman A: Recurrent urinary tract infections in women. Prevention by topical application of anti-microbial ointment to urethral meatus. *J Urol* 104:749, 1970

Moore T, Hira N: The role of the female urethra in infections of urinary tract. *Br J Urol* 37:25, 1965

Stamey T, Timothy M: Studies of introital colonization in women with recurrent urinary incontinence. I. The role of vaginal pH. *J Urol* 114:261, 1975

62

Management of Stress Urinary Incontinence

CHARLES A. BALLARD, M.D.

Urinary incontinence in the female is very common and not necessarily pathologic. Questionnaires given to large numbers of young, nulliparous women reveal that half have experienced incontinence at one time or another and 16% suffer from this problem daily. Parous women in their 30s or 40s would give positive replies even more frequently. Only when the incontinence has progressed to the point where it is socially embarrassing should it be considered pathologic.

DIAGNOSIS

Before the management of stress incontinence can be discussed, it is important to make the correct diagnosis. Not infrequently a patient undergoes surgery for incontinence when in fact medical therapy is necessary because she is suffering from an unstable bladder. A complete history and physical examination are required in all patients. A history of urgency, urge incontinence, frequency, nocturia, enuresis, pyelitis, brain tumor, or radical pelvic surgery suggests a nonsurgical approach. Minimum additional work-up should consist of a urinalysis, culture, cystoscopy, urethroscopy, cystometry, and measurement of residual urine. It is also important to rule out a fistula or urethral diverticulum.

Patients with anatomic stress incontinence may give a history of loss of urine with coughing, sneezing, lifting, laughing, or running. A cystocele may or may not be present. On cystometric studies the opening urethral pressure is low, the bladder capacity is normal, there is no residual or detrusor activity, and the intravesicular pressure is normal. The major defect seen is a drop and opening of the vesicle neck with straining. Once the diagnosis of stress incontinence is made, management depends on its severity.

TREATMENT

Mild Incontinence

An exercise program aimed at strengthening the pelvic diaphragm can achieve a medical cure of mild incontinence and—more important—prevent the incontinence from becoming so severe as to necessitate surgery. The muscles of the pelvis most responsible for maintaining continence are the pubococcygeus and deep transverse perineal (muscle of the urogenital diaphragm). The latter muscle is also the main component of the "external sphincter" of the urethra. Improving the tonus of these muscles during the early reproductive years can avert the later development of true stress incontinence.

The patient is instructed to squeeze the examiner's fingers while in the lithotomy position. A perineometer may be used to obtain more objective information, but its use is not necessary. Once the examiner is satisfied that the patient understands how to perform the exercise she is instructed to perform it at home. She is advised to begin with 50 repetitions each time and work up to 100 repetitions twice daily, and more often if she wishes. Frequent return visits to the office early in the course of therapy will maximize patient cooperation and understanding.

All women who develop stress incontinence after the menopause should undergo a trial of estrogen therapy. Often the estrogen stimulus at the vascular cuff surrounding the urethra is adequate to improve urethral resistance and restore continence.

Severe Incontinence

Once a patient has progressed to a severe degree of incontinence, perineal exercise alone will usually not suffice and surgical intervention will be required. Since many of these patients also have pelvic relaxation, it has been the habit of most gynecologists to perform a vaginal hysterectomy and anterior and posterior colporrhaphy. Unfortunately, the anterior repair does not always provide an adequate cure and should no longer be automatically selected as the initial procedure for women with true stress incontinence. If the incontinence is mild and the prolapse significant, a vaginal approach is often warranted. However, if stress incontinence is the main problem and prolapse is of secondary concern (or no problem at all), a retropubic suspension is the procedure of choice.

Green performed chain cystourethrograms on patients with stress urinary incontinence and divided them into two groups. In type I, the anatomic defect involved loss of only the normal posterior urethrovesical angle. He found vaginal repair highly successful in correcting the anatomic defect and achieving complete cure of stress incontinence in 85-90% of such patients. In type II incontinence, in addition to obliteration of the posterior urethrovesical angle, there was also inferior and posterior rotational descent of the urethra and bladder neck with a resulting characteristic abnormal urethral axis. The urethral axis angle was increased to more than 45°. Here the surgery of choice is suprapubic urethrovesical suspension. Unfortunately, chain cystourethrograms give at least 25% false-positive and 25% false-negative results.

The various procedures available for severe stress incontinence include the Marshall-Marchetti-Krantz, Burch, and Pereyra operations and a fascial sling. If a vaginal approach is necessary for uterine descensus plus a cystocele and a rectocele, one may do a Pereyra procedure. The endopelvic fascia is detached from the pubic rami bilaterally. A helical suture is placed through this fascia, incorporating the pubourethral ligament, and then tied over the rectus fascia.

If there is no need for a vaginal repair or if a primary abdominal hysterectomy is to be performed, a Marshall-Marchetti-Krantz (MMK) or Burch procedure is carried out. The MMK is a vesicourethral suspension. The space of Retzius is entered, with sutures placed in the periurethral tissue and the posterior periosteum of the pubis. This procedure has had widespread use with a high success rate. It has been especially useful as a secondary procedure in patients who have failed a prior operation for stress incontinence.

We feel that the Burch procedure offers some technical advantages over the original MMK procedure. Cooper's ligament is a more reliable tissue than the periosteum, and the vagina allows a more sturdy purchase than the periurethral tissue. After the space of Retzius has been entered, using a nonabsorbable suture, the vagina lateral to the bladder neck is transfixed to the iliopectineal ligament. This effectively creates a sling out of the patient's anterior vagina and leaves the bladder neck and urethra alone so that excessive scarring will not interfere with the delicate mechanism of voiding and continence. The bladder neck is identified with a large transurethral Foley catheter, and if there is any doubt as to the placement of the sutures in relationship to the bladder, the bladder is opened. We have achieved a very high success rate using the Burch procedure as the primary approach in women with severe incontinence.

The fascial sling operation has been performed as the ultimate effort where other procedures have failed. Numerous modifications in materials and the placement of the support sling have been made. The most successful versions are those using homologous tissues such as the anterior abdominal fascia or fascia lata.

SUGGESTED READING

Aldridge AH: Transplantation of fascia for relief of urinary stress incontinence. *Am J Obstet Gynecol* 44:398, 1942

Burch JC: Cooper's ligament urethrovesical suspension for stress incontinence. *Am J Obstet Gynecol* 100:764, 1968

Green TH: Development of a plan for the diagnosis and treatment of urinary stress incontinence. *Am J Obstet Gynecol* 83:632, 1962

Marshall VF, Marchetti AA, Krantz KE: The correction of stress incontinence by simple vesicourethral suspension. *Surg Gynecol Obstet* 88:509, 1949

Pereyra AJ, Lebherz TB: Combined urethrovesical suspension and vaginourethroplasty for correction of urinary stress incontinence. *Obstet Gynecol* 30:4, 1967

Robertson JR: Urethroscopy—The neglected gynecologic procedure. *Clin Obstet Gynecol* 19:318, 1976

Zacharin RR: The suspensory mechanism of the female urethra. *J Anat* 97:423, 1963

63

Bladder Injuries and Vesicovaginal Fistulas

LESTER T. HIBBARD, M.D.

BLADDER INJURIES

Bladder injuries are common complications of pelvic surgery despite the best of operative techniques. Fortunately, such injuries heal rapidly and securely if promptly recognized and appropriately repaired.

Injuries to the Bladder Dome

The dome of the bladder can be either lacerated or deliberately opened during the course of an abdominal operation. Accidental lacerations are commonly associated either with an anatomical distortion as a result of previous operations or tumors, or with adhesions as a result of surgery, infection, or endometriosis. Elective cystotomy is usually performed to assist in dissecting the bladder free of dense adhesions, or as an aid in evaluating suspected ureteral injury. Cystotomy can also be utilized in techniques to correct urinary stress incontinence. While accidental bladder injury can be minimized by good technique, including intrafascial rather than extrafascial hysterectomy and sharp rather than blunt dissection, it is equally important to disprove a suspected injury by filling the bladder with dye or even opening the dome of the bladder to inspect its mucosal surface.

Closure of accidental or intentional cystotomy is best accomplished utilizing 2-0 chromic suture, which holds its tensile strength better than polyglycolic or polyglactin suture, particularly in the presence of infected urine. While several closure techniques are satisfactory, animal experimentation has demonstrated that continuous sutures produce a better closure. Paradoxically, continuous locking sutures result in excessive leakage and should be avoided. If a two-layer closure is employed, the first layer should include both the mucosa and muscularis. There is no advantage in attempting to avoid the mucosa because chromic sutures that penetrate this layer will be covered by epithelium in 3 days. In addition, closure of the mucosa eliminates the possibility of subsequent bleeding from its free edge as a result of the lytic action of urine. A second layer of continuous inverting suture provides reinforcement.

Testing a two-layer continuous closure by distending the bladder with 500 ml of fluid is reassuring but probably not necessary, because such a repair is invariably watertight. Prolonged postoperative decompression of the bladder by catheter drainage is also unnecessary; we find 5 days of catheter drainage more than adequate. Drainage of the space of Retzius is not required.

Injuries to the Bladder Base

Accidental injuries to the bladder base are more complicated, for several reasons. First, they are apt to be unrecognized. Second, healing may be impeded because the immediate operative field is infected. Third, one or both ureters may be involved by either the injury or the repair.

The most common cause of injury to the bladder base is a laceration occurring during vaginal entry of the anterior cul-de-sac. Such a misadventure is likely to be due to forceful blunt dissection by jabbing with a gauze-wrapped finger. The site of injury is usually in the midline, permitting repair without encroaching on the ureters. A two-layer repair as described above should be utilized. The second layer of suture may be interrupted rather than continuous. If there is any question of ureteral involvement, cystoscopy should be performed following closure and the ureteral orifices observed for the prompt bilateral appearance of indigo carmine dye after intravenous administration. Because of the uncertainty of healing, postoperative urethral or suprapubic catheter drainage should be continued for at least 10 days. In addition, transvaginal drainage of the proximal area of the repair can be considered. If the closure is less than satisfactory, the area of repair should be reinforced with a bulbocavernous fat pad (Martius) graft. Injury to the bladder base during the course of an abdominal procedure, if recognized, should be managed in a similar fashion.

VESICOVAGINAL FISTULAS

Vesicovaginal fistulas can be categorized as being due to surgery, radiation, obstetric trauma, or a miscellany of rare causes such as tuberculosis, syphilis, trauma, electrocautery, malignancy, or bladder neck resection. Obstetric trauma is no longer a significant factor in developed countries, and the incidence of radiation fistulas has been greatly reduced with the advent of more sophisticated techniques. At the M. D. Anderson Hospital, the incidence of vesicovaginal fistulas resulting from radiation therapy for cervical carcinoma is only 1.2%. The great majority of vesicovaginal fistulas currently encountered are the result of pelvic surgery for benign disease.

Three-quarters of vesicovaginal fistulas follow an abdominal operation, and the vast majority of these are the results of unrecognized trauma at the time of operation. The most common error is misplacement of a suture through the bladder wall at the time of closure of the vaginal cuff. The resulting focal devascularization, supplemented by an inflammatory response, results in a small vesicovaginal fistula just anterior to the line of vault closure. Vesicocervical or vesicouterine fistulas can occur if these structures have not been removed.

Fistulas can also result from the presence of a foreign body draining an open vaginal cuff or from an infected vault hematoma.

The diagnosis of a postoperative vesicovaginal fistula can be suspected by unexplained fever, persistent bloody urine, or heavy vaginal discharge. If the diagnosis is suspected, cystoscopy can be considered, although the additional trauma of the procedure may make matters worse. Constant or intermittent leakage of urine is usually observed on the fifth postoperative day or later, depending on the size and length of the fistula tract.

Once the fistula has developed, the diagnosis may be obvious, depending on its size and location. Even so, excretory urography is mandatory to rule out coincidental involvement of the upper urinary tract. If the opening is small or the tract is long or tortuous, cystoscopy and the instillation of methylene blue dye into the bladder may not be adequate to confirm the diagnosis, particularly in the presence of mucosal edema. In this event, the triple-swab test of Moir is helpful. Following dye instillation into the bladder, three dry cotton swabs are inserted deep into the vagina, and the patient is instructed to ambulate for 20-30 minutes. If at the end of this period only the innermost swab is wet but not blue, the diagnosis is ureterovaginal fistula. If only the outermost swab is wet (and blue), the diagnosis is urinary incontinence. If the upper swabs are both wet and blue, the diagnosis is a vesicovaginal or high urethrovaginal fistula. Occasionally, ingenious methods must be employed to locate an elusive fistula. As recommended by Robertson, the "flat tire test" consists of placing the patient in the knee-chest position, filling the vaginal vault with water, insufflating the bladder with CO_2, and observing the water for the appearance of bubbles.

Whenever a diagnosis of vesicovaginal fistula is strongly suspected or established, prolonged bladder drainage is indicated, in the hope of spontaneous closure. Suprapubic drainage may be more convenient, particularly if the patient is sent home. In addition, the urine is acidified by means of ascorbic acid 500 mg twice daily, and sterilized utilizing an appropriate antibiotic. Once it is apparent that the tract is epithelialized, the possibility of spontaneous closure no longer exists.

While cauterization of a small, persistent fistulous tract is occasionally successful, the majority will require a surgical repair. Immediate combined transabdominal-transvesical repair has its advocates, but risks failure with a resulting larger defect and a more difficult secondary repair. Early closure following a 10-day course of glucocorticoids has been recommended by Collins, but the majority opinion is that it is better to wait at least 3-6 months to allow all inflammatory changes to subside before attempting a repair. Experience proves that delayed closure has the greatest chance of success.

When the optimal time for surgical repair is reached, preoperative preparation should include acidification and sterilization of the urine, local estrogens when indicated, and correction of any coexisting vaginal infection. A regimen of prophylactic antibiotics, such as cefoxitin (Mefoxin) 2 gm on call to surgery and 6 and 12 hours later, may enhance the chances of successful closure.

In 95% of cases, or better, vaginal repair of a fistula is preferable. Indwelling ureteral catheters should be placed prior to surgery if the fistula is in close proximity to a ureter. As an aid to palpation, the wire stints should then be replaced in the catheters. Principles of repair include adequate mobilization, excision of the fistulous tract, and a three-layer closure using absorbable sutures. For fistulas at the apex of the vaginal vault, Latzko's technique, including a partial colpocleisis, is particularly effective.

When poor healing is a possibility, the area of repair should be reinforced with a Martius graft. In cases of large radiation fistulas, even better reinforcement is provided by a myocutaneous graft utilizing the gracilis muscle. While a Martius graft is a simple procedure that should be in the repertoire of every pelvic surgeon, a gracilis muscle graft is a relatively formidable undertaking.

SUGGESTED READING

Collins CG, Collins JH, Harrison BR, et al: Early repair of vesicovaginal fistula. *Am J Obstet Gynecol* 111:524, 1971

Everett HS, Mattingly RF: Urinary tract injuries resulting from pelvic surgery. *Am J Obstet Gynecol* 71:502, 1956

Latzko W: Postoperative vesicovaginal fistulas. *Am J Surg* 58:211, 1942

Moir JC: Personal experience in treatment of vesicovaginal fistulas. *Am J Obstet Gynecol* 71:471, 1956

Robertson JR: *Disorders of the Female Urethra and Urinary Incontinence.* Baltimore: Williams & Wilkins, 1982

64

Surgical Injury to the Ureter

LESTER T. HIBBARD, M.D.

Accidental injury of a ureter is the bugaboo of the pelvic surgeon. In some cases, surgical pathology such as interligamentous tumors, extensive endometriosis, dense surgical adhesions, or inflammatory masses serve as a warning; in other cases, operative complications such as uncontrolled hemorrhage deep in the pelvis or inadequate exposure of the operative field are red flags. But if the operator is able to anticipate an injury, the damage can almost always be successfully repaired. On the other hand, most injuries undetected at surgery are not associated with difficult operations but rather with procedures that were thought to be relatively straightforward and routine.

The incidence of ureter injury during operations for benign conditions lies somewhere between 0.5% and 2.5%, with the higher figure being more likely because many ureteral injuries are asymptomatic and go undetected. Between 80% and 90% of ureteral fistulas are secondary to gynecologic operations; 70% to 75% are related to abdominal hysterectomy. The most common site of injury is at the level of the ureterosacral ligaments. Other common injury sites are at the vaginal angle and pelvic brim.

PREVENTION

As a means of reducing ureteral injury, preoperative excretory urography has been widely recommended. While these studies are useful in identifying ureteral obstruction, or anomalies such as double ureters or the rare pelvic kidney, the surgeon is still obligated to expose and identify the ureters to prevent surgical damage. The only circumstance where urography is of special value is to detect anterior ureteral displacement by a retroperitoneal mass. Unless a lateral film is taken, such displacement may not be detected.

Preoperative placement of ureteral catheters has also been recommended for difficult cases. But this procedure is not particularly rewarding because preoperative selection of appropriate patients for catheterization is most difficult. In addition, ureteral catheters have been criticized on the grounds that they give a false sense of security, increase ureteral trauma, and often cannot be palpated at their lowest (and most critical) point.

The mainstay in prevention of ureteral trauma is adequate operative exposure combined with positive identification of the ureters when indicated. This includes not only an appropriate surgical incision but also cautious dissection of adherent or broad ligament masses, removal of large myomas before proceeding to hysterectomy, and opening the broad ligaments to expose the ureters in all difficult cases. While palpation has limited usefulness in locating a ureter, positive identification can be made only by observing its peristaltic action. If a structure does not exhibit peristalsis, it cannot be a ureter.

Even in the easiest of cases there is virtue to dissecting out the ureters, not only as a safeguard but also as a means of becoming thoroughly familiar with the anatomy involved. Easy cases also demand precision, since a substantial percentage of ureteral injuries involve seemingly innocuous steps such as re-peritonealization of the bladder flap.

DIAGNOSIS

When ureteral injury is suspected but not certain during an abdominal procedure, either the ureter must be positively identified and traced to the point of potential injury or, in the event exposure is unsatisfactory, its patency must be demonstrated. Patency is most easily demonstrated by a retroperitoneal cystotomy in the dome of the bladder followed by the intravenous injection of 10 ml of indigo carmine dye. Using the uninvolved side as a control, the ureteral orifices are observed for active spurting of urine and bilateral appearance of the dye. If ureteral function appears in any way to be impaired, a No. 4 or No. 5 ureteral catheter should be passed in retrograde fashion to make sure no obstruction exists. If patency is established, the bladder is closed. If the catheter can be passed only with difficulty, it should remain in situ and its distal end secured to an indwelling urethral catheter.

As an alternative, ureteral patency can be tested by passing a ureteral catheter down to the bladder through a longitudinal slit in the proximal ureter. The catheter can then be left as a splint or removed and the ureteral slit closed with one or two 5-0 catgut sutures and drained retroperitoneally.

OPERATIVE MANAGEMENT

In the operative management of ureteral injuries, the most important step is to deal with the threat of urinary extravasation around the site of injury. Unless extravasated urine is drained, the result is a periureteral fibrosis that can cause subsequent ureteral stricture and obstruction. Thus, any significant damage will require a Penrose or suction drain placed near but not touching the injured segment and brought retroperitoneally through the flank. This drain should be left in place either until all drainage has stopped or it is demonstrated that no extravasation has occurred. In addition, a ureteral catheter can assist in draining urine and reducing (but not eliminating) extravasation.

A ureter can be clamped, crushed, ligated, lacerated, transected, or denuded of its sheath. The management of these injuries depends principally upon their extent and location. Other factors to be considered are mobility of the ureter and bladder, the condition of the tissues, associated pelvic pathology, and the general condition of the patient.

Apparent minor injuries, such as small tears in the ureteral sheath, light clamping, or ligatures that have been in place for a short period of time, can be treated conservatively by removing the clamp or ligation, observing for ureteral peristalsis, and repairing the sheath with chromic 5-0 catgut.

But if there has been an apparent loss of viability or definite injury, such as crushing, ureteral laceration, or extensive denudation that strips away a large segment of blood supply, active measures must be instituted. These injuries must be protected by extraperitoneal drainage and, in most cases, by a ureteral catheter. In addition, lacerations are repaired over a catheter by several sutures of 5-0 catgut. If a segment of ureter is devitalized, resection or implantation may be necessary.

When a ureter has been transected, it usually can be either reunited by end-to-end anastomosis or implanted in the bladder dome. In unusual situations, ligation or external drainage may be necessary as dictated by pelvic pathology and the general condition of the patient. The choice between anastomosis and implantation depends on the site and extent of injury as well as the preference of the surgeon.

Transections of the ureter in the middle or upper pelvis are preferably handled by end-to-end anastomosis. The cut ends of the ureter are spatulated and reapproximated over a ureteral splint by five or six loose sutures of 5-0 catgut. No attempt is made to achieve a watertight anastomosis, and the area is drained by a retroperitoneal flank drain as previously described. The ureteral catheter can be left in situ for 10-12 days; as an alternative, the catheter can be removed, a longitudinal slit made in the ureter approximately 5 cm proximal to the damage site, and a second extraperitoneal drain inserted. When this drain is removed, the ureteral slit will close spontaneously.

Transection or devitalization of the lower ureter is treated either by bladder implantation or, in favorable cases, by anastomosis. The advantage of an anastomosis is the avoidance of subsequent ureteral reflux. On the other hand, implantation reduces the risk of poor healing accompanied by ureteral stricture. When bladder implantation has been selected, the distal ureteral stump is ligated with nonabsorbable suture and the proximal ureter is brought through a stab wound and its spatulated ends fixed to the bladder wall with fine chromic suture. A reinforcing outer layer of suture unites the adventitia of the ureter to the bladder surface. More elaborate methods of implantation to reduce the threat of reflux are also available. Whenever possible, the implantation should be placed retroperitoneally and, if necessary, tension on the line of anastomosis can be reduced by hitching the bladder dome to the psoas muscle. Retroperitoneal drainage at the site of union is also established.

POSTOPERATIVE MANAGEMENT

Unfortunately, the majority of ureteral injuries are not recognized at the time the injury occurs. This reduces the available options for their correction. It also prolongs the period of disability, and dims the expectation of eventual complete recovery.

Postoperative manifestations depend on the nature of the injury and include an otherwise unexplained fever, flank pain, ileus, abdominal distension, peritonitis, and urinary leakage from the vaginal vault. In the case of ligation, the patient is sometimes asymptomatic. Excretory urography can show nonfunction, delayed excretion, hydronephrosis, or extravasation.

If the problem is ligation, an early deligation followed by a short period of ureteral catheterization may suffice. Or if vaginal drainage of urine from a low injury has been established, spontaneous closure may occur. Most cases are less favorable, and the question will be whether to attempt a primary repair or to establish urinary diversion until the primary inflammatory insult has subsided. This decision requires fine judgment and expert consultation. Ureteral implantation is often needed, and more complicated procedures, such as tube bladder grafts, ileal grafts, or transposition by anastomosis to the opposite ureter, may be necessary.

SUGGESTED READING

Freda VC, Tachi D: Ureteral injury discovered after pelvic surgery. *Am J Obstet Gynecol* 80:406, 1962

Higgins CC: Ureteral injuries during surgery: A review of 87 cases. *JAMA* 199:82, 1967

Symmonds RE: Ureteral injuries associated with gynecologic surgery: Prevention and management. *Clin Obstet Gynecol* 19:623, 1976

FIVE

GYNECOLOGIC
ONCOLOGY

65

Evaluation and Management of the Patient With Vulvar and Urethral Carcinoma

C. PAUL MORROW, M.D.

Vulvar carcinoma is predominantly a disease of postmenopausal women; the average age at diagnosis is 68 years. Although the etiology is unknown, vulvar cancer tends to occur in women with a history of chronic vulvar disease, including lymphogranuloma venereum, lichen sclerosus, and condyloma acuminatum. There also appears to be an increased frequency of this malignancy among women who are obese. The most common symptoms are vulvar pruritus, pain, and a lump or mass. Occasionally the patient with vulvar malignancy presents with bleeding or spotting, burning with urination, or vaginal discharge. Burning results from the urine's passing over the ulcerated tumor.

PATHOPHYSIOLOGY

Approximately 90% of all carcinomas of the vulva are squamous. They usually arise from the clitoral prepuce, the labia minora, the interlabial sulcus, the Bartholin's gland area, or the posterior fourchette. The growth pattern of vulvar squamous carcinoma may be endophytic and ulcerative, or exophytic and polypoid. As the tumor enlarges, it extends to the adjacent vagina, urethra, anus, rectum, levators, or pubic ramus. There may be a concurrent invasive carcinoma or carcinoma in situ of the cervix or vagina. The lymphatics of the vulva, from the perineal body to the clitoral prepuce, drain in an orderly fashion anteriorly to the mons pubis and then laterally to the inguinal and femoral lymphatics. Under normal circumstances the vulvar lymphatics do not cross the labial crural fold onto the medial thigh. From the inguinal nodes, the lymphatics drain to the pelvic wall nodes and then to more distant sites. The orderly lymphatic spread of squamous vulvar carcinoma is one of its most characteristic features.

DIAGNOSIS

The diagnosis of vulvar carcinoma depends on patient cooperation and physician alertness. Management of this disease still suffers from patients' reluctance to seek medical attention and from physicians' delay in making the diagnosis. When a mass is present, directed biopsy is indicated immediately. Patients with a diffuse lesion of the vulva may require multiple biopsies. If a mass is small (1-2 cm), *excision* rather than incision biopsy is done. The workup begins with a careful physical examination. Since many of these patients are elderly, medical problems are common and may require attention before definitive treatment for the malignancy is carried out. In addition to a detailed evaluation of the primary lesion and the peripheral lymph nodes, colposcopic and cytologic study of the cervix and vagina is necessary. Chest x-ray and IVP will complete the diagnostic survey for evidence of distant metastasis.

TREATMENT

Broadly speaking, the treatment of choice for invasive squamous carcinoma of the vulva is radical vulvectomy and bilateral groin lymphadenectomy. If the groin nodes are positive, pelvic lymphadenectomy should be carried out on the side of the involved groin nodes. There are many indications for modifying this procedure. When it extends to the vagina, urethra, anus, levators, or pubic ramus, more extensive local surgery is necessary. If the lesion is too advanced to resect, radiation therapy often provides satisfactory control of the disease. In elderly or debilitated patients, wide resection alone may be warranted. Malignant melanoma is treated the same as squamous carcinoma if the lesional thickness is greater than 1 mm. Certain sarcomas and basal-cell carcinoma of the vulva can be managed by wide local excision.

PROGNOSIS

As with other malignancies, the prognosis for squamous carcinoma of the vulva is related to the extent of disease at the time of diagnosis. Lesions greater than 3 cm in size, particularly if they extend to the urethra, vagina, or anus, are associated with a significant risk of local recurrence. Patients with inguinal and/or pelvic node metastases are likely to have both local recurrence and distant metastases. Most recurrences are identified within 2 years after treatment. The corrected 5-year survival rate for patients with squamous carcinoma of the vulva and negative groin nodes is approximately 90%. Patients with positive groin nodes have a 5-year cure rate of about 40%. Women with pelvic node metastases have a 20% probability of surviving 5 years.

COMPLICATIONS

Although the operation of radical vulvectomy and bilateral groin dissection is relatively extensive and disfiguring, it is surprisingly well tolerated by even elderly, frail patients. Operative mortality has been less than 5% and usually results from pulmonary thromboembolism, stroke, or myocardial infarction. Pulmonary embolism can be minimized by the prophylactic use of low-dose heparin. Other postoperative complications include infection and necrosis of the groin skin flaps, and lymphocysts. Rupture of the femoral artery has been eliminated as a problem by transposing the proximal head of the sartorius muscle over the femoral vessels. Long-term postoperative problems include chronic lymphedema, genital prolapse, and urinary incontinence. Chronic lymphedema may be complicated by intermittent bouts of streptococcal cellulitis if long-term antibiotic prophylaxis is not utilized.

MICROINVASIVE CARCINOMA

The recent literature has several reports on the prognosis and treatment of so-called microinvasive carcinoma of the vulva. It is unclear whether there exists an early invasive lesion that is adequately treated electively by partial vulvectomy (wide excision) without lymph node dissection. It is our practice to do partial vulvectomy for lesions with less than 1 mm of invasion and no vascular space involvement. Lateralized lesions exhibiting confluent tongues of invasion no more than 3 mm deep are managed by partial vulvectomy and ipsilateral groin dissections. More extensive lesions are treated as frankly invasive carcinoma.

CARCINOMA IN THE DISTAL URETHRA

Carcinoma in the distal urethra deserves special consideration. It may be squamous, transitional, or glandular in histology. It is frequently confused with urethral prolapse or caruncle. The lymphatics from the distal third of the urethra drain predominantly to the inguinal nodes, while the lymphatics of the proximal two-thirds drain to the bladder and pelvic nodes. Preoperative evaluation should include cystoscopy and urethroscopy to determine the extent of the lesion. If the lesion is small and confined to the distal urethra, resection with bilateral groin lymphadenectomy followed by interstitial radiation is recommended. For all other cases, external radiation and anterior exenteration are recommended.

SUGGESTED READING

Benson RC, Tunca JC, Buchler DA, Uehling DT: Primary carcinoma of the female urethra. *Gynecol Oncol* 14:313, 1982

Krupp PJ, Bohm JW: Lymph gland metastases in invasive squamous cell cancer of the vulva. *Am J Obstet Gynecol* 130:943, 1978

Magrina JF, Webb MJ, Goffey TA, et al: Stage I squamous cell cancer of the vulva. *Am J Obstet Gynecol* 134:453, 1979

Morley GW: Infiltrative carcinoma of the vulva: Results of surgical treatment. *Am J Obstet Gynecol* 124:874, 1976

Morrow CP, Townsend DE: Vulvar cancer. In *Synopsis of Gynecologic Oncology*, ed 2, ch 8. New York: Wiley, 1981

Parry-Jones E: Lymphatics of the vulva. *J Obstet Gynaecol Br Commonw* 70:751, 1963

Rutledge F, Smith JP, Franklin EW: Carcinoma of the vulva. *Am J Obstet Gynecol* 106:1117, 1970

66

Carcinoma of the Vagina

OTIS GADDIS JR., M.D.

A primary vaginal malignancy is one arising de novo in the vagina without evidence of continuity of the lesion with the vulva inferiorly or with the cervix superiorly. Before a vaginal lesion can be considered a primary malignancy, metastases from the cervix, endometrium, ovary, gastrointestinal tract, and urinary tract must be excluded. This is very important, since metastases to the vagina are much more common than primary vaginal carcinoma. By this definition, the vagina ranks fifth among genital organ sites, following uterine, cervical, ovarian, and vulvar carcinomas, and accounts for 1-2% of all gynecologic malignancies.

INCIDENCE

Approximately 90% of vaginal lesions are of the squamous-cell variety. Adenocarcinoma, sarcoma, melanoma, and rare miscellaneous lesions make up the remaining 8-10%. There appears to be a predominant histologic cell type for a given age level. Squamous-cell carcinoma and melanoma frequent the postmenopausal age group, while sarcoma botryoides and rare endodermal sinus tumor occur in infancy. The diethylstilbestrol-related clear-cell adenocarcinoma is commonly found in the teen-age years, with a peak age of 19, while leiomyosarcoma frequents the 30-50 age group.

ETIOLOGY

Most epidemiologic studies of vaginal carcinoma have sought to outline the etiology of squamous-cell disease, since it is the most common cell type. While many predisposing factors have been suggested and numerous etiologic agents incriminated, no cause-effect documentation is known to date. There is, however, a strong association between maternal DES ingestion and clear-cell adenocarcinoma of the vagina in young female offspring.

DIAGNOSIS

The diagnosis of vaginal carcinoma is usually entertained because of abnormal cytology or patient symptomatology. Abnormal vaginal cytology is investigated in the same way as abnormal cervical cytology (see Chapter 69). Vaginal bleeding and vaginal discharge of various quantities and characteristics are the most common symptoms. Less frequent symptoms include dyspareunia, urinary frequency, pelvic pain, and postcoital spotting. Few patients are asymptomatic at the time of diagnosis. The more severe the symptoms, usually the greater the stage and extent of tumor spread.

Actual diagnosis is made by vaginal inspection, palpation, and direct biopsy of any gross lesion. The most common tumor location is the upper posterior vagina. The lesions are usually exophytic, papillary, spongy, and friable. In the absence of a gross lesion, areas of colposcopic abnormalities as well as epithelium that does not stain after application of Lugol's iodine should also be biopsied.

STAGING

Once malignancy is confirmed, the disease should be staged. Minimum investigation should include a detailed pelvic exam, cystoscopy, proctoscopy, sigmoidoscopy, intravenous pyelography, and chest x-ray. The pelvic examination should include meticulous inspection and palpation of the vulva, perineal area, vagina, and cervix. In addition to outlining uterine and ovarian pathology, the bimanual examination should detail any tumor infiltration of the paravaginal and parametrial tissues.

Further radiologic studies, such as full lung tomography or CT scan, are indicated when the lesion is sarcomatous. Radionuclide scans of the liver, brain, and bones should be done as clinical presentation dictates.

The stage indicates the extent of the disease spread. Stage I carcinoma is limited to the vaginal mucosa; stage II carcinoma involves the subvaginal tissues but has not extended onto the pelvic wall; stage III carcinoma has extended onto the pelvic wall; stage IV carcinoma has extended beyond the true pelvis or has involved the mucosa of the bladder and/or the rectum. Bullous edema or extrinsic tumor compression of the bladder or rectum is not acceptable evidence of invasion of these organs.

TREATMENT

The treatment modality depends on the histologic cell type, tumor location, volume, potential for spread, the patient's age, desire to retain sexual function, and the tumor's proximity to the bladder and rectum. Surgery is the treatment of choice for melanoma, sarcoma, and adenocarcinoma, including the DES-related clear-cell variety. Surgical procedures range from partial vaginectomy to total pelvic exenteration. Irradiation therapy is the treatment of choice for squamous-cell carcinoma because of large lesion size, advanced patient age, and poor operative risk. Irradiation treatment usually entails 4,000-5,000 rads of whole-pelvis teletherapy and two brachytherapy applications. The brachytherapy applications consist of tandem and ovoids, or volume interstitial vaginal implants, or a combination of both. The two applications deliver between 3,000 and 4,000 rads to the vaginal tumor, depending on the duration of treatment time. When deemed necessary, a radiation booster dose via a smaller treatment field is given to the involved area.

Chemotherapy is used as an adjuvant to surgery and irradiation therapy. It is also used in the treatment of recurrent disease.

PROGNOSIS

Prognostic data indicate an overall 5-year survival rate of 5% for melanoma, 35% for sarcoma, 60% for clear-cell adenocarcinoma, and 35-45% for squamous-cell carcinoma. The 5-year survival rates for early-stage clear-cell adenocarcinoma and squamous-cell carcinoma are significantly higher than the collective survival rate.

SUGGESTED READING

Gusberg SB, Frick HC II: *Corscaden's Gynecologic Cancer,* ed 5. Baltimore: Williams & Wilkins, 1978

McGowan L: *Gynecologic Oncology*. New York: Appleton-Century-Crofts, 1978

Morrow CP, Townsend DE: *Synopsis of Gynecologic Oncology,* ed 2. New York: Wiley, 1981

Rutledge F, Boronow RC, Wharton JT: *Gynecologic Oncology*. New York: Wiley, 1976

67

Clear-Cell Carcinoma and Adenosis Due to Diethylstilbestrol Exposure

RICHARD H. NALICK, M.D.

As we advance through the early 1980s, the DES exposure continues to provoke controversy: from the cancer precursor status of offspring exposed in utero to the management of this supposed benign condition, from the primary treatment of early clear-cell carcinoma to the care of the patient with recurrent or metastatic disease, and from the effects of DES exposure on female reproductive function to those seen in the exposed male.

HISTORY OF DES USE

Widespread interest in this problem was initiated by the now classic report of Herbst, Ulfelder, and Poskanzer published in 1971. This thoughtful, retrospective, case-matched study provided statistically significant evidence for the association between DES exposure in utero and the development of clear-cell adenocarcinoma of the cervix and/or vagina.

DES was synthesized in 1938 by Sir Charles Dodd as the first inexpensive, orally effective estrogen. Although it was initially recommended to prevent fetal loss in high-risk pregnancy, potential dangers were recognized through animal studies, resulting in delay in its widespread use. However, in 1945 its use was approved by the AMA and FDA, and it was then widely prescribed from the early 1950s to 1971, even though Dieckmann and colleagues had shown it to be ineffective in the prevention of threatened abortion in 1953. Following the report of Herbst et al, Greenwald et al confirmed the DES-vaginal cancer relationship in 1971 and the FDA recommended that the drug not be used in pregnancy. In 1975, the National Cancer Institute initiated a $2 million, four-center, 5-year cooperative study, the DESAD Project, which has resulted in the accumulation of much significant data.

CLEAR-CELL CARCINOMA

Incidence

It is estimated that over 2 million women were exposed to DES in utero between 1941 and 1971. At least 50,000 females were exposed each year between 1960 and 1970, and as many as 4 million individuals under the age of 35 may have been exposed. To date, over 430 cases of vaginal and cervical clear-cell carcinoma have been reported from the United States alone. The number of cases diagnosed each year increased in the 1960s to 25-30/year in the early 1970s and has now appeared to have reached a plateau or slightly decreased. Among DES-exposed female offspring, the risk of developing this cancer is estimated to be 0.14-1.4:1,000. However, a more accurate figure, based on known cases and estimated numbers exposed, is 1:4,760, or 0.21:1,000.

Of patients with clear-cell carcinoma, 65% have had a history of intrauterine exposure to nonsteroidal synthetic estrogens, 10% were treated with an unidentified drug, and 25% have had no history of DES or DES-like exposure. Clear-cell carcinomas of the cervix and vagina were, of course, also reported to occur prior to the synthesis and widespread use of DES.

In 100% of the cancer cases associated with DES, drug exposure occurred in the first 18 weeks of gestation. Over 90% of these cancer patients have been 14 years of age or older. The age range is 7-31 years, with a peak at 19 years at the time of diagnosis. The dose and duration of maternal DES therapy varied from 1.5 mg to 21,400 mg daily, and from 1 week to 8 months. The duration and dosage appear unimportant, but the stage of gestation at which DES was administered is directly related to the drug's observed effects.

Histopathology

Clear-cell cancer may be flat, nodular, polypoid, papillary, or, occasionally, ulcerated, but most often is submucosal when diagnosed early. Lesions have averaged 1-3 cm (range, 0.3-10 cm) and have been found most often in the upper third of the vagina, with a predilection for the anterior wall. Over 90% have been found in association with adenosis or ectopic columnar epithelium.

Histologically, the patterns vary. Clear-cell carcinomas may be solid, tubulocystic, or papillary, and may occur in pure or mixed forms. The tubulocystic type is the most common, and the papillary pattern the least. The cell type ranges from clear to a hobnail or endometrioid type.

The incidence of lymph node metastases is quite high—approximately 16-18% in stage I disease, and ranging from 30% in vaginal to 60% in cervical stage II disease. It correlates somewhat with lesion size. Spread to regional nodes is uncommon if the primary lesion is less than 1 cm or the depth of invasion is less than 3 mm.

Diagnosis

The diagnosis of clear-cell carcinoma depends on cytology, iodine staining, palpation, and adequate biopsy. Above all, a significant degree of suspicion is necessary. Patients may present with the complaint of vaginal bleeding or discharge; however, 20% are asymptomatic because of the common submucosal position of this tumor. Colposcopy is inadequate as a screening technique for clear-cell carcinoma, and cytology yields a false-negative rate of 20% or more. Thus, non-iodine-staining areas and palpable submucosal nodules must be biopsied.

With a positive diagnosis, the patient should be referred to a gynecologic oncologist for complete oncologic evaluation and definitive treatment. After treatment of clear-cell carcinoma, close follow-up is mandatory and should include chest x-ray, palpation of all nodal areas (especially supraclavicular), rectovaginal pelvic examination, abdominal palpation, Pap test, IVP, and liver scan and/or CT scan as indicated. Colposcopy is useful in the evaluation of mucosal lesions, and for directing biopsies in abnormal areas of the transformation zone, especially when the cytology indicates the presence of squamous dysplasia (CIN).

Management

The management of clear-cell cancer of the cervix and vagina depends on tumor size, depth of invasion, stage, location, and need to preserve fertility. As this tumor tends to remain superficial, some have suggested that it can be treated locally, especially with small, stage I lesions. On this basis, local excision with interstitial or transvaginal radiation has been recommended. However, we are not comfortable with this form of "conservative" therapy, as the nodes are untreated, the ovaries are at risk of radiation damage, the peripheral tumor field may be undertreated, and a high recurrence rate has been noted. Furthermore, our cumulative experience indicates that many of these lesions may be radiation resistant. Thus we consider such conservative management only if there is a strong desire to preserve reproductive function, the lesion is at stage I and smaller than 3 cm, and therapy is preceded by a staging laparotomy to include washings for cytology and selective pelvic lymph node evaluation.

If the lesion is confined to the cervix or upper vagina, the treatment of choice is radical hysterectomy with proximal vaginectomy, pelvic lymphadenectomy, conservation of the ovaries, and reconstruction of the vagina with a split-thickness skin graft. The ovaries may be relocated high and laterally by ovariopexy in order to preserve their function should postoperative pelvic irradiation become necessary to treat positive nodes found on final pathologic evaluation. In such young patients, it is desirable to avoid the late effects of irradiation such as obliterative arteritis, radiation-induced carcinogenesis, bowel and bladder injury, and diminished vaginal function, and this should be carefully considered in planning treatment.

Patients with more extensive lesions—i.e., those larger than 3 cm, stage II-IV lesions, or multifocal tumors—should undergo staging laparoscopy and radical surgical extirpation with or without preoperative irradiation. Primary pelvic exenteration may be considered in selected cases and in those failing to respond to radiation therapy. For cases involving lesions in the distal vagina, radical vulvectomy, inguinal node dissection, and total vaginectomy followed by reconstruction of the vagina by split-thickness skin graft can be considered, although the surgical margins in the region of the bladder may be found to be inadequate, and either anterior exenteration or postoperative radiation may prove necessary.

Prognosis

Survival is related to stage, lesion size, node status, and treatment provided, although follow-up data are still inadequate to determine ideal therapy. Results have been best in patients over 19 years of age and those with the tubulocystic pattern. DES registry data from 1979 and 1980 indicated a 5-year survival rate of 87% and 91% for stage I carcinoma of the vagina and cervix, respectively; 76% and 70% for stage II; 30% for stage III; and one survival for 27 months out of five cases of stage IV disease. A total of 346 patients were followed for as long as 15.3 years (mean, 4.0 years) with a combined (cervical and vaginal) 4-year survival rate of 78%. Of the 346, 68 had died (19.7%). Survival for all stages combined was worse for vaginal cancers (30-35%) than for cervical lesions (55%). However, survival was better for clear-cell adenocarcinoma than for squamous-cell carcinoma of the cervix and vagina.

The majority of recurrences occur in the pelvis (53%), lungs (22%), and supraclavicular nodes (13%). Recurrences have been highest in patients treated by local excision and those with extensive lesions treated by radiation only. To date, chemotherapy has not proven effective in the management of metastatic disease. No complete responses have been reported with cytotoxic drugs, and no objective responses were seen in nine cases treated with progestational agents. 5-Fluorouracil, actinomycin, the *Vinca* alkaloids, and doxorubicin (Adriamycin) have not been of benefit, but results with cisplatin (Platinol) may prove of interest. Increasing experience with the clonogenic assay may reveal single agents or drug combinations of significant benefit.

ADENOSIS

Clinical Picture

In addition to clear-cell carcinoma, structural and epithelial changes are frequently observed in DES-exposed females. Adenosis is defined as the presence of endocervical-like epithelium (mucus-secreting columnar epithelium) in an ectopic position on the ectocervix or vagina. In actuality, adenosis may also consist of nonmucinous epithelium of the tubal or endometrial type, which may be ciliated. To the naked eye, adenosis may appear as areas of friable, red, velvety tissue on the cervix or vagina that do not stain with iodine. These lesions bleed easily and may be covered by mucus. The anterior cervical lip and proximal anterior vagina are most often affected. The endocervical (mucinous) type of cell is seen most often in the proximal vagina; the endometrial or tubal (ciliated) type is usually in the middle or distal third.

In about 20-25% of DES-exposed females, other non-neoplastic structural abnormalities will be found, including so-called transverse ridges, cervical collar, a "cockscomb," concentric cervical rings, a pseudopolypoid appearance of the cervix, obliteration of the vaginal fornices, and a hypoplastic cervix. These structural changes often make delineation of the cervical-vaginal boundaries difficult. They often resolve over time, and appear to be of little importance by themselves. They do seem to be associated with uterine or tubal abnormalities that may adversely affect reproductive function.

Adenosis occurs more often on the cervix than on the vagina, although the vagina is involved in 73% of cases if DES exposure occurred before 8 weeks. The incidence of adenosis in fetuses exposed to DES after 18 weeks is only 7-10%. This is related to the effect of DES on embryogenesis and to more distal placement of the squamocolumnar junction, since vaginal embryogenesis takes place between the 5th and 20th weeks of gestation.

Vaginal adenosis has been seen in women with no history or chance of DES exposure. However, the findings are usually minimal in these cases and may be secondary to high levels of endogenous estrogen during pregnancy.

Patients with adenosis may or may not have a documented history of DES exposure, and may or may not have specific symptoms. The most common complaint is a heavy, mucoid discharge, although vaginal spotting is frequently noted. Of great importance is the presence of these symptoms in the prepubertal child, especially with a DES history.

Risk of Malignancy

Although the development of clear-cut adenocarcinoma from adenosis remains to be proven, there have been several recent reports of carcinoma diagnosed in patients previously noted to have adenosis alone. Progression from the benign to the malignant state may have occurred, but it is more likely that an early, submucosal tumor was missed. In any event, patients with adenosis are at risk of developing carcinoma and must be carefully examined and followed closely.

It has been suggested that the larger transformation zones seen in these patients place them at greater risk for cervical/vaginal dysplasia, but this has not proven to be the case. Interestingly, one often sees abnormal colposcopic patterns suggestive of severe dysplasia or carcinoma in situ, most frequently represented by a coarse mosaic pattern. However, the Pap test is usually negative, and the directed biopsy proves consistent with atypical or immature squamous metaplasia. Obviously, histologic evaluation of an abnormal Pap smear or colposcopic lesion is mandatory before any treatment is initiated. Of 1,275 DES-exposed females reviewed, only 14 (1.1%) had mild or moderate dysplasia, an incidence similar to the unexposed population.

Screening and Examination

We recommend that any young woman exposed to DES in utero be examined when she begins to menstruate or by age 14. Any DES-exposed prepubertal child with vaginal bleeding, staining, or discharge should undergo immediate examination under anesthesia. Women exposed early in their mothers' pregnancies (7-18 weeks) and/or with cervical/vaginal adenosis and/or structural change should be examined every 6 months; others yearly.

Examination of the DES-exposed patient is comprehensive. A routine history is obtained, and a complete physical examination is then performed with inspection of the entire vagina and the cervix. Direct cytologic scraping of all four walls of the upper vagina, the ectocervix, and the endocervical canal is done. The vaginal and cervical samples are obtained separately. One-half-strength Lugol's solution is then liberally painted over the cervix and entire vagina. Nonstaining areas are biopsied. Colposcopy may be employed before iodine staining, but it is not mandatory, rather adjunctive, especially if the Pap test is abnormal.

The entire vagina is palpated, preferably before the speculum examination. Any nodular or polypoid areas are biopsied, especially if associated with non-staining or colposcopic abnormality. A bimanual rectovaginal pelvic examination completes the evaluation process.

If the initial examination is negative for adenosis and/or structural changes, the patient should be re-examined annually. If these changes are noted later, examination should then be carried out every 6 months.

Treatment

Although a variety of modalities have been utilized for the treatment of symptomatic adenosis, none is recommended other than such conservative measures as douching with vinegar solutions, use of acidic vaginal creams, and close observation. If the mucous discharge is particularly bothersome to the patient, cryosurgery may be used to treat a large cervical zone of adenosis. However, there is absolutely no place for surgery, hot cautery, or hormone therapy in this setting. With the passage of time, squamous metaplasia usually replaces the ectopic mucinous epithelium, with an accompanying reduction in vaginal discharge and friability.

There is no evidence that use of oral contraceptives is either beneficial or harmful. These products may increase the degree of mucous discharge, which may prove to be a relative drawback. Microspectrophotometric study of nuclear DNA can be utilized to differentiate neoplastic (aneuploid) from immature metaplastic (euploid) cells.

EFFECTS OF DES ON FEMALE REPRODUCTIVE FUNCTION

Problems of infertility and pregnancy have been noted in DES-exposed women. These include morphologic defects: the "DES" uterus with abnormal cavity, hypoplasia, synechiae, and patulous cervix as well as transverse vaginal septa and a narrowed vagina. Physiologic abnormalities—oligomenorrhea, hypomenorrhea, and primary dysmenorrhea—are also seen, in addition to functional problems. Effects on pregnancy outcome include abortion, premature labor due to incompetent cervix, and ectopic pregnancy.

Studies at Chicago Lying-In Hospital, reported in May 1981, indicated that DES daughters are less likely to conceive and have a lower chance of delivering full-term infants. These conclusions were based on a double-blind study of 226 DES-exposed pregnancies. However, a second study, at Massachusetts General Hospital as part of the DESAD Project, contradicts the Chicago findings in that fertility was not affected. Although more DES-exposed daughters had unfavorable outcomes, 81% who did become pregnant achieved at least one full-term birth.

When pregnant, the DES-exposed daughter should be followed closely and considered at high risk for either early or late pregnancy loss. The cervix should be examined frequently and cerclage considered if there is a history of prior loss or evidence of premature cervical ripening or dilation. Sonography should be considered at 5-6 weeks' gestation to rule out ectopic pregnancy. Prolonged bed rest may be required, and drugs such as ritodrine (Yutopar) may be beneficial.

EFFECTS OF DES ON MALE OFFSPRING

Collected studies now indicate that transplacental effects of DES do indeed occur in the male, including structural and functional changes that may impair fertility. More recently, evidence is accumulating that implies a possible association with testicular carcinoma.

Related abnormalities include "small penis," cryptorchidism, epididymal cysts, urethral stenosis, hypospadias, and varicocele. Functional changes include low sperm counts, decreased motility, abnormal sperm forms, and resultant impaired fertility. A 1979 study by Henderson indicated that a relative excess of endogenous or exogenous hormone (including estrogen) at the time of testicular differentiation (seventh week of gestation) is related to cryptorchidism and may be a major risk factor in testicular cancer. Of course, much more information is required before this hypothesis can be substantiated.

Certainly, the full impact of intrauterine exposure to DES and other nonsteroidal synthetic estrogens remains to be elucidated. In the interim, all known exposed individuals should be closely observed and the appropriate diagnostic studies utilized as indicated. The DES-exposed male should be followed by an interested and well-informed pediatrician, pediatric urologist, or urologist.

SUGGESTED READING

Barnes AB: Reduced fertility in women exposed to DES in utero. *N Engl J Med* 302:609, 1980

Berger MJ, Goldstein DP: Impaired reproductive performance in DES-exposed women. *Obstet Gynecol* 55:25, 1979

Bibbo M, Gill WB, Azizi F, et al: Follow-up study of male and female offspring of DES-exposed mothers. *Obstet Gynecol* 49:1, 1977

Cosgrove M, Benton B, Henderson B: Male genitourinary abnormalities and maternal diethylstilbestrol. *J Urol* 117:220, 1977

Dieckmann WJ, Davis MD, Rynkiewiez LM, Pottinger RE: Does administration of diethylstilbestrol during pregnancy have therapeutic value? *Am J Obstet Gynecol* 66:1062, 1953

Forsberg JG: Cervicovaginal epithelium: Its origin and development. *Am J Obstet Gynecol* 115:1025, 1973

Fowler WC Jr, Schmidt G, Edelman DA, Kaufman AG, Fenoglio CM: Risks of cervical intraepithelial neoplasia among DES-exposed women. *Obstet Gynecol* 58:720, 1981

Gill WB, Schumacher GFB, Bibbo M: Pathological semen and anatomical abnormalities of the genital tract in human male subjects exposed to diethylstilbestrol in utero. *J Urol* 117:220, 1977

Greenwald P, Nasca PC, Burnett WS, Polan WS: Prenatal stilbestrol experience of mothers of young cancer patients. *Cancer* 31:568, 1973

Henderson BE, Benton B, Jing J, Yu MC, Pike MC: Risk factors for cancer of the testis in young men. *Int J Cancer* 23:598, 1979

Herbst AL, Cole P, Colton T, Robboy SJ, Scully RE: Age incidence and risk of diethylstilbestrol-related clear cell adenocarcinoma of the vagina and cervix. *Am J Obstet Gynecol* 135:876, 1979

Herbst AL, Hubby MN, Azizi F, Makii MM: Reproductive and gynecologic surgical experience in diethyl-stilbestrol-exposed daughters. *Am J Obstet Gynecol* 141:1019, 1981

Herbst AL, Norusis MJ, Rosencro PJ, Welsh WR, Scully RE: An analysis of 346 cases of clear cell adeno-carcinoma of the vagina and cervix with emphases on recurrence and survival. *Gynecol Oncol* 1:111, 1979

Herbst AL, Scully RE: Update on DES daughters. *Contemp Ob/Gyn* 17:55, 1981

Herbst AL, Ulfelder H, Poskanzer DC: Adenocarcinoma of the vagina: Association of maternal stilbestrol therapy with tumor appearance in young women. *N Engl J Med* 284:878, 1971

Kaufman RH, Binder GC, Gray PM, Adam E: Upper genital tract change associated with exposure in utero to DES. *Am J Obstet Gynecol* 128:51, 1977

Mangan CE, Borow L, Burtnett-Rubin MM, Egam V, Giuntoli RL, Mikuta JJ: Pregnancy outcome in 98 women exposed to diethylstilbestrol in utero, their mothers and unexposed siblings. *Obstet Gynecol* 59:315, 1982

Sandberg EC: Benign cervical and vaginal changes with exposure to stilbestrol in utero. *Am J Obstet Gynecol* 125:777, 1976

Sandberg EC, Riffle NL, Higdon JV, Getman CE: Pregnancy outcome in women exposed to diethylstilbes-trol in utero. *Am J Obstet Gynecol* 140:194, 1981

Scully RE, Robboy SJ, Welch WR: Pathology and pathogenesis of diethylstilbestrol-related disorders of the female genital tract. In Herbert AL, ed: *Intrauterine Exposure to Diethylstilbestrol in the Human.* Chicago: American College of Obstetricians and Gynecologists, 1978, pp 8-22

Stafl A, Mattingly RF: Vaginal adenosis: A precancerous lesion? *Am J Obstet Gynecol* 120:666, 1977

Stilman RJ: In utero exposure to diethylstilbestrol: Adverse effects on the reproductive tract and reproduc-tive performance in male and female offspring. *Am J Obstet Gynecol* 142:905, 1982

Veridiano NP, Tancer ML, Deike I, Gal D, Giannatasio C: Delayed onset of clear cell adenocarcinoma of the vagina in DES-exposed pregnancy. *Obstet Gynecol* 57:395, 1981

Welch WR, Robboy SJ, Townsend DE, Barnes AB, Scully RE, Herbst AL: Comparison of histologic and colposcopic findings in DES-exposed females. *Obstet Gynecol* 52:457, 1978

Wharton JT, Rutledge GN, Gallagher SH, Fletcher GH: Treatment of clear cell adenocarcinoma in young females. *Obstet Gynecol* 45:365, 1975

68

The Pap Test: Significance, Frequency, and Technique

RICHARD H. NALICK, M.D.

INCIDENCE OF CIN

American Cancer Society data, as well as general large-scale cytologic screening programs, have documented a significant decline in the incidence of cervical cancer and modest decreases in the associated death rate. Projections for 1980 indicated that approximately 20,000 new cases would be diagnosed, and that 6,800-7,000 women would die from their disease. Although newer techniques of radical surgery and megavoltage radiation therapy have played an important part in decreasing the death rate, the majority of improvement can be clearly attributed to cytologic screening for the precursor lesions, which form a continuum from mild dysplasia to carcinoma in situ (cervical intraepithelial neoplasia, or CIN). Appropriate obliteration of these lesions prevents progression to malignancy, while cytologic screening also increases the odds of detecting existing invasive cancer at early stages in the screened population. These findings are manifested in the results of the Canadian Task Force on Cervical Cancer Screening Programs, as well as in the analysis by Boyes et al of the British Columbia Screening Program.

However, as the overall incidence of invasive cancer has fallen, the number of cases of both preinvasive and invasive disease has rapidly increased in the younger population. In fact, the spectrum has shifted to the left, with a lower average age for all lesions of the CIN spectrum. In 1978, 40,000 cases of CIN were reported, and the trend continues upward. Several studies have shown a substantial incidence of dysplasia in sexually active but asymptomatic 14-16-year-olds, with a marked increase in the late teens and early 20s.

These data, in addition to other epidemiologic evidence, suggest that squamous-cell carcinoma and its precursors (CIN) represent a venereal disease, with all that this implies. Thus, a woman's risk is related to young age (<18 years) at first intercourse, early pregnancy, contact with multiple partners at an early age, and promiscuity of her male contacts. Changing sexual habits have led not only to a decrease in age at first coitus and early contact with multiple partners, but also, with increasing use of oral contraceptives and IUDs, to more frequent direct contact between penis and cervix. Thus, whatever the etiologic agent—herpesvirus type 2, sperm DNA, condyloma virus, or other carcinogen—frequent sexual exposure of the "young" cervix increases the risk of cervical cancer and its precursors.

SCREENING FREQUENCY AND TECHNIQUE

Epidemiologic information should be taken into consideration in determining the frequency of cytologic screening. Yet at a time when the incidence of CIN is approaching epidemic proportions, we see publications that discredit annual cytologic screening as not being cost-effective, and the American Cancer Society advocating a departure from annual screening for the majority of women. They do not clearly define low-risk versus high-risk women, nor do they take into consideration ethnic, socioeconomic, and geographic factors. In addition, they ignore the changing sexual habits of the young women of today.

What, then, is the ideal screening frequency and technique? The answer depends on two important considerations: the false-negative rate of the routine Pap test and high-risk versus low-risk factors. The overall false-negative rate for a Pap smear of the ectocervix is at best 12-14%. If a smear of the vaginal pool alone is obtained, it may be as high as 25-50%. For samples obtained by bulb aspiration or a saline-moistened cotton swab from the endocervical canal, however, the false-negative rate is 8%, and a sample combining both an ectocervical scrape and an endocervical smear or aspirate will result in a false-negative rate of 4-6%. Thus, we recommend the latter two-sample technique, with the material combined on one slide. The slide must be clean, the smear must not be too thick or thin, and it should be fixed rapidly.

The clinician should choose a laboratory that employs an experienced cytopathologist who will report the cytologic results in a narrative style using histologic terminology (e.g., "atypical cells present, consistent with moderate dysplasia") rather than in a numerical format (e.g., class II) or a cursory "negative," "suspicious," or "positive."

In 1976, the Canadian Task Force on Cervical Cancer Screening Programs recommended (1) an initial Pap test by age 18 or whenever the woman becomes sexually active, (2) a repeat smear 1 year later to rule out a previous false-negative result, and (3) if both were negative, repeat cytology every 3 years until age 35, and then every 5 years until age 60, after which no further screening is necessary. A subgroup of "high-risk" patients, having had early coitus with multiple partners, would receive an annual smear. The American Cancer Society recommendations are essentially a modification of this scheme.

However, in dealing with the United States population today, which increasingly falls within the high-risk category, the data of Fox take on great significance for the frequency of cytologic sampling. Fox reported on 547 patients with abnormal cytology and CIN of varying degrees of severity. Of these, 195 had had three prior negative reports; 141 developed their atypia less than 2 years after their last smear, with one patient found to have stage I invasive carcinoma 14 months after her last negative Pap test; finally, 53 of 140 patients developed significant changes within 6 months of a negative smear. This study makes a strong argument for an annual Pap test in all women, and perhaps a smear every 6 months for high-risk patients.

Although we may identify a high-risk group, we must remember that these women do not readily identify themselves. Furthermore, the clinical history in regard to sexual activity is generally unreliable. Thus, the Pap test may be more cost-effective than the in-depth interview necessary to identify the high-risk patient.

It also should not be forgotten that a yearly Pap test provides the stimulus for the majority of women to obtain a yearly check-up, which should include palpation of the breasts, bimanual rectovaginal examination of the uterus and ovaries, and digital examination of the anus and rectum—all organ sites that harbor a significant proportion of the malignancies afflicting women.

Finally, in view of Fox's data, the clinician should consider the medicolegal implications of missing an early invasive cervical carcinoma on the basis of a prolonged interval between Pap tests in a supposedly "low-risk" patient.

SUMMARY

The following are our recommendations:

1. Obtain an initial Pap test in all women by age 18. Repeat it 1 year later to rule out a false-negative result, and then do the test annually in all sexually active women.
2. A Pap test should be done as soon as any young girl begins an active sexual life, regardless of age, and repeated annually.
3. A Pap test should be part of an annual physical that also includes breast examination, rectovaginal palpation of the ovaries, and digital anorectal examination.
4. Perform an annual Pap test in all high-risk women regardless of age; consider a Pap smear every 6 months in women with previous CIN and other high-risk factors:
   a. First coitus under age 18; multiple partners.
   b. First pregnancy under age 18.
   c. History of herpesvirus type 2 or condyloma acuminatum.
   d. Contact with a promiscuous male, with a male previously married to a woman with cervical carcinoma, or a male with a history of carcinoma of the penis.
5. Low-risk women who may undergo a Pap test at longer intervals while still having a yearly examination include the following:
   a. Those not falling in any category above.
   b. Those with a history of three consecutive negative annual Pap tests, and over age 35: recommend a Pap test every 2 years.
   c. Those with no history of CIN and over age 50: recommend a Pap test every 3 years unless at risk for endometrial cancer, i.e., on estrogen, obese, history of D&Cs for abnormal bleeding or late menopause: recommend Pap to assist in detection of endometrial carcinoma.

6. Obtain Pap smear as follows:
   a. Use only vaginal secretions to lubricate the speculum; avoid trauma to ectocervix.
   b. Gently remove *excess* exudate or mucus with sponge or cotton balls.
   c. Have fixative jar open and clean slides ready.
   d. Rotate saline-moistened, cotton-tipped applicator in endocervical canal for 5 seconds, rapidly spread over two-thirds of glass slide, and immediately place in fixative.
   e. Firmly scrape ectocervix circumferentially several times with wooden or plastic spatula and spread over two-thirds of a second slide and place in fixative.
   f. Both samples may be placed on one slide if the procedure is performed rapidly.
7. Choose a lab with an experienced cytopathologist who reports results utilizing a narrative form and histologic criteria. The lab should process a minimum of 25,000 smears per year and employ at least three qualified cytotechnologists. There should be a high degree of correlation between the smear reports and any subsequent histology as seen on biopsy.

SUGGESTED READING

American Cancer Society Report on Cytologic Screening. New York: American Cancer Society, 1980

Boyes DA, Nichols TM, Milner AM, Worth AJ: Recent results from the British Columbia Screening Program for Cervical Cancer. *Am J Obstet Gynecol* 128:692, 1977

Canadian Task Force: Cervical Cancer Screening Programs: The Walton report. *Can Med Assoc J* 114:1003, 1976

Fox CH: Time necessary for conversion of normal to dysplastic cervical epithelium. *Obstet Gynecol* 31:749, 1968

Nalick RH: The Pap test: How often? *West J Med* 233, March 1980

69

Preinvasive Cancer of the Cervix and Vagina

OTIS GADDIS JR., M.D.

A report from the pathology laboratory indicating an abnormal Papanicolaou smear suggestive of cervical or vaginal dysplasia should always arouse suspicion of possible genital tract malignancy. It is the physician's duty to ferret out the etiology of the abnormal smear with the ultimate goal of ruling out invasive carcinoma of the cervix or vagina. Exfoliative cytology is the primary tool used to identify patients with preinvasive or invasive neoplasia. Fewer than 5% of smears showing dysplasia will lead to a diagnosis of invasive cervical or vaginal cancer. Many more abnormal smears will be secondary to cervical inflammation, vaginitis, or immature squamous metaplasia. Nevertheless, all abnormal cytologic smears, even those showing mild dysplasia, must be evaluated to the maximum, since invasive cancer has been found with very early changes in the Pap smear and, on rare occasions, even with a normal Pap smear report.

The characteristics of the high-risk patient include teen-age marriage and childbirth, first coitus in teen-age years, multiple sexual partners or marriages, high parity, and herpes type 2 infections. Investigations of abnormal smears in such patients are more likely to reveal significant cervical or vaginal neoplasia.

EVALUATION SCHEME

A step-by-step evaluation of the patient with an abnormal Pap smear should include repeat cytology, gross inspection of the cervix and vagina, colposcopy of the cervix and vagina using 3-5% acetic acid, staining with Lugol's solution, endocervical curettage if the patient is not pregnant, and colposcopically directed biopsy.

Repeat Cytology

When an abnormal smear is obtained, the first step is to repeat the cytology. This is best performed by os aspiration combined with ectocervical scrape. If an os aspirator is unavailable, a saline-moistened cotton-tipped applicator serves as a good second choice. Pap smears in posthysterectomy patients should include a 360-degree vaginal scrape from apex to introitus. A second abnormal smear confirms the initial cytology and decreases the possibility of initial lab error. Nevertheless, a single abnormal smear should receive aggressive investigation.

Gross Inspection
The cervix and vagina should now be cleansed of mucus and debris and inspected for possible gross lesions. If found, these lesions should be biopsied.

Colposcopy
Without evidence of gross lesions, colposcopy is employed. A solution of 3-5% acetic acid is applied copiously to the cervix and vagina. The cervicovaginal epithelium is then inspected colposcopically for patterns consistent with dysplasia. Frequently noted abnormal patterns include white epithelium, punctation, mosaic structure, and abnormal blood vessels. If found, such lesions are biopsied under direct colposcopic vision. It is of utmost importance to examine the total limits of the lesion and evaluate the entire transformation zone—the area of columnar epithelium that has been replaced by squamous metaplasia. When the lesion extends into the endocervical canal, an endocervical speculum will aid in its evaluation.

The advent of the colposcope has made four-quadrant cervical biopsy obsolete. Colposcopy has also decreased the necessity for conization to fewer than 10% of cases. However, failure to outline the limits of lesions with the colposcope, or the presence of dysplastic cells on endocervical curettage, mandates a cone biopsy. It is also of note that the accuracy of colposcopy decreases when used to evaluate previously manipulated lesions. Such manipulations include previous hot cautery or cryosurgery, multiple biopsies, previous cone biopsy, and endocervical curettage.

Staining With Lugol's Solution
Occasionally the colposcope will not reveal any lesion. In such cases, Lugol's iodine solution is helpful in identifying neoplastic epithelium. Glycogen-rich normal epithelium stains a deep mahogany, whereas dysplastic tissue does not take up the stain and appears pale yellow or gold. Lugol's solution is extremely helpful in evaluating vaginal lesions in posthysterectomy patients, in whom multiple vaginal folds and furrows make colposcopy extremely difficult.

Endocervical Curettage
There is a continued controversy as to which patients should undergo endocervical curettage. Because of varying levels of colposcopic expertise, it is recommended that endocervical curettage be performed on all nonpregnant patients, regardless of lesion location, to minimize the possibility of mismanagement secondary to insufficient data. Failure to perform pretreatment endocervical curettage is a major breach in the work-up schema, which has occasionally resulted in inappropriate cryotherapy of invasive cervical carcinoma.

Also, early endocervical adenocarcinoma, which does not lend itself well to colposcopic techniques, is sometimes diagnosed by endocervical curettage.

TREATMENT

Outpatient treatment modalities for intraepithelial neoplasia consist of excision biopsy for small isolated vaginal or cervical lesions, cryosurgery or carbon dioxide laser for diffuse ectocervical disease without canal involvement, and 5-fluorouracil chemotherapy for diffuse vaginal disease. Inpatient treatment may consist of irradiation or surgery. Irradiation can be used to treat inoperable cervical and/or vaginal intraepithelial lesions. Surgical modalities consist of partial or complete vaginectomy with split-thickness skin graft for diffuse vaginal disease, and conization for inadequately evaluated cervical lesions.

Cryosurgery is an ideal treatment for cervical dysplasia in young women with low parity because cervical damage is minimal, fertility is unaltered, and significant complications are rare. Compared with conization, the procedure is quite economical and requires no hospital stay. A cryosurgery cure rate of approximately 90% in the mild to moderate dysplasia groups is comparable to that achieved with conization. However, recent data suggest that conization is superior to cryosurgery for advanced dysplasia and carcinoma in situ. The recurrence of dysplasia following cryosurgery ranges from 3% to 6%.

Another controversy concerns conization-associated infertility. Cone biopsy is a more morbid procedure than cryotherapy, with postcone hemorrhage and infection leading the list of potential complications. And while there is a suggestive relationship, it has not been possible to verify a direct causal relationship between cone biopsy and infertility because of concomitant uncontrollable reproductive factors. Recent data do suggest a direct correlation between pregnancy wastage and increasing size of cone biopsy, and a positive correlation between cervical stenosis and increasing cone size.

Literature review indicates that cone biopsy with clear margins is as effective as hysterectomy in preinvasive disease. Hysterectomy is thus reserved for patients with postcone residual endocervical lesions or associated gynecologic pathology, or for patients requesting sterilization by hysterectomy. Patients with stage Ia microinvasion of the cervix should also be treated with simple hysterectomy.

SUGGESTED READING

Benedet JL, Nickerson KG, Anderson GH: Cryotherapy in the treatment of cervical intraepithelial neoplasia. *Obstet Gynecol* 58:725, 1981

Hatch KD, Shingleton HM, Austin JM Jr, et al: Cryosurgery of cervical intraepithelial neoplasia. *Obstet Gynecol* 57:692, 1981

Ostergard DR: Cryosurgical treatment of cervical intraepithelial neoplasia. *Obstet Gynecol* 56:231, 1980

Townsend DE, Richart RM, Marks E, et al: Invasive cancer following outpatient evaluation and therapy for cervical disease. *Obstet Gynecol* 57:145, 1981

70

Invasive Carcinoma of the Cervix

RICHARD H. NALICK, M.D.

INCIDENCE

Although carcinoma of the endometrium has now surpassed cervical carcinoma as the most common gynecologic malignancy, cervical cancer annually accounts for more than twice as many deaths as endometrial carcinoma in the United States. Approximately 16,000 new cases of cervical carcinoma were diagnosed in 1981, and 6,800 women succumbed to this neoplasm. Today this malignancy ranks sixth in incidence among all cancers in American women. However, there are varying incidence rates in different populations: 12:100,000 in Israeli women, 180:100,000 in Colombian women, and 50:100,000 in Connecticut women 45-65 years old.

Although a simple vaginal speculum makes the uterine cervix clearly accessible for inspection, cytologic evaluation, and tissue biopsy, thus allowing diagnosis of the precursor lesions of dysplasia and carcinoma in situ, the incidence data indicate that those individuals most at risk are not being screened. Clearly, all precursor lesions of cervical intraepithelial neoplasia (CIN) should be diagnosed and treated before progression to invasive carcinoma. Although exceptions may exist, the majority of advanced CIN lesions persist for months to years before becoming invasive, and are entirely curable; yet 75-80% of patients present with advanced disease (stages IIb-IVb) and the number of deaths from this form of cancer has decreased only imperceptibly over the past 10-15 years. Improved techniques of radical surgery and megavoltage irradiation have prolonged survival and decreased morbidity.

Although initially confined to the cervix, cervical carcinoma is an aggressive malignancy that may spread to the vagina, tissues adjacent to the cervix, pelvic and aortic lymph nodes, bladder, rectum, vulva, liver, peritoneal cavity, supraclavicular nodes, lungs, and bones. Advanced disease thus may result in severe hemorrhage, pelvic, low back, and leg pain, multiple fistulas involving the vagina, rectum, bladder, ureters, and small bowel, foul necrotic discharge, widespread metastases, uremia, sepsis, and, mercifully, death.

EPIDEMIOLOGY

Most studies indicate a relationship between the incidence of cervical cancer and sexual activity, including first intercourse at an early age (<18 years), first pregnancy at an early age, and coitus with multiple partners. In one study, 23% of controls and 45% of cervical cancer patients had married before age 20. Other studies have shown that cervical cancer occurs five times more frequently among women starting intercourse by age 16 than among those starting at the age of 24. Other factors directly or indirectly related to sexual activity include low socioeconomic status, prostitution, divorce, poor genital hygiene, marriage to a man previously married to a woman with cervical cancer, and a history of herpes simplex type 2 genital infection.

The rate of dysplasia and carcinoma in situ is increasing among young teenagers and women in their early 20s—a finding related to the increased rate of frequent intercourse at a young age and with multiple sexual partners. The young cervix is exposed to a potential carcinogen (herpesvirus, condyloma virus, abnormal sperm DNA, etc.), often in the absence of a barrier method of contraception, at a time when it is most vulnerable, i.e., when rapidly undergoing the physiologic changes of squamous metaplasia. It is estimated that 45,000 new cases of carcinoma in situ of the cervix were reported in 1981, and a significant proportion was found in young girls and women.

Factors such as chronic cervicitis, diethylstilbestrol exposure, use of oral contraceptives, *Trichomonas* infection, and lack of circumcision in male partners are now felt to be unimportant in the etiology of this malignancy. Cervical carcinoma is more prevalent among women with syphilis than among controls, in a ratio of 3:1, but this is more likely a function of sexual activity.

Orthodox Jewish women may have a degree of immunity to cervical cancer. The ratio of incidence of squamous-cell cervical carcinoma between non-Jewish and Jewish populations varies from 5.3:1 to 9:1. In fact, an Orthodox Jewish woman with squamous-cell carcinoma of the cervix represents a reportable case. However, these women do develop adenocarcinoma of the cervix.

Although the condyloma virus has recently been suggested as a possible etiologic agent, herpesvirus type 2 remains the most likely infectious agent. Approximately 24% of women with active herpes infection of the external genitalia have abnormal Pap tests, as compared with 1.6% of controls. Furthermore, 80-100% of patients with invasive cancer have positive HSV-2 titers, compared with 20% of controls. However, research has yet to firmly establish herpesvirus type 2 as a direct cause of cervical carcinoma. Epidemiologic evidence has accumulated over the past few years, suggesting that the histone:protamine ratio in sperm may be an important factor in the development of this neoplasm.

SCREENING

At present, cervical carcinoma is the sole cancer for which long-term, widespread screening has been carried out. According to a 1976 report, almost 61% of women (in the U.S.) aged 18-34 had had a Pap test during the preceding year and 82% reported having had at least one during their lives. With increasing emphasis on the annual Pap test, a significant proportion of informed women have availed themselves of it. However, this leaves a sizable segment of the population that does not get routine screening and, in some cases, has never had a Pap test: mostly women in the lower socioeconomic, high-risk group, who present most often with advanced cancer. Obviously, more effort must be expended to bring these women into screening programs such as the Porta-Pap program sponsored by the Community Cancer Center of Los Angeles (CCCLA), which concentrates its screening efforts in low socioeconomic neighborhoods. Clearly, the women *least* at risk for cervical cancer are the ones most likely to obtain routine screening, and vice versa.

There is no morbidity related to the Pap test. The only risks revolve around the accuracy of the technique and the potential for undertreatment or overly aggressive therapy. A Pap smear taken from the vaginal pool of secretions is essentially worthless in diagnosing cervical neoplasia. A smear obtained from the ectocervix alone (as practiced by most physicians) may miss or underestimate a lesion in as many as 14-33% of cases. This degree of inaccuracy may be significantly diminished by sampling the endocervical canal with a saline-moistened cotton swab. This technique, combined with an ectocervical scrape, yields the best results—a false-negative rate of <5%. Other factors leading to inaccuracy are thick smears, too much blood or mucus, speculum lubrication, and recent douching or application of vaginal medications. In addition, different cytologists often reach different conclusions about the same slides, which emphasizes the need to base therapy on histologic information (directed biopsy) and not on cytology alone.

SIGNS AND SYMPTOMS

Early invasive cancer produces few symptoms, even when as much as two-thirds of the ectocervix is involved. Endocervical tumors are also notoriously asymptomatic. However, as the tumor progresses, it may outgrow its own blood supply, resulting in necrosis and a foul vaginal discharge. Friable exophytic lesions may bleed spontaneously or after douching or coital contact, although patients more often complain of abnormal menstrual bleeding. In fact, in hospitals dealing with indigent populations, postmenopausal bleeding may be the most common presenting symptom of cervical carcinoma rather than endometrial carcinoma.

As the tumor spreads laterally into the paracervical tissues, the ureters, lymphatics, and pelvic veins and nerves become involved, with resultant back pain, leg swelling, sciatic pain, and uremia if the ureteral obstruction is bilateral. Alternatively, the bladder or rectum may be invaded, with resultant fistula formation, although this is distinctly less common in primary disease and is rare in the absence of lateral spread. When present, symptoms may include dysuria, hematuria, incontinence, diarrhea, or rectal bleeding. Symptoms of advanced or metastatic disease include significant weight loss (>15 lb), anorexia, anemia, bone pain, jaundice, hemoptysis, and cough.

Exophytic lesions originating on the ectocervix are classically cauliflower-like and friable and may become massive, replacing the cervix, involving the vagina, and later ulcerating by sloughing centrally. Endocervical lesions, on the other hand, most often produce a hard, nodular, expanded cervix, with deep stromal invasion resulting in a so-called barrel-shaped cervix. Often the surface appears deceptively benign, frequently leading to missed diagnosis and delayed or inappropriate therapy.

PRINCIPLES OF DIAGNOSIS AND MANAGEMENT

Whether the lesion is occult, confined to the cervix, or massive and fixed to the pelvic sidewall, causing vaginal hemorrhage, the principles of diagnosis and management remain the same: histologic diagnosis with careful review of the slides, gynecologic oncology work-up, clinical staging, management of medical complications such as hemorrhage, anemia, infection, uremia, and fistulas, and appropriate treatment, including irradiation, surgery—either radical or conservative, and/or chemotherapy.

Diagnostic errors can occur when vaginal bleeding is assumed to be caused by an endocrinologic abnormality, "erosion," cervicitis, threatened abortion, placenta previa, condyloma acuminatum, or cervical polyps. The Pap test often is not performed in the presence of vaginal bleeding, resulting in delayed diagnosis. However, if the cervix is abnormal in appearance, *it must be biopsied regardless of the Pap test result*. In fact, the Pap test may be reported as class I or II in the presence of an exophytic, fungating tumor! Both the center and the periphery of the cervical lesion should be biopsied.

Bleeding is controlled by firm pressure alternating with application of Monsel's solution (ferric subsulfate). Monsel's solution kept exposed to the air in an open jar and allowed to become yellow and soupy is a far more effective hemostatic substance than silver nitrate sticks, acetone, or sponge packs.

If the cervix is grossly normal with an abnormal Pap test, an endocervical curettage and endometrial biopsy or D&C are indicated. A cone biopsy may prove necessary if the ectocervix is grossly normal, if the canal cannot be evaluated by colposcopy, or if endocervical curettage is abnormal. Cone biopsy is contraindicated if there is obvious carcinoma, as it is unnecessary and may lead to hemorrhage, tumor dissemination, and treatment complications.

HISTOLOGY

In 90% of cases, biopsy will reveal squamous-cell (epidermoid) carcinoma. This tumor is felt to arise from dysplastic epithelium originating in the transformation zone at the advancing active squamocolumnar junction. The subgroup classification of Wentz and Reagan divides these lesions into large-cell nonkeratinizing, large-cell keratinizing, and small-cell squamous carcinoma, but does not appear to correlate well with biologic behavior, response to therapy, or prognosis. Table 70-1 lists the histologic variants of cervical cancer.

Glandular variants account for 5-15% of cervical cancers, arise in the endocervical canal, and often lead to endophytic growth. They also may be found more often in the older, obese woman of low parity. The prognosis in these tumors, especially those of mixed types (adenosquamous), is said to be worse, but this may not be true if the data are corrected for stage and age.

TABLE 70-1. HISTOLOGIC VARIANTS OF CERVICAL CANCER

Squamous-cell carcinoma
    Large-cell, keratinizing
    Large-cell, nonkeratinizing
    Small-cell
    Mucoepidermoid
    Verrucous
Sarcoma
    Mixed müllerian
    Leiomyosarcoma
    Rhabdomyosarcoma
    Lymphoma

Glandular carcinoma
    Endocervical (mucinous, colloid)
    Endometrioid (adenoacanthoma)
    Clear-cell (mesonephric)
    Adenoid cystic
    Adenosquamous (mixed)
    Glassy-cell
Apudoma
    Melanoma
    Carcinoid (argentaffin-cell)
    Others (oat-cell)

STAGING

As with all neoplasms, treatment programs must take into consideration both the primary tumor and its potential routes of spread. This is the basis of clinical staging and the oncologic evaluation. Cervical carcinoma spread patterns include contiguous spread to the vaginal membrane, parametrium, pelvic sidewall, uterosacral ligaments, bladder, rectum, and endometrium; lymphatic spread to the regional nodes of the pelvis and inguinal region as well as to distant nodes of the para-aortic chain and supraclavicular region; and hematogenous spread to the lungs, liver, bones, brain, and other distant organs.

Oncologic Work-Up

Cervical cancer is staged clinically as proposed by the General Assembly of the International Federation of Gynecology and Obstetrics (FIGO) in September 1961 and modified in 1976. On this basis, the oncologic work-up should include a CBC, platelet count, liver and renal function tests, PA lateral and oblique chest x-rays, IVP, cystoscopy, sigmoidoscopy, and an adequate rectovaginal examination. Although studies such as colposcopy, venography, and lymphangiography are helpful, they do not form an intrinsic part of the work-up as they are not universally available and their accuracy is variable. A skeletal survey or bone scan is obtained only in the presence of bone pain or lesions seen on chest x-ray or IVP. A barium enema is necessary only in the case of a large pelvic mass, rectal bleeding, or a rectovaginal fistula. A liver scan is ordered only if the liver is enlarged or liver function tests are abnormal. On occasion, if the clinical examination is equivocal, examination under anesthesia may clarify the clinical stage. Lymphangiography appears to have been replaced in many centers by the CT scan, but neither these nor venography are accepted as valid adjuncts for clinical staging. In particular, lymphography is not without complications and has a high rate of false-negative results. Most important, its accuracy is lowest in the presence of small nodal metastases—just the case in which radiation therapy would be most effective. Table 70-2 lists clinical studies to consider in a patient with cervical carcinoma.

TABLE 70-2. CLINICAL STUDIES SUGGESTED FOR PATIENTS WITH CERVICAL CARCINOMA

All patients	Stages II-IV and stage I with bulky disease
Physical exam	Cystoscopy
Biopsy	Sigmoidoscopy
Chest x-ray	Liver scan (also with adenocarcinoma or
Intravenous pyelogram	adenosquamous carcinoma)
Urinary cytology	Liver function tests
Test for occult blood in stool	Serum calcium
Carcinoembryonic antigen (CEA)	CT scan
Routine laboratory tests	Surgical staging laparotomy (IIb, IIIb)

Staging Laparotomy

In recent years, surgical staging laparotomy has been intensively evaluated at major academic centers by gynecologic oncologists under the auspices of the Gynecologic Oncology Group (GOG). These studies have indicated gross inaccuracies in clinical staging, ranging from 15% to 25% in stage Ib and II lesions. A higher than expected incidence of para-aortic node metastases, as well as intra-abdominal seeding and liver metastases, has been found. The frequency of positive pelvic nodes averages 1.5-2% in stage Ia, 10-15% in Ib, 20-25% in II, 35% in III, and 50% in IV. Pelvic node metastases are also closely related to the size of the cervical lesion, as noted by Piver and Chung: <1 cm in 18%, 2-3 cm in 22%, 4-5 cm in 36%, and >6 cm in 50%. Between 10% and 15% of stage II patients have positive para-aortic nodes, and 35-40% of patients with advanced disease (bulky IIIb and IVa) have para-aortic node metastases.

Preradiation laparotomy may uncover large pelvic nodes (>2 cm), which if removed could improve the 30-50% survival figures for patients with positive nodes, but whether or not the same holds true for para-aortic node involvement is debatable, as survival figures for these patients are generally dismal. However, the major cause of treatment failure, other than bulky cervical lesions, does appear to be extrapelvic spread, outside the conventional field of irradiation—i.e., the para-aortic nodes. Therefore, some large institutions are carrying out prospective studies to evaluate the practical efficacy of pretreatment staging laparotomy with para-aortic node evaluation. It would seem logical to assume that a small but definite percentage of patients with palpably negative nodes, but with microscopic disease, may be curable by 4,500-5,000 rads of extended-field irradiation; results of these ongoing studies should soon clarify this point.

MANAGEMENT

Large institutions, such as the Los Angeles County/University of Southern California Medical Center, evaluate 1,000-1,200 new abnormal Pap tests and manage 75-100 fresh cases of invasive cervical cancer per year, while the *busy* clinician may encounter only 10-20 class III Pap tests and 0-2 invasive cancers yearly. However, the private physician must remain cognizant of the correct management of these lesions, both preinvasive and invasive. The benefit of colposcopy in the evaluation of abnormal Pap tests has been well publicized. However, when the diagnosis of invasive carcinoma of the cervix is made on punch biopsy or conization, the clinician may not feel competent to evaluate and manage this malignancy and may seek the assistance of a radiotherapist. Furthermore, when the clinician is confronted in the emergency room with a large, friable lesion and vaginal hemorrhage, panic may be the response, and silver nitrate cauterization and packing inadequate. In both instances, consultation with an experienced gynecologic oncologist may be in the best interests of the patient.

Radiation Therapy

Radiation therapy remains the standard treatment choice for carcinoma of the cervix. Although nearly every large community has a radiation therapist with megavoltage equipment, gynecologic oncologists capable of providing radical surgical treatment are generally found only in large cities, major treatment centers, and university hospitals. Furthermore, radical surgery is indicated as primary treatment only in patients with early invasive disease, i.e., small stage I lesions.

Modern radiation can cure over 50% of patients, all stages combined. At M. D. Anderson Hospital the 5-year survival rate for 2,000 patients was 91.5% for stage I, 83-85% for IIa, 66.5% for IIb, 45% for IIIa, 36% for IIIb, and 14% for IV. The use of radium or cesium is emphasized in early disease, while pelvic irradiation with megavoltage machines (cobalt, linear accelerator, or betatron) provides the major form of treatment in more advanced lesions. In most cases both techniques are utilized, the isotope providing local treatment to the cervix, parametrium, and proximal vaginal membrane, and pelvic irradiation covering these structures as well as other pelvic tissues at risk, such as the pelvic lymph nodes. Sample treatment plans are listed in Table 70-3.

Although the early complications from radiation are generally mild (diarrhea, dysuria, watery vaginal discharge), the late complications may be significant, ranging from vaginal stenosis to sigmoid obstruction, small-bowel injury, and fistulas involving the gastrointestinal, genitourinary, or genital tract. However, radiation therapy is applicable to all patients regardless of age, stage, or medical condition, and with skillful application, morbidity can be minimized.

Radical Hysterectomy

For years the question of radical hysterectomy versus radiation for patients with stage Ib and IIa disease has been controversial. Certainly the cure rates of both modalities are similar for stage Ib disease. Therefore, other factors

TABLE 70-3. SAMPLE RADIATION TREATMENT PLANS
FOR CERVICAL CANCER

Stage	Regimen
Ib	2,000 rads to whole pelvis
	2,000 rads to parametrium (midline block)
	Two 48-hour radium implants* 2 weeks apart
IIb	4,000 rads to whole pelvis; possible 1,000-rad boost to involved side
	Two radium implants* 2 weeks apart for 72 and 48 hours
IIIb	4,000 rads to whole pelvis
	1,000 rads to involved side (parametrium)
	Two radium implants* 2 weeks apart for 72 and 48 hours
IVa	5,000-6,000 rads to whole pelvis
	One 72-hour radium implant*

*Implants average 1,200 to 1,500 mg-hours/24 hours.

must be considered in making the decision. Not least important is the necessity for the services of an experienced gynecologic oncologist if a surgical procedure is contemplated. Second is the need for an adequate supportive facility such as an intensive-care unit. Third is the patient herself: The ideal candidate for radical hysterectomy would be a young, thin woman with a small stage Ib lesion; conversely, a short, obese patient may make the procedure difficult, resulting in potential compromise of the surgical resection. Large cervical lesions may often prove unresectable when positive nodes are found on pelvic lymphadenectomy—a finding that in the minds of many gynecologic oncologists contraindicates radical hysterectomy.

Indications for radical hysterectomy:

Desire to preserve ovarian function

Patient's refusal to accept radiation therapy

History of pelvic inflammatory disease or diverticulitis

Undiagnosed pelvic mass or large uterine fibroids

Geometry of lesion precluding adequate radium placement

Stage Ib lesion in association with early pregnancy

Patient's desire for rapid, definitive therapy.

Advantages of radical hysterectomy:

Preservation of the ovaries

Removal of infected adnexa

Preservation of a functional, though shortened, vagina

Prevention of central recurrence

Avoidance of radioresistance

Shorter treatment

Avoidance of late irradiation complications

Clear estimation of prognosis.

Disadvantages of radical hysterectomy:
Limitation to certain patients
Greater risk of early morbidity and mortality
Higher incidence of urinary fistulas (<1%)
High incidence of bladder dysfunction (usually only short-term)
Shortened vagina
Need for postoperative irradiation if positive pelvic nodes are diagnosed on
final pathologic analysis.

"Barrel Cervix"

Radiation and surgery are often combined for improved results. An example is seen in the management of the large (5-6-cm), barrel-shaped stage Ib cervical lesion. Studies at M. D. Anderson Hospital have shown that the incidence of local recurrence in these cases may be significantly decreased if an extrafascial hysterectomy is performed 4-6 weeks after 4,000-rad whole-pelvis irradiation and one 72-hour radium implant. With this technique, morbidity is acceptable, the central recurrence rate is decreased, and the para-aortic nodes, omentum, and peritoneal cavity can be sampled for cytology at the time of surgery. Appropriate postoperative radiation and/or chemotherapy is then given as indicated.

Pregnancy

Although rare, carcinoma of the cervix is occasionally found in a pregnant woman. Stage for stage, the cure rates are identical with those in nonpregnant women, although curability appears to be lower for patients whose disease is diagnosed in the third trimester or postpartum. The choice between primary surgery and primary irradiation depends on the stage of disease, the stage of gestation, the age of the patient, and her medical condition. Radiation therapy is the same as for nonpregnant patients except that it must be initiated with external therapy and hysterotomy is required in patients beyond the early second trimester of pregnancy. In either case, after extraction or delivery of the fetus, treatment is completed by further irradiation and/or radium implant after uterine involution and cessation of uterine drainage.

Specifically, in the first trimester radical hysterectomy is performed for a stage Ib tumor with the fetus in situ. In the second trimester, hysterotomy may facilitate radical hysterectomy. In the period of viability, a classical cesarean section is performed first. When carcinoma of the cervix is diagnosed between the 26th and 32nd weeks, treatment can be delayed until fetal maturity is reached, as indicated by L/S ratio and other tests. In all cases, pelvic lymphadenectomy is an essential part of the surgical treatment.

Carcinoma of the Cervical Stump

Carcinoma of the cervical stump occurs in 1-10% of patients with cervical cancer. Stage I and IIa disease can be managed by radical cervicectomy, but the operation is made more difficult by adhesions, fibrosis, an absent corpus, and an adherent bladder or rectum. Results are comparable to those achieved with an intact uterus. Although intracavitary radiation therapy is necessarily suboptimal because of the lack of a fundus to hold a tandem, the use of increased external radiation, interstitial implants, or transvaginal orthovoltage therapy can compensate for this disadvantage. Complications of radiation therapy may be higher than with radical surgery.

"Inappropriate" Hysterectomy

Most important is the problem of the "cut-through" hysterectomy. On occasion, a woman undergoing surgery for a benign condition will be found to have invasive cervical carcinoma. Most often such a woman will have been diagnosed as having abnormal uterine bleeding, complications of pregnancy or labor, or a tubo-ovarian abscess. Although some of these women are operated upon on an emergency basis, the majority have elective procedures.

In most cases, adequate preoperative evaluation of the cervix has not been carried out. Not uncommonly, a Pap test has been performed but read as negative. More often, no test has been done within 12 months. Also reported are cases where an irregular cervix is simply assumed to represent chronic cervicitis or cervical "erosion" and has not been biopsied. Unfortunately, in others the Pap test was not normal—i.e., was read as class II or class III—but the cervix was not properly evaluated preoperatively by endocervical curettage, D&C, or cone biopsy. In the majority of these cases the ectocervix is normal and the lesion originated within the endocervical canal.

As tumor is seldom found at the cervical margins (no vaginal or parametrial involvement), the term "cut-through" is too often inaccurate. "Inappropriate hysterectomy" would be more in keeping with surgical or histologic findings.

When carcinoma is unexpectedly found in a simple hysterectomy specimen, postoperative radiation therapy is required. If the disease is localized and the surgical margins are negative, the vagina may be treated by two 48-hour colpostat applications 2 weeks apart or 4,000-rad whole-pelvis irradiation and one 48- or 72-hour colpostat. If the vaginal vault is too narrow for colpostats, treatment may consist of 5,000-rad whole-pelvis irradiation with the port covering the upper third of the vagina. If there is gross tumor in the specimen or tumor transected at the surgical margins (i.e., clinical residual disease), 5,000-5,500 rads may be given to the whole pelvis followed by a vaginal radium implant of 2,000-3,000 mg-hours.

Survival in these cases is excellent (80-100% at 5 years) if there is no tumor at the margins of resection. However, if clinical residual cancer is present or treatment is begun more than 6 months postoperatively, the survival at 5 years is halved (35-40%) in spite of appropriate radiation therapy. In addition, the risk of complications involving the small bowel is greater in the absence of an intervening uterus, intracavitary radium treatment gives suboptimal results (because a tandem cannot be utilized), and the risk of intraperitoneal tumor dissemination is greater following inappropriate hysterectomy. Clearly, the cervix must be adequately evaluated preoperatively by cytology and further investigated by punch biopsy, endocervical curettage, or cone biopsy should results prove other than normal.

POST-TREATMENT FOLLOW-UP

Following initial treatment, close observation is extremely important. Fifty percent of recurrences will be diagnosed within 1 year after treatment, and 75% in 2 years. Ninety-five percent of deaths due to treatment failure occur within 5 years after therapy. Each visit should include review of the stage, grade, and treatment; review of systems with attention to weight loss, vaginal bleeding or discharge, pelvic and leg pain, bladder and bowel function, leg swelling, groin or neck lumps, cough, and chest pain; complete physical examination with particular attention to left supraclavicular and inguinal nodes, abdomen, and pelvis (especially the vulva, suburethral area, clitoris, vagina, cervix, and parametrium); and a Pap test. A chest x-ray is obtained annually, and an IVP at 6 months and 2 years. Any patient with a swollen leg and/or sciatic pain should be assumed to have recurrence until proven otherwise, and an IVP should be obtained immediately. If leg swelling, sciatic pain, and ureteral obstruction on IVP occur on the same side, this triad is essentially pathognomonic of recurrent cervical carcinoma. Often much time is lost in treating such patients for phlebitis or deep vein thrombosis with anticoagulation without obtaining an IVP or a venogram.

RECURRENT CERVICAL CARCINOMA

Recurrent cervical carcinoma is an aggressive disease with a poor prognosis: a 1-year survival rate of 15% and a 5-year survival rate of less than 5%. Basically, only local, resectable disease is really curable, including central pelvic recurrences after primary treatment with radiation. These patients may be treated by anterior or total exenteration, occasionally supplemented by adjunctive chemotherapy.

Patients treated initially by radical hysterectomy who have pelvic recurrences may be salvaged by aggressive radiation. Lower vaginal recurrences may be treated surgically or by radioactive interstitial implants. Unifocal bone metastases may be radiated; a solitary lung nodule may be resectable.

All patients with recurrent cervical carcinoma should be immediately referred to an experienced gynecologic oncologist—not to a medical oncologist, radiation therapist, or general surgeon. The gynecologic oncologist will be able to determine most accurately the best plan of management, whether radical surgery, radiation, or chemotherapy, and will coordinate therapy as indicated. The 2-year survival rate with untreated recurrent cervical cancer is essentially zero, while combined series for pelvic exenteration reveal a 5-year survival of approximately 35%.

CHEMOTHERAPY

If exenteration is determined not to be possible on the basis of metastatic work-up or exploratory laparotomy, chemotherapy may offer significant palliation. Cure rates will be low (<5%), but objective responses have been reported in 13-50% of patients treated with single or multiple agents. Recent results with cisplatin (Platinol), either alone or in combination with such drugs as doxorubicin (Adriamycin) and cyclophosphamide (Cytoxan), are very encouraging. Bleomycin (Blenoxane), mitomycin-C (Mutamycin), vincristine (Oncovin), and methotrexate have also produced reasonable response rates.

Chemotherapy in advanced cervical carcinoma or metastatic disease is best administered by a gynecologic oncologist when possible, as this subspecialist is ideally suited to manage such common problems as complicated fistulas, bowel obstruction, radiation necrosis, pelvic hemorrhage, and chronic pain.

SUMMARY

The ideal management of cervical carcinoma is based on these principles:
- Early diagnosis
- Comprehensive oncologic pretreatment evaluation
- Accurate clinical staging (which may soon include retroperitoneal staging laparotomy for advanced cases, i.e., stages IIb and IIIb)
- A tailor-made plan of management, which may include radical surgery, radiation therapy, and chemotherapy
- Close post-treatment surveillance
- Coordination and management of therapy by a gynecologic oncologist—the "general practitioner" for the woman with gynecologic malignancy.

SUGGESTED READING

Andras EJ, Fletcher GH, Rutledge FN: Radiotherapy of carcinoma of the cervix following simple hysterectomy. *Am J Obstet Gynecol* 115:647, 1973

Averette HE, Dudan RC, Ford JH Jr: Exploratory celiotomy for surgical staging of cervical cancer. *Am J Obstet Gynecol* 113:1090, 1972

Baker LH, Opipari MI, Izbicki RM: Phase II study of mitomycin-C, vincristine, and bleomycin in advanced squamous cell carcinoma of the uterine cervix. *Cancer* 38:2222, 1976

Ballon SC, Berman ML, Lagasse LD, Petrilli ES, Castaldo TW: Survival after extraperitoneal pelvic and paraaortic lymphadenectomy and radiation therapy in cervical carcinoma. *Obstet Gynecol* 57:90, 1981

Buchsbaum HJ: Extrapelvic lymph node metastases in cervical carcinoma. *Am J Obstet Gynecol* 133:814, 1979

Creasman WT, Rutledge FN, Fletcher GH: Carcinoma of the cervix associated with pregnancy. *Obstet Gynecol* 36:495, 1970

Davy M, Bentzen H, Jahren R: Simple hysterectomy in the presence of invasive cervical cancer. *Acta Obstet Gynecol Scand* 56:105, 1977

Delgado G: Stage Ib squamous cancer of the cervix: The choice of treatment. *Obstet Gynecol Surv* 33:174, 1978

DiSaia PJ, Creasman WT: *Clinical Gynecologic Oncology.* St Louis: Mosby, 1981

Fletcher GH: Basic principles of the combination of irradiation and surgery. *Int J Radiat Oncol Biol Phys* 5:2091, 1979

Fletcher GH, ed: *Textbook of Radiotherapy*, ed 3. Philadelphia: Lea & Febiger, 1980

Grumbine FC, Rosenshein NB, Serhouni EA, Siegelman SS: Abdominopelvic computed tomography in the pre-operative evaluation of early cervical cancer. *Gynecol Oncol* 12:286, 1981

Gusberg SB, Frick HC II: *Corscaden's Gynecologic Cancer*, ed 5. Baltimore: Williams & Wilkins, 1978

Hughes RR, Brewington KC, Hanjani P, et al: Extended field irradiation for cervical cancer based on surgical staging. *Gynecol Oncol* 9:153, 1980

Kessler II: On the etiology and prevention of cervical cancer: Status report. *Obstet Gynecol Surv* 34:790, 1979

Kolbenstvedt A: Lymphography in the diagnosis of metastases from carcinoma of the uterine cervix stages I and II. *Acta Radiol Diagn* 16:81, 1975

Kottmeier HL, ed: *Annual Report on the Results of Treatment in Gynecologic Cancer*, vol 17. Stockholm, 1979

Lagasse LD, Creasman WT, Shingleton HM, et al: Results and complications of operative staging in cervical cancer: Experience of the Gynecologic Oncology Group. *Gynecol Oncol* 9:90, 1980

Lu T, Macasaet MA, Nelson JH Jr: The barrel-shaped cervical carcinoma. *Am J Obstet Gynecol* 124:596, 1976

McGowan L: *Gynecologic Oncology*. New York: Appleton-Century Crofts, 1978

Miyamoto T, Takabe Y, Watanabe M, et al: Effectiveness of a sequential combination of bleomycin and mitomycin-C on an advanced cervical cancer. *Cancer* 41:403, 1978

Morley GW, Seski JC: Radical pelvic surgery versus radiation therapy for stage I carcinoma of the cervix. *Am J Obstet Gynecol* 126:785, 1976

Morrow CP, Townsend DE: *Synopsis of Gynecologic Oncology*, ed 2. New York: Wiley, 1981

Nelson AJ III, Fletcher GH, Wharton JT: Indications for adjunctive conservative extrafascial hysterectomy in selected cases of carcinoma of the cervix. *Am J Radiol* 123:91, 1975

O'Quinn AG, Fletcher GH, Wharton JT: Guidelines for conservative hysterectomy after irradiation. *Gynecol Oncol* 9:68, 1980

Piver MS, Chung WS: Prognostic significance of cervical lesion size and pelvic node metastases in cervical carcinoma. *Obstet Gynecol* 46:507, 1975

Prempree T, Patanaphan V, Scott RM: Radiation management of carcinoma of the cervical stump. *Cancer* 43:1262, 1979

Reagan JW, Fu YS: Histologic types and prognosis of cancers of the uterine cervix. *Int J Radiat Oncol Biol Phys* 5:1015, 1979

Rutledge FN, Boronow RC, Wharton JT: *Gynecologic Oncology*. New York: Wiley, 1976

Rutledge FN, Smith JP, Wharton JT, et al: Pelvic exenteration: An analysis of 296 patients. *Am J Obstet Gynecol* 129:881, 1977

Schellhas HF: Extra-peritoneal node dissection through an upper abdominal incision. *Obstet Gynecol* 46:444, 1975

Shingleton HM, Fowler WC Jr, Koch GG: Pretreatment evaluation in cervical cancer. *Am J Obstet Gynecol* 110:385, 1971

Thigpen T, Shingleton H, Homesley H, et al: cis-Dichlorodiammineplatinum(II) in the treatment of gynecologic malignancies: Phase II trials by the Gynecologic Oncology Group. *Cancer Treat Rep* 63:1549, 1979

VanNagell JR Jr, Donaldson ES, Parker JC, et al: The prognostic significance of cell type and lesion size in patients with cervical cancer treated by radical surgery. *Gynecol Oncol* 5:142, 1977

Wentz WB, Reagan JW: Survival in cervical cancer with respect to cell type. *Cancer* 12:384, 1959

Wolff JP, Lacour J, Chassagne D, et al: Cancer of the cervical stump: A study of 173 patients. *Obstet Gynecol* 39:10, 1972

71

Endometrial Hyperplasia

JOHN B. SCHLAERTH, M.D.

The endometrial hyperplasias comprise a spectrum of alterations of the endometrial glands and stroma, from the physiologically normal endometrium to endometrial carcinoma. The terminology for these disorders is not standardized. Most generally accepted are the categories of cystic hyperplasia, adenomatous hyperplasia, atypical adenomatous hyperplasia, and carcinoma in situ. It is felt that these various grades of hyperplasia constitute a continuum of increasing risk for endometrial carcinoma.

The endometrial hyperplasias are clinically important because they are associated with bleeding, which can be severe, infertility, estrogen-producing neoplasms of the ovaries, and endometrial cancer. The management of endometrial hyperplasia depends on the woman's age relative to her reproductive life and the histologic severity of the endometrial lesion.

POSTPUBESCENT WOMEN

In the postpubescent woman, endometrial hyperplasia usually presents as menstrual cycle irregularities and may culminate in heavy vaginal bleeding. If the bleeding is severe, a therapeutic D&C should be done. Otherwise, an endometrial biopsy is the indicated diagnostic test. However, if the biopsy reveals cystic or adenomatous hyperplasia, a diagnostic D&C should be done to evaluate the hyperplasia completely and exclude carcinoma. Then monthly cyclic progestins, such as medroxyprogesterone acetate (Amen, Provera) 10 mg or norethindrone acetate (Norlutate) 10 mg daily for 5-7 days, will prevent further episodes of heavy bleeding and ensure regular withdrawal bleeding.

For the rare patient in this age group with atypical adenomatous hyperplasia or carcinoma in situ of the endometrium, the therapy is more extended. Again, a D&C is recommended to exclude carcinoma. We then favor long-term progestin therapy to reverse the hyperplasia. Many regimens have been used with some success. Our preference is to use megestrol (Megace) 20 mg bid. We obtain a follow-up endometrial biopsy after 3 and 6 months of progestin therapy to confirm regression of the hyperplastic lesion. Megestrol is stopped after 6 to 12 months. If a normal menstrual pattern does not return, it would be well to maintain these women on monthly cyclic progestin therapy, using medroxyprogesterone acetate 10 mg daily for 10-14 days.

WOMEN OF CHILDBEARING AGE

Another group of patients presenting with endometrial hyperplasia comprises women in the reproductive age group in whom infertility is a problem. The association of infertility, anovulation, and endometrial hyperplasia makes an endometrial biopsy an important step in the evaluation of these patients. For patients with cystic or adenomatous hyperplasia, the routine therapy is to induce ovulation after a D&C to exclude carcinoma. For patients with atypical adenomatous hyperplasia or carcinoma in situ diagnosed on biopsy and D&C, it is well to document regression before attempting to induce ovulation. This is preferred because ovulation may not occur for several months and during this time the endometrium would continue to be stimulated by endogenous estrogens. Also, pregnancy can occur even if the premalignant lesion does not revert to a normal pattern. Suppression can be accomplished with megestrol 20 mg bid for 6 months. The endometrium is biopsied at 3 and 6 months to confirm regression.

PERIMENOPAUSAL WOMEN

As a woman ends her reproductive years and ovulation tends to become less regular, endometrial hyperplasia may occur. Any abnormal bleeding in perimenopausal women should be evaluated by a fractional D&C to rule out the presence of endometrial or endocervical carcinoma. With a fractional D&C diagnosis of cystic or adenomatous hyperplasia, the patient is maintained on monthly progestins such as medroxyprogesterone acetate 10 mg for 5-7 days to ensure regular withdrawal bleeding. However, at times perimenopausal patients with cystic or adenomatous hyperplasia may have difficulties complying with progestin therapy, which they may have to continue for several years. In addition, these patients may be a high-risk group for treatment with estrogens after the menopause. Because of these circumstances, hysterectomy may be a suitable alternative for these patients. If atypical adenomatous hyperplasia or carcinoma in situ is present, hysterectomy is indicated in the medically suitable patient. These women appear to be at high risk for eventually developing endometrial carcinoma even after cessation of menses. Hormonal treatment alone is often not curative, and long-term progestin therapy is of unproven value.

POSTMENOPAUSAL WOMEN

Postmenopausal patients not on estrogen therapy who present with vaginal bleeding should have a fractional D&C to rule out endometrial and endocervical carcinoma. Proliferative endometrium or cystic hyperplasia, especially in women who have ceased menses in the last 3-5 years, may be followed expectantly by biopsy every 4-6 months until regression is documented.

Proliferative endometrium and cystic hyperplasia in a woman more than 5 years after menopause should not be followed expectantly. D&C and hysterectomy with bilateral salpingo-oophorectomy are indicated. Endogenous estrogen sources (granulosa-theca-cell tumors, ovarian cortical stromal thecosis, other gonadal stromal or metastatic neoplasms to the ovary) should be considered in this setting. The presence of adenomatous hyperplasia or carcinoma in situ in this age group implies that cancer may already be present or may soon develop if the source of stimulation to the endometrium is endogenous. Long-term continuous progestin therapy may well convert the lesions to an atrophic pattern and abolish the cancer risk, but the data in this regard are scanty. The standard therapy for adenomatous or more severe hyperplasia in this age group should be hysterectomy and bilateral salpingo-oophorectomy.

The postmenopausal patient on estrogen replacement therapy who has endometrial hyperplasia should also have a fractional D&C to rule out endometrial carcinoma. In the absence of significant hyperplasia, the estrogen replacement therapy can be resumed with medroxyprogesterone acetate 10 mg/day for the last 10 days of each month of treatment. Significant hyperplasias (adenomatous, atypical adenomatous, carcinoma in situ) occurring during postmenopausal estrogen replacement therapy are best treated by hysterectomy and bilateral salpingo-oophorectomy.

BASIC PRINCIPLES

The management of all patients presenting with endometrial hyperplasia is facilitated by keeping in mind a few principles. The cause of endometrial hyperplasia is unopposed estrogen. Before definitive therapy is undertaken, a firm understanding of the source of and indications for estrogen should be known. Patients with endometrial hyperplasia may be harboring an endometrial carcinoma, and until the endometrial cavity is thoroughly evaluated by D&C, one cannot disregard this possibility. Last, the synthetic oral progestins play a large role in the management of these patients and in most instances can, over a period of time, restore most endometrial hyperplasia to an atrophic pattern.

SUGGESTED READING

Eichner E, Abellera M: Endometrial hyperplasia treated by progestins. *Obstet Gynecol* 38:739, 1971

Gambrell RD: The prevention of endometrial cancer in postmenopausal women with progestins. *Maturitas* 1:107, 1978

Kistner RW: Hormonal treatment of premalignant lesions. In Lewis GC Jr, Wentz WB, Jaffers RM, eds: *New Concepts in Gynecological Oncology*. Philadelphia: FA Davis, 1966, p 287

Wentz WB: Progestin therapy in endometrial hyperplasia. *Gynecol Oncol* 2:362, 1974

72

Evaluation and Management of Early Endometrial Carcinoma

C. PAUL MORROW, M.D.

INCIDENCE

Endometrial carcinoma is the most common malignancy of the female genital tract in the United States. Among all malignancies in women, it is exceeded in frequency only by breast and colorectal cancer. According to American Cancer Society projections for 1982, 39,000 new cases of endometrial carcinoma are expected annually, and each year 3,000 women will die from it. The average age at the time of diagnosis is 58 years. The incidence at age 40 is less than 10 cases per 100,000 population per year. The incidence rises to 50:100,000 at age 50 and reaches a peak of 85:100,000 at age 70.

RISK FACTORS

Constitutional factors associated with an approximately two-fold increase in the risk of developing endometrial cancer are: obesity, infertility, late menopause, and diabetes mellitus. Several studies have shown an association between the use of postmenopausal estrogens and a two- to six-fold increased risk for developing endometrial cancer. Although over 90% of cases occur in postmenopausal women, the obese, infertile, premenopausal woman characterized by the sclerocystic ovary syndrome is also in a relatively high-risk group.

Endometrial carcinoma is predominantly a disease of middle- and upper-class women, and studies have suggested an associated risk with breast and ovarian carcinoma. There have been few reported instances of the familial occurrence of endometrial cancer.

DIAGNOSIS AND EVALUATION

The first sign of endometrial carcinoma is usually abnormal vaginal bleeding after or around the time of the menopause. Methods of evaluation are discussed in detail in Chapter 54. Any woman with abnormal perimenopausal or postmenopausal bleeding requires a careful evaluation for genital tract cancer.

Common presumptions regarding postmenopausal bleeding that can lead to delay in diagnosis are: (1) that the bleeding is due to supplemental estrogens in women receiving such therapy; (2) that the bleeding is of vaginal origin in women with atrophic vaginitis; (3) that the bleeding is from the endometrium, when it may be arising from vaginal or ovarian carcinoma; and (4) that the bleeding is not sufficient to require evaluation. Less commonly the patient with endometrial carcinoma may present with enlargement of the uterus without bleeding, or with chronic vaginal discharge.

Prognosis and, therefore, survival are related to the histologic degree of differentiation, the extent of disease at the time of diagnosis, the quality of the therapy, and the patient's medical status. Pretreatment evaluation is directed toward the definition of these factors.

The histology of endometrial carcinoma is often not straightforward. Distinguishing between severe atypical hyperplasia and very well-differentiated adenocarcinoma is a frequent problem. At the other end of the spectrum, it can be difficult to distinguish between poorly differentiated endometrial carcinoma and endometrial sarcoma. Finally, as with many cancers, the degree of histologic differentiation may vary from one area of tumor to another. The grade assigned should be that of the least differentiated area. If the tumor is not adequately sampled, an error in assessing the histologic grade may occur.

The selection of tests that will complement the physical examination in determining the extent of disease must be based on knowledge of its spread pattern. Endometrial carcinoma usually arises in the fundus and tends to remain localized. Initially, it spreads by extension within the endometrium and then invades the myometrium, advancing towards the isthmus and cervix. It can invade the full thickness of the uterine musculature and disseminate within the peritoneal cavity. Occasionally, it presents with parametrial invasion or metastases to the vagina, particularly the suburethral area.

Less well appreciated is the proclivity of this disease to spread via the lymphatics. Approximately 10% of patients with clinical stage I endometrial carcinoma have pelvic lymph node metastasis. The probability of pelvic node involvement increases as the tumor becomes less differentiated, and also increases as the tumor invades the myometrium more deeply. Other common, clinically occult sites of spread are the adnexa, cervix, para-aortic nodes, and peritoneal cavity.

Based on this information, the preoperative evaluation should include the following: a general physical examination with special attention to the supraclavicular and inguinal lymph nodes and abdominal masses. After inspection and palpation of the introitus, the suburethral area, the vaginal walls, and the cervix, a Papanicolaou smear is taken. On bimanual rectovaginal examination, the uterus, adnexa, and parametrium are evaluated. The uterine cavity is sounded. A fractional curettage is performed, submitting the endocervical and endometrial specimens separately.

In terms of a metastatic survey, only a chest x-ray is needed unless the patient has specific symptoms, such as bone pain, suggesting metastases. Many of these patients have medical problems related to age and obesity; evaluation for diabetes, hypertension, and renal disease is required.

MANAGEMENT

Surgery

The cornerstone in the management of stage I endometrial carcinoma (confined to the uterine fundus) is total hysterectomy, including removal of the tubes and ovaries. In most instances, an abdominal procedure should be done in order to further evaluate the extent of disease. The aortic and pelvic areas are palpated for evidence of retroperitoneal node metastases. Enlarged or suspicious nodes should be removed or biopsied. Cytologic washings are taken from the pelvis, and the abdomen is carefully explored.

Removal of the adnexa is part of the therapy, as they may be sites of occult metastases. In addition, the ovaries may contain occult ovarian tumors or produce estrogen that might stimulate residual, occult disease. It is not necessary to remove a margin of vaginal cuff, nor does there appear to be any benefit to freeing up the ureters and taking extra parametrial tissue. The entire cervix, however, should be excised with the uterus.

The pathologist's evaluation of the specimen is very important. He must identify the least differentiated area of the tumor, the greatest depth of myometrial invasion, and the proximity of the tumor to the isthmus or cervix. Each of these factors has prognostic as well as therapeutic implications. In addition, accurate study of the peritoneal cytology, lymph nodes, and adnexa is crucial. To acquire the optimal information, it is often required that the surgeon and pathologist discuss their respective needs.

Radiation

The role of radiation therapy in the management of stage I adenocarcinoma of the endometrium is the subject of a long-standing controversy. The primary issue in dispute is whether radiation must be administered preoperatively to exert its optimal effect. The major demonstrated benefit from adjuvant radiation therapy is a reduction in vaginal cuff recurrences. It appears, however, that radiation therapy is equally effective in preventing cuff recurrences when given preoperatively or postoperatively. For this reason, the issue of preoperative versus postoperative therapy is not as important as a plan of treatment suitable to both the surgeon and the radiation therapist.

Although the focus for adjuvant therapy has been on the vaginal cuff, this site of recurrence undoubtedly reflects lymphatic involvement rather than operative spill. Thus, it is recommended that adjuvant radiation therapy consist of whole-pelvis irradiation of 4,000-5,000 rads with or without additional intracavitary therapy, rather than intracavitary or cuff radiotherapy alone.

Most authorities agree that the woman with a small uterus and a well-differentiated endometrial carcinoma will not need adjuvant radiation therapy unless there is invasion greater than one-third of the thickness of the uterine wall, occult extension to the isthmus or cervix, adnexal metastases, positive peritoneal cytology, or poorly differentiated areas found on the hysterectomy specimen. Since these features occur in only a small percentage of grade 1 cases, preoperative radiation therapy for such patients usually constitutes unnecessary treatment. The grade 1 cases with deep myometrial invasion, adnexal spread, or extension to the cervix, and all other grades of stage I endometrial carcinoma should receive adjuvant radiation therapy.

PROGNOSIS AND FOLLOW-UP

The 5-year survival rate for stage I endometrial carcinoma varies from 75-95% in reported series in the literature. The variation in results reflects more differences in study groups than differences in therapy. The patient with a very well-differentiated adenocarcinoma confined to the endometrium probably has a 5-year survival expectancy of 95% with simple hysterectomy alone. In contrast, the patient with a deeply invading, poorly differentiated endometrial carcinoma may have an expected 5-year survival of less than 50%. Thus, prognostic estimates need to be individualized.

The follow-up of endometrial cancer patients should include routine evaluation of the peripheral lymph node areas and abdomen, a bimanual pelvic examination, and a Pap smear every 2-4 months for 2 years, and every 6 months thereafter. An annual chest x-ray is also recommended. It should be remembered that these women are epidemiologically similar to those who are at high risk for developing breast and colon carcinoma.

SUGGESTED READING

Aalders J, Abeler V, Kolstad P, et al: Postoperative external irradiation and prognostic parameters in stage I endometrial carcinoma. *Obstet Gynecol* 56:419, 1980

Boronow RC, Morrow CP: Adenocarcinoma of the body of the uterus. In Goldsmith HS, ed: *Practice of Surgery,* ch 29. Hagerstown, Md: Harper & Row, 1979

Gusberg SB: The individual at high risk for endometrial carcinoma. *Am J Obstet Gynecol* 74:31, 1957

Joelsson I, Sandri A, Kottmeier HL: Carcinoma of the uterine corpus: A retrospective survey of individualized therapy. *Acta Radiol Suppl* 334, 1973

Jones HW III: Review: Treatment of adenocarcinoma of the endometrium. *Obstet Gynecol Surv* 30:147, 1975

Morrow CP, Townsend DE: Cancer of the uterine corpus. In *Synopsis of Gynecologic Oncology*, ed 2, ch 5. New York: Wiley, 1981

Prem KA, Adcock LL, Okagaki T, et al: The evolution of a treatment program for adenocarcinoma of the endometrium. *Am J Obstet Gynecol* 133:803, 1979

73

Advanced Endometrial Carcinoma

RICHARD H. NALICK, M.D.

The estrogen controversy and an apparent relative increase in the annual incidence of new cases of adenocarcinoma of the endometrium have rekindled interest in the diagnosis and management of this disease. The American Cancer Society projected that 39,000 new cases would be diagnosed and 3,000 women would succumb to this malignancy in 1982.

Endometrial cancer tends to remain localized to the uterine cavity for some time and frequently is manifested by postmenopausal bleeding early in its clinical course. As a result, approximately 75% of cases are diagnosed as stage I. Modern therapy combining irradiation with total abdominal hysterectomy and bilateral salpingo-oophorectomy has resulted in excellent survival statistics for patients with early disease. As a result, there has been no sense of urgency to re-evaluate treatment until recently. However, the efforts of such investigators as Morrow, Creasman, Boronow, and Lewis have now brought this neoplasm, its associated prognostic parameters, and new concepts in management into sharp focus.

PATTERNS OF SPREAD

Reviews of large series of patients reveal that in 25% of cases, the disease has spread beyond the endometrium at the time of diagnosis. Basic spread patterns include:

1. Retrograde spread into the uterine isthmus, endocervix, and vagina via surface spread and/or lymphatic channels
2. Parametrial and pelvic sidewall involvement
3. Adnexal spread by lymphatics
4. Pelvic and para-aortic lymph node involvement
5. Spread from the round ligament to inguinal lymph nodes
6. Hematogenous spread to lungs, liver, and bone
7. Deep myometrial invasion through the serosa with intraperitoneal dissemination.

CLINICAL STAGING

Involvement of the cervix (stage II) is found in 5-10% of cases. With delay in diagnosis, especially in grade 3 lesions, parametrial, adnexal, or vaginal involvement (stage III) occurs in about 10% of cases. In 5%, the disease will involve bladder and/or rectal mucosa or distant sites (stage IV). As with other gynecologic tumors, stage correlates well with prognosis; corrected 5-year survival rates are: stage I—85%; stage II—60%; stage III—25%; and stage IV—8%. Clearly, carcinoma of the endometrium can behave in a virulent fashion and deserves the utmost respect.

MANAGEMENT

Stage III Disease

In stage III, the carcinoma has spread outside the uterus, but not outside the true pelvis. Here, as defined by FIGO (International Federation of Gynecology and Obstetrics), clinical examination may reveal parametrial nodularity, an adnexal mass, or vaginal extension below the level of the levator muscles. A pelvic mass could represent extrauterine spread involving the sigmoid colon, ileum, or pelvic omentum and would also lead to a stage III classification.

The accepted management of stage III endometrial carcinoma is preoperative irradiation and intracavitary radium or cesium, followed by total abdominal hysterectomy and bilateral salpingo-oophorectomy. However, this may not always represent the best course. For example, cases with evidence of intraperitoneal dissemination (ascites, adnexal or abdominal masses) would benefit from exploratory laparotomy with reductive surgery, node sampling, extrafascial abdominal hysterectomy, bilateral salpingo-oophorectomy, and omentectomy to be followed by postoperative irradiation, i.e., whole-pelvis, vaginal cuff, extended-field, or whole-abdomen therapy as indicated. Strong consideration would also be given to the use of adjunctive hormonal and non-hormonal cytotoxic chemotherapy. This mode of treatment should also be considered in cases with pyometra resistant to drainage and appropriate antibiotics, large fibroids, or a history of chronic pelvic inflammatory disease or diverticulitis.

Suggested plans of management for stage III include:

1. Standard
   a. External-beam, whole-pelvis irradiation with 4,500-5,000 rads to the midpelvis in daily fractions of 200 rads in 5 weeks, followed by
   b. A single application of radium or cesium by Heyman's capsules and/or Fletcher-Suit afterloading applicator to a dose of 6,000 rads to the endometrial surface and 4,000 rads to the vaginal surface by colpostats. Usually a 48-72-hour application is used, although if indicated, a second application may be required
   c. As soon as the patient has recovered from the effects of the pelvic radiation (after 4-6 weeks), surgical completion of therapy is carried out. This includes careful exploration, with special attention paid to the liver, bowel, diaphragm, and parietal peritoneum. Washings for cytology and random omental biopsies are obtained. The para-aortic nodes should be palpated and any suspicious nodes biopsied; alternatively, para-aortic biopsy may be performed routinely.

2. Alternative
  a. 5,400-5,500 rads of pelvic irradiation to include the proximal vagina; intracavitary brachytherapy is omitted
  b. Surgery as above in 4-6 weeks.
3. Alternative
  a. Primary exploratory laparotomy as discussed above
  b. Postoperative whole-pelvis irradiation to 5,000 rads; if grade 3, deep myometrial invasion, or occult isthmus or endocervical extension, vaginal radium (by colpostats) to 4,000 rads surface dose. Extended-field irradiation to 4,500 rads is indicated for microscopically positive (or <2 cm) para-aortic nodes.

Notes: Vaginal lesions may benefit from interstitial brachytherapy. Adjuvant hormonal therapy or chemotherapy should be considered if any of the following is present:
1. Grade 3 disease
2. Deep myometrial invasion
3. Positive cytology (consider radioactive ^{32}P instillation)
4. Intraperitoneal dissemination
5. Positive para-aortic nodes > 2 cm.

Stage IV Disease

The rare patient who presents with stage IV disease on the basis of bladder and/or rectal mucosal involvement, without fistulas, can be treated primarily with 5,000-6,000 rads of whole-pelvis irradiation and intracavitary radium. Treatment in this stage must be individualized. To prevent persistent or recurrent symptomatic uterine disease, postradiation total abdominal hysterectomy and bilateral salpingo-oophorectomy should be considered in the plan of management.

If the patient presents with a rectovaginal fistula, a preradiation colostomy should be performed. A vesicovaginal or ureterovaginal fistula usually requires diversion prior to initiation of irradiation. Although pelvic exenteration can be considered as primary treatment, or following preoperative pelvic irradiation, it is not recommended. Stage IV patients are usually not surgical candidates; the incidence of extrapelvic node involvement and occult distant metastases is so great that ultraradical surgery is not justified. Exenteration can be considered only if all the following criteria are present:
1. Relatively young patient (under 50)
2. Histologic grade 1 or 2 disease
3. Negative comprehensive metastatic work-up
4. Medically operable patient
5. Vesicovaginal and/or rectovaginal fistulas
6. En bloc surgical extirpation possible at exploratory laparotomy
7. Negative para-aortic nodes on frozen section.

Obviously, these criteria would rarely be encountered in patients with stage IV disease.

On occasion a stage IV patient will present with distant metastases involving the lungs, liver, bones, distal vagina, or inguinal lymph nodes. Here again, treatment must be individualized. In most cases local radiation to the pelvis, vagina, or inguinal nodes will provide worthwhile palliation. Hormonal and/or cytotoxic chemotherapy is indicated for distant metastases.

Although, theoretically, disease classified as stage IV on the basis of bladder and/or rectal invasion and vulvar involvement could be treated by exenteration plus radical vulvectomy, this is not recommended unless the seven criteria listed above are present. Experience in these cases indicates that appropriate radiation and hormonal therapy and/or cytotoxic chemotherapy provide the best results. The latter two modalities are thoroughly discussed in the following chapter.

SUGGESTED READING

Antoniades J, Brady LW, Lewis GC: The management of stage III carcinoma of the endometrium. *Cancer* 38:1838, 1976

Coppleson M, ed: *Gynecologic Oncology: Fundamental Principles and Clinical Practice*, vol 2. New York: Churchill Livingstone, 1981, pp 581-582

Creasman WT, Boronow RC, Morrow CP, et al: Adenocarcinoma of the endometrium: Its metastatic lymph node potential. *Gynecol Oncol* 2:130, 1974

Lewis CG, Slack NH, Mortel R, et al: Adjuvant progestogen therapy in the primary definitive treatment of endometrial cancer. *Gynecol Oncol* 2:368, 1974

Morrow CP, DiSaia PJ, Townsend DE: Current management of endometrial carcinoma. *Obstet Gyneco* 42:399, 1973

74

Recurrent Endometrial Carcinoma

RICHARD H. NALICK, M.D.

Approximately one-third of all patients with adenocarcinoma of the endometrium (all stages) develop recurrent disease. Persistent, recurrent, and metastatic endometrial carcinoma is a malignant disease in the true sense of the word. Even with the best treatment, survival rates average less than 10%, and 85% of deaths from endometrial cancer occur within the first 3 years following initial therapy.

Finn has reported that 42% of recurrent endometrial cancer is diagnosed within 6 months of primary therapy, 56% within 1 year, 69% within 2 years, and 85% by 3 years. It is clear that post-therapy surveillance is of great importance during the first 3 years. Patients should be seen monthly for the first 6 months, every 2 months for the next 6 months, at 3-month intervals the second year, 4-month intervals the third and fourth years, 6-month intervals the fifth year, and yearly thereafter.

Autopsy data and clinical information indicate that although pelvic, lung, and liver metastases are common, any parenchymal organ and all nodal groups are at risk. At each visit a careful review of systems is necessary, and should include questioning as to the presence of weight loss, anorexia, chest pain, dyspnea, hemoptysis, nausea, abdominal pain, jaundice, constipation, back pain, vaginal bleeding, pelvic pain, leg swelling, or bone pain.

The physical examination should emphasize left supraclavicular and inguinal lymph nodes, lungs, abdomen (presence of ascites, hepatomegaly, or mass), suburethral region, vagina, rectovaginal septum, cul-de-sac, central pelvis, pelvic sidewall, rectum, and extremities. A complete blood count, liver and renal function tests, and a chest x-ray should be obtained at regular intervals. An intravenous pyelogram, barium enema, liver scan, and bone scans should be ordered when indicated by examination, symptoms, or review of systems.

Recurrent disease is related to: (1) extent (stage) of primary disease, (2) histologic grade, (3) depth of myometrial invasion, (4) host factors such as age and immunocompetence, and (5) adequacy of primary therapy. In the majority of cases, the patient's initial treatment will have been surgery and (preoperative or postoperative) radiation, which will usually preclude additional pelvic radiotherapy.

Therapy for recurrent disease must be individualized. Selection of therapy is based on: (1) location of recurrence, (2) extent and volume of tumor, (3) history of previous irradiation, (4) treatment goals (cure or palliation), and (5) availability of an experienced gynecologic oncologist, adequate support facilities, and assistance.

Isolated vaginal vault lesions are uncommon, occurring most often in association with pelvic, abdominal, and/or distant metastases. However, if the vaginal vault is the only site of recurrence and primary treatment was with surgery alone, 4,000-5,000 rads of whole-pelvis irradiation and vaginal brachytherapy may be used successfully.

Recurrent tumor in a previously radiated field requires exenteration and/or hormonal therapy or chemotherapy. These patients are rarely candidates for ultraradical surgery. However, total pelvic exenteration should be considered if all the following criteria are present:

1. Recurrent disease apparently confined to the pelvis
2. Recurrence following irradiation
3. Well-differentiated tumor
4. Tumor-free interval of at least 1 year
5. Medically operable patient
6. Resectable disease and negative para-aortic nodes.

Collected series have indicated a 5-year survival rate of approximately 20% in operable cases.

In cases where surgery alone was the primary therapy, large inoperable pelvic recurrences may be temporarily controlled by 6,000 rads of whole-pelvis irradiation. Only rarely can a small central recurrence be completely resected and the bladder and rectum preserved. In most cases, whole-pelvis irradiation should be given to a dose of 5,000 rads in conjunction with vaginal radium or interstitial implants.

Clinical experience indicates that what may appear to be local vaginal recurrence is usually associated with intrapelvic, abdominal, or distant metastases. Thus, systemic therapy is theoretically indicated in most cases of recurrent endometrial carcinoma.

PROGESTIN THERAPY

Traditionally, progestin therapy has been the most widely used approach to the management of recurrent corpus cancer. In a classic paper, Kelly and Baker (1961) reported remissions lasting 9 months to 4.5 years in 21 cases of pulmonary metastases treated with progesterone in oil. Later evaluation of their data indicated a 32% objective response, including three complete responses. Since their report, numerous studies have substantiated that 30-37% of patients will experience an objective response to progestins, with a median remission duration of 24-30 months in cases with well-differentiated lesions.

Although a number of progestins have been evaluated, the greatest experience has been gained with 17α-hydroxyprogesterone caproate (Delalutin). In 1974, Reifenstein collected data from various studies of a total of 314 patients with advanced or recurrent metastatic endometrial carcinoma. The treatment regimen consisted of 1 gm or more of Delalutin per week for at least 12 weeks. There was an objective response rate of 37% and a complete response rate of 6-8%.

The best results were noted in patients under 50 years of age, with well-differentiated lesions, long tumor-free intervals, slowly growing lesions, and in those who survived long enough to receive at least 12 weeks of therapy. Survival averaged 27 months in responders, but only 6 months in nonresponders. Initially, as reported by others, pulmonary lesions were thought to respond best. However, analysis of Reifenstein's data as well as that of Smith (1975, at M. D. Anderson Hospital and Tumor Institute, Houston) indicates that pelvic and lymph-node metastases may respond as well as lung lesions.

Smith's study also found that histologic grade was associated with progestin response. Of 25 patients with well-differentiated adenocarcinoma, 24 responded to progestin. There were no responders among the four patients with undifferentiated tumors.

Although many reports indicate that patients under 50 respond more often than those over 50, other reports do not substantiate this allegation. Younger patients tend to have more well-differentiated tumors, and this may explain the differences.

The size of a recurrent lesion is also an important predictive factor. Large masses are anoxic; this may lead to radioresistance as well as drug resistance. The majority of large masses are not resectable, but they may respond to systemic chemotherapy, especially if their blood supply has not been compromised by prior radiotherapy. This is particularly true of pulmonary lesions.

To summarize, the best progestin responses are seen with:
1. Well-differentiated lesions
2. Long tumor-free intervals
3. Slowly progressive disease
4. A treatment course of at least 12 weeks
5. Patients under 50 years of age
6. Pulmonary and pelvic metastases.

Delalutin was used in the majority of earlier studies of progestin therapy. But recent studies have evaluated other progestins, such as medroxyprogesterone acetate (Depo-Provera, Provera) and megestrol acetate (Megace). In general, response rates have been similar regardless of the type of progestin, dosage, or dosage schedule; no statistically significant differences have been noted. The most commonly used regimens include: Delalutin 750-3,000 mg IM weekly; Depo-Provera 200-800 mg IM weekly; Provera 100-300 mg daily PO; and Megace 40-320 mg daily PO.

The following objective response rates, reported by Smith et al (1975) in a study comparing Depo-Provera and Megace, are characteristic of average rates reported elsewhere: 10% complete responses, 25% partial responses, and a 5-10% incidence of stable disease. Approximately 55-60% experienced progressive disease.

From 50% to 75% of patients report a subjective response to progestins—increased feeling of well-being and improved appetite. This subjective response alone may be a sufficient reason for offering progestin therapy.

In summary, progestins are relatively inexpensive, nontoxic, easy to administer, produce a sense of well-being and increased appetite, and produce an objective response rate ranging from 30% to 40%. It is therefore recommended that progestins be used in all cases of advanced, recurrent, or metastatic endometrial carcinoma, in conjunction with surgery, radiotherapy, and nonhormonal chemotherapy. Results of current studies of progesterone receptors may soon prove reliable enough to indicate the probability of progestin response in a given patient.

CYTOTOXIC CHEMOTHERAPY

Cytotoxic chemotherapy has, until recently, been used infrequently in the management of recurrent or metastatic endometrial cancer. This has probably been due to: (1) the relatively good response of this disease to radiation therapy, (2) the demonstrated response to progestin therapy, and (3) the lack of a truly effective cytotoxic agent. In addition, most reports have involved few patients, a variety of cytotoxic agents, and few objective responses of only short duration.

Until a few years ago, only three drugs had been adequately evaluated: 5-fluorouracil (5-FU), cyclophosphamide (Cytoxan), and, later, doxorubicin (Adriamycin). In collected series, the combined (complete and partial) response rates for these drugs were: Cytoxan—22%; 5-FU—34%; and Adriamycin—38%.

In reviewing the literature in 1974, Donovan cited a number of studies using a total of 16 different agents in 126 patients. The objective response rate was 27% (34/126). Chlorambucil (Leukeran), 6-mercaptopurine (Purinethol), and nitrogen mustard have not seemed to be of much value, while a 33% objective improvement rate (10/30) was reported for cytembena by Dvorak.

Adriamycin appears to be the most effective single agent. De Vita (at the National Cancer Institute) reported seven responses in 18 patients (38.9%). In a phase II study of 43 patients given Adriamycin, sponsored by the Gynecologic Oncology Group (GOG), Thigpen noted that 37.2% of patients showed an objective response, 30.2% had stable disease, and only 32.6% had progressive disease. This latter study was most instrumental in demonstrating the benefit of Adriamycin in endometrial carcinoma.

Since then, most studies have evaluated drug combinations including Adriamycin. One exception was a study by Horton and the Eastern Cooperative Oncology Group, comparing Adriamycin and Cytoxan. There were no objective responses with Cytoxan, but a 19% response rate with Adriamycin.

In 1977, Bruckner and Deppe reported excellent response rates to melphalan (Alkeran)-5-FU-medroxyprogesterone acetate and to Adriamycin-Cytoxan-5-FU-medroxyprogesterone acetate. Objective responses were seen in 11 of 26 (42%) patients with five complete responses in the first instance, and in four of seven (57%) patients with the latter combination. In 1980, Piver treated 13 patients with Alkeran-5-FU-medroxyprogesterone acetate. There was an objective response in six of 11 (54.4%) evaluable women with recurrent or metastatic corpus cancer, with two complete and four partial responses.

As a result of these studies, a popular combination has evolved: 5-FU-Adriamycin-Cytoxan with megestrol acetate (Megace) or medroxyprogesterone acetate (Depo-Provera). A typical schedule would include: 400 mg/m^2 of 5-FU, 40 mg/m^2 of Adriamycin, and 400 mg/m^2 of Cytoxan IV every 3 weeks, *or* the same regimen, but with 5-FU given again on day 8, and the whole combination repeated every 28 days. In both cases, 400 mg of medroxyprogesterone acetate is given IM 1-3 times per week or 160-320 mg of megestrol acetate is given PO daily.

In the mid-1970s, it became apparent that cis-platinum (cisplatin, Platinol) was effective in the management of ovarian cancer. Bruckner and co-workers summarized the evidence in 1977. Since then, several papers have addressed the role of cisplatin in advanced endometrial cancer. Tropé noted four objective responses in 11 patients (36%) with recurrent disease. Deppe, Cohen, and Bruckner reported an objective response in four of 13 (30%) patients with advanced disease, using high-dose (3 mg/kg) cisplatin as a second-line agent (after failure of previous intensive combination chemotherapy).

Initial GOG phase II trials showed only a 4% partial response to cisplatin. But in 1982, Seski et al (at M. D. Anderson Hospital) treated 26 women with advanced or recurrent endometrial cancer with relatively high-dose cisplatin (50-100 mg/m^2) every 4 weeks. An objective response was obtained in 11/26 patients (42%). There were 10 partial responses and one complete response. Better response rates occurred with higher doses: 57% with 70 mg/m^2 and 40% with 100 mg/m^2.

A new tumor antibiotic, aclacinomycin A, has shown promise in corpus cancer, as has metronidazole-bleomycin (Flagyl-Blenoxane), but details are lacking. Also of interest are preliminary data reported by Swenerton et al, indicating a response to tamoxifen (Nolvadex) in advanced corpus cancer, especially in patients with well-differentiated tumors and longer disease-free intervals.

It has been shown that both hormonal therapy and cytotoxic therapy can be beneficial in recurrent and metastatic endometrial adenocarcinoma. It seems logical to evaluate response to a progestin first, especially for tumors shown to have adequate levels of progesterone receptors. Depo-Provera (parenteral), Provera (oral), or Megace (oral) can be utilized. Few studies have adequately attempted to compare these drugs or to determine the minimal dose.

However, cytotoxic chemotherapy should be considered in the following situations:

1. Cases not treatable by radiation or surgery and:
    a. Tumors negative for progesterone receptors or
    b. Previous failure of an adequate trial of progestin therapy.
2. Early recurrences (<1 year) with multiple-site involvement, grade 3 histology, and rapid progression

3. As adjuvant therapy in:
   a. Surgical stage I and II with:
      1) Grade 3 histology (poor differentiation)
      2) Grade 2 histology with deep (outer $\frac{1}{3}$) myometrial invasion
      3) Gross ectocervical extension.
   b. All cases with:
      1) Peritoneal implants or omental metastases
      2) Adnexal metastases
      3) Pelvic or aortic lymph-node metastases
      4) Positive peritoneal cytology.

Patients with widespread metastases such as in the lungs and/or liver with intraperitoneal implants or aortic-node disease will require intensive combination chemohormonal therapy to realize a high objective response rate, significant palliation, or a chance for cure. Selection of agents depends on renal/hepatic function, cardiac status, amount/region of prior irradiation, age, tumor receptor status, and perhaps a clonogenic tumor chemosensitivity assay.

On the basis of the foregoing, a plan of management for advanced recurrent or metastatic endometrial cancer is suggested as follows:

1. If at all possible, obtain tumor tissue for:
   a. Estrogen and progesterone receptor determination
   b. Clonogenic chemosensitivity assay.
2. Hormonal therapy:
   a. Progesterone-receptor positive:
      1) Megace 320 mg/day × 3 months, then 160 mg/day, or
      2) Depo-Provera 400 mg IM weekly.
   b. Estrogen-receptor positive: Nolvadex 10 mg PO bid.
3. Intensive combination chemotherapy, modified as indicated by the clonogenic chemosensitivity assay:
      1) Cisplatin 40-60 mg/m^2 IV infusion
      2) Adriamycin 40-60 mg/m^2 IV push
      3) Cytoxan 400-600 mg/m^2 IV push
      4) 5-FU 400-600 mg/m^2 IV push.
   5-FU could be administered on days 1 and 8 of a 28-day program, or all four drugs could be given every 3 weeks at the lower-dose levels.

Other drugs indicated effective by clonogenic assay in individual cases include mitomycin-C (Mutamycin), vinblastine (Velban), hexamethylolmelamine, and melphalan (Alkeran). Of the drugs mentioned here, only cisplatin requires inpatient therapy—for hydration and prolonged antinauseant therapy. The rest can be given to outpatients without undue difficulty.

CONCLUSION

The above aggressive plan offers an excellent chance for response and even cure. However, only well-controlled, prospective, randomized studies with sufficient numbers of patients can provide statistically meaningful data that can support the recommendation of any one drug, dose, or combination.

SUGGESTED READING

Barber HRK, Brunschwig M: Treatment and results of recurrent cancer of the corpus uteri in patients receiving anterior and total exenteration. *Cancer* 22:949, 1968

Beck RP, Latour JPA: Necropsy reports on 36 cases of endometrial carcinoma. *Am J Obstet Gynecol* 185:307, 1963

Bruckner HW, Cohen CJ, Gusberg SB, et al: Chemotherapy of gynecological tumors with platinum II. *J Clin Hematol Oncol* 1:619, 1977

Bruckner HW, Deppe G: Combination chemotherapy of advanced endometrial adenocarcinoma with Adriamycin, cyclophosphamide, 5-fluorouracil and medroxyprogesterone acetate. *Obstet Gynecol* 50:105, 1976 (suppl 1)

Cohen CJ, Deppe G, Bruckner HW: Treatment of advanced adenocarcinoma of the endometrium with melphalan, 5-fluorouracil and medroxyprogesterone acetate. *Obstet Gynecol* 50:415, 1977

Dede JA, Plentl AA, Moore JG: Recurrent endometrial carcinoma. *Surg Gynecol Obstet* 126:553, 1968

Deppe G, Cohen CJ, Bruckner HW: Treatment of advanced endometrial adenocarcinoma with cis-dichlorodiammine platinum (II) after intensive prior therapy. *Gynecol Oncol* 10:51, 1980

De Vita VT, Wasserman TH, Young RC, et al: Perspectives on research in gynecologic oncology. Treatment protocols. *Cancer* 38:161, 1976

De Vita VT, Wasserman TH, Young RC, Carter SK: Perspectives on research in gynecologic oncology. Treatment protocols. *Cancer* 38:509, 1976

Donovan JF: Nonhormonal chemotherapy of endometrial adenocarcinoma: A review. *Cancer* 34:1587, 1974

Dvorak O: Cytembena treatment of advanced gynecological carcinomas. *Neoplasma* 18:461, 1971

Finn WF: Time, site and treatment of recurrence of endometrial carcinoma. *Arch Intern Med* 121:236, 1968

Horton J, Begg CB, Arseneault J, et al: Comparison of Adriamycin with cyclophosphamide in patients with advanced endometrial cancer. *Cancer Treat Rep* 62:159, 1978

Kelly RM, Baker WH: Progestational agents in the treatment of carcinoma of the endometrium. *N Engl J Med* 264:216, 1961

Muggia FM, Chia G, Reed LJ, Romney SL: Doxorubicin-cyclophosphamide: Effective chemotherapy for advanced endometrial carcinoma. *Am J Obstet Gynecol* 128:314, 1977

Muggia FM, Perloff M, Chia GA, et al: Adriamycin (NSC-123127) in combination with cyclophosphamide (NSC-26271): A phase I and II evaluation. *Cancer Chemother Rep* 58:919, 1974

Piver MS, Shashikant L, Barlow JJ: Melphalan, 5-fluorouracil and medroxyprogesterone acetate in metastatic or recurrent endometrial carcinoma. *Obstet Gynecol* 56:370, 1980

Reifenstein EC Jr: Hydroxyprogesterone caproate therapy in advanced endometrial cancer. *Cancer* 27:485, 1971

Reifenstein EC Jr: The treatment of advanced endometrial cancer with hydroxyprogesterone caproate. *Gynecol Oncol* 2:380, 1974

Seski JC, Edwards CL, Copeland LJ, et al: Hexamethylmelamine chemotherapy for disseminated endometrial cancer. *Obstet Gynecol* 58:361, 1981

Seski JC, Edwards CL, Herson J, Rutledge FN: Cisplatin chemotherapy for disseminated endometrial cancer. *Obstet Gynecol* 59:225, 1982

Smith JP: Hormone therapy for adenocarcinoma of the endometrium. In *Cancer of the Uterus and Ovary*. Chicago: Year Book, 1969, pp 73-83

Smith JP, Rutledge FN: Gynecologic tumors. In *Cancer Chemotherapy*. Chicago: Year Book, 1975, pp 505-522

Swenerton KD, Shaw D, White GW, Boyes DA: Treatment of advanced endometrial carcinoma with tamoxifen. *N Engl J Med* 301:105, 1979

Thigpen T, Vance RB, Balducci L, Blessing J: Chemotherapy in the management of advanced or recurrent cervical and endometrial carcinoma. *Cancer* 48:658, 1981

Tropé C, Grundsell H, Johnsson JE, Cavallin-Stahl E: A phase II study of cis-platinum for recurrent corpus cancer. *Eur J Cancer* 16:1025, 1980

75

Neoplastic Disease of the Fallopian Tube: Diagnosis and Management

RICHARD H. NALICK, M.D.

INCIDENCE

Review of the current literature continues to indicate that primary carcinoma of the fallopian tube is the rarest tumor of the female genital tract. Its average reported incidence is 0.3%. It is responsible for 1:15,000-20,000 gynecologic hospital admissions, 0.34-1.33% of all operations for tubal disease (not including chronic pelvic inflammatory disease or tubo-ovarian abscess), and 0.16-1.11% of gynecologic cancers. Although reported only sporadically as isolated cases and in small series, as of 1977 approximately 950 cases had been documented. The largest series are those of Benedet et al (1977) and Fogh (1969), who reported series of 41 and 34 cases, respectively.

Benign neoplasms of the tube are rare, occurring less frequently than malignant tumors, and include benign cystic teratomas (most common), hemangiomas, lymphangiomas, mesonephromas, solid teratomas, neurilemmomas, and lipomas. Endometriosis may present as a small nodule and must be differentiated from metastatic adenocarcinoma. Interestingly, dysgerminoma or granulosa-cell tumors have been reported to occur in the fallopian tube, arising from misplaced primordial germ cells or ovarian remnants. Leiomyomata of the tube are very rare. When found, they vary in size from very small to up to 2 kg, are unilateral, involve the left tube more often than the right, and are found in the interstitial portion of the tube. The differential diagnosis includes salpingitis isthmica nodosa and adenomatoid tumors.

Adenomatoid tumors of the fallopian tube are rare (0.4%), small (<3 cm), circumscribed, unencapsulated benign neoplasms of the tube, which usually represent an incidental finding. Microscopically, small glandular or vascular spaces are seen, lined by mesothelial, endothelial, or epithelial-like cells within a fibromuscular stroma. Most authors consider this lesion to be of peritoneal (mesothelial) origin. Occasionally, differentiating adenomatoid tumors from adenocarcinoma may be somewhat difficult, although this tumor usually is found to involve the subserosal or muscular tissues of the fallopian tube, not the mucosa.

DIAGNOSIS AND ETIOLOGY

As primary carcinoma of the fallopian tube is so uncommon, an accurate pre-operative diagnosis is rarely made. Although there is no dependable clinical syndrome, the following triad should lead to strong consideration of this lesion, especially if seen in a perimenopausal woman: (1) pelvic mass, (2) pelvic pain, and (3) intermittent, profuse, watery, blood-tinged, clear-yellowish vaginal discharge occurring with partial or complete disappearance of the mass and relief of pain.

The age range is reported to be from 18 to 80, with the majority of cases occurring between 40 and 65. The average age is 51-52. A history of chronic salpingitis is often found retrospectively, as is decreased fertility. Chronic tubal infection is often noted in the affected tube. However, it is more logical to assume that salpingitis is secondary to tubal obstruction and not an etiologic factor. Profuse vaginal discharge can occur with hydrosalpinx and thus is clearly not pathognomonic.

Why this neoplasm is so rare is unknown, but speculation suggests it may be due to the relative stability of the tubal epithelium during the menstrual cycle. Transformation from a benign lesion is unlikely; only two cases of tubal carcinoma in situ have been reported to date. Tuberculosis does not appear to be important as an etiologic factor.

Only rarely has this tumor been suggested by the appearance of malignant cells in the Papanicolaou smear. More often the diagnosis revolves about the investigation of a persistent vaginal discharge or scant abnormal bleeding in a postmenopausal woman. Cytologic smears should be performed; however, a negative Pap test should not lead to complacency. The majority of these carcinomas occur postmenopause, when the cervix may be stenotic, preventing exfoliation of abnormal cells into the vaginal pool. Careful examination and colposcopy of the vagina and cervix are required. Examination under anesthesia and laparoscopy should be considered. Unexplained malignant cells on the cytologic smear following the above diagnostic studies should definitely be followed by exploratory laparotomy.

CLINICAL DESCRIPTION, GRADING, AND STAGING

In 75-80% of cases of tubal carcinoma, only one tube is involved. Appearance depends on size of the tumor and patency of the fimbriated end. If occluded, it may present as a hydro- or pyosalpinx. The absence of adhesions (free-floating tubal mass) should suggest tubal carcinoma, especially if papillary projections are noted intraluminally and the tube contains blood-tinged serous fluid. Careful surgical removal and opening the tube in the operating room should be followed by frozen section.

The tumor itself may range from 1 to 15 cm, appearing purple to grayish-yellow. Consistency varies from firm to doughy. Most often the distal one-third of the tube is involved. Metastatic involvement of the tube is common. If it is a primary carcinoma, the tumor mass should grossly appear to be confined to the tube and microscopically appear to have arisen in the mucosal lining. The wall of the tubal mass may be quite thin due to distension with fluid. Great care should be exercised to prevent rupture and dissemination of tumor cells, which may affect prognosis.

Microscopically, primary tubal carcinoma reveals the endosalpinx to be replaced by adenocarcinoma cells of the tubal type, usually papillary in architecture, which invade the submucosal tissue and grow along the tubal lumen, replacing normal tubal epithelium.

Histologic grade may be assigned as follows (as suggested by Hu et al): grade 1—well-differentiated papillary tumor confined to the mucosa with few mitoses; grade 2—papillary-alveolar, moderately differentiated (papillary or glandular); and grade 3—alveolar-medullary, poorly differentiated, with cells in solid sheets around gland-like spaces, loss of papillary pattern, frequent mitoses, and lymphatic invasion. Within any given tumor, marked histologic variation may be seen.

Prognosis is related to grade, but extent of tubal involvement and extratubal spread appears to be the most important prognostic factor. No staging protocol has been officially accepted. However, since the spread pattern, treatment, and prognosis are similar to those of serous cystadenocarcinoma of the ovary, most gynecologic oncologists have adopted the staging criteria for ovarian carcinoma used by FIGO (International Federation of Gynecology and Obstetrics):

Stage I	Growth limited to the tube
Stage Ia	Growth limited to one tube; no ascites
Stage Ib	Growth limited to both tubes; no ascites
Stage Ic	Growth limited to one or both tubes; ascites present with malignant cells in fluid
Stage II	Growth involving one or both tubes with pelvic extension
Stage IIa	Extension and/or metastasis to the uterus or ovary
Stage IIb	Extension to other pelvic tissues
Stage III	Growth involving one or both tubes with widespread intraperitoneal metastasis to the abdomen (the omentum, the small intestine, and its mesentery)
Stage IV	Growth involving one or both tubes with distant metastasis outside the peritoneal cavity.

The usual mode of spread is along the tubal mucosa and via the lymphatics. As the fimbriated end is often occluded, intraperitoneal spill does not occur early. However, with tubal distension and rupture, or serosal invasion, intraperitoneal spread soon occurs, with resultant peritoneal involvement not unlike that seen in ovarian cancer. Lymphatic or hematogenous metastases may occur before invasion of the tubal wall. Hematogenous dissemination often leads to liver metastases, particularly with poorly differentiated lesions. In view of the above, it is easy to see why in the majority of cases (>90%), the diagnosis is first made at the operating table, and then often after advanced stages have been reached.

INTRAOPERATIVE MANAGEMENT

Intraoperatively, meticulous exploration of the pelvis and abdomen should be performed and the disease surgically staged in a fashion similar to that used for ovarian cancer. If an intact tubal mass is found, it should be handled gently, excised, and opened in the surgical suite. Appropriate tissue samples should be sent for frozen section. Suspicion of cancer, rather than hydro- or pyosalpinx, should be entertained when a unilateral, distal tubal mass without adhesions is found.

The treatment of fallopian tube carcinoma should include total abdominal hysterectomy and bilateral salpingo-oophorectomy with infracolic omentectomy, especially if postoperative intraperitoneal radionuclide therapy is contemplated. An aggressive effort should be made to remove all gross disease, short of radical procedures that would add to postoperative morbidity and delay early adjunctive chemotherapy or radiation. However, if the tube is found to be adherent to a loop of small bowel, an en bloc dissection with primary anastomosis should be considered. In apparent stage I disease, a generous omental biopsy (or omentectomy), washings for cytology, examination of the lateral gutters, diaphragm, etc., and selective node biopsies are indicated, in addition to definitive surgery. If ^{32}P is to be used, Silastic or polyethylene catheters should be placed intraoperatively in the right upper quadrant and cul-de-sac.

ADJUNCTIVE CHEMOTHERAPY AND RADIATION

Whole-abdomen or strip radiation with a pelvic boost has been recommended for some years, especially in patients with minimal residual disease or positive cytology. Response has been variable and usually short-term. When residual tumor exceeds 2 cm, therapy of less than 5,000 rads is generally ineffective.

It appears that a colloidal suspension of radioactive chromic phosphate (^{32}P), placed intraperitoneally, is the best form of treatment for microscopic disease (positive cytology). Systemic chemotherapy should be used for gross residual disease. Pelvic radiation should be considered for residual pelvic disease, to a midpelvic dose of 5,000 rads.

Tubal carcinoma has been shown to respond to progestins, as well as to nonhormonal chemotherapeutic agents such as thiotepa, 5-fluorouracil (5-FU), melphalan (Alkeran), and cyclophosphamide (Cytoxan). The use of newer agents such as doxorubicin (Adriamycin) and cis-platinum (cisplatin, Platinol) should be considered for advanced disease, especially in combination with Cytoxan.

Prognosis is generally poor, reflecting advanced disease at diagnosis. Schiller and Silverberg in a series of 76 cases found that 5-year survival correlated well with extent of tubal penetration: lumen only—91%; serosa—53%; and beyond the tube and/or distant metastases—25%. Benedet noted similar results: 88% 5-year survival if disease was confined to the tube and 20% with advanced disease. Hayden and Potter reported a 5-year survival of 27% at all stages, while Hanton noted 12 (44%) of 27 cases surviving 5 years.

SUMMARY

The following are the key factors in the diagnosis and management of primary tubal carcinoma:

1. Causes of suspicion
   a. Unilateral mass associated with pelvic pain and watery discharge
   b. Abnormal Pap test result; if cervix, vagina, and endometrium negative to colposcopy, biopsy, and D&C, proceed to laparoscopy and/or laparotomy.
2. Meticulous intraoperative exploration and staging
3. Aggressive reductive surgery
4. Total abdominal hysterectomy and bilateral salpingo-oophorectomy (TAH-BSO)
5. ^{32}P for small (<1 cm) residual disease or positive cytology
6. Whole-pelvis irradiation of 5,000 rads for gross residual pelvic disease; modify to 4,000 rads if used in conjunction with ^{32}P
7. Postoperative chemotherapy
   a. Alkeran + progestins—minimum treatment
   b. Consider combination therapy for stages III or IV, large residual, or recurrent disease.
      1) 5-FU-Adriamycin-Cytoxan + progestin, or
      2) Adriamycin-Cytoxan-cisplatin + progestin.

OTHER MALIGNANT TUBAL DISEASE

Metastatic carcinoma of the tube is far more common than primary tubal carcinoma, occurring in 1:650 gynecologic hospital admissions. In the majority of cases, the primary tumor is ovarian or endometrial (ovarian two times more often than endometrial). The microscopic pattern usually mirrors that of the primary tumor, as does the prognosis. Treatment is as recommended for the primary tumor.

Sarcoma of the fallopian tube is extremely rare. Fewer than 20 cases have been reported to date. Grossly, sarcoma tumors tend to be firmer, but they may be soft and papillary. Microscopically, the predominant cells may be spindle cells, round cells, or represent mixed müllerian elements. The prognosis is poor, but we recommend aggressive treatment. This would include: reductive surgery, TAH-BSO, omentectomy, and pelvic irradiation, followed by chemotherapy with progestins + VAC (vincristine-dactinomycin-cyclophosphamide) or Adriamycin + dacarbazine (DTIC-Dome) or cisplatin.

SUGGESTED READING

Benedet JL, White GW, Fairey RN, Boyes DA: Adenocarcinoma of the fallopian tube. *Obstet Gynecol* 50:654, 1977

Boronow RC: Chemotherapy for disseminated tubal cancer. *Obstet Gynecol* 42:62, 1973

Boutselis JG, Thompson JM: Clinical aspects of primary carcinoma of the fallopian tube. *Am J Obstet Gynecol* 111:98, 1971

Deppe G, Bruckner H, Cohen CJ: Combination chemotherapy for advanced carcinoma of the fallopian tube. *Obstet Gynecol* 56:530, 1979

Finn WF, Javert CT: Primary and metastatic cancer of the fallopian tube. *Cancer* 2:803, 1949

Fogh I: Primary carcinoma of the fallopian tube. *Cancer* 23:1332, 1969

Hanton EM, et al: Primary carcinoma of the fallopian tube. *Am J Obstet Gynecol* 94:832, 1966

Hayden GE, Potter EL: Primary carcinoma of the fallopian tube. *Am J Obstet Gynecol* 79:24, 1960

Hu CY, Taymor ML, Hertig AT: Primary carcinoma of the fallopian tube. *Am J Obstet Gynecol* 50:58, 1950

Kinzel GF: Primary carcinoma of the fallopian tube. *Am J Obstet Gynecol* 125:816, 1976

Phelps HM, Chapman KE: Role of radiation therapy in the treatment of primary carcinoma of the uterine tube. *Obstet Gynecol* 43:669, 1974

Schiller HM, Silverberg SG: Staging and prognosis in primary carcinoma of the fallopian tube. *Cancer* 28:389, 1971

Yoonessi M: Carcinoma of the fallopian tube. *Obstet Gynecol Surv* 34:257, 1979

76

Management of Ovarian Germ-Cell Tumors

JOHN B. SCHLAERTH, M.D.

Proper management of germ-cell tumors of the ovary is important because many are malignant, they occur in young women, and they can be curable without loss of fertility. The dermoid cyst may be the most common ovarian neoplasm. The malignant germ-cell tumors are distinctly uncommon: immature teratoma, dysgerminoma, endodermal sinus tumor, embryonal carcinoma, and choriocarcinoma.

TERATOMAS

Dermoid Cyst

Over 95% of teratomas are mature cystic teratomas, commonly referred to as dermoid cysts. These tumors can occur throughout a woman's reproductive life and can frequently give rise to symptoms of an acute abdomen secondary to either rupture or torsion. More commonly, dermoid cysts are detected on routine pelvic examination or during investigation of minor complaints. Over half of dermoids can be diagnosed by x-ray or ultrasonography through the identification of calcification, tooth formation, or a particular fat-halo sign.

The surgical procedure of choice for a dermoid cyst in a young woman is enucleation with preservation of as much ovarian tissue as possible. The opposite gonad should also be evaluated for the presence of a dermoid tumor. Dermoid cysts have an overt bilaterality rate approaching 15%. However, bilaterality is not always expressed at the time of laparotomy and may not be detected until months or years later. Consideration has been given to bivalving the opposite, normal-appearing ovary and removing a wedge for biopsy. But if the contralateral ovary is normal to inspection and palpation, we do not recommend that it be bivalved. The risk of infertility from bivalving the ovary probably outweighs the benefit.

Approximately 1% of dermoid cysts will contain a malignancy. Usually these malignancies occur in postmenopausal women and are squamous-cell carcinomas. However, a variety of other malignancies may also occur. These tumors are usually found in the solid papilla on the inside of the cyst, the so-called Rokitansky's protuberance.

Immature Teratoma

Malignant ovarian teratomas are called immature teratomas because their malignant behavior is exhibited by tissues that are embryonic or fetal in appearance. The more immature the tissue, the more malignant its behavior.

A microscopic grading system for immature teratomas has been proposed by Norris and seems to correlate well with prognosis. In the past, confusion has arisen from use of the terms "solid" or "cystic" to describe teratomas. But these terms are purely descriptive. Whether a tumor is solid, cystic, or both has no bearing on its degree of malignancy.

Most immature teratomas occur in adolescent girls and involve only one ovary. In these patients, the operative treatment consists of unilateral salpingo-oophorectomy. Bilateral extension or metastatic spread requires hysterectomy, bilateral salpingo-oophorectomy, and removal of as much tumor as possible.

A patient with higher-grade or metastatic immature teratoma needs additional therapy after surgery. Radiotherapy has not been shown to be of benefit. Impressive results have been obtained with combination chemotherapy using vincristine (Oncovin), dactinomycin (Cosmegen), and cyclophosphamide (Cytoxan). Equally good, possibly superior, results have occurred with vinblastine (Velban), bleomycin (Blenoxane), and cisplatin (Platinol).

DYSGERMINOMA

The dysgerminoma is the most common malignant germ-cell tumor of the ovary. It usually occurs under the age of 30, often in females with dysgenetic gonads. Most often, it is confined to one ovary at the time of diagnosis. In 15% of cases the dysgerminoma is not a pure tumor. Therefore, it is important that dysgerminomas be sampled extensively for microscopic study, particularly in areas of hemorrhage or necrosis, to rule out the presence of a more malignant element.

A suggested treatment plan for dysgerminoma is as follows: If a patient is young and desirous of childbearing, and the dysgerminoma involves only one ovary and is less than 10 cm in diameter, unruptured, and without malignant ascites or positive peritoneal cytology, a unilateral salpingo-oophorectomy should be done. A wedge biopsy of the opposite, normal-appearing ovary should be done, as the opposite ovary can contain a subclinical focus of tumor. At laparotomy, particular attention should be paid to pelvic and para-aortic lymph nodes, as this is the primary route of metastasis. Any enlarged nodes should be removed. Routine postoperative radiation is unnecessary.

A karyotype should be obtained to rule out the presence of a Y chromosome. The presence of a uterus and a nonstreak gonad does not necessarily rule out the presence of a Y chromosome and dysgenetic gonads. If a Y chromosome is found, bilateral gonadectomy is indicated; prospects for fertility are nil and malignant risk is present in both gonads.

If the tumor is bilateral, larger than 10 cm, or accompanied by rupture, hysterectomy and bilateral salpingo-oophorectomy should be performed.

Surgery should be followed by radiation therapy to the abdomen with a boost to the pelvis. The radiation dosage considered curative in this disease is within the range that is tolerable for the abdomen and pelvis. If metastases are found in the aortic nodes, radiation therapy should be extended to include the mediastinum and supraclavicular areas. Postoperative lymphangiography or computerized tomography should be done to monitor for retroperitoneal lymph node metastases or recurrence.

Follow-up of dysgerminoma patients should include chest x-rays every 3 months and consideration of a repeat lymphangiogram or computerized tomography of the chest, abdomen, and pelvis at 1 year. Serum studies of α-fetoprotein (AFP) and human chorionic gonadotropin (hCG) should be performed every 3 months to monitor for the appearance of another type of metastatic germ-cell tumor missed on the initial examination of the tumor. Its presence would be an indication for chemotherapy. Essentially, all recurrences become manifest within 5 years.

ENDODERMAL SINUS TUMOR

The endodermal sinus tumor (or yolk-sac carcinoma) is perhaps the most malignant ovarian neoplasm. It is rare, occurring usually in female children or young adults, and is characterized by rapid growth. AFP is secreted by most, if not all, endodermal sinus tumors.

When only one ovary is involved, a unilateral salpingo-oophorectomy is appropriate. When intra-abdominal metastases are encountered, it seems most reasonable to remove as much as possible without risking delayed postoperative recovery. The ultimate fate of these patients, whether the tumor seems confined to one ovary or not, rests on the success of chemotherapy, and it should be initiated as quickly as possible postoperatively. The same chemotherapeutic agents recommended for immature teratomas should be used for endodermal sinus tumors.

The diagnosis of this rare tumor can challenge the most experienced pathologist. There should be no hesitation in confirming the diagnosis by pathologic consultation with acknowledged experts in the field. But keep in mind that delay in starting therapy may be fatal.

Follow-up should be very frequent, even after chemotherapy has been terminated, to detect recurrence as soon as possible. Serial assays for hCG and AFP should be included in the management of these patients to confirm tumor progression or regression.

EMBRYONAL CARCINOMA

This neoplasm has only recently been recognized as a distinct entity in women. It shares many features with endodermal sinus tumors, with which it had undoubtedly been grouped in the past. But it differs most significantly from endodermal sinus tumors in that it usually produces both hCG and AFP. Aggressive behavior is the rule for this neoplasm. The same treatment guidelines apply here as for endodermal sinus tumors.

CHORIOCARCINOMA

Pure choriocarcinoma arising in the ovary is indeed a rare tumor. It is virulent and is reported to have a high death rate. Because of this, most patients have been treated postoperatively with chemotherapy regimens similar to those used in gestational choriocarcinoma, i.e., a combination of methotrexate, dactinomycin, and an alkylating agent—cyclophosphamide or chlorambucil (Leukeran). These tumors secrete hCG, which should be used as a tumor marker.

GONADOBLASTOMA

The gonadoblastoma occurs almost exclusively in dysgenetic gonads. The affected females usually have a Y chromosome. The gonadoblastoma is included here because nearly 30% are associated with the development of malignant germ-cell tumors. The gonadoblastoma is a benign tumor composed of two cell types: primitive germ cells and a sex cord stromal element. There may also be cells resembling luteinized theca cells or Leydig cells. Because of the high risk for dysgerminomas, endodermal sinus tumors, etc., to develop in gonadoblastomas, appropriate therapy is bilateral gonadectomy.

MIXED GERM-CELL TUMORS

Not uncommonly, malignant germ-cell tumors contain more than one histologic type. Usually, routine examinations of the primary tumor and sampling of metastases, if present, will make the mixture apparent. However, the detection of a mixture of elements may be difficult due to small foci in a large tumor mass. Therefore, it is recommended that thorough and painstaking microscopic investigation be carried out for all germ-cell malignancies.

The detection of a mixed germ-cell tumor may also be indirect. The presence of elevated hCG or AFP levels in the serum of a patient presumed to have an immature teratoma or a dysgerminoma is evidence for the presence of choriocarcinoma or embryonal or endodermal sinus tumor elements as well.

One example of a situation in which precise diagnosis may be critical: the patient with an apparently pure dysgerminoma. Postsurgical management for pure dysgerminoma consists of either radiation therapy or no further treatment. But if the tumor is actually a mixture of dysgerminoma and one or more other germ-cell elements, these therapy choices could prove to be fatal errors. In this setting, chemotherapy, not radiation, should be considered.

SUGGESTED READING

Einhorn LH, Donohuf J: Cis-diammine, dichloroplatinum, vinblastine, and bleomycin combination chemotherapy in disseminated testicular cancer. *Ann Intern Med* 87:293, 1977

Krepart G, Smith JP, Rutledge F, et al: The treatment for dysgerminoma of the ovary. *Cancer* 41:986, 1978

Kurman RJ, Norris HJ: Malignant mixed germ cell tumors of the ovary. *Obstet Gynecol* 48:579, 1976

Norris HJ, Zirkin HJ, Benson WL: Immature (malignant) teratoma of the ovary. *Cancer* 37:2359, 1976

Smith JP: The treatment of embryonal carcinoma of the ovary. In De Watteville H, ed: *Diagnosis and Treatment of Ovarian Neoplastic Alterations*. Amsterdam-Oxford: Excerpta Medica, 1975, p 214

77

Postoperative Management of Ovarian Epithelial Carcinoma

C. PAUL MORROW, M.D.

INITIAL POSTSURGICAL EVALUATION

Although surgery is the primary component of the management of ovarian carcinoma, most patients will need adjuvant radiation therapy or chemotherapy. There are two prerequisites to selecting the best treatment for each patient. First is exact information regarding the location and volume of *residual disease*. In the case of completely resectable ovarian carcinoma, and especially if the malignancy was apparently confined to the ovaries, it is important to know if the search for extraovarian disease at the time of surgery included omentectomy or biopsy, peritoneal cytology, evaluation of the retroperitoneal nodes and right hemidiaphragm, and biopsies of the cul-de-sac and gutter peritoneum.

The second prerequisite is an accurate *histologic diagnosis* based on an adequate sampling of the ovarian neoplasm and the tissue excised with it. The clinician must know if the tumor is primary in the ovary or represents a metastasis from another organ. This is a particularly important consideration in cases of mucinous carcinoma.

The histologic type may be epithelial carcinoma, i.e., a mucinous, endometrioid, clear-cell, or poorly differentiated carcinoma. Or it may be a germ-cell tumor. The latter occur almost exclusively in women under the age of 30. In contrast, malignant epithelial tumors are uncommon before age 30 and rare before age 20. Ovarian tumors of the stromal type should be suspected whenever there is evidence of hormonal activity.

The majority of ovarian malignancies belong to one of the common epithelial varieties for which histologic grade is of prognostic importance. (The other types of ovarian cancer are discussed in Chapter 76.) Tumors of borderline malignant potential are far more limited in biologic behavior than are true carcinomas. Furthermore, well-differentiated true carcinomas are less aggressive than the more undifferentiated forms.

Each of these factors—volume of residual disease, location of residual disease, histologic type, and grade—has important implications for prognosis and treatment. The 5-year survival rate for patients with ovarian epithelial carcinoma limited to the ovaries (stage I) and histologically borderline or grade 1 is 90% or better, compared with a 50% or less 5-year survival for other stages and grades. It is this latter group who require postsurgical therapy.

SELECTION OF ADJUVANT THERAPY

For resectable ovarian carcinoma requiring adjuvant therapy, the minimum treatment field is the entire abdominal cavity and the retroperitoneal lymphatics. This large field is necessitated by the early spread of ovarian carcinoma to the peritoneal surfaces. Patients with residual abdominal disease after surgery are at high risk for subclinical, extra-abdominal metastasis. They need systemic, not just abdominal, therapy.

Based on these considerations, the recommended postoperative management of patients with ovarian epithelial carcinoma is the following:

When disease is limited to the ovaries, ascites is absent, peritoneal cytology is negative, and histologic grade is borderline or well differentiated, no further treatment is indicated.

When disease is apparently limited to the ovaries but ascites is present, peritoneal cytology is positive, or the tumor is grade 2 or 3, intraperitoneal colloidal chromic phosphate therapy is recommended. A dose of 10 to 15 mc is administered through an intraperitoneal catheter placed either at the time of surgery or postoperatively.

When intraperitoneal adhesions contraindicate such therapy, external whole-abdomen irradiation by strip technique or chemotherapy with an alkylating agent may be used instead. Both these treatments appear to have higher incidences of complications than intraperitoneal chromic phosphate therapy. Alkylating agent chemotherapy is inexpensive, well tolerated, and easy to administer, but it may be followed by leukemia in 5-10 years. This risk may be reduced by treating the patient for 6 rather than 12 months. At present, none of these three methods seems to have a significantly better cure rate than the other two.

For patients with ovarian epithelial carcinoma involving pelvic structures but with no extrapelvic disease, or for patients with unresectable or incompletely resected ovarian epithelial carcinoma involving the abdomen, recommended postoperative treatment is combination chemotherapy. Therapy is started in the early postoperative period and continued for 12-18 months if the patient is doing well and the disease is stable or responding to therapy. A second-look operation is often indicated before stopping chemotherapy.

Single-drug (alkylating agent) therapy for advanced disease has been replaced by combination therapy with the following drugs: cisplatin (Platinol), doxorubicin (Adriamycin), and cyclophosphamide (Cytoxan). Normal-tissue toxicity as well as tumor response is increased with multiple-drug therapy, but improvement of response rates from 35% to 80% seems to justify the added morbidity. The efficacy of the newer regimens has all but eliminated abdominal radiation as a treatment modality for advanced ovarian carcinoma.

Serous effusions are commonly associated with advanced ovarian carcinoma. Clinically apparent ascites occurs in about one-third of cases. The abdominal fluid should be withdrawn to relieve respiratory embarrassment or pain. Improved gastrointestinal function and relief of nausea, vomiting, and constipation may also result from paracentesis.

Control of ascites is one of the earliest and most reliable indications of response to chemotherapy. Patients with unresectable ovarian carcinoma often reaccumulate ascites rapidly in the immediate postoperative period. Serious fluid and electrolyte disturbance, oliguria, and other management problems may result. These patients often benefit from immediate institution of intravenous chemotherapy. Ascites and pleural effusions unresponsive to systemic chemotherapy may be controlled by instilling radioactive chromic phosphate into the serous cavity. Intractable serous effusions have also been managed successfully with intracavitary bleomycin (Blenoxane), tetracycline, or quinacrine (Atabrine).

SECOND-LOOK SURGERY

The second-look operation has received much attention in the management of ovarian carcinoma. It is generally agreed that certain patients may benefit from a second laparotomy at the completion of a year of chemotherapy. The primary objective is to document as accurately as possible, prior to discontinuing chemotherapy, that no carcinoma remains, or to remove resectable residual carcinoma.

Only patients with residual disease following initial surgery or a relatively high risk of early recurrence are candidates for second-look surgery. Patients treated with whole-abdomen radiotherapy or intraperitoneal nuclides are not candidates because of the risk of bowel complications. Patients with stage I ovarian tumors of low malignant potential or grade 1 differentiation are not benefited by a second-look operation.

Second-look surgery involves numerous biopsies of the peritoneal surfaces and retroperitoneal nodes, resection of the residual omentum, and multiple cytologic specimens. It is most appropriately done in a treatment center.

FOLLOW-UP

Follow-up evaluation of ovarian carcinoma patients should be frequent during the first 2 years; the majority of recurrences will appear during this time. Long-term follow-up is also recommended since this malignancy may recur 10, 15, or even 20 years post-treatment.

History and physical examination are of primary importance in follow-up evaluation, since few laboratory tests or x-rays are useful. Recurrences are often heralded by partial large- or small-bowel obstruction, indigestion, a palpable pelvic mass, an enlarged peripheral lymph node, or evidence of ascites. It should be remembered that these women are epidemiologically similar to high-risk breast cancer patients. Adequate breast examination should be part and parcel of follow-up care.

SUGGESTED READING

Abell MR, Johnson VJ, Holtz F: Ovarian neoplasms in childhood and adolescence. II. Tumors of non-germ cell origin. *Am J Obstet Gynecol* 93:850, 1965

Aure JC, Hoeg K, Kolstadt P: Clinical and histologic studies of ovarian carcinoma: Long term follow-up of 990 cases. *Obstet Gynecol* 37:1, 1971

Dembo AJ, Bush RS, Beale FA, et al: Ovarian carcinoma: Improved survival following abdominopelvic irradiation in patients with a complete pelvic operation. *Am J Obstet Gynecol* 134:793, 1979

Hreshchyshyn MM, Park RC, Blessing JA, et al: The role of adjuvant therapy in Stage I ovarian cancer. *Am J Obstet Gynecol* 138:139, 1980

Morrow CP, Townsend DE: Tumors of the ovary. In *Synopsis of Gynecologic Oncology*, ed 2, ch 6. New York: Wiley, 1981

Smith JP, Delgado G, Rutledge F: Second-look operation in ovarian carcinoma. *Cancer* 38:1438, 1976

78

Diagnosis and Management of Molar Pregnancy

C. PAUL MORROW, M.D.

Hydatidiform or hydatid mole is an abnormal pregnancy characterized by gross vesicular swelling of the placental villi and the absence of a fetus or embryo. In the United States, its prevalence is approximately 1:1,500 live births. Typically the patient presents with a clinical picture of threatened abortion with a uterus larger than 12 weeks' gestational size. In addition to absence of fetal heart tones, other evidence supporting the diagnosis of hydatid mole includes hyperemesis gravidarum, a uterus large for gestational age, and toxemia.

Because molar pregnancy is uncommon, the diagnosis is often overlooked until the patient aborts the pathognomonic vesicles. However, the patient with a molar pregnancy is at high risk for serious complications that tend to worsen with time, making an early diagnosis desirable. Chronic and acute blood loss, hypervolemia, toxemia, and thyrotoxicosis are some of the likely complications of molar pregnancy. High-output heart failure accompanied by acute pulmonary edema may result. Another serious potential complication is infection of the uterine contents accompanied by sepsis, occurring in approximately 10% of cases.

When there is suspicion of a molar pregnancy, an ultrasound examination will usually confirm or rule out the diagnosis. If ultrasound is unavailable or equivocal, a transabdominal amniocentesis with amniography is employed to confirm the diagnosis. Ultrasound examination is also very useful in the unusual case in which a fetus coexists with a molar pregnancy. This condition is characterized by toxemia and a large uterus.

In the past, measurement of urinary hCG was often used to help identify patients with molar pregnancies. However, while a urinary concentration exceeding 500,000 IU/l is highly suggestive of the presence of hydatid mole, it is not diagnostic. A multifetal gestation may also be associated with very high levels of urinary hCG.

The differential diagnosis of hydatid mole includes multifetal gestation, polyhydramnios, uterine fibroids (which may enlarge rapidly during early pregnancy), and ovarian tumor during early pregnancy.

MANAGEMENT

Termination of Molar Pregnancy

As soon as the diagnosis of hydatid mole is confirmed, the pregnancy should be terminated by vacuum curettage. Conventional sharp curettage is adequate in those patients who have spontaneously evacuated part of the mole so that the uterus is less than 12 weeks' gestational size. Oxytocin or prostaglandin induction is indicated only in the case with a coexistent fetus. Vacuum curettage is carried out under general anesthesia in the operating room. If the patient is bleeding heavily on admission, an oxytocin infusion is started at that time; otherwise none is given until the curettage is completed.

Complications

During the immediate postoperative period the most common and important complications are sepsis and acute pulmonary crisis. The latter is due to trophoblastic embolization or fluid overload with heart failure. This syndrome appears within 4 hours postevacuation and is characterized by dyspnea, tachycardia, and hypotension.

Unilateral or bilateral enlargement of the ovaries due to multiple theca-lutein cysts is clinically detectable in approximately 30% of patients with hydatid moles, although in our experience they are not usually noted until the first or second week after evacuation. These cysts apparently result from the high levels of hCG. They regress slowly as the hCG titer diminishes postevacuation. The presence of these cysts should not lead to surgical intervention on the mistaken belief that they represent an ovarian neoplasm. It is recommended that RhoGAM be given to Rh-negative mothers, although hydatid mole has not been documented as a cause of Rh-sensitization.

Surveillance for Trophoblastic Neoplasia

Approximately 15% of patients with molar pregnancies will have either invasive mole or choriocarcinoma. Invasive mole is histologically similar to noninvasive mole, but is distinguished by its ability to invade the uterine muscle and metastasize, usually to the lungs or lower genital tract. Uterine perforation and hemorrhage may occur with invasive mole or choriocarcinoma.

Evaluation for neoplastic complications begins during initial hospitalization when a chest x-ray and pelvic examination are performed. Mole patients with a uterus large for dates or clinically detectable theca-lutein cysts are more likely to have invasive mole or choriocarcinoma than other mole patients.

The high incidence of postmolar trophoblastic disease and its potentially serious sequelae requires follow-up surveillance for every patient. Weekly measurements of serum hCG by radioimmunoassay for the β-subunit should begin 1 week after the mole is delivered and continue until the titer becomes normal (<1 mIU/ml). A normal value should occur within 15 weeks postevacuation. Titers are then repeated monthly for a year. If no rise occurs, no further follow-up is necessary. Pregnancy should be prevented during follow-up to avoid difficulties in interpreting a rise in hCG titer.

There are three indications for treatment: (1) the presence of metastases, (2) a titer rising or unchanged over a 3-week period, and (3) a rise in titer after it has returned to normal. A tissue diagnosis from uterine curettings of chorio-carcinoma or invasive mole is not an indication for treatment (nor is it neces-sary to have a tissue diagnosis prior to initiating treatment). A diagnosis of trophoblastic neoplasia is based on clinical history and hCG titer. Early detec-tion based on postevacuation serial hCG titers assures a virtually 100% cure rate of these potentially lethal growths.

During the period of surveillance with serial hCG titers, no other tests or examinations need to be carried out unless the patient develops symptoms or the hCG titer fails to fall. The most common associated problem is vaginal bleeding, which may require curettage. In the absence of vaginal bleeding or an enlarging uterus, uterine curettage is not indicated and is of neither diag-nostic nor therapeutic value.

The patient who develops stable or rising hCG titers should be evaluated for evidence of metastasis by physical examination and chest x-ray. The most common sites of metastases are the lungs and lower genital tract. If metastases are noted on these studies, additional work-up is necessary. This work-up and the management of metastatic disease are discussed in the next chapter.

Treatment of Nonmetastatic Trophoblastic Disease

The treatment of choice for postmolar nonmetastatic disease is simple hyster-ectomy for those women who wish to be sterilized. The ovaries need not be removed. Patients treated by hysterectomy must still be monitored postop-eratively by monthly hCG titers until the titers have been normal for 12 months. Titer remission, as this is called, must be confirmed by β-hCG serum radioimmunoassay, because it is the most sensitive and specific means avail-able of measuring chorionic gonadotropin.

Most women with a molar pregnancy wish to retain their childbearing ca-pacity. For them, the treatment of choice is systemic chemotherapy. Chemo-therapy should be carried out only by a physician experienced in its use and in the treatment of trophoblastic disease. Single-agent therapy, using metho-trexate, 0.4 mg/kg/day IV or IM, or dactinomycin (Cosmegen), 10-12 μg/kg/day IV, is the treatment of choice. These drugs are given in 5-day courses, repeated after a rest period of 9 days.

Chemotherapy is continued to one course past the first normal hCG titer. The average number of treatments required to induce titer remission is four. Patients must use effective means of contraception during treatment to avoid the confusion of a rising hCG titer due to an intercurrent pregnancy. Follow-ing titer remission, patients are monitored by monthly hCG assays until a minimum of 1 year in remission has been observed.

Chemotherapy has not been associated with a detectable increase in con-genital anomalies in subsequent pregnancies, but these women may have a higher probability of spontaneous abortions. In general, patients with a histo-ry of molar gestation seem to have a greater frequency of infertility and spontaneous abortions than women without such a history. Any woman who has had one molar pregnancy has an approximately 3% risk of having another molar pregnancy during her reproductive life.

SUGGESTED READING

Curry SL, Hammond CB, Tyrey L, et al: Hydatidiform mole: Diagnosis, management, and long term follow-up of 347 patients. *Obstet Gynecol* 45:1, 1975

Llewellyn-Jones D: Management of benign trophoblastic tumors. *Am J Obstet Gynecol* 128:424, 1977

Morrow CP, Kletzky OA, DiSaia PJ, et al: Clinical and laboratory correlates of molar pregnancy and trophoblastic disease. *Am J Obstet Gynecol* 128:424, 1977

Morrow CP, Townsend DE: Gestational trophoblastic neoplasia. In *Synopsis of Gynecologic Oncology*, ed 2, ch 10. New York: Wiley, 1981

Schlaerth JB, Morrow CP, Kletzky OA, et al: Prognostic characteristics of the serum human chorionic gonadotropin titer regression following molar pregnancy. *Obstet Gynecol* 58:479, 1981

Twiggs LB, Morrow CP, Schlaerth JB: Acute pulmonary complications of molar pregnancy. *Am J Obstet Gynecol* 135:189, 1979

79

Diagnosis and Management of Metastatic Trophoblastic Disease

C. PAUL MORROW, M.D.

In contrast to trophoblastic neoplasia confined to the uterus, metastatic trophoblastic disease is, in the great majority of cases, choriocarcinoma rather than invasive mole. Because of the important differences in prognosis and management, these two clinical situations are presented separately. The management of nonmetastatic trophoblastic disease is discussed in the previous chapter.

DIAGNOSIS

Metastatic trophoblastic disease usually has a latency period of several months following the culpable pregnancy. During this time the patient invariably has low but detectable levels of hCG, which neither cause symptoms nor interfere with normal, cyclic menstruation. She may, in fact, ovulate and conceive during this latency period. Occasionally, metastases from choriocarcinoma appear during a molar or nonmolar gestation, particularly during a normal intrauterine pregnancy.

Metastatic choriocarcinoma is a great mimic, usually presenting with symptoms entirely unrelated to the genital tract. It must be considered in women of reproductive age who have any of the following presumptive diagnoses: stroke, intracerebral hemorrhage, brain or spinal cord tumor, hepatitis, cholecystitis, gastrointestinal bleeding, hematuria, and nodular or diffuse pulmonary disease. It is a good policy to screen all women admitted with these diagnoses with a sensitive pregnancy test.

The patient with choriocarcinoma may also present with signs and symptoms of eclampsia, hemoperitoneum, threatened or missed abortion, or delayed postpartum hemorrhage. The patient with intrauterine choriocarcinoma presenting with symptoms of threatened or missed abortion has a typical history of amenorrhea followed by uterine enlargement, vaginal spotting, and a positive pregnancy test. A high suspicion should be aroused if there is a history of molar pregnancy. Diagnosis is made when the uterus fails to enlarge further; curettage is performed, and trophoblast without fetal or placental tissue is obtained.

Hemoperitoneum may be secondary to a ruptured liver, bleeding ovarian metastases, ruptured theca-lutein cysts, or perforation of the uterus by tumor. Understandably, these patients often undergo laparotomy, with a presumptive diagnosis of ruptured ectopic pregnancy.

Every patient with delayed postpartum bleeding should be screened for choriocarcinoma by pregnancy testing, even though the yield will be small.

The importance of the hCG titer in the diagnosis of choriocarcinoma cannot be overemphasized. This test and the medical history are sufficient to make the diagnosis in virtually every case. Tissue diagnosis is almost always unnecessary, sometimes dangerous, and often misleading. On physical examination, special attention is given to the genital tract since choriocarcinoma often metastasizes to the cervix, vagina, urethra, and vulva. There may be parametrial extension and ovarian metastases.

In addition to a chest x-ray, a radionuclide or CAT scan of the brain, liver, and spleen should be performed as part of the work-up. If the chest x-ray is negative, whole-lung tomograms may identify sites of metastases. An intravenous pyelogram (IVP) is performed to evaluate renal function and assess the kidney and urinary tract for metastases. This is of special importance in the patient with gross or microscopic hematuria.

MANAGEMENT

The management of metastatic choriocarcinoma will depend to some extent upon the site of the metastases. Patients with metastases only in the lung have the most favorable prognosis; those with metastases in the liver are the most difficult to cure.

All cases require combination chemotherapy, usually employing dactinomycin (Cosmegen), 8-10 μg/kg/day IV; methotrexate, 0.3 mg/kg/day IV; and chlorambucil (Leukeran), 0.2 mg/kg/day PO for 5 days each treatment cycle. Intravenous cyclophosphamide (Cytoxan), 3-5 mg/kg/day, may be substituted for chlorambucil if nausea and vomiting make oral therapy difficult. The 5-day course is repeated approximately every other week.

Often the patient with metastatic choriocarcinoma presents in poor condition and will not tolerate combination drug therapy immediately. When this situation arises, it has been our practice to initiate treatment with dactinomycin alone.

The most common reason for treatment failure has been bone-marrow and gastrointestinal toxicity, rather than drug resistance. Toxicity can result in prolonged intervals between treatment courses, during which the tumor recovers along with the normal tissues. If the 5-day regimen cannot be given more frequently than every 3 weeks, cure is unlikely.

hCG titers are obtained weekly to monitor tumor response. The drugs are continued on an every-other-week schedule until three consecutive weekly β-hCG serum values < 1 mIU/ml are reported. Because of an approximately 10% relapse rate after titer remission, continuing treatment is recommended for a minimum of three courses after the first normal titer.

The presence of CNS metastases requires special management because of the threat of intracranial hemorrhage. The brain is also a sanctuary for cancer, because the blood-brain barrier protects it from cytotoxic agents. Although choriocarcinoma is sometimes initially diagnosed at craniotomy, surgery can usually be avoided if the diagnosis is made earlier. Nevertheless, decompression craniotomy may be a necessity.

As soon as the presence of brain metastases has been demonstrated by clinical symptoms, physical examination, or computerized tomography, whole-brain irradiation should be initiated. A total dose of 2,000-3,000 rads should be delivered over 2 weeks. This has the immediate effect of preventing hemorrhage, and it is therapeutic as well.

Liver metastases are a most difficult problem to contend with. To prevent hemorrhage and eradicate tumor some authorities have recommended whole-liver irradiation to approximately 2,000 rads. However, this has not been proven to be effective. We reserve it for cases with extensive or subcapsular metastases. We recommend chemotherapy alone for all other cases with liver involvement.

The prognosis is excellent for patients with lung metastases only. Approximately 90% can be expected to have a sustained remission. For those with CNS metastases, a 50% cure rate can be anticipated, while those with liver metastases have a significantly poorer prognosis—perhaps 25% will survive.

The curability of metastatic choriocarcinoma is to a great extent dependent upon the therapist's understanding of this cancer; the role of surgery, radiation, and chemotherapy in its management; and the nuances of hCG testing. Consequently, referral to a treatment center may be advisable. Metastatic trophoblastic disease is so extraordinarily uncommon that few physicians, even specialists, have the experience required to optimally manage this potentially lethal malignancy.

SUGGESTED READING

Bagshawe KD: *Choriocarcinoma: The Clinical Biology of the Trophoblast and Its Tumors*. Baltimore: Williams & Wilkins, 1969

Brewer JI, Halpern B, Torok ED: Gestational trophoblastic disease: Selected clinical aspects and chorionic gonadotropin test methods. In Hickey RC, Clark RL, Benfield JR, et al, eds: *Current Problems in Cancer*, vol 3. Chicago: Year Book, 1979, p 1

Hammond CB, Borchert LG, Tyrey L, et al: Treatment of metastatic trophoblastic disease: Good and poor prognosis. *Am J Obstet Gynecol* 115:451, 1973

Hertz R: *Choriocarcinoma and Related Gestational Trophoblastic Tumors in Women*. New York: Raven, 1978

Morrow CP, Townsend DE: Gestational trophoblastic neoplasia. In *Synopsis of Gynecologic Oncology*, ed 2, ch 10. New York: Wiley, 1981

Weed JC Jr, Hammond CB: Cerebral metastatic choriocarcinoma: Intensive therapy and prognosis. *Obstet Gynecol* 55:89, 1980

SIX

REPRODUCTIVE ENDOCRINOLOGY AND INFERTILITY

80

Diagnosis and Management of
Sexual Ambiguity in the Newborn

DANIEL R. MISHELL JR., M.D.

The sex of an individual can be identified by four anatomic characteristics: (1) sex chromosomes, (2) gonadal histology, (3) morphology of the external genitalia, and (4) morphology of the internal genitalia. When all these characteristics are not consistently male or female, the condition of hermaphroditism, or intersexuality, exists. The psychological characteristics of sex, which include sex of rearing, are usually related to the morphology of the external genitalia. When intersexuality exists in a newborn, it is very important to determine and designate the individual's future sex soon after birth to avoid future psychological problems. A sex assignment decision should be made before the infant leaves the hospital to avoid a change in gender role later in life with its accompanying psychological trauma.

Whenever intersexuality exists, the Krebs classification is used to provide definitions. When there is inconsistency among the four morphologic essential characteristics just described and the gonads are masculine, the individual is designated a male pseudohermaphrodite. Likewise, when the histology of the gonads is feminine, the individual is designated a female pseudohermaphrodite. If both male and female elements are present in one or both gonads, the individual is classified as a true hermaphrodite.

Disorders of sexual ambiguity can be further divided into two major categories on the basis of their etiology: (1) disorders of gonadal development, in which the basic defect is usually a major chromosomal lesion that occurs by chance and is not hereditary, and (2) disorders of fetal endocrinology, in which the individual has normal chromosomes but usually has a genetic defect that in many instances is hereditary.

DISORDERS OF GONADAL DEVELOPMENT

When a disorder of gonadal development occurs, the major chromosomal lesion can be due to an error in either meiosis or mitosis. Since these lesions occur by chance, they are neither hereditary nor more likely to occur in siblings. Errors in meiotic division can cause aneuploidy, which produces an incorrect number of sex chromosomes or structural abnormalities in sex chromosomes. Abnormalities in mitotic division can also occur. In this instance, both divided cells remain in the organism and mosaicism results. Mosaicism is a condition in which the individual has cells of different karyotypes but of one genetic origin.

The most common disorders of gonadal development, Klinefelter's syndrome and gonadal dysgenesis, do not cause problems of sexual differentiation in the newborn. Klinefelter's syndrome with a 47,XXY karyotype produces aspermia, and infertility is the most common presenting complaint.

Gonadal dysgenesis may have several karyotypes, all of which are associated with failure of the germ cells to migrate into the undifferentiated gonads during embryonic life. The gonads fail to develop and persist only as bilateral streaks. Phenotypically, individuals with gonadal dysgenesis appear as females with normal external and internal genitalia. With the lack of estrogen production, they fail to develop secondary sex characteristics and present with the complaint of primary amenorrhea.

The other disorders of gonadal development include true hermaphroditism and male pseudohermaphroditism. These disorders will cause problems in identifying the sex of the newborn. In true hermaphroditism, there are both male and female elements in the gonads. A uterus is nearly always present, and the differentiation of the internal genitalia corresponds closely to the histology of the adjacent gonads. Cryptorchidism is frequently present, together with some deficiency in labial-scrotal fusion. The external genitalia are generally more male than female, but at puberty about three-fourths of true hermaphrodites develop gynecomastia and more than half menstruate. Therefore, it is important to make the diagnosis at birth.

There are two types of male pseudohermaphrodites with problems of gonadal development. The first has a primary gonadal defect with no gonads present and a normal 46,XY karyotype. The external genitalia are ambiguous, a vagina is present, and there is no evidence of female internal genitalia. The other is a Y chromosomal defect, which causes the syndrome of mixed gonadal dysgenesis. These patients have a testis on one side and a streak on the other. The external genitalia are ambiguous, ranging from a normal male type with hypospadias to a normal female type with clitorimegaly. The internal genitalia usually are normal female.

DISORDERS OF FETAL ENDOCRINOLOGY

Female Pseudohermaphroditism With Partial Virilization

The second major category, disorders of fetal endocrinology, can be subdivided into female pseudohermaphroditism with partial virilization and male pseudohermaphroditism with some degree of failure of virilization. Female pseudohermaphroditism is usually due to congenital adrenal hyperplasia (CAH), although some forms have a nonadrenal etiology. CAH is the most frequent cause of ambiguous genitalia in the newborn. This is the only type of intersexuality with the possibility of entirely normal sexual function, including the capability of conception, as the virilization involves only the external genitalia. The gonads and internal genitalia are completely normal female, and the external genitalia can be surgically reconstructed as those of a normal female. This is the only intersex disorder that can jeopardize survival, and it is imperative to make the diagnosis at birth.

CAH is a recessive disorder that produces one of three enzyme deficiencies, which in turn cause lack of cortisol synthesis with a resultant increase in ACTH production. The increased ACTH causes increased production of adrenal androgens, which masculinize the external genitalia. Because the androgen production can vary according to the enzymatic defect, the virilization seen in these patients is variable in degree and can range from clitorimegaly with minimal labial fusion to complete scrotal fusion with the urethra ending at the tip of the phallus. In the latter case, the infant may resemble a completely normal male with cryptorchidism. It is therefore very important for the obstetrician to examine every male newborn and palpate the scrotum. If no testes are palpable, CAH should be suspected and appropriate diagnostic tests should be performed as soon as possible.

11β-Hydroxylase deficiency is the form of CAH least dangerous to the patient's life but is associated with hypertension. 21-Hydroxylase deficiency with salt wasting and 3β-ol dehydrogenase deficiency may cause death. Once the diagnosis of CAH is suspected, it can be confirmed by measuring the levels of 17-hydroxyprogesterone in the serum. This steroid is elevated in all forms of CAH. The nonadrenal type of female pseudohermaphroditism is caused by excess exogenous or endogenous androgen stimulation of the fetus during pregnancy. Exogenous androgen can come from maternal ingestion of androgenic drugs, including oral contraceptives. Endogenous androgen can be produced by a virilizing ovarian tumor such as a luteoma.

Male Pseudohermaphroditism With Partial Failure of Virilization

There are three categories of male pseudohermaphroditism with partial failure of virilization. The most common is due to a defect in testosterone action. This is most frequently caused by a complete or partial defect of the androgen cellular receptor in the target organs. The terms "androgen insensitivity syndrome" and "testicular feminization syndrome" have been applied to this disorder. These individuals are genetically gonadal males with complete, normal external female appearance and normal growth and development, including breast development. They usually present to the clinician after puberty with primary amenorrhea, scanty or absent body hair, absent internal genitalia, and female external genitalia with a short or absent vagina. These individuals have to be differentiated from females with normal ovaries and congenital absence of the uterus. The latter have normal body hair. If there is only a partial defect in the receptor protein, there may be varying degrees of ambiguity in the external genitalia, ranging from females with partial labial-scrotal fusion through males with only minimal hypospadias. All of these individuals develop breasts at puberty, and varying degrees of development of the male internal genitalia are also seen.

Another type of defect of testosterone action is a deficiency of the 5α-reductase enzyme. This defect is an autosomal recessive disorder found in certain families. Males with this disorder are born with ambiguity of the external genitalia with bilateral undescended testes and lack of a phallus. Puberty brings marked virilization, phallic growth, and descent of the testes into the scrotum. Gynecomastia does not occur. In certain instances, individuals with this disorder can be raised as males, as they can ultimately have adequate male sexual function.

The second category of male pseudohermaphroditism is abnormality of müllerian inhibitory factor synthesis, which leads to males with bilateral testes and normal male internal and external genitalia; however, they also have a uterus and oviducts. The latter are frequently present in an inguinal hernia.

The third category includes those rare patients with various defects of biosynthesis of testosterone due to an autosomal recessive deficiency of certain enzymes. They have male gonads, ambiguous external genitalia, and no female internal genitalia, and may develop breasts at puberty. They constitute the nonvirilizing form of the adrenogenital syndrome.

DIFFERENTIAL DIAGNOSIS

In order to establish the differential diagnosis of sexual ambiguity at birth, a complete physical examination should be done with special attention to determining the size of the phallus, the position of the urethral orifice, the degree of hypospadias, the amount of labial-scrotal fusion, and the presence or absence of scrotal testes as well as a uterus. X-rays, laboratory tests, and, not infrequently, exploratory laparotomy are necessary to make the diagnosis.

The sex of an apparently male neonate should not be pronounced until testes are palpated in the scrotum. If the infant does have ambiguous genitalia, the parents should be informed immediately that the baby's sex organs are incompletely developed and it has a congenital anomaly. The parents should also be informed that diagnostic studies will commence at once for evaluation of the problem and that the infant should not be assigned a sex before evaluation has been completed. In talking to the parents, it is important to use understandable, nontraumatizing language and convey hope. It helps to have the parents examine the genitalia along with the physician.

If the external genitalia are ambiguous but the phallus is in normal position relative to the labial-scrotal region, the differential diagnosis includes (1) a virilized genetic female (most likely CAH), (2) a nonvirilized or incompletely virilized male, and (3) a true hermaphrodite. If gonads are present in the labial-scrotal inguinal area, they are virtually always testes and rule out virilization of a genetic female. If the testes are bilateral, the differential diagnosis includes (1) incomplete forms of testicular feminization, (2) 5α-reductase deficiency, and (3) defects in testosterone biosynthesis. If there is a unilateral testis, the differential diagnosis includes mixed gonadal dysgenesis and true hermaphroditism. If gonads are absent from the labial-scrotal and inguinal area, the differential diagnosis includes (1) undescended testes with normal or abnormal hormonal function, (2) a virilized genetic female, (3) mixed gonadal dysgenesis, and (4) some type of true hermaphroditism. If a uterus and cervix are present with no palpable testes, the differential diagnosis includes (1) virilized genetic female, (2) mixed gonadal dysgenesis, and (3) true hermaphroditism. If a uterus and cervix are not present and testes are not palpable, the differential diagnosis includes (1) a male without gonads and (2) cryptorchidism with defects in testosterone production or action, i.e., incomplete forms of testicular feminization or 5α-reductase deficiency.

In order to make the differential diagnosis among these disorders after physical examination, it is very helpful to measure 17α-hydroxyprogesterone in neonates in whom congenital adrenal hyperplasia is suspected. If this metabolite is elevated, i.e., above 2 ng/ml, the diagnosis of CAH can be made and appropriate corticosteroid therapy should be initiated. Chromosomal karyotypes are helpful in confirming the clinical and anatomic findings, but they may not be necessary to formulate a treatment plan or to decide the sex of rearing.

MANAGEMENT

The sex that should be assigned to the infant should be based primarily on the potential of the external genitalia for coital adequacy, since these patients—except for those with CAH and 5α-reductase deficiency—are infertile. Since it is easier to surgically create functional female external genitalia than male external genitalia, most patients with more than a mild form of ambiguity of the external genitalia, with the exception of 5α-reductase deficiency, should be raised as female. The phallus should be amputated soon after birth in order to avoid psychological trauma to the infant and parental concern.

All intra-abdominal gonads in hermaphrodites with a Y chromosome have a relatively high potential of becoming malignant, with the two most common tumors being dysgerminomas and gonadoblastomas. The incidence of tumors increases markedly at the time of puberty in all intersex disorders with a Y chromosome except testicular feminization. Therefore, the gonads should be removed before puberty from individuals who have mixed gonadal dysgenesis and male hermaphroditism. In individuals with testicular feminization, tumors are uncommon before the age of 25. Since the gonadal secretion of these individuals induces normal pubertal feminization, including breast development, removal of the gonads should be delayed until age 20. Individuals with intersexuality without a Y chromosome rarely develop gonadal tumors, so their gonads or streaks should not be removed. Individuals with gonadal dysgenesis without a Y chromosome in their peripheral white blood cells do not need to have their streak gonads removed.

SUGGESTED READING

Donahoe PK, Hendran WM: Evaluation of the newborn with ambiguous genitalia. *Pediatr Clin North Am* 23:361, 1976

Imperato-McGinley J, Peterson RE: Male pseudohermaphroditism. The complexities of male phenotypic development. *Am J Med* 61:251, 1976

Manuel M, Katayama KP, Jones HW: The age of occurrence of gonadal tumors in intersex patients with a Y chromosome. *Am J Obstet Gynecol* 124:293, 1976

Park IJ, Aimakhu VE, Jones HW: An etiologic and pathogenic classification of male hermaphroditism. *Am J Obstet Gynecol* 123:505, 1975

Walsh PC, et al: Pseudohermaphroditism type II. *N Engl J Med* 291:944, 1974

Wilson JD, et al: Familial incomplete male pseudohermaphroditism, type I. Evidence of androgen resistance and variable clinical manifestations in a family with the Reifenstein syndrome. *N Engl J Med* 290:1097, 1974

81

Differential Diagnosis of Primary Amenorrhea

OSCAR A. KLETZKY, M.D., and VAL DAVAJAN, M.D.

The diagnosis of primary amenorrhea is made when a patient has had no spontaneous uterine bleeding by the age of 17. However, a diagnostic work-up should be initiated at age 15 if the patient has no secondary sex characteristics or if 2 years or more have elapsed following the onset of secondary sexual development without menarche.

Patients with primary amenorrhea are classified into four groups, based on the presence or absence of breast development and uterus. Group 1 consists of patients without breast development but with a palpable uterus; group 2, patients with breast development but no uterus; group 3, patients with neither breast development nor uterus; group 4, patients with breast development and a palpable uterus.

GROUP 1

Patients without breast development but with a palpable uterus may have either hypogonadotropic hypogonadism or gonadal dysgenesis. The correct differential diagnosis can easily be made by measuring serum follicle-stimulating hormone (FSH), which is consistently elevated in patients with gonadal dysgenesis. Although serum luteinizing hormone (LH) is usually elevated, it can be within the normal range. Patients with hypogonadotropic hypogonadism will have either low or normal serum levels of both LH and FSH. Some of these patients also have anosmia (Kallmann's syndrome). Therefore, all patients in this group without elevated FSH should have at least a qualitative test for olfaction with coffee, tobacco, orange, and cocoa.

Hypothalamic or higher CNS disorders are probably the most common cause of hypogonadotropic primary amenorrhea. Additional causes can be craniopharyngioma, tuberculous granuloma, sequelae of meningoencephalitis, thalassemia major, or a rare case of nonsecreting pituitary adenoma. Therefore anteroposterior and lateral cone views of the sella turcica should be obtained. To pursue the etiology of the hypogonadotropic hypogonadism, patients may be tested with gonadotropin-releasing hormone (GnRH). A karyotype is not necessary, since all these patients are 46,XX. Patients with hypogonadotropic hypogonadism have good potential for successful reproduction with the administration of exogenous gonadotropins. If pregnancy is not desired, low doses of estrogen—i.e., 0.625 mg of conjugated estrogen daily—should be given to induce breast development.

Patients with gonadal dysgenesis who have elevated gonadotropins do need chromosome analysis. Karyotype is important, since the presence of a Y chromosome is an indication to remove the gonads surgically. It has been estimated that the risk of developing a gonadal tumor with a Y chromosome present is over 25% by age 30. However, if the peripheral karyotype does not contain a Y chromosome, the gonads need not be removed unless there is clinical evidence of excessive androgen production.

Patients with gonadal dysgenesis are sterile and need estrogen replacement to induce breast development and prevent osteoporosis. In short patients, the daily conjugated estrogen dose should not be more than 0.3 mg in order to avoid premature closure of the epiphyses. Patients of normal height should be given 0.625 or 1.25 mg/day. This dosage of estrogen is sufficient to produce adequate breast development. Higher doses of estrogen do not render better results. It is recommended that estrogen be given in cycles of 25 days, from the 1st to the 25th day of each calendar month. In the last 10 days of treatment (days 16 through 25), 5-10 mg of oral medroxyprogesterone acetate (Provera) are added in order to differentiate and cause sloughing of the endometrium.

GROUP 2

Patients with primary amenorrhea with normal breast development but no uterus have either congenital absence of the uterus or the complete form of androgen insensitivity syndrome (testicular feminization). Patients with congenital absence of the uterus ovulate and have normal body hair. Patients with androgen insensitivity syndrome do not ovulate and have no pubic hair. The presence of ovulation can be determined by taking the basal body temperature or weekly measurements of serum progesterone. If ovulation is documented, no further testing is necessary, since the patient obviously does not have androgen insensitivity. Since patients with congenital absence of the uterus still have normal ovarian function, no hormone replacement therapy is necessary.

Another way to differentiate these two types of patients is to measure serum testosterone. In patients with congenital absence of the uterus, serum testosterone levels are within the normal female range. In patients with androgen insensitivity, serum testosterone levels are within the normal male range. The testosterone does not act on target tissues because of the congenital absence of testosterone receptors. Only patients with elevated testosterone levels need a karyotype examination. An individual with this syndrome has 46,XY chromosomes, testes, and a female phenotype. The abnormal clinical features in patients with androgen insensitivity include lack of axillary and pubic hair with normal breast development and a blind vaginal pouch with absence of the uterus.

All patients with androgen insensitivity should have the gonads surgically removed after puberty because of the high incidence of malignancy (dysgerminoma). The incidence of gonadal tumors in patients over 30 years of age with this syndrome is approximately 25%. Since gonadal malignancy has rarely been reported in patients under 20 years, it is recommended that the testes not be removed until the patient has undergone full sexual development and normal epiphyseal closure with her own endogenous testicular steroids. Following surgery, the patient should be placed on 0.625 mg of conjugated estrogen replacement for the first 25 days of each month in order to prevent osteoporosis. Progestins do not have to be used in these patients, as they do not have a uterus.

It is our recommendation to tell patients with this syndrome that there is an abnormal sex chromosome and not to refer specifically to the abnormality as a Y chromosome, since most patients know that an XY karyotype is indicative of being male. The term gonad should be used instead of testis when referring to the gonadal abnormality. The patient should also be told that she cannot become pregnant and that she may require vaginoplasty in order to have normal sexual function. Patients with congenital absence of the uterus may also need a vaginoplasty, as they usually have no vagina.

GROUP 3

Patients with primary amenorrhea who have neither breast nor uterine development are very rare. These patients have a male karyotype, elevated gonadotropin levels, and testosterone values in the normal female range. They differ from patients with gonadal dysgenesis because they do not have a uterus, and from patients with testicular feminization because they do not have breast development and their serum testosterone levels are in the normal female range. It has been reported that the etiology in these patients can be a 17,20-desmolase deficiency or testicular regression. If the patient has gonads, they should be surgically removed. If no gonads were ever present, or after the gonads have been removed, estrogen replacement therapy should be given in the doses and form previously recommended, in order to induce the development of the breasts.

GROUP 4

The presence of primary amenorrhea in patients with spontaneous breast development and a normal uterus indicates that a disturbance of the hypothalamic-pituitary-ovarian axis has occurred after the initiation but before the completion of puberty. It is recommended that all patients with primary amenorrhea with breast development and an intact uterus have a careful breast examination to detect the presence of galactorrhea, and a serum prolactin determination to rule out a prolactin-secreting pituitary adenoma. Patients with normal serum prolactin levels have the same features as patients with secondary amenorrhea, and their work-up is discussed in detail in the following chapter.

SUGGESTED READING

Kletzky OA, Marra RP, Costin G, Bernstein G, March CM, Mishell DR Jr: Gonadotropin insufficiency in patients with thalassemia major. *J Clin Endocrinol Metab* 48:901, 1979

Kletzky OA, Nicoloff JT, Davajan V, Mims R, Mishell DR Jr: Idiopathic hypogonadotrophic hypogonadal primary amenorrhea. *J Clin Endocrinol Metab* 46:808, 1978

Manuel M, Katayama KP, Jones HW Jr: The age of occurrence of gonadal tumors in intersex patients with a Y chromosome. *Am J Obstet Gynecol* 124:293, 1976

Mashchak CA, Kletzky OA, Davajan V, Mishell DR Jr: Clinical and laboratory evaluation of patients with primary amenorrhea. *Obstet Gynecol* 57:715, 1981

Wentz AC, Jones GS: Prognosis in primary amenorrhea. *Fertil Steril* 29:614, 1978

82

Differential Diagnosis of Secondary Amenorrhea

OSCAR A. KLETZKY, M.D., and VAL DAVAJAN, M.D.

If the onset of secondary amenorrhea is acute, a 6-month interval is considered sufficient for the diagnosis. If the patient gives a history of oligomenorrhea, a 12-month interval is used to make the diagnosis of secondary amenorrhea. Patients with amenorrhea and no clinical evidence of excess cortisol (Cushing's syndrome), androgen production, or galactorrhea can be first divided into two groups, based upon whether or not they have uterine bleeding following intramuscular injection of 100 or 200 mg of progesterone in oil.

The positive or negative response of the endometrium to progesterone correlates well with the levels of serum estradiol. No uterine bleeding will occur if the level of estradiol is below 40 pg/ml. Any amount of uterine bleeding is considered a positive test (from minimal dark brown staining to a normal menstrual flow). When uterine bleeding does occur, it usually occurs between 3 and 14 days after the intramuscular injection. Amenorrhea in individuals with normal breast development and an intact uterus without evidence of androgen or cortisol excess or galactorrhea can be due to a uterine, hypothalamic, pituitary, or ovarian factor.

UTERINE CAUSES

The integrity of the endometrium should always be considered first, before initiating an endocrine evaluation. Causes affecting the uterus are pregnancy and intrauterine synechiae (Asherman's syndrome). Therefore, any patient with amenorrhea who has had a prior curettage, especially in pregnancy or postpartum, should have a hysterosalpingogram and/or hysteroscopy. If synechiae are found, appropriate therapy should be performed as discussed in Chapter 101. These patients will have a biphasic basal body temperature, indicating normal hypothalamic-pituitary-ovarian function.

HYPOTHALAMIC CAUSES

Hypothalamic Dysfunction With/Without History of Drugs and/or Stress

One of the most common causes of amenorrhea is anovulation secondary to hypothalamic dysfunction without any history of stress or drug intake. Drugs most commonly associated with amenorrhea are the phenothiazine derivatives and contraceptive steroids used previously. Some patients will develop amenorrhea when a stressful situation is encountered (e.g., going away to school, divorce in the family). These patients have levels of estradiol of at least 40 pg/ml and therefore will have uterine bleeding following progesterone administration. Random samples of luteinizing hormone (LH) and follicle-stimulating hormone (FSH) levels are in the normal range.

Hypothalamic Failure Secondary to Hypothalamic Lesions or Lack of Synthesis of Gonadotropin-Releasing Hormone

These disorders may manifest themselves as either primary or secondary amenorrhea. Lesions of the hypothalamus that have been associated with amenorrhea include craniopharyngioma, tuberculous granuloma, and the sequelae of meningoencephalitis.

These patients have a low estradiol level and will not have uterine bleeding after progesterone administration. Random serum FSH and LH levels in these patients are either very low or in the low normal range—insufficient to stimulate the ovarian follicles to synthesize estradiol.

Hypothalamic Amenorrhea Secondary to Weight Loss

This category includes simple weight loss and anorexia nervosa. Patients with simple weight loss who become amenorrheic after losing 15-20% of their ideal body weight are usually referred to as being underweight; those who have lost more than 25% of their ideal weight are labeled severely underweight. These individuals may have normal or low gonadotropins and normal or low estrogen, depending on the degree of weight loss.

Patients with anorexia nervosa, in addition to having severe weight loss (more than 25% of ideal body weight), have constipation, hypotension, bradycardia, and hypothermia. These individuals invariably have an abnormal ideation concerning their body image and an aversion to food intake. They have low serum gonadotropin and estrogen levels. In addition, almost every patient with anorexia nervosa, in contrast to women with simple weight loss, has a low serum triiodothyronine by radioimmunoassay.

The treatment of these two groups of patients appears to be related primarily to promoting weight gain. Patients with anorexia nervosa also need psychiatric therapy.

PITUITARY CAUSES

Patients with amenorrhea due to a pituitary etiology may have either nonneoplastic lesions or tumors.

Non-neoplastic Lesions of the Pituitary

This group includes patients with a destructive process of the pituitary, such as seen in Sheehan's or Simmonds's disease. The pituitary cells are damaged by anoxia, thrombosis, or hemorrhage, which frequently occurs postpartum.

These patients have low serum levels of LH, FSH, and estradiol and therefore will not bleed following intramuscular progesterone.

Pituitary Tumors

Amenorrhea may be the first sign of a pituitary tumor (non-prolactin-secreting chromophobe adenoma). Patients with amenorrhea due to pituitary tumors usually have low estradiol levels and therefore do not have uterine bleeding following administration of intramuscular progesterone. Random serum levels of FSH and LH may be either low or normal. However, repeated sampling at 15-minute intervals for 4 hours will reveal less than normal amounts of these hormones being secreted. Repeated sampling is not clinically practicable, and therefore a "normal" value should be considered low.

OVARIAN CAUSES

Three different ovarian causes of amenorrhea are discussed. Two result in ovarian failure and include premature ovarian failure and loss of ovarian function secondary to castration, infection, hemorrhage, or compromised blood supply. The third cause is polycystic ovarian disease (PCO). Patients in the first two groups have elevated FSH levels; patients in the third group have elevated LH levels.

Premature Ovarian Failure

This diagnosis is made when ovarian failure occurs at any age between menarche and age 35. Since the ovaries of these patients do not secrete sufficient amounts of estradiol to maintain negative feedback to the hypothalamus, gonadotropins are found to be elevated into the postmenopausal range. Although gonadotropin levels do fluctuate, they are consistently elevated and therefore a single serum FSH determination is adequate to make the diagnosis. These patients will not have uterine bleeding following intramuscular progesterone. With rare exceptions, ovulation cannot be induced in these patients with drug therapy, and therefore they should be considered sterile and receive estrogen replacement.

Loss of Ovarian Function Secondary to Castration, Intraovarian Infection, or Interference With Blood Supply

Loss of ovarian function following surgical castration is self-explanatory. On rare occasions, patients with severe bilateral tubo-ovarian abscesses have responded well to antibiotic therapy and did not require surgical treatment. In some of these patients the infection completely destroys the ovarian tissue, resulting in ovarian failure. Following hysterectomy, the ovarian blood supply may be compromised, resulting in "cystic degeneration." Usually this process is unilateral and therefore does not manifest itself with amenorrhea. However, it may occur bilaterally or in the only remaining ovary, resulting in loss of ovarian function. These patients are sterile and need estrogen replacement therapy.

Polycystic Ovarian Disease

PCO is a multiglandular disease and is included here because in 60% of cases it is possible to palpate enlarged ovaries. Hirsutism, obesity, and infertility may also be present. Patients with PCO usually have oligomenorrhea but many have primary or secondary amenorrhea. These patients secrete normal amounts of estradiol and therefore have uterine bleeding following intramuscular progesterone. Management of this disease is discussed in Chapter 89.

DIAGNOSTIC EVALUATION

The initial work-up of patients with secondary amenorrhea includes history and physical examination, CBC, thyrotropin, VDRL, chest x-ray, and at least one fasting blood sugar. If the patient has any signs and symptoms of hyperthyroidism, triiodothyronine and thyroxine levels should be obtained by radioimmunoassay. A D&C and laparoscopy are not indicated or necessary to work up patients with secondary amenorrhea.

Withdrawal uterine bleeding following an injection of progesterone in oil has made it possible to divide patients with amenorrhea into two major categories. In individuals with uterine bleeding, a single serum LH value of over 30 mIU/ml is indicative of polycystic ovarian disease. LH values below 30 represent hypothalamic dysfunction. In these patients, serum prolactin levels should be determined even in the absence of galactorrhea and, if they are elevated, an x-ray of the sella turcica should be performed to rule out a pituitary tumor. In addition, a thyrotropin-releasing hormone stimulation test and CT scan may be indicated, as discussed in Chapter 84.

If the prolactin level is normal, uterine withdrawal bleeding should be induced with medroxyprogesterone (10 mg for 10 days) or 100 mg progesterone IM at least once every 3 months if the patient does not desire pregnancy. If pregnancy is desired, these patients should be treated with clomiphene citrate (Clomid, Serophene). If pregnancy is not desired, it is recommended that these patients use a barrier method of contraception, since spontaneous recovery and ovulation can occur and be masked by use of oral contraceptives. It is unnecessary to perform x-rays of the sella turcica in patients in this group unless they have an elevated serum prolactin.

A single serum FSH (but not LH) measurement in patients who do not have withdrawal uterine bleeding can identify two distinct populations. One group will have a low or normal FSH, and the other an elevated value. The low or normal FSH represents hypothalamic-pituitary failure, while the elevated FSH represents ovarian failure.

All patients with hypothalamic-pituitary failure without a history of drugs or weight loss should have further evaluation to demonstrate the presence or absence of a pituitary tumor. This evaluation should include a serum prolactin followed by anteroposterior and lateral cone views of the sella turcica. If the prolactin is not elevated, neither a polytomogram nor a CT scan of the sella is indicated. If no tumor is demonstrated, cone view x-rays of the sella turcica should be repeated every 24 months. In addition, patients with a possible history of Sheehan's disease should have an insulin-induced hypoglycemia test in order to determine the pituitary growth hormone, prolactin, and ACTH reserve. If cortisol fails to rise by 10 μg/dl above baseline, 10 mg bid of hydrocortisone should be given as a maintenance dose. Since these patients have low levels of estradiol, they rarely respond to clomiphene citrate. If no tumor is found, it is recommended that induction of ovulation be first attempted with clomiphene citrate 250 mg/day for 5 days. If they fail to ovulate following treatment, therapy with human menopausal gonadotropins should be initiated.

Patients with ovarian failure are easily diagnosed since they invariably fail to respond to progesterone challenge and have elevated FSH values. These patients will not respond to any form of ovulatory drug therapy, and therefore are sterile and should be given estrogen replacement therapy in order to prevent osteoporosis since they do not have adequate endogenous levels of estrogen. The recommended regimen of estrogen replacement is 0.625 mg of conjugated estrogen given days 1 through 25 of each month. Medroxyprogesterone acetate (Provera) 5.0 mg/day should be given on days 16 through 25 in order to avoid an unopposed estrogen effect on the endometrium.

SUGGESTED READING

diZerega G, Kletzky OA, Mishell DR Jr: Diagnosis of patients with Sheehan's syndrome using a sequential pituitary stimulation test. *Am J Obstet Gynecol* 132:348, 1978

Kletzky OA, Davajan V, Nakamura RM, Mishell DR Jr: Classification of secondary amenorrhea based on distinct hormonal patterns. *J Clin Endocrinol Metab* 41:660, 1975

Kletzky OA, Davajan V, Nakamura RM, Mishell DR Jr: Clinical categorization of patients with secondary amenorrhea using progesterone induced uterine bleeding and measurement of serum gonadotropin levels. *Am J Obstet Gynecol* 121:695, 1975

Kletzky OA, Mishell DR Jr, Davajan V, Nicoloff JT, Mims R, Nakamura RM: Pituitary stimulation test in amenorrheic patients with normal or low serum estradiol. *Acta Endocrinol* 87:456, 1978

Kletzky OA, Nakamura RM, Thorneycroft IA, Mishell DR Jr: The log-normal distribution of gonadotropins and ovarian steroid values in the normal menstrual cycle. *Am J Obstet Gynecol* 121:688, 1975

Mishell DR Jr, Kletzky OA, Brenner PF, Roy S, Nicoloff JT: The effect of contraceptive steroids on hypothalamic-pituitary function. *Am J Obstet Gynecol* 128:60, 1977

83

Postpill Amenorrhea

CHARLES M. MARCH, M.D.

Approximately 30% of women who practice contraception use oral contraceptives. Most will experience a slight delay in the resumption of menses following oral contraceptive use, but 95% resume spontaneous menstrual cycles within 3 months. Postpill amenorrhea is defined as the absence of spontaneous menses for more than 6 months following the discontinuation of oral contraceptives. The incidence of this condition is approximately 1:500 pill users. A cause-and-effect relationship has not been established. It is most likely that these preparations merely conceal the existence of an unrelated endocrinopathy that is manifested only following the withdrawal of oral contraceptives.

Investigators have sought to answer three questions: (1) Do women who develop postpill amenorrhea have any predisposing factors? (2) What is the nature of the endocrinologic defect? (3) What treatment is most appropriate for these patients?

PREDISPOSING FACTORS

All reports that have included data collected from a large number of women with postpill amenorrhea have included a disproportionately high number of subjects with oligomenorrhea prior to the use of oral contraceptive steroids— three to four times higher than would be expected. From these data, it may be inferred that a relationship does exist: Patients who have abnormalities of the hypothalamic-pituitary-ovarian axis manifested as oligomenorrhea prior to pill use are more likely to develop amenorrhea following the removal of oral contraceptive steroids. During use, these agents specifically suppress all components of the hypothalamic-pituitary-ovarian axis.

Oral contraceptive steroids are frequently prescribed for women with oligomenorrhea for the purpose of "regulating their periods." This practice is illogical. Monthly bleeding occurs because of the effect of pills on the endometrium, but the endocrinopathy cannot be reversed by this therapy. This practice might be reflected in the high number of women with previous oligomenorrhea among those who develop postpill amenorrhea. However, in a large series of amenorrheic women studied at LAC/USC (Los Angeles County/University of Southern California) Medical Center, the frequency of prior oligomenorrhea was identical irrespective of exposure to oral contraceptives.

Therefore, it appears that the underlying defect may become progressive in some oligomenorrheic women and that pill use may be coincidental.

Prolonged use of oral contraceptives has not been associated with the subsequent development of amenorrhea, nor has the use of pills at an early age. On the other hand, neither prior pregnancy nor childbearing seems to have a protective effect against the development of postpill amenorrhea.

UNDERLYING ENDOCRINOLOGIC DEFECT

Investigation of patients with postpill amenorrhea should proceed like investigation of women with secondary amenorrhea unrelated to pill use. Therefore, if a patient presents with postpill amenorrhea and galactorrhea, she would be investigated like any other patient with amenorrhea/galactorrhea.

In a large series of patients studied at LAC/USC Medical Center, approximately two-thirds of those with amenorrhea following discontinuation of oral contraceptives also had galactorrhea. If a relationship between pill use and the subsequent development of amenorrhea exists at all, it seems to lie in the causation of hyperprolactinemia and galactorrhea in a high number of these patients. Among all our patients, galactorrhea occurred in only 32% of those who developed secondary amenorrhea without prior exposure to oral contraceptive steroids. The more frequent association of galactorrhea and hyperprolactinemia with the amenorrhea seems to be the only underlying endocrinologic defect that is more common to patients whose amenorrhea follows pill use. However, our findings must be confirmed by other investigators before we are certain that this association is valid.

THERAPY

Therapy for patients with postpill amenorrhea is the same as for women whose amenorrhea does not follow oral contraceptive use. Following a complete investigation, the patient who has amenorrhea without galactorrhea may be categorized as having a normal estrogen status or a low estrogen status by use of the progesterone challenge test. Patients who have withdrawal uterine bleeding after IM administration of progesterone in oil have circulating estradiol levels in the follicular-phase range. Estrogen-deficient women will not have withdrawal bleeding. The serum level of follicle-stimulating hormone should be determined to rule out ovarian failure in the low-estrogen group.

Patients who have normal estrogen status and who do not wish to conceive should be treated on a monthly basis with medroxyprogesterone acetate (Amen, Provera) 5 mg daily for 10 days beginning on the first of the month. This should permit the endometrium to be differentiated to a secretory type and desquamated every month to prevent the excessive proliferation that follows unopposed estrogen stimulation. These patients are advised to use mechanical methods of contraception, such as an IUD, or barrier techniques.

Patients who have amenorrhea only, are in the normal estrogen group, and wish to conceive may be treated with clomiphene citrate (Clomid, Serophene). Approximately three-quarters can be expected to ovulate. Those with amenorrhea and low estrogen status (excluding those with ovarian failure) who do not wish to conceive should also use mechanical methods of contraception and receive estrogen replacement with conjugated estrogens 0.625 mg daily for the first 25 days of each month plus medroxyprogesterone acetate 5 mg daily from day 16 through day 25. For amenorrheic, low-estrogen patients who wish to conceive, clomiphene citrate will induce ovulation in only a small number. Most will require human menopausal gonadotropins.

Patients with amenorrhea and galactorrhea should also have a complete investigation, consisting of serum prolactin and thyrotropin levels, x-rays of the sella turcica, and an estimation of estrogen status by the progesterone challenge test. Whether conception is desired or not, bromocriptine (Parlodel) may be given. About 80% will experience resumption of normal ovulatory cycles and remission of galactorrhea. Patients desiring contraception should use a mechanical method. Most patients treated with bromocriptine will require it for an indefinite period; most will relapse after it is stopped.

SUMMARY

We do not yet know whether oral contraceptive use can induce amenorrhea or amenorrhea/galactorrhea following drug withdrawal. There may be a cause-and-effect relationship between oral contraceptive use and galactorrhea accompanying amenorrhea. However, these steroids may merely mask symptoms of a non-pill-related endocrinopathy. Oral contraceptives induce regular bleeding, and their estrogenic component acts directly on the breasts to inhibit milk secretion in women with hyperprolactinemia. Thus the symptoms of amenorrhea and amenorrhea/galactorrhea may be noted only after pill withdrawal. Until final answers are available, it is wise to withhold oral contraceptives from women with oligomenorrhea and to investigate all postpill amenorrhea that persists for 6 months. Those with amenorrhea and galactorrhea should be evaluated as soon as diagnosis is established.

SUGGESTED READING

Kletzky OA, Davajan V, Mishell DR Jr, Nicoloff J, Mims R, March CM, Nakamura RM: A sequential pituitary stimulation test in normal subjects and in patients with amenorrhea-galactorrhea with pituitary tumors. *J Clin Endocrinol Metab* 45:631, 1977

Kletzky OA, Davajan V, Nakamura RM, Mishell DR Jr: Classification of secondary amenorrhea based on distinct hormonal patterns. *J Clin Endocrinol Metab* 14:660, 1975

Kletzky OA, Davajan V, Nakamura RM, Mishell DR Jr: Clinical categorization of patients with secondary amenorrhea using progesterone induced uterine bleeding and measurement of serum gonadotropin levels. *Am J Obstet Gynecol* 121:695, 1975

March CM, Kletzky OA, Davajan V: Clinical response to CB-154 and the pituitary response to thyrotropin-releasing hormone-gonadotropin-releasing hormone in patients with galactorrhea-amenorrhea. *Fertil Steril* 28:521, 1977

March CM, Mishell DR Jr, Kletzky OA, Israel R, Davajan V, Nakamura RM: Galactorrhea and pituitary tumors in postpill and non-postpill secondary amenorrhea (pituitary tumors in secondary amenorrhea). *Am J Obstet Gynecol* 134:45, 1979

84

Galactorrhea and Hyperprolactinemia

OSCAR A. KLETZKY, M.D., and VAL DAVAJAN, M.D.

Galactorrhea is defined as nonpuerperal lactation noted either spontaneously or following manual expression from one or both breasts. To detect galactorrhea, the breast examination should be performed by compressing the glands from the periphery of the breast toward the nipple concentrically. Galactorrhea fluid appears as either a milky or watery substance. The observation of microscopic fat globules in the fluid is a simple and accurate diagnostic test of galactorrhea.

The exact incidence of galactorrhea in women of the reproductive age group is unknown.

PATHOPHYSIOLOGY

Prolactin (PRL) is the most important hormone involved in the pathophysiology of galactorrhea. It is now evident that prolactin secretion is controlled mainly by the hypothalamus. The predominant action of the hypothalamus on PRL release in mammals seems to be inhibitory, probably through dopamine acting as a prolactin-inhibiting factor (PIF). There is also some evidence in animals for the existence of a PRL-releasing factor (PRF), probably related to serotonin.

In humans, PRL is stimulated by sleep, stress, exercise, nipple stimulation, thyrotropin-releasing hormone (TRH), insulin-induced hypoglycemia, and phenothiazines. PRL is inhibited by L-dopa, dopamine, and certain ergot alkaloids, including bromocriptine mesylate (Parlodel). While TRH directly stimulates the pituitary to release prolactin, chlorpromazine (Thorazine) and L-dopa seem to influence PRL secretion indirectly by affecting PIF production by the hypothalamus. Bromocriptine, in addition to inhibiting prolactin secretion by a direct action on the pituitary, also has a dopaminergic effect on the hypothalamus.

DIFFERENTIAL DIAGNOSIS

Galactorrhea and hyperprolactinemia have been associated with the use of drugs, prolactin-secreting pituitary adenomas, hypothyroidism, acromegaly, Cushing's disease, chest trauma, surgery, herpes zoster, and extensive breast manipulation.

Drugs

Drugs appear to be the most common etiologic factor. Drugs associated with galactorrhea include the major and minor tranquilizers, antihypertensive agents, and narcotics. Oral contraceptive steroid formulations and estrogen stimulate PRL secretion but also prevent PRL action on the breast, thus inhibiting galactorrhea.

Pituitary Tumors

The term microadenoma has been used to describe pituitary tumors smaller than 10 mm in diameter. Those larger than 10 mm in diameter are called macroadenomas.

The major effort in the work-up of patients with galactorrhea is directed toward the diagnosis of a pituitary tumor because of its serious endocrinologic and ophthalmologic implications. Between 60% and 70% of patients with galactorrhea have serum PRL levels greater than the upper limit of normal (20 ng/ml). An unknown, but probably small, percentage of women with menstrual dysfunction will also have hyperprolactinemia without galactorrhea. Approximately 50% of these patients with elevated levels of PRL will have radiographic changes of the sella turcica compatible with the presence of a pituitary adenoma. In approximately 10% of galactorrheic patients with an abnormal x-ray, the serum PRL levels have been reported to be normal. Nearly all of these patients have empty sella syndrome, but the etiology of the galactorrhea is obscure.

Gonadotropin levels would be expected to be low in patients with pituitary tumors. However, many of these patients have normal baseline levels and normal or exaggerated LH and FSH responses to the administration of gonadotropin-releasing hormone.

The lack of response of PRL following hypoglycemia or chlorpromazine or TRH administration suggests independent secretion of this hormone. However, bromocriptine (in most patients) and L-dopa (in some patients) can induce a fall in circulating levels of PRL in patients with amenorrhea/galactorrhea and pituitary adenomas. It appears that in most patients with pituitary tumors, the stimulatory and not the inhibitory effect of various agents is lost.

Hypothyroidism

In approximately 2-5% of patients with galactorrhea, the etiology has been determined to be primary hypothyroidism. These patients have diminished thyroid function and therefore lack negative feedback on the hypothalamic-pituitary axis. This failure results in increased secretion of endogenous TRH, which then overstimulates the thyrotrophs as well as the lactotrophs, causing an increase in the release of TSH and PRL.

The diagnosis of primary hypothyroidism is made by measuring serum TSH by radioimmunoassay (RIA). In these patients, the value of TSH is elevated above the normal range (the upper limit of normal TSH varies in different laboratories, from 5 to 10 μU/ml). In addition to TSH, measurement of serum thyroxine by RIA and the free thyroxine index (FTI) is used in order to rule out the rare case of TSH-producing pituitary adenoma and to confirm the diagnosis of primary hypothyroidism.

Acromegaly and Cushing's Disease
Galactorrhea in these diseases is of secondary importance, and treatment is directed toward the primary disease.

Chest Trauma, Surgery, Herpes Zoster, Extensive Breast Manipulation
The exact mechanism by which these conditions cause galactorrhea has not been clearly defined. It is known that breast manipulation increases the serum levels of PRL in normal women. If the manipulation or irritation is constant, the resultant hyperprolactinemia may lead to galactorrhea. If no other causes of hyperprolactinemia and galactorrhea are established, the patient should be advised to avoid excessive breast manipulation.

Galactorrhea, Menstrual Patterns, and Prolactin Levels
Galactorrhea can be present in patients with either normal or abnormal menses. In fact, galactorrhea associated with a pituitary tumor has been reported in postmenopausal women. Therefore, the menstrual history alone cannot be used to select patients who need a complete work-up. However, the menstrual history in conjunction with a single serum PRL value has been used to identify patients with low or high risk of having a pituitary adenoma.

The high-risk group of patients were found to be those with PRL levels greater than 200 ng/ml and those with amenorrhea/galactorrhea and low circulating levels of estrogen as determined by failure to have uterine bleeding following progesterone administration. Two-thirds of these patients were found to have abnormal x-rays compatible with pituitary adenomas.

The low-risk group of patients are those with galactorrhea, normal menses, and serum PRL levels of less than 20 ng/ml. In a recent study, none of the patients with these findings had abnormal hypocycloidal tomograms of the sella turcica. However, in galactorrheic patients with normal menses and PRL levels over 20 ng/ml, abnormal tomograms compatible with microadenomas were found; thus, it is recommended that all patients with galactorrhea, normal menses, and normal PRL need no further diagnostic evaluation.

WORK-UP AND TREATMENT

Patients with galactorrhea who are using tranquilizers, amphetamines, or oral contraceptives should be encouraged to stop the medication for at least 3 months. After a period free of medication, the patient should be re-evaluated; if galactorrhea continues, the following systematic work-up is recommended.

If the patient is taking a major tranquilizer or antihypertensive and cannot interrupt the medication, the work-up should be initiated immediately, because an underlying cause of galactorrhea may be present. These patients' serum PRL should be measured and a cone view of the sella turcica obtained if the PRL is less than 100 ng/ml. If serum PRL is higher than 100 ng/ml, a CT scan is recommended, since medications rarely induce hyperprolactinemia greater than 100 ng/ml.

Serum TSH
As an initial test, serum TSH identifies patients who may have primary hypothyroidism as the etiology of their galactorrhea. The diagnosis is confirmed by measurement of the free thyroxine index (FTI). Patients with primary hypothyroidism will have elevated TSH and low FTI values. These patients should be given thyroxine replacement therapy, starting at a low daily dose of 0.05 mg for 2 weeks. Then the dose should be increased by 0.05 mg every 2 weeks, up to a maintenance dose of 0.15 or 0.2 mg/day. This dose will lower the elevated TSH and PRL levels into the normal range; however, it may take as long as 6 months.

Serum PRL and Radiography
All patients with galactorrhea and a normal serum TSH value should have a serum PRL measurement. If it is elevated, or normal with an abnormal menstrual pattern, anteroposterior (AP) and lateral x-rays of the sella turcica (cone view) should be obtained.

A recent study revealed that with a single serum PRL determination and AP and lateral plain radiographs of the sella turcica, it is possible to identify patients with galactorrhea who do not need sella tomography to establish the diagnosis of pituitary microadenoma. Patients who have normal AP and lateral plain films of the sella turcica and a normal serum PRL do not need tomograms even if they have amenorrhea. Also, patients with abnormal plain films do not need tomograms, only CT scans with cuts every 2 mm. Patients with galactorrhea, normal plain films, serum PRL greater than 60 ng/ml, or PRL less than 60 ng/ml with an abnormal PRL response to TRH need tomograms or CT scans with 2-mm cuts. A CT scan is not necessary for a patient with a serum PRL of 20-60 ng/ml whose PRL level triples 20 minutes after intravenous administration of 500 μg of TRH.

Neurologic Studies
Patients with abnormal x-rays should have neurologic studies to determine whether the tumor has escaped beyond the sella turcica. These tests include visual field examination and CT scan. ACTH and growth hormone reserve, using insulin-induced hypoglycemia, should also be measured in patients with large pituitary tumors.

Surgery
At LAC/USC (Los Angeles County/University of Southern California) Medical Center, surgical therapy is recommended only for patients with macroadenomas or evidence of extrasellar extension of the tumor who fail to respond to bromocriptine therapy. Following surgery, if the pituitary tumor is thought

to be incompletely resected, these patients should be given bromocriptine therapy. For patients with microadenomas, conservative management has been used. These patients are being followed every 6 months with PRL measurements and every 24 months with CT scan. Only if there is enlargement of the adenoma should surgery be performed.

Pregnancy

Because the physiologic increase in the size of the pituitary gland during pregnancy may not be applicable to a microadenoma and because surgical removal of pituitary tumors has been performed during pregnancy without added morbidity, patients with microadenomas who desire to conceive and who are willing to take the risk of having a sudden growth of the tumor during pregnancy are being managed conservatively in many medical centers. While pregnant, these patients should have visual field examinations every month. Utilizing this approach, nearly all patients have been delivered at term without complications. There is no contraindication to breast-feeding. The general consensus is that a macroadenoma should be removed before a patient undertakes pregnancy. An alternative method of treatment could be continuation of bromocriptine during pregnancy to prevent a sudden increase in size of the adenoma. Such treatment has been used in other countries without apparent detriment to the fetus.

Drug Therapy

Bromocriptine mesylate has been found to be successful in lowering serum PRL to normal levels, stopping galactorrhea, and establishing normal ovulatory menstrual cycles. In accordance with FDA recommendations, this agent can be administered to patients who desire pregnancy and have amenorrhea/galactorrhea and hyperprolactinemia without evidence of a pituitary adenoma. For patients with a pituitary adenoma, bromocriptine continues to be an investigational drug that can be used with informed consent. The recommended dose is 2.5-7.5 mg/day for 6 months, followed by re-evaluation of the patient. The effects of this drug appear to be only temporary, since the majority of patients revert to amenorrhea, hyperprolactinemia, and galactorrhea after discontinuing it. No definitive information is yet available as to bromocriptine's long-term effects in patients with known PRL-secreting pituitary adenomas, although some reports of tumor regression have been published.

Although estrogen therapy is successful in suppression of postpartum lactation by its direct effect on the breasts, it is not recommended for use in the galactorrheic patient, since estrogen is known to stimulate both the growth of the pituitary and the release of prolactin.

SUGGESTED READING

Davajan V, Kletzky OA, March CM, Roy S, Mishell DR Jr: The significance of galactorrhea in patients with normal menses, oligomenorrhea and secondary amenorrhea. *Am J Obstet Gynecol* 130:894, 1978

Kletzky OA, Davajan V, Mishell DR Jr, Nicoloff JT, Mims R, March CM, Nakamura RM: A sequential pituitary stimulation test in normal subjects and in patients with amenorrhea-galactorrhea with pituitary tumors. *J Clin Endocrinol Metab* 45:631, 1977

March CM, Kletzky OA, Davajan V, Teal J, Weiss M, Apuzzo ML, Marrs RP, Mishell DR Jr: Longitudinal evaluation of patients with untreated prolactin-secreting pituitary adenomas. *Am J Obstet Gynecol* 139:835, 1981

March CM, Mishell DR Jr, Kletzky OA, Israel R, Davajan V: Galactorrhea and pituitary tumors in post-pill and non-post-pill amenorrhea. *Am J Obstet Gynecol* 134:45, 1979

Marrs RP, Bertolli SJ, Kletzky OA: The use of thyrotropin releasing hormone in distinguishing prolactin-secreting pituitary adenoma. *Am J Obstet Gynecol* 138:620, 1980

Marrs RP, Kletzky OA, Teal J, Davajan V, March CM, Mishell DR Jr: Comparison of serum prolactin, plain radiography and hypocycloidal tomography of the sella turcica in patients with galactorrhea. *Am J Obstet Gynecol* 135:467, 1979

85

Therapy With Bromocriptine

CHARLES M. MARCH, M.D.

INDICATIONS

The ergot alkaloid bromocriptine (Parlodel) may currently be prescribed for the short-term management of amenorrhea, galactorrhea, and hyperprolactinemia in women who do not have evidence of a pituitary tumor. It may be used for all women who meet these criteria, whether or not they wish to conceive. It is also indicated specifically for treatment of infertility. Another indication is the suppression of puerperal lactation. This agent's ultimate impact on gynecologic practice is not yet clear. Its role in the treatment of male infertility and/or hypogonadism, and in the short- and long-term management of patients with prolactin-secreting pituitary adenomas, is also uncertain.

Over the past 10 years, there have been many reports of hyperprolactinemia and galactorrhea, with or without menstrual abnormalities, and of prolactin-secreting pituitary adenomas. Various drugs, primarily tranquilizers and some antihypertensives, have been associated with hyperprolactinemia, amenorrhea, and menstrual abnormalities. Thus the number of candidates for bromocriptine therapy appears to be growing exponentially. It is uncertain whether hyperprolactinemia is a new disease or is being diagnosed more frequently today because of more sophisticated techniques.

More recently, bromocriptine was approved for the inhibition of postpartum lactation. The medications previously available for suppressing puerperal and nonpuerperal lactation are only moderately effective. Additionally, the fears of estrogen-related side effects have grown steadily. In addition to current guidelines for the use of bromocriptine, some indications for which bromocriptine may be used in the future will be discussed briefly in this chapter. The use of bromocriptine for the treatment of men and for therapy of women with evidence of pituitary adenomas has not been approved and must be considered investigational.

TREATMENT OF HYPERPROLACTINEMIA

Hyperprolactinemia may result from a number of physiologic disturbances. The two organs central to this disorder are the hypothalamus and the pituitary. The hypothalamus produces prolactin-inhibiting factor and thereby prevents the release and/or synthesis of prolactin by the pituitary. If this mechanism is inoperative, the bridling effect of the hypothalamus on the pituitary will be lost and the uninhibited pituitary lactotrophs will produce and release an excessive amount of prolactin.

Another possible cause of the defect is the pituitary gland. It may become autonomous; hyperplasia or neoplasia could result. Pituitary hyperplasia would be similar to the physiologic hyperplasia of the lactotrophs that occurs in pregnancy, and the end result would be hyperprolactinemia. Although it is certain that higher centers are responsible for control of the hypothalamus and pituitary, these mechanisms have not yet been defined and our understanding of the cerebral control of endocrine function is minimal.

If hyperprolactinemia develops, the cyclic discharge of follicle-stimulating hormone (FSH) and luteinizing hormone (LH) from normal gonadotrophs is usually inhibited. Therefore, although FSH and LH levels may remain within the normal range, total FSH and LH production is reduced and consequently estrogen production by the ovaries is also reduced. Depending on the degree of suppression, circulating levels of estradiol (E_2) may remain in the normal follicular phase range or may be markedly reduced. The level of estrogen determines the menstrual pattern. Patients may have oligomenorrhea or amenorrhea with normal E_2 levels (either measured by radioimmunoassay or evidenced by progesterone-induced withdrawal bleeding). If estrogen levels are markedly reduced, the administration of progesterone in oil will not result in withdrawal bleeding.

The estrogen status of a patient with amenorrhea-galactorrhea and hyperprolactinemia does not seem to play a role in her response to bromocriptine. Bromocriptine differs in this respect from clomiphene citrate (Clomid, Serophene), which is rarely successful in women who are estrogen-deficient. The mechanism of action of bromocriptine appears to be two-fold: It directly affects the pituitary to inhibit the release of prolactin and also works through hypothalamic receptors, possibly to stimulate the release of prolactin-inhibiting factor. These two mechanisms result in a return of serum prolactin levels to normal and thus remove the block to spontaneous release of FSH and LH. Normal cyclic pituitary and ovarian function is subsequently restored.

With return of prolactin levels to normal, ovulatory menstrual cycles resume and lactation ceases in approximately 80% of patients. In most women, menstrual periods resume 4-6 weeks following the initiation of therapy, and the galactorrhea ceases approximately 4 weeks thereafter. Because the menstrual cycles are likely to be ovulatory, women who do not wish to conceive should use a mechanical method of contraception during therapy. Following the discontinuation of bromocriptine, most patients will have a relapse and the hyperprolactinemia, amenorrhea, and galactorrhea will recur.

Serious side effects occur very rarely during therapy with bromocriptine. More than one-half of patients experience nausea, which is usually mild and transient. The severity of the nausea may be reduced by beginning therapy with one 2.5-mg tablet ingested with the evening meal. If this dose is tolerated, it should be doubled within 4-7 days and maintained. A serum prolactin

(PRL) level should be obtained in about 1 month. If it is not normal, the dose may be increased to thrice daily. Although higher doses have not been approved, they are necessary on occasion.

The frequency and severity of nausea may be reduced by instructing the patient to take the medication with meals. Other gastrointestinal side effects, such as abdominal pain, vomiting, diarrhea, and constipation, have also been reported. Headaches, dizziness, lightheadedness, and nasal congestion have occurred in 5-10% of patients. These have usually been mild and transient. Orthostatic hypotension, a serious side effect, has occurred in a very small number of patients, almost all of whom were treated at much higher doses than recommended for the management of amenorrhea-galactorrhea syndrome.

INDUCTION OF OVULATION

Most women who have amenorrhea, galactorrhea, and hyperprolactinemia have estrogen deficiency. These women rarely ovulate when treated with clomiphene citrate and, in the past, required treatment with human menopausal gonadotropins (hMG, Pergonal), which is more complex than bromocriptine. When the outcome of more than 1,200 bromocriptine-induced pregnancies was summarized, there was no increase in the rate of multiple gestation, abortion, or major or minor congenital abnormalities. Because the mechanism of action involves the removal of an inhibitor to gonadotropin secretion rather than direct ovarian or pituitary stimulation, as occurs with hMG and clomiphene, no increase in multiple births would be expected. Bromocriptine is more convenient to use than hMG and will probably play an intermediate role between clomiphene citrate and gonadotropin therapy.

A barrier method of contraception is prescribed during the first month of treatment, and the patient records her basal body temperature (BBT). Following the first menstrual period, contraception is discontinued and the patient continues to record her BBT. If the luteal-phase shift is maintained for 17 days, a rapid, sensitive serum pregnancy test is performed and, if positive, the medication is discontinued.

Recent reports have described intermittent therapy with bromocriptine. With this method, treatment is continued until a shift in BBT is maintained for 3 days. The medication is discontinued and is restarted only if menses occur. In this way, the drug is not ingested during the critical phases of implantation and early embryogenesis. If these reports are substantiated, this regimen will provide a significant advance for the management of anovulatory infertility. Bromocriptine currently appears to be of no benefit in amenorrheic and/or infertile women who do not have hyperprolactinemia.

SUPPRESSION OF POSTPARTUM LACTATION

Bromocriptine is effective in preventing postpartum lactation and will also suppress established lactation. Although estrogens are highly effective in the inhibition of postpartum lactation, there is concern about their potential neoplastic effects and alterations in clotting factors, with a subsequent increased rate of postpartum thromboembolism. Finally, there is a high rebound rate following the discontinuation of estrogens, especially when these drugs are used in an attempt to inhibit established lactation.

The postpartum patient appears to be especially resistant to the side effects of bromocriptine, the rebound rate is low, and clotting factors remain unchanged. The dose is 2.5 mg bid for 14 days. Some patients may require a third week of treatment, usually with a daily dose of 2.5 mg. This prolonged regimen may be used with safety even for patients in whom estrogenic treatment is contraindicated and those at higher risk of puerperal thromboembolism because of operative delivery. As more data accumulate, bromocriptine may become the drug of choice for inhibiting postpartum lactation.

FUTURE INDICATIONS

Bromocriptine is effective in reducing serum prolactin levels, in restoring regular ovulatory menstrual cycles, and in eliminating galactorrhea. However, its beneficial effects are temporary in most patients.

In the future, bromocriptine may be utilized for a variety of other indications. These include amenorrhea and galactorrhea without hyperprolactinemia, luteal-phase defects in association with hyperprolactinemia, galactorrhea without menstrual disturbances, prolactin-secreting pituitary tumors, mastodynia, premenstrual tension, acromegaly, and Parkinson's disease.

The prospects of using bromocriptine in women who have prolactin-secreting pituitary tumors are most exciting. Both large tumors and microadenomas have been shown to shrink during treatment, and studies in vitro have demonstrated tumor cell destruction. Preliminary studies have shown long-term (5-10-year) control of tumor growth; however, more data are necessary because these tumors grow very slowly even without treatment.

Multiple reports have been published on the efficacy and safety of ovulation induction and pregnancy in women with prolactin-secreting microadenomas, but bromocriptine has not been approved for this indication. Because of recurrences following surgery, with their occasional complications, bromocriptine may replace transsphenoidal surgery as the treatment of choice for microadenomas. Additionally, it may be utilized to treat breast carcinoma.

Some men with hypogonadotropic hypogonadism also respond favorably; however, as with women, one key to a favorable response to treatment appears to be hyperprolactinemia. The symptom complex in men often includes loss of libido and impotence. Dosages are similar to those in women.

Bromocriptine is a highly effective drug for a wide variety of conditions. It is more effective than other currently available medications or modalities of therapy for many of these indications. Bromocriptine has few side effects, especially in postpartum patients. However, the induction of ovulation in women not interested in pregnancy or in whom pregnancy is contraindicated must be considered a serious side effect. The occasional catastrophic complications that occur during the pregnancy of a patient with a large pituitary tumor may limit bromocriptine's applicability in patients with macroadenomas.

SUGGESTED READING

Corenblum B, Hanley DA: Bromocriptine reduction of prolactinoma size. *Fertil Steril* 36:716, 1981

Davajan V, Kletzky OA, March CM, Roy S, Mishell DR Jr: The significance of galactorrhea in patients with normal menses, oligomenorrhea and secondary amenorrhea. *Am J Obstet Gynecol* 130:894, 1978

March CM: The role of bromocriptine in gynecologic practice. *West J Med* 132:232, 1980

March CM: The use of bromocriptine in the treatment of hypogonadism and male infertility. *Drugs* 17:349, 1979

March CM, Kletzky OA, Davajan V: Clinical response to CB-154 and the pituitary response to TRH-GnRH in patients with galactorrhea-amenorrhea. *Fertil Steril* 28:521, 1977

86

Androgen Excess:
Differential Diagnosis

ROGERIO A. LOBO, M.D.

Signs and symptoms of androgen excess are both defeminizing (oligomenorrhea, amenorrhea, decreased breast tissue, decreased cervical mucus, decreased vaginal rugae) and virilizing (hirsutism, temporal balding, deepening of the voice, clitorimegaly, increased muscle mass, increased libido, acne). Although these terms are not synonymous, the presence of virilism—defined as hirsutism and other physical signs of masculinization and defeminization—or the progression of hirsutism to virilism implies a more severe form of androgen excess.

HIRSUTISM

Hirsutism is increased hair growth in a central body location or the appearance of hair in an area where it does not normally occur. This term has to be distinguished from hypertrichosis, which is a generalized increase in body hair. Hirsutism has been graded by several techniques. We have adopted the classification of Casey in order to categorize patients into four groups for the purpose of their evaluation and follow-up: Group I patients have increased hair on the face only; group II, increased hair on the face and abdomen; group III, increased hair on the face, abdomen, and intermammary area; group IV, increased hair on the face, abdomen, intermammary area, and back. Increased hair on the face is further classified as: a, upper lip; b, sideburns; c, chin; d, male-type beard, neck. Hirsutism and menstrual irregularity are the earliest and most common signs of androgen excess.

Idiopathic Hirsutism

The most common cause of androgen excess has been thought to be constitutional. As many as one-third of all women have cosmetic complaints pertaining to excess hair growth. Women of Mediterranean ancestry have been thought to be more likely to appear hirsute, usually with no disruption of their ovulatory menstrual pattern or evidence of virilization.

Some women with constitutional hirsutism have increased levels of one or several androgens (testosterone, androstenedione, dehydroepiandrosterone, and dehydroepiandrosterone sulfate) in their peripheral circulation. Indeed, only a minority of women will have no elevated androgen levels, particularly if several androgens are measured. Many women have an increased clearance rate of testosterone and/or an increased daily production rate of testosterone, and most women will have an increase in unbound, or free, testosterone in the peripheral circulation. These changes suggest that perhaps these women should not be considered to have "idiopathic" hirsutism, because they may have subtle changes in androgen metabolism. Furthermore, it has recently been shown that women with "idiopathic" hirsutism have abnormally high androgen metabolism in peripheral tissues such as skin and hair. Under these circumstances, normally circulating androgens like testosterone are converted more efficiently to more potent androgens like dihydrotestosterone and androstanediol. At present we use the term "idiopathic hirsutism" to refer to patients who have hirsutism and minimal changes in menstrual function without a firm diagnosis such as polycystic ovary syndrome or congenital adrenal hyperplasia.

Physiologic Changes in Hair Growth

It must be remembered that at three times during a woman's life (puberty, pregnancy, postmenopause) hair may appear at an accelerated rate as the result of physiologic changes in circulating sex steroids. At puberty, adrenal androgen increases prior to an increase in ovarian estrogen. During the postmenopausal years, the ovaries secrete virtually no estrogen while androgens continue to be produced by both the ovaries and the adrenal glands. During pregnancy, total circulating testosterone levels are increased, and this may be associated with an increase in the unbound fraction of testosterone as well.

ANDROGEN EXCESS

Ovarian Causes of Androgen Excess

Functional ovarian disease and ovarian tumors can both cause androgen excess. Following "idiopathic" hirsutism, polycystic ovary syndrome (PCO) is the most common cause of clinical androgen excess. This topic is presented in Chapters 87 and 89.

Hyperthecosis syndrome. Women with hyperthecosis are more likely than women with PCO to have virilizing signs and symptoms and are less likely to ovulate in response to clomiphene citrate (Clomid, Serophene). Most often the history is one of long-standing, progressive hirsutism and virilization. Patients with hyperthecosis syndrome are usually older than those with the diagnosis of PCO. The diagnosis of hyperthecosis is confirmed histologically when nests of theca cells are found in the ovarian stroma at a considerable distance from the follicles. With the decline in popularity of surgical wedge resection, the diagnosis of hyperthecosis is rarely documented.

Androgen-producing ovarian tumors. Androgen-producing ovarian tumors are rare. The largest and most common are the Sertoli-Leydig cell tumors, formerly referred to as arrhenoblastomas. Sertoli-Leydig cell tumors occur most often in the second, third, and fourth decades of life, are usually palpable on pelvic examination, and have a low-grade malignant potential.

Hilus-cell tumors occur most commonly in postmenopausal women, usually are not palpable on pelvic examination, and have a low-grade malignant potential. Lipoid-cell tumors can also secrete androgens. They are more common in premenopausal women and have a somewhat greater malignant potential than the others. Seventy-five per cent of women with lipoid-cell tumors are virilized, and 10% have Cushing's syndrome. These tumors are usually cystic. Granulosa-theca-cell tumors usually secrete estrogens but infrequently have been associated with excess androgen secretion.

The diagnosis of an androgen-producing ovarian tumor should be considered whenever a woman has male levels of total serum testosterone, usually above 200 ng/dl. The lipoid-cell tumor is an exception and behaves endocrinologically as an adrenal androgen-producing tumor. Other ovarian tumors may also cause androgen excess by a mechanism other than secretion of androgen by the tumor cells. Any ovarian tumor has the potential of being associated with androgen secretion. Mucinous cystadenomas, Brenner tumors, cystadenocarcinomas, and Krukenberg tumors have all been associated with a functioning ovarian stroma that elaborates increased amounts of androgen.

Adrenal Causes of Androgen Excess

Congenital adrenal hyperplasia—adult onset. The postpubertal manifestation of hirsutism and/or virilization as the result of congenital adrenal hyperplasia is now an established diagnostic entity. These patients are taller than their peers early in life, but the excess sex steroids cause the distal epiphyses to close prematurely and the patients are ultimately shorter than their peers and other members of their families. Anovulation with either oligomenorrhea or amenorrhea is a frequent finding.

Most women with an adult-onset enzyme deficiency in the cortisol pathway have an incomplete 21-hydroxylase deficiency. This usually does not result in salt wasting. A few have an incomplete 11β-hydroxylase deficiency. Both enzyme defects produce an increase in serum 17α-hydroxyprogesterone or its urinary metabolite, pregnanetriol, and inefficient cortisol production. The 11β-hydroxylase deficiency also causes an increase in 11-deoxycortisol (substance S) and clinical hypertension. Both enzyme defects may be accentuated by the administration of intravenous ACTH, which causes a marked increase in the 17α-hydroxyprogesterone level. Serum levels of adrenal androgens such as dehydroepiandrosterone sulfate (DHEA-S) are usually increased, but the most commonly elevated androgen is androstenedione. Administration of dexamethasone 0.5-0.75 mg/day suppresses androgen levels and relieves the clinical signs and symptoms. Spontaneous ovulation and pregnancy often occur. Recently a 3β-ol dehydrogenase defect has also been diagnosed in adult women presenting with androgen excess. This is probably extremely rare.

Androgen-producing adrenal tumors. Adrenal adenomas or carcinomas that produce androgens are rare causes of clinical androgen excess. Adrenal carcinomas are usually large enough to be detected on an intravenous pyelogram by the time they produce signs and symptoms of androgen excess. Androgen-producing adrenal adenomas may be macro or micro in size. The extent of symptoms bears no relation to the size of the adenomas. Patients with androgen-producing adrenal tumors have extremely high levels of adrenal androgens, with serum dehydroepiandrosterone sulfate levels usually over 9 μg/ml. Adrenal tumors rarely produce testosterone, but may secrete increased levels of estrogen.

Cushing's syndrome. Centripetal obesity, thinning of the skin, facial flushing, supraclavicular and dorsal neck fat pads, purple striae, muscle wasting, weakness, easy bruisability, ecchymoses, osteoporosis, hypertension, diabetes, alkalosis, hypokalemia, amenorrhea, and hirsutism are the clinical signs in women with Cushing's syndrome. The hirsutism is usually increased growth of the fine hairs of the face and extremities, rather than the coarse hairs. Whenever signs and symptoms of Cushing's syndrome are present, this life-threatening diagnosis must be investigated.

Iatrogenic Causes

Drugs may cause hirsutism. Some of these include phenytoin (Dilantin), diazoxide (Proglycem), corticosteroids, ACTH, 19-nortestosterone-derived progestins, anabolic steroids, danazol (Danocrine), and some nonprescription medications that have been found to contain androgens.

Genetic Causes

Rare cases of gonadal dysgenesis in which a Y chromosome is present and incomplete forms of testicular feminization may produce clinical evidence of androgen excess and primary amenorrhea. This combination of androgen excess and primary amenorrhea requires a karyotype examination for the detection of a Y chromosome. The presence of a Y chromosome in a female patient mandates surgical extirpation of the gonadal tissue because of the increased risk of neoplasia. Any woman with primary amenorrhea, gonadal failure, and clinical evidence of excess androgen should have her gonads removed for the same reason.

Rare Causes

Extremely rare causes of androgen excess include acromegaly and porphyria. These diagnoses have usually been confirmed prior to the investigation of androgen excess.

VIRILIZATION IN PREGNANCY

Virilization in pregnancy is a rare phenomenon. The endogenous source of the excess androgen is thought to be the ovaries in virtually all cases. The most common cause of virilization in pregnancy is the luteoma of pregnancy, which usually regresses spontaneously postpartum. Conservative management is recommended. Other causes include ovarian androgen-producing tumors, ovarian tumors associated with a functional stroma, polycystic ovary syndrome, and hyperthecosis. Half the female infants born to mothers with virilization in pregnancy have ambiguous external genitalia.

SUGGESTED READING

Casey J: Chronic treatment regimens for hirsutism in women: Effect on blood production rates of testosterone and on hair growth. *Clin Endocrinol* 4:313, 1975

Horton R, Dawks D, Lobo RA: Idiopathic hirsutism. *J Clin Invest* 69:1203, 1982

Kirschner MA, Zucker R, Jespersen D: Idiopathic hirsutism—An ovarian abnormality. *N Engl J Med* 294:637, 1976

Lobo RA, Goebelsmann U: Adult manifestation of congenital adrenal hyperplasia due to incomplete 21-hydroxylase deficiency mimicking polycystic ovarian disease. *Am J Obstet Gynecol* 138:720, 1980

Lobo RA, Paul WL, Goebelsmann U: Serum levels of DHEA-S in gynecologic endocrinopathy and infertility. *Obstet Gynecol* 57:607, 1981

87

Androgen Excess: Evaluation

ROGERIO A. LOBO, M.D.

HISTORY

In evaluating a woman with the signs and symptoms of androgen excess, a careful history is mandatory to narrow down the differential diagnosis. Iatrogenic causes and medical illnesses such as porphyria or acromegaly may be excluded. Rapidly progressive hirsutism and virilization would suggest a neoplastic cause such as an androgen-producing ovarian tumor. In addition, it is important to determine whether hair has been removed by shaving or other means, at what age the symptoms were first noticed, and whether any menstrual irregularities are present.

PHYSICAL EXAMINATION

On physical examination, the presence of virilism (increased muscle mass, decreased breast size, clitorimegaly) and signs suggestive of Cushing's syndrome (central obesity, striae, bruisability) should be noted. If Cushing's syndrome is suspected clinically, it may be ruled out by an overnight dexamethasone (DEX) suppression test. DEX (1 mg) is ingested at 11 pm. If the patient's cortisol is suppressed (<5 μg/dl) at 8 o'clock the next morning, the diagnosis of Cushing's syndrome is effectively ruled out. If the cortisol level is >5 μg/dl, the diagnosis may be made only by a more prolonged DEX suppression test, as described by Liddle.

Weight loss, a unilateral adnexal mass, or bilaterally enlarged ovaries may be helpful in making the diagnosis of ovarian neoplasm or polycystic ovary syndrome (PCO). If the patient is shorter than her peers and has significant androgen excess, the diagnosis of adult-onset congenital adrenal hyperplasia (CAH) may be entertained.

DIAGNOSTIC APPROACH

Adrenal and Ovarian Androgen Levels

The diagnostic approach is based on whether ovarian androgens or adrenal androgens are elevated. Adrenal androgen secretion is best assessed by the measurement of serum dehydroepiandrosterone sulfate (DHEA-S). Over 90% of DHEA-S is derived from the adrenals, and its measurement is more useful and sensitive than measurements of urinary 17-ketosteroids.

Serum testosterone (T) is the best indicator of ovarian androgen production because about two-thirds of serum T in women is derived from the ovaries and it is rarely produced by the adrenals. Measurement of free, or unbound, T (defined in Chapter 88) allows a more sensitive estimation of T production, as sex hormone-binding globulin is often decreased in androgen excess. The only other test to be considered is the measurement of 17α-hydroxyprogesterone. This should be done to rule out CAH if the patient is shorter than her peers, has significant hirsutism or virilization, has a strong family history of hirsutism, and has high measured androgen levels regardless of the degree of hirsutism.

Neoplasms
If total serum T is in the male range (>200 ng/dl), an ovarian neoplasm should be evaluated by ultrasound or, rarely, by ovarian venous catheterization studies. If DHEA-S is above 8-9 μg/ml, an adrenal neoplasm should be suspected and IVP, ultrasonography, a CT scan, or venous catheterization studies should be carried out.

Functional Diagnoses: PCO and CAH
If ovarian or adrenal neoplasms are ruled out by the combination of clinical and laboratory assessment, the remaining diagnoses fall into a functional class. Adrenal and/or ovarian androgen excess can occur in PCO as well as in some women who have been thought to have "idiopathic" hirsutism. Therefore, further evaluation of these patients depends on whether there is increased adrenal androgen production (reflected by DHEA-S) and/or ovarian androgen production (reflected by unbound T). The specific diagnosis of PCO will not be discussed here. However, in a patient who is suspected of having adult-onset CAH, measurement of 17α-hydroxyprogesterone is very helpful. If this level is greater than 10 ng/ml, the diagnosis is almost certain. If it is elevated ($\geq$3.3 ng/ml) but less than 6 ng/ml, a diagnosis of CAH cannot be made without ACTH stimulation. Many women with PCO or adrenal androgen excess may have slight elevations of 17α-hydroxyprogesterone.

ACTH testing is carried out by giving 1 mg of DEX at 11 pm as is done to rule out Cushing's syndrome. At 8 am the next day, 0.25 mg of cosyntropin ACTH is given IV as a bolus. Since adrenal function has been suppressed by DEX, the 8 am level of 17α-hydroxyprogesterone will be low, usually <3 ng/ml. If the 60-minute level is elevated, usually >10 ng/ml, the diagnosis of CAH can be made. Women with PCO who have elevated basal levels of 17α-hydroxyprogesterone will not have an exaggerated response to ACTH.

Without regard to the specific functional diagnosis, if total or unbound T is elevated but below the male range, the diagnosis of ovarian androgen excess can be made. If DHEA-S is between 2.8 and 9 μg/ml, adrenal androgen excess is diagnosed. We have used a level above 5 μg/ml to diagnose a moderate to severe form of adrenal androgen excess, and patients with DHEA-S levels between 2.8 and 5 μg/ml are diagnosed to have mild adrenal androgen excess.

Women who have elevated unbound T levels in combination with elevations in DHEA-S have a mixed form of androgen excess. In our studies, the mixed group is the most common group, with the ovarian androgen excess group being next most frequent (elevated unbound T, normal DHEA-S), and adrenal androgen excess being the least common abnormality (elevated DHEA-S, normal total or unbound T).

Idiopathic Hirsutism

Hirsutism in association with completely normal levels of unbound T and DHEA-S may be termed "idiopathic." This term may be used in a practical way to categorize patients. However, careful study of these women indicates that most do have subtle androgen abnormalities—specifically, increased androgen action in their peripheral tissues (skin and hair follicles). A new hormonal marker of this peripheral androgen action is serum 3α-androstanediol glucuronide, although it is not clinically available at present.

SUGGESTED READING

Abraham G: Ovarian and adrenal contributions to peripheral androgens during the menstrual cycle. *J Clin Endocrinol Metab* 39:340, 1979

Abraham G, Chakmakjian ZH, Buster JE, Marshall JR: Ovarian and adrenal contributions to peripheral androgens in hirsute women. *Obstet Gynecol* 46:169, 1975

Kirschner MA, Zucker IR, Jespersen D: Idiopathic hirsutism—An ovarian abnormality. *N Engl J Med* 294:637, 1976

Liddle GW: Tests of pituitary adrenal suppressibility in the diagnosis of Cushing's syndrome. *J Clin Endocrinol Metab* 20:1539, 1960

Lobo RA, Goebelsmann U: Adult manifestation of congenital adrenal hyperplasia due to incomplete 21-hydroxylase deficiency mimicking polycystic ovarian disease. *Am J Obstet Gynecol* 138:720, 1980

Lobo RA, Paul W, Goebelsmann U: Dehydroepiandrosterone sulfate (DHEA-S) as an indicator of adrenal androgen function. *Obstet Gynecol* 57:69, 1980

Lobo RA, Paul WL, Goebelsmann U: Serum levels of DHEAS in gynecologic endocrinopathy and infertility. *Obstet Gynecol* 57:607, 1981

88

Management of Hirsutism

ROGERIO A. LOBO, M.D.

Physiologic hirsutism at the time of puberty, pregnancy, or the postmenopausal years obviously requires no treatment. It is frequently difficult to discover iatrogenic causes of androgen excess but, once one is detected, treatment is simply removal of the offending agent. The treatment of androgen
excess associated with Cushing's syndrome, acromegaly, or porphyria is directed at the primary disease. Genetic causes of excess androgen and tumors
producing androgens are managed by surgical intervention. Patients with virilization of a short duration have a better prognosis when the source of the
androgen is removed than those with long-standing virilization. Hirsutism
secondary to a tumor may respond dramatically when the tumor is excised.

SOURCE OF ANDROGEN

Stimulation-suppression testing of ovarian and adrenal androgens has been
suggested to define the source of the excess androgen as ovarian, adrenal, or
both. We do not feel that this testing adds important information or distinguishes completely between androgens secreted by the two sets of glands.
Serum dehydroepiandrosterone sulfate (DHEA-S) is used to reflect adrenal
androgen excess, and serum testosterone (T), together with T not bound to
sex hormone-binding globulin (SHBG), or unbound T, is used to reflect primarily ovarian androgen excess.

Testosterone is a potent androgen in the peripheral circulation. Approximately 90% of the circulating T is bound to a high-affinity protein referred to
as testosterone-estradiol-binding globulin, or sex-hormone-binding globulin
(SHBG). Testosterone bound to SHBG is biologically and physiologically inactive. The remaining 10% of the testosterone in the circulation is not bound
to SHBG. Of this 10%, 9% is bound to albumin and the remaining 1% is free,
not bound to any protein. The portion of testosterone in the circulation bound
to the low-affinity protein albumin is available to the androgen receptors and
is therefore biologically active and considered "unbound." As the majority of
women with androgen excess have a decreased level of SHBG, serum unbound T is often elevated and gives more information than the measurement
of total serum T. Unbound T levels have been used to monitor the treatment
of androgen excess. We currently base the treatment of hirsutism on basal

determinations of serum DHEA-S, serum total T and unbound T, and serum 17α-hydroxyprogesterone if indicated.

MEDICAL MANAGEMENT

Hirsutism may be treated with corticosteroids, combination oral contraceptives (OCs), combinations of corticosteroids and OCs, and receptor-blocking agents. Receptor-blocking agents include cyproterone acetate (Androcur; not available in the United States), cimetidine (Tagamet), cyproheptadine (Periactin), and spironolactone (Aldactone). Each will be discussed below.

Corticosteroids

Corticosteroids are indicated if serum DHEA-S is elevated above 3 μg/ml and/or for the diagnosis of congenital adrenal hyperplasia (CAH). We have used dexamethasone (DEX), although other corticosteroids, such as prednisone, may also be used. DEX inhibits ACTH secretion from the pituitary and in addition may exert a direct inhibitory effect on steroidogenesis. We use 0.5 mg each night and re-evaluate treatment at 3-month intervals. The dose may be lowered to 0.25 mg/night in order to keep the 8 am cortisol around 5 μg/dl. In patients who have CAH, 0.75 mg is often necessary for treatment, although many women may be adequately maintained on 0.5 mg.

Oral Contraceptives

To select the proper OC, it is necessary to understand the effects of sex hormones on SHBG. Estrogens increase SHBG, resulting in an increase in total testosterone but a decrease in the biologically active unbound fraction of testosterone in the peripheral circulation. Androgens decrease SHBG, resulting in an increase in the biologically active unbound testosterone in the peripheral circulation. The progestin in OCs decreases luteinizing hormone-dependent production of ovarian testosterone and androstenedione. When OCs are used for the management of hirsutism, they should not contain levonorgestrel, which has androgenic properties of its own and decreases SHBG. An oral combination contraceptive containing norethindrone 0.5 mg and ethinylestradiol 35 μg has a very favorable estrogen/gestagen ratio for the treatment of hirsutism and can be administered cyclically.

Receptor-Blocking Agents

Receptor-blocking agents are effective antiandrogens. Cyproterone acetate is a progestin derivative that has been effectively used together with estrogen for the treatment of hirsutism as well as for contraception. In this country, cimetidine, cyproheptadine, and spironolactone have been used effectively to treat hirsutism. More is known about spironolactone than about the other two drugs. In addition to its effect on decreasing steroidogenesis (primarily ovarian), spironolactone increases the clearance of testosterone and also blocks the action of androgens at their target tissues, i.e., hair follicles. Doses of 50-250 mg/day have been used and have been found to be effective for most patients.

Combination Treatment

We have utilized a therapeutic approach based on abnormalities in serum total T, unbound T, and DHEA-S. If only serum total T or unbound T is elevated, OCs are used. This is also the case even if DHEA-S is mildly elevated—less than 5 μg/ml. However, if the elevation in serum total T or unbound T is associated with DHEA-S levels over 5 μg/ml, DEX 0.5 mg nightly is added to the OC regimen. If DHEA-S is moderately elevated (5 μg/ml or more) without any increase in serum total T or unbound T, DEX is used alone. It is unusual for women to have marked elevations in DHEA-S (e.g., 6-8 μg/ml) without any elevation in unbound T. Therefore, most of our patients with higher levels of DHEA-S receive DEX and OCs in combination.

Women with hirsutism and no increases in serum total T, unbound T, or DHEA-S are given spironolactone 100 mg/day. This dose has been used effectively and without side effects. Effectiveness is usually noted within 3 months. This therapy is also used if hirsutism is not improved after 6 months of conventional therapy, as discussed above.

MONITORING

Patients being followed on therapy should have their serum DHEA-S, total T, and unbound T monitored. We have recently been able to assess the peripheral, or androgen receptor-blocking, effects of the treatment by measuring an androstanediol metabolite, 3α-androstanediol glucuronide. This is not clinically available at present, but it offers significant promise as a means of evaluating and treating women who benefit from receptor-blocking therapy such as spironolactone.

SURGERY

Wedge resection of the ovaries has been recommended previously for the treatment of hirsutism due to polycystic ovary syndrome. Because ovaries that have been invaded surgically are prone to adhesions and there is no evidence of a long-term reduction in circulating androgens by this procedure, it is not recommended in the management of hirsutism. Oophorectomy may be considered in women with markedly elevated serum levels of T and normal serum DHEA-S levels. Many of these women will have long histories of hirsutism and virilization, and often the histologic diagnosis is hyperthecosis. The closer these women are to spontaneous menopause, the more reasonable surgical extirpation of the ovaries would be.

EFFICACY OF TREATMENT

It may take 6-12 months before the patient notices a decrease in hair growth due to hormonal therapy. Hormonal therapy inhibits the growth of new hair follicles, but follicles that are already present will not disappear. Temporary methods of removing or concealing excess hair include tweezing, clipping, shaving, waxing, bleaching, and depilatories. Electrolysis is the only method of permanent hair removal. This procedure is limited, in that only 100 hair follicles can be removed at each session and the process can result in hyperpigmentation and folliculitis. This treatment is recommended only after hormonal levels are normalized and new hair growth has been arrested.

Women with hirsutism have to be treated for many months. However, approximately 1 year after the cessation of hair growth and the normalization of hormone levels, we have attempted to discontinue therapy and re-evaluate the patient. The problem often recurs, but in some women treatment has had a long-lasting effect.

SUGGESTED READING

Boissells A, Tremblay RR: New therapeutic approach to the hirsute patient. *Fertil Steril* 32:276, 1979

Casey JH: Chronic treatment regimens for hirsutism in women: Effect on blood production rates of testosterone and on hair growth. *Clin Endocrinol* 4:313, 1975

Cumming DC, Yang JC, Rebar RW, Yen SSC: Treatment of hirsutism with spironolactone. *JAMA* 247:1295, 1982

Givens J, Andersen RN, Wisner WL, Umstot ES, Fish SA: The effectiveness of two oral contraceptives in suppressing plasma androstenedione, testosterone, LH, and FSH, and in stimulating plasma testosterone-binding capacity in hirsute women. *Am J Obstet Gynecol* 124:333, 1976

Judd HL, McPherson RA, Rakoff JS, Yen SSC: Correlation of the effects of dexamethasone administration on urinary 17 ketosteroid and serum androgen levels in patients with hirsutism. *Am J Obstet Gynecol* 128:408, 1977

Lobo RA, Paul WL, Goebelsmann U: Serum levels of DHEA-S in gynecologic endocrinopathy and infertility. *Obstet Gynecol* 57:607, 1981

89

Therapy of Polycystic Ovarian Disease

UWE T. GOEBELSMANN, M.D.

Polycystic ovarian disease (PCO), also referred to as Stein-Leventhal syndrome, is characterized by the presence of menstrual irregularities such as amenorrhea, oligomenorrhea, and dysfunctional (anovulatory) uterine bleeding, infertility, and hirsutism. Therapy depends on the patient's chief complaint. By and large, it can be stated that amenorrhea and oligomenorrhea are treated with intermittent administration of a progestin, infertility is treated with clomiphene citrate (Clomid, Serophene), and hirsutism is treated with oral contraceptive steroids.

ETIOLOGY

PCO is associated with prolonged periods of anovulation and extraovarian estrogen production, largely by peripheral conversion of androstenedione to estrone. This derangement leads to persistent acyclic estrogen overproduction associated with a lack of progesterone, which would normally be produced by the corpus luteum. Persistent acyclic estrogen overproduction in conjunction with the absence of luteal-phase progesterone causes prolonged estrogenic stimulation of the endometrium and may lead to cystic hyperplasia, atypical hyperplasia, or even endometrial carcinoma. The untreated PCO patient risks development of endometrial carcinoma earlier than women with regular menstrual cycles. All therapeutic modalities for PCO must eliminate the persistent acyclic estrogen overproduction or counteract its consistent mitogenic effect on the endometrium by administering an appropriate progestogen dose for a sufficient length of time.

MANAGEMENT

Medroxyprogesterone Acetate
PCO patients with oligo- or amenorrhea who neither desire fertility in the immediate future nor complain about increased hair growth should receive a 10-day course of medroxyprogesterone acetate (Provera) 10 mg/day orally—conveniently given for the first or last 10 days of a calendar month. This regimen is repeated each month in patients with PCO who present with oligo- or amenorrhea because they are unlikely to resume regular ovulatory cycles spontaneously.

Dilation and Curettage

Dysfunctional uterine bleeding may require D&C to stop the acute bleeding episode. This procedure also permits histologic examination of the endometrium in women who are at a higher risk for developing endometrial carcinoma at an earlier age. Actually, all PCO patients who present with a history of long-standing untreated amenorrhea, oligomenorrhea, or anovulatory bleeding should undergo endometrial biopsy to rule out a malignancy.

Dysfunctional uterine bleeding will be prevented by medroxyprogesterone 10 mg/day taken daily for 10 consecutive days each month. Cyclic administration, as this regimen is called, does not inhibit ovulation. Spontaneous ovulation may occur occasionally in PCO, so women who desire contraceptive protection should be advised to use an intrauterine device or barrier method of contraception.

Clomiphene Citrate

On the other hand, if the patient desires to conceive, she should be treated with clomiphene citrate. In order to avoid clomiphene citrate administration in early pregnancy, it is imperative to rule out an existing pregnancy in any oligo- or amenorrheic patient by history, examination, pregnancy test, and particularly the progesterone withdrawal test—intramuscular injection of 100 or 200 mg of progesterone in oil (only progesterone, no other progestogen). Uterine bleeding, even if minimal, within 14 days after progesterone injection indicates the absence of pregnancy and the presence of sufficient amounts of endogenous estrogens for endometrial stimulation. On the fifth day after the onset of bleeding, clomiphene citrate therapy is begun. We use the individualized graduated clomiphene citrate regimen described by Rust, Israel, and Mishell and discussed in detail in Chapter 92.

Combined Drug Therapy

If clomiphene citrate fails to induce ovulation, dexamethasone in combination with clomiphene citrate may be tried, as may human menopausal gonadotropins (hMG, Pergonal). Dexamethasone is indicated in patients who fail to ovulate on clomiphene citrate alone if their serum dehydroepiandrosterone sulfate (DHEA-S) is elevated. DHEA-S is an indicator of adrenal androgen production, which is controlled by ACTH and suppressed by as little as 0.5 mg of dexamethasone given daily at bedtime, ideally at 11 pm. Dexamethasone is given in conjunction with the same dose of clomiphene citrate given before dexamethasone was started. Dexamethasone therapy should be started 2 weeks prior to the first clomiphene citrate dose and continued until a β-human chorionic gonadotropin radioimmunoassay is positive.

Wedge Resection

Wedge resection to induce ovulation is rarely indicated, because the overwhelming majority of patients will ovulate when treated with clomiphene citrate and some of those who don't ovulate on clomiphene citrate alone may do so when it is given in combination with dexamethasone or when they are treated with hMG. Wedge resection may result in ovulation in women who fail to respond to clomiphene citrate. However, wedge resection may also cause tubo-ovarian adhesions and thus may decrease the chances for fertility. Therefore, clomiphene citrate is the method of choice for induction of ovulation in the PCO patient.

MANAGEMENT OF HIRSUTISM

Hirsutism results from excessive androgen production of adrenal and/or ovarian origin. Adrenal and ovarian catheterization studies in PCO patients have shown that the androgen excess is predominantly of ovarian origin in the majority. Ovarian androgen overproduction in PCO patients is stimulated by elevated serum luteinizing hormone (LH) concentrations and is compounded by a decrease in circulating sex hormone-binding globulin (SHBG). The latter results in an increase in non-SHBG-bound (i.e., androgenically active) testosterone. When combination oral contraceptive steroids with norethindrone as the progestogenic compound are given, serum LH is suppressed while ovarian androgen production is reduced, and the ethinylestradiol present in combination oral contraceptives increases circulating SHBG through its effect on the liver. Norgestrel, but not norethindrone, counteracts the desired effect. Thus, combination oral contraceptive steroids containing norethindrone will decrease both the absolute amount of circulating testosterone and the relative proportion of free (i.e., androgenically active) testosterone. We prescribe combination oral contraceptives that contain 35 μg of ethinylestradiol in combination with 500 μg of norethindrone. This amount of ethinylestradiol suffices to induce hepatic SHBG production, and the combination of norethindrone and ethinylestradiol suppresses serum LH.

Corticosteroids such as dexamethasone suppress adrenal androgen production, as indicated by increased serum DHEA-S levels above 5 μg/ml. Corticosteroids are indicated only in those hirsute patients with elevated serum DHEA-S whose non-SHBG testosterone does not respond to combination oral contraceptives, because corticosteroids have potentially more dangerous side effects and some patients may ingest larger doses than recommended.

Excess body hair will not disappear even when androgen excess has been corrected. On the other hand, hair will not regrow as quickly or be as coarse as it was before. Thus, additional mechanical methods of hair removal are indicated.

Wedge resection is followed by an immediate decrease in serum testosterone and androstenedione levels. However, the drop in serum androstenedione is only temporary, and there is no conclusive evidence as to how long the decreased serum testosterone levels will persist after wedge resection. Clinical experience teaches that wedge resection is not an effective therapy for hirsutism. In older women who do not desire further childbearing and are severely affected by androgen excess of primarily ovarian origin, oophorectomy should be considered.

SUGGESTED READING

Givens JR, Andersen RN, Wiser WL, Umstot ES, Fish SA: The effectiveness of two oral contraceptives in suppressing plasma androstenedione, testosterone, LH, and FSH, and in stimulating plasma testosterone-binding capacity in hirsute women. *Am J Obstet Gynecol* 124:333, 1976

Goldzieher JW, Axelrod LR: Clinical and biochemical features of polycystic ovarian disease. *Fertil Steril* 14:631, 1963

Judd HL, Rigg LA, Anderson DC, Yen SSC: The effects of ovarian wedge resection on circulating gonadotropin and ovarian steroid levels in patients with polycystic ovary syndrome. *J Clin Endocrinol Metab* 43:347, 1976

Kirschner MA, Jacobs JB: Combined ovarian and adrenal vein catheterization to determine the site(s) of androgen overproduction in hirsute women. *J Clin Endocrinol Metab* 33:199, 1971

Lobo RA, Paul W, March CM, Granger L, Kletzky OA: Clomiphene and dexamethasone in women unresponsive to clomiphene alone. *Obstet Gynecol* 60:497, 1982

Rust LA, Israel R, Mishell DR Jr: An individualized graduated therapeutic regimen for clomiphene citrate. *Am J Obstet Gynecol* 120:785, 1974

90

Work-Up of the Infertile Couple

VAL DAVAJAN, M.D.

It has been stated that approximately 10-15% of all married couples in the United States are infertile. The diagnosis of infertility is usually made when conception has not occurred after 1 year of unprotected sexual exposure in a couple trying to achieve a pregnancy. The term primary infertility is used when no conception has ever taken place. In contrast, secondary infertility implies that at least one previous conception has been either hormonally or histologically documented. The diagnosis of sterility should be made only when the etiology of infertility is established and no possible therapy can be instituted.

The etiology of infertility can be divided into three major categories: (1) the female factor, (2) the male factor, and (3) undetermined etiology. It is difficult to assign exact percentages to each of these three categories. It is reported that approximately 40% of infertility cases are due to a female factor and 40% to a male factor, and in 10-20% no diagnosis can be made after a complete investigation. It has also been reported that in as many as 35% of couples the infertility may be of multiple origins.

PROCEDURE FOR INVESTIGATION

Investigation of infertility should be designed to be complete and as rapid as possible. The approach of "buying time" by having a patient record her daily basal body temperature (BBT) for three to six cycles before starting a work-up is unproductive. It is true that some women do conceive soon after the initial visit to the physician's office, but the percentage is small and does not warrant deliberate delay of the investigation.

All couples should have a complete history and physical. Routine laboratory tests include complete blood count, urinalysis, VDRL, and a fasting blood sugar (FBS). A sexual history should be obtained, with special emphasis on the frequency and timing of intercourse and the use of lubricants.

Investigations of infertility should be initiated in the following manner: (1) semen analysis, (2) documentation of ovulation (presumptive), (3) postcoital test, and (4) investigation of the female upper genital tract. If all these tests are normal, the following additional tests should be performed: (5) immunologic tests, (6) *Mycoplasma* cultures, (7) endometrial biopsy to establish the

TABLE 90-1. NORMAL SEMEN ANALYSIS*

Volume	3-5 ml
Sperm count	>20 million/ml
Motility	60-80%
Normal morphology	80%
Cytology	<5 WBC/high-power field
Viscosity	Total liquefaction within 20 minutes

*Results from LAC/USC Medical Center.

diagnosis of inadequate luteal phase, and (8) measurement of thyroid-stimulating hormone (TSH) to detect hypothyroidism.

EXAMINATION OF SEMEN

Examination of semen is obviously an integral part of the clinical investigation of infertility. In fact, since obtaining a specimen and performing a routine semen analysis are relatively easy, it should be the first step in the investigation of the infertile couple.

Semen specimens are best collected at home and should be obtained by masturbation if at all possible, since in withdrawal the first portion of the ejaculate may be lost. The semen should be collected in a clean glass container. The interval of abstinence should be determined by the frequency of intercourse routinely practiced by the couple. In areas where the weather is mild, the specimen need not be kept warm en route to the laboratory. Since most of the spermatozoa are found in the first milliliter of the ejaculate, the man should be instructed to take extreme precautions not to spill any portion of the specimen. Semen should be examined within the first 1-2 hours after collection (Table 90-1).

PRESUMPTIVE DOCUMENTATION OF OVULATION

An infertile woman who gives a history of regular monthly menstrual cycles is probably ovulating. Nevertheless, ovulation should be documented at least once in the work-up of the infertile patient. Any one of the following three tests can be used as presumptive evidence of ovulation: BBT, serum progesterone, or endometrial biopsy.

Basal Body Temperature

Under the influence of circulating progesterone, the BBT rises in the luteal phase of the cycle. A mean increase of at least 0.4°F over the proliferative-phase temperature is considered normal. The patient should be instructed to take her temperature each morning prior to getting out of bed. Oral temperatures are just as accurate as rectal temperatures and are much easier for the patient to take. The length of the luteal phase should be at least 10 days.

Serum Progesterone

A single serum progesterone value above 3 ng/ml obtained between days 20 and 24 of the menstrual cycle can be considered indicative of ovulation. However, it has been reported that a midluteal-phase level of 8 ng/ml is necessary for pregnancy to occur. If the sample is obtained too early or too late in the luteal phase, a false-negative result may be obtained because of the rise and fall of serum progesterone in a normal cycle.

Endometrial Biopsy

The biopsy should be obtained with a single swipe of the endometrium high on the anterior wall of the uterine fundus. A biopsy obtained between days 20 and 22 of the cycle should reveal histologic evidence of ovulation by the presence of secretory changes in the endometrial glands.

Following documentation of ovulation, the investigation should proceed to the next step outlined. However, if the patient is not ovulating, an endocrine work-up should be instituted to determine the etiology of anovulation.

Ovulation-Inducing Drugs

Some 10-15% of all infertile women are anovulatory. These patients should be completely evaluated and, if possible, treated with ovulation-inducing drugs. Anovulatory patients with adequate levels of circulating serum estradiol should be treated with clomiphene citrate (Clomid, Serophene). Patients with low levels of estradiol should be treated with human menopausal gonadotropins (hMG, Pergonal). Anovulatory patients with hyperprolactinemia should be treated with bromocriptine mesylate (Parlodel).

Clomiphene therapy is started on the fifth day of the cycle at 50 mg/day and is continued for 5 days. Semen analysis should be done before therapy is begun. If the patient fails to ovulate at 50 mg/day, the dose should be increased to 100 mg/day and, if necessary, to 150, 200, and finally 250 mg/day for 5 days. At the 250-mg dose, 10,000 units of human chorionic gonadotropin (hCG) can be given 7 days after the last dose of clomiphene. If the patient fails to ovulate on this regimen, the clomiphene should be given at 250 mg/day for 8 days and the hCG added 1 week later.

With an intact hypothalamic-pituitary axis, clomiphene has been successful in over 90% of cases. If clomiphene fails to induce ovulation, hMG therapy should be given; this method has been close to 100% effective in women with intact ovaries. Documentation of ovulation by either a BBT record or a serum progesterone determination should be obtained in each treatment cycle. Patients receiving clomiphene and hMG are at risk of developing ovarian cysts and therefore should always have a pelvic exam before taking the next dose. The exact mode of administration of hMG with steroid monitoring is discussed in Chapter 93.

The couple should try to achieve pregnancy for at least three ovulatory cycles before any further diagnostic procedures are instituted. Eighty per cent of patients treated with clomiphene who get pregnant do so within three cycles of therapy. If no conception occurs after the first ovulatory cycle, a post-coital test should be done in the second cycle and hysterosalpingography should be performed after three ovulatory cycles. If these tests are normal, the patient should be allowed at least six ovulatory cycles before undergoing laparoscopy. If the patient successfully ovulates with clomiphene and if no other factors for infertility can be found, she should be continued on this drug as long as she desires.

POSTCOITAL TESTING

This subject is covered in Chapter 91.

INVESTIGATION OF THE FEMALE UPPER GENITAL TRACT

Along with the male factor, pelvic abnormalities (tubal occlusion, adhesions, and endometriosis) account for the majority of infertility. In most clinics, 30-40% of female infertility can be attributed to the pelvic factor. With indigent populations, tubal disease will be much more prevalent than endometriosis. Although the diagnosis of tubal and pelvic disease is relatively straightforward, not all of the various therapeutic modalities available for these problems yield satisfying results.

The diagnostic techniques for evaluating tubal function, and the pelvis in general, indicate only patency, obstruction, and/or distortion, but not the degree of physiologic impairment that exists. The capacity for evaluating true reproductive function remains unrealized.

Hysterosalpingography

Evaluation of the patency of the fallopian tubes involves transuterine dye instillation under fluoroscopic and x-ray visualization. The study should be performed in the follicular phase of the cycle, prior to ovulation. If a radiologist performs the hysterosalpingography (HSG), the gynecologist should at least review the x-rays. If at all possible, the gynecologist should be present during the procedure, since fluoroscopy adds to the interpretation of the final x-rays. The contrast medium should be water-soluble.

HSG is extremely valuable in the work-up of the infertile patient. In a population prone to pelvic disease, an HSG should be obtained relatively early in the infertility investigation. We delay the test until the semen is evaluated and at least one ovulatory cycle is documented.

Laparoscopy

Laparoscopy has been a significant addition to the gynecologist's diagnostic and therapeutic armamentarium. It should always be performed even if the patient has a normal HSG, since as many as 25% of patients with a normal HSG have been reported to have abnormal findings at laparoscopy.

In addition to its value in diagnosing unsuspected pelvic pathology, laparoscopy is an essential primary step when the x-rays reveal abnormalities and surgery is contemplated. In cases where the x-rays are inaccurate, the laparoscope will reveal a normal pelvis, thus eliminating the need for further surgery. The laparoscope also makes it possible for the infertility surgeon to define and categorize the degree of pelvic disease and distortion. In some instances, major surgery can be deferred and the medical work-up and/or therapy continued on a more solid basis. And when the laparoscope reveals extremely severe tubal disease, laparotomy can be avoided and the patient advised to abandon further infertility studies and consider adoption.

As with any study of tubal function, laparoscopy should be performed in the follicular phase of the menstrual cycle. The accessory probe must be utilized for a thorough, accurate examination of the pelvic organs. In some patients, adequate evaluation requires a double-probe technique, which also permits the use of scissors and cautery. Prior pelvic surgery is usually not a contraindication to laparoscopic examination.

OTHER FACTORS

It has been reported that in approximately 10-20% of couples no abnormalities can be found after establishing that ovulation is occurring, obtaining a semen analysis, performing a postcoital test, and investigating the upper female genital tract with HSG and laparoscopy. The following additional investigations should then be performed: (1) immunologic tests, (2) cultures of the cervical mucus and semen, (3) endometrial biopsy to establish adequacy of the luteal phase, and (4) measurement of serum TSH to evaluate thyroid status.

Infertility Secondary to Immunologic Factors

Immunologic incompatibility may be the cause of infertility in some patients. The exact incidence of this phenomenon is not known. The fact that antibodies can be induced in laboratory animals by injecting semen has been known for over 75 years. In humans, two different systems have been implicated in the etiology of infertility: autoimmunity in men and the presence of circulating sperm-agglutinating and -immobilizing antibodies in women.

Autoimmunity in the male. In 1959, it was reported that in 3% of 2,000 infertile couples the etiology was autoimmunity in the husband. Most of these men showed spontaneous agglutination of spermatozoa in their own seminal plasma. A significant number had a history of genital tract infection, surgery, or trauma. In addition to autoagglutination, autoantibodies in men may decrease the ability of sperm to penetrate the cervical mucus. No successful therapy has yet been found, although some investigators have recommended high doses of corticosteroids. Artificial insemination using donor semen may be the only treatment.

Sperm-agglutinating and -immobilizing antibodies in the female. Agglutination of sperm by the woman's serum has been reported to be a factor in infertility. Most authors have not found the incidence of sperm-agglutinating antibodies in infertile women as high as reported originally by Franklin and Dukes. At the present time, therefore, it can be stated only that sperm-agglutinating antibodies appear to exist in the serum of women in a small percentage of infertile couples and that if they are a cause of infertility, the relationship is probably titer-dependent. Another test for detecting sperm-agglutinating antibodies in female serum is the Kibrick test. The usual incidence of positive tests using this technique has varied between 5% and 20%.

Isojima et al reported a complement-dependent serum sperm-immobilization technique. Their incidence of positive tests has varied between 12% and 19%, with an incidence of 0% in controls.

Since the role of immune reactions as a cause of infertility has not been totally disproven, the Kibrick and Isojima tests should be performed if all other tests outlined previously prove to be negative. If an immunologic test is positive at greater than 1:4 titer, condom therapy should be recommended for 3 months. At the end of this time, the tests should be repeated. If they remain positive, another 3 months of condom use should be advised. If at the end of 6 months the tests are still positive, condom therapy should be discontinued.

Genital Mycoplasma and Its Role in Infertility

Mycoplasma, previously known as PPLO organisms, and now referred to as *Ureaplasma urealyticum,* has been reported to be a possible factor in patients with undiagnosed infertility. The T strain of *Mycoplasma* has been reported to be the significant organism. Both cervical mucus and semen should be cultured for this organism. The treatment recommended is doxycycline 200 mg on the seventh day of the cycle, followed by 100 mg/day for 9 days. Both partners should be treated for two to three cycles. If the cultures remain positive, the dose should be doubled and treatment continued for 2 months.

Pregnancy rates of 42% after 3 months and 84% after 1 year have been reported following antibiotic therapy, even though published and unpublished studies have shown little or no relationship between the incidence of T *Mycoplasma* infection and infertility. However, until further results are published, T *Mycoplasma* cultures should be obtained in infertile couples, and if the cultures are positive, treatment should be instituted. In addition to *Mycoplasma*, organisms such as *Chlamydia* may play a role in infertility.

Inadequate Luteal Phase

Inadequate luteal phase is a histologic diagnosis made in a small number of infertile women in whom an endometrial biopsy shows a histologic maturational lag of 2 days or more compared with chronologic dating. Inappropriate maturation of the endometrium may be due to inadequate production of progesterone from the corpus luteum. It is assumed that poorly developed endometrium prevents successful implantation of the fertilized ovum.

It is important to differentiate between inadequate luteal phase and short luteal phase. In a short luteal phase, the interval between the peak level of luteinizing hormone and the onset of menses is less than 10 days. Short luteal phase does not seem to cause infertility.

Inadequacy of the luteal phase must be documented in two cycles, since normal fertile women may occasionally have an out-of-phase endometrial biopsy. A BBT chart cannot be used in making the diagnosis. The daily progesterone values obtained in inadequate luteal phases appear to be somewhat lower than in normal women; however, the differences in the absolute values are debatable.

The therapy for inadequate luteal phase has been a 25-mg progesterone vaginal suppository inserted twice daily during the luteal phase or a daily IM dose of 12.5 mg of progesterone in oil starting with the rise in BBT until the onset of menses. If the patient becomes pregnant, it has been recommended that the therapy be continued until the second trimester.

Thyroid-Stimulating Hormone

In rare instances, subclinical hypothyroidism may be the cause of infertility. The treatment of choice is L-thyroxine (Levothroid, Synthroid) 0.1-0.15 mg/day. TSH should be maintained in the normal range.

SUGGESTED READING

Ansbacher R, Keung-Yeung K, Behrman SJ: Clinical significance of sperm antibodies in infertile couples. *Fertil Steril* 24:305, 1973

Davajan V, Kharma K, Nakamura RM: Spermatozoan transport in cervical mucus. *Obstet Gynecol Surv* 25:1, 1970

Davajan V, Kunitake GM: Fractional in vivo and in vitro examination of post-coital cervical mucus in the human. *Fertil Steril* 20:197, 1969

Davajan V, Nakamura RM, Mishell DR Jr: A simplified technique for evaluation of the biophysical properties of cervical mucus. *Am J Obstet Gynecol* 109:1042, 1971

Davajan V, Nakamura RM, Saga M: Role of immunology in the infertile human. *Biol Reprod* 6:443, 1972

Dukes CD, Franklin RR: Sperm agglutinins and human infertility: Female. *Fertil Steril* 19:263, 1968

Franklin RR, Dukes CD: Antispermatozoal antibody and unexplained infertility. *Am J Obstet Gynecol* 89:6, 1964

Friberg J, Gnarpe H: Mycoplasma and human reproductive failure. III. Pregnancies in "infertile" couples treated with doxycycline for T-mycoplasmas. *Am J Obstet Gynecol* 116:23, 1973

Gnarpe H, Friberg J: Mycoplasma and human reproductive failure. I. The occurrence of different mycoplasmas in couples with reproductive failure. *Am J Obstet Gynecol* 114:727, 1972

Horne HW Jr, et al: The role of mycoplasma infection in human reproductive failure. *Fertil Steril* 25:380, 1974

Isojima S, Li TS, Ashitake Y: Immunologic analysis of sperm-immobilizing factor found in sera of women with unexplained sterility. *Am J Obstet Gynecol* 101:677, 1968

Jones GS: The luteal phase defect. *Fertil Steril* 27:351, 1976

Jones GS, Aksel S, Wentz AC: Serum progesterone values in the luteal phase defects. Effect of chorionic gonadotropin. *Obstet Gynecol* 44:26, 1974

Jones GS, Madrigal-Castro V: Hormonal findings in association with abnormal corpus luteum function in the human: The luteal phase defect. *Fertil Steril* 21:1, 1970

Kunitake GM, Davajan V: A new method of evaluating infertility due to cervical mucus-spermatozoa incompatibility. *Fertil Steril* 21:706, 1970

Mishell DR Jr, Davajan V, eds: *Reproductive Endocrinology, Infertility and Contraception*. Philadelphia: FA Davis, 1979

Mycoplasmas in human infertility. *Lancet* 1:1162, 1973

Scott JZ, Nakamura RM, Mutch J, et al: The cervical factor in infertility. Diagnosis and treatment. *Fertil Steril* 28:1289, 1977

Tredway DR, Settlage DS, Nakamura RM, et al: The significance of timing for the post-coital evaluation of the cervical mucus. *Am J Obstet Gynecol* 121:387, 1975

91

Postcoital Testing: The Cervical Factor as a Cause of Infertility

VAL DAVAJAN, M.D.

The incidence of infertility secondary to abnormal midcycle cervical mucus-spermatozoa interaction is estimated to be about 10%. Microscopic examination of preovulatory postcoital cervical mucus specimens obtained from these patients reveals few or no sperm, or only immobilized sperm. These findings are believed to be incompatible with normal reproductive processes. In the evaluation of infertility, the postcoital test (PCT) is the only in vivo test that brings together both partners in a testing system.

TECHNIQUE

Before the cervical mucus is aspirated, the portio vaginalis is cleansed using a moistened sponge. Then the cervical mucus is aspirated with a large syringe attached to a polyethylene suction catheter. The catheter may be sizes 8-14 French, depending on the diameter of the external os. The tubing is grasped 2.5 cm from the distal end with an atraumatic clamp. The aspiration must be initiated just as the tip of the catheter is inserted into the external os. A constant negative pressure is maintained with the syringe as the catheter is advanced to the internal os level (2.5 cm). The aspiration should then be terminated and the clamp closed completely.

The catheter is withdrawn gently, and the trailing mucus is cut away with scissors in order to prevent the sample from being pulled out of the catheter. The catheter segment containing the mucus is then cut into three segments. The segment from the tip of the catheter contains mucus from the internal os level, and the segment closest to the clamp represents mucus from the level of the external os. A smear of the posterior vaginal fornix should always be obtained to make sure that spermatozoa were deposited in the vaginal vault.

The PCT should be performed within 2 hours of coitus, since it has been reported that the number of sperm present in the cervical canal is at a maximum 2-2½ hours after coitus. The examination should be scheduled 1-3 days prior to the expected rise in BBT as determined by reviewing previous temperature graphs. A "mini-BBT," taken from the end of menses until the temperature has been elevated for 3 days, should be performed in every cycle in which a PCT is performed. If the PCT is abnormal, it should be repeated every 2 days until there is a temperature rise to make sure it is performed during the time of maximal estrogen stimulation—1-3 days *before* the rise in BBT. Before each PCT, the couple should observe their usual period of abstinence so the test will provide an accurate evaluation of what has occurred in the past.

For a test to be considered normal, there should be at least 5 motile sperm per high-power field at the internal os level. The spinnbarkeit measured in the same mucus sample should be no less than 6 cm (Table 91-1).

ABNORMAL PCT WITH ANATOMIC DEFECTS

Cervical Stenosis

Conization of the cervix is still the most common etiology of cervical stenosis. The diagnosis is made when attempts to pass a size 5 French catheter into the endocervical canal encounter resistance. Neither estrogen therapy nor attempts to recanalize the endocervix with dilators or cryosurgery have been successful. Small *Laminaria* has been employed in our clinic and an occasional pregnancy has been achieved.

Intrauterine insemination using washed sperm obtained from the patient's husband is being evaluated extensively. At LAC/USC Medical Center, the specimen of semen is collected in a sterile jar and allowed to liquefy. The semen is placed in a sterile tapered centrifuge tube and the volume tripled by the addition of Ham's F-10 solution (37°C). The specimen is mixed on a Vortex mixture set at a reading of 4 and then centrifuged for 5 minutes at 1,000 rpm. The supernatant is then discarded and 1 ml of Ham's solution is added to the "button" of sperm found at the bottom of the centrifuge tube. The specimen is mixed again on the Vortex mixer and then centrifuged for 3 minutes at 1,000 rpm. The supernatant is discarded, and 0.5 ml of Ham's solution is added to the "button." The specimen is mixed again and drawn up in a sterile 3-ml syringe. Using a size 8 French feeding tube, the specimen is gently deposited high in the fundus of the uterus. Approximately 1 cc of air is gently pushed through the catheter to make sure that the entire specimen is placed inside the uterine cavity.

TABLE 91-1. NORMAL POSTCOITAL TEST

Days of abstinence	Usual pattern
Day of exam	$-3, -2, -1$ before ↑BBT
Hours from coitus to exam	2-$2\frac{1}{2}$
Sperm/high-power field ($\times 400$) (internal os level)	$\geqslant 5$
Spinnbarkeit	$\geqslant 6$ cm

Varicosities of the Hypoplastic Endocervical Canal

There are patients in whom any attempt to collect cervical mucus leads to immediate bleeding. These patients have poorly developed columnar epithelium with prominent superficial varicosities. The diagnosis has been made by colposcopy. The treatment for this type of cervical problem has been cryosurgery, and in a small number of patients this therapy has improved the quality of mucus. A newer technique, using laser cautery, is being attempted, but no published information is available as to its efficacy.

ABNORMAL PCT WITH ABNORMAL CERVICAL MUCUS

Poor Quality of Mucus

There are patients who secrete abnormally thick, cellular cervical mucus at midcycle. In some patients a daily dose of 0.1 mg of diethylstilbestrol (DES) given on days 5-15 of a 28-day menstrual cycle markedly improves the quality of mucus and may result in a normal PCT. If there is no improvement, the DES dose should be increased to 0.2 mg/day. With improvement, the appropriate dose should be given for no less than 1 year.

In all patients undergoing treatment for any type of cervical problem, the treatment should result in an improved PCT. Therefore all treatment efforts should be evaluated by performing a repeat PCT during a treatment cycle. If improvement still is not noted, the abnormal mucus should be removed by aspiration, and if clear mucus is trailing behind the thick mucus, the thick mucus should be cut away from the clear mucus and the clear mucus allowed to remain in the canal. Following this "unplugging" procedure, the patient may either have artificial insemination or be instructed to return home to have intercourse.

Conjugated estrogens at doses of 1.25-5 mg/day can be given to patients in whom the DES therapy is ineffective. However, the 2.5-5-mg/day dosage of conjugated estrogens may suppress or delay ovulation. Therefore, all patients receiving high doses of conjugated estrogens must monitor ovulation using a BBT graph. If ovulation is suppressed with conjugated estrogens, clomiphene citrate (Clomid, Serophene) can be prescribed. If this fails to induce ovulation, the estrogen therapy should be discontinued and the patient can receive midcycle intrauterine inseminations using the washed sperm technique.

Low Quantity of Mucus

Some women secrete only minimal amounts of mucus at midcycle. In some of these patients, DES therapy (0.1 mg/day on days 5-15 of a 28-day cycle) increases mucus secretion. If there is an increase in mucus production with DES, the PCT should be repeated at midcycle; if the test is normal, the therapy should be continued for at least 1 year. In unresponsive patients, the dose of DES should be increased to 0.2 mg/day. If no mucus is produced at this dose level, the higher dose of conjugated estrogens, described above, should be prescribed. If this also fails, the patient should be treated with midcycle intrauterine inseminations as already described.

ABNORMAL PCT WITH NORMAL CERVICAL MUCUS

Faulty Coital Technique

In some infertile patients, no spermatozoa can be seen in the cervical mucus following intercourse. If a smear taken from the posterior vaginal fornix contains no sperm and the husband is known to have sperm, a faulty coital technique is highly likely (Chapter 90). If the patient is extremely obese, the fault may be the husband's failure to penetrate into the vagina. In such patients, careful review of coital technique is all that is necessary to correct the abnormality. Artificial insemination using the husband's semen can be performed if the couple cannot correct a faulty technique.

"Vaginal Factor," or "Weak Sperm Factor"

If the semen analysis is normal and no sperm are seen in the cervical mucus but are found in the vagina, cervical cup insemination followed by a PCT in 1 hour should be performed in order to rule out a "hostile vaginal factor" or "weak sperm factor." A specially designed cup (Milex Products, Chicago) is placed on the cervix. Semen is then introduced through the stem and exposed to the cervix for 1 hour. The cup is then removed, the portio vaginalis is cleansed, and an in vivo PCT is performed. If motile sperm are seen at the internal os level, the procedure can be instituted as therapy in the ensuing cycles. The exact etiology of the vaginal factor, or weak sperm factor, has not yet been established.

Oligospermia

Oligospermia is considered to be a sperm concentration of less than 20 million/ml. If an abnormal PCT is due to oligospermia, cervical cup therapy as outlined above should be attempted. If an improvement is noted on the post-cup PCT, cup insemination should be used as therapy for at least four cycles. If no improvement is noted, washed sperm intrauterine inseminations should be performed; if possible, two per cycle. The best days for performing insemination are the 3 days prior to the expected rise in BBT.

Low Semen Volume

In a certain number of couples with an abnormal PCT, lack of sperm penetration into the cervical canal may be due to an abnormally low volume of semen (less than 2 ml). If semen specimens are found to be consistently smaller than 2 ml and the low volume is not due to fault in the collection method, a cervical cup insemination should be tried as therapy. It is essential to follow the first insemination in 1 hour with a PCT as described previously in order to prove the efficacy of such therapy. If the cup method does not improve the PCT, washed sperm intrauterine insemination should be done.

Immobilized Sperm in the Endocervical Canal

Not infrequently an abnormal PCT is due to immobilization of sperm. In such cases, immunologic tests (Kibrick, Isojima) should be done, although in most of these patients there is no correlation between positive immunologic tests and immobilization of sperm in the cervical canal. Immobilization of sperm in the cervical mucus may be due to some as yet undetermined factors, or due to locally secreted antibodies not detected by the Kibrick or Isojima tests. The presence of *Mycoplasma* (*Ureaplasma urealyticum*) or other organisms in either the semen or cervical mucus may play a role in this finding. If immunologic tests and *Mycoplasma* cultures are both negative, cup insemination should be attempted. If the postcup PCT shows motile sperm at the internal os level, the cup technique should be tried as therapy for at least four cycles.

Large Volume of Semen

If a PCT is abnormal and the only finding is a large volume of semen (more than 8 ml), a split ejaculate specimen should be collected and cup insemination performed using the first 2 ml of ejaculate. If the PCT 1 hour later is normal, this therapy should be continued for at least four cycles. An alternative to this technique is washed sperm intrauterine inseminations.

IN VITRO METHODS

In vitro methods of evaluating sperm-cervical mucus interaction have not been routinely used in this clinic. The two most popular methods are the Miller-Kurzrok slide test and the capillary tube method of Kremer. For detailed descriptions of these methods, refer to the suggested reading.

SUGGESTED READING

Davajan V, Kharma K, Nakamura RM: Spermatozoa transport in cervical mucus. *Obstet Gynecol Surv* 25:1, 1970

Davajan V, Kunitake GM: Fractional in vivo and in vitro examination of post-coital cervical mucus in the human. *Fertil Steril* 20:197, 1969

Davajan V, Nakamura RM, Mishell DR Jr: A simplified technique for evaluation of the biophysical properties of cervical mucus. *Am J Obstet Gynecol* 109:1042, 1971

Kremer J: A simple sperm penetration test. *Int J Fertil* 10:201, 1965

Kunitake GM, Davajan V: A new method of evaluating infertility due to cervical mucus-spermatozoa incompatibility. *Fertil Steril* 21:706, 1970

Miller EG Jr, Kurzrok R: Biochemical studies of human semen. *Am J Obstet Gynecol* 24:19, 1932

Mishell DR Jr, Davajan V: *Reproductive Endocrinology, Infertility and Contraception*. Philadelphia: FA Davis, 1979

Scott JZ, Nakamura RM, Mutch J, et al: The cervical factor in infertility. Diagnosis and treatment. *Fertil Steril* 28:1289, 1977

Tredway DR, Settlage DS, Nakamura RM, et al: The significance of timing for the postcoital evaluation of cervical mucus. *Am J Obstet Gynecol* 121:387, 1975

92

Ovulation Induction With Clomiphene Citrate

CHARLES M. MARCH, M.D.

Induction of ovulation with clomiphene citrate (Clomid, Serophene) should be restricted to patients with oligomenorrhea or with primary or secondary amenorrhea who do not have ovarian failure and who wish to conceive. The administration of clomiphene citrate to an anovulatory patient who does not desire pregnancy is not warranted. Such therapy is often given to learn information regarding the dynamics of the hypothalamic-pituitary-ovarian defect responsible for the anovulation, but the results do not give prognostic information regarding the patient's ability to respond to the drug at a later date, when she may wish to conceive. In addition, there is a small risk of side effects and complications during clomiphene therapy, and these occurrences would obviously be inappropriate in someone not interested in conception.

Clomiphene citrate should be used as therapy in patients with either anovulation or oligo-ovulation. The latter group should be treated with clomiphene because it will induce ovulation more often, i.e., monthly. More important, ovulation will occur at a relatively predictable time; therefore, the chance of conception will increase. Clomiphene is the pharmacologic agent of choice for ovulation induction in most anovulatory patients. It is safer and more effective than the administration of glucocorticoids or gonadotropins for ovulation induction and is cheaper and easier to use than gonadotropins.

PHARMACOLOGY

Clomiphene citrate is both an antiestrogen and a weak estrogen. It acts by competitively displacing endogenous estradiol from estrogen-binding sites in the hypothalamus. By blocking the static negative feedback of estradiol on the hypothalamus, it permits an increased release of gonadotropin-releasing hormone, which stimulates the pituitary to increase the production and release of follicle-stimulating hormone (FSH) and luteinizing hormone (LH). In turn, the gonadotropins cause follicular development, with an increasing release of estradiol. The estradiol initially produces negative feedback on the hypothalamus and pituitary to reduce gonadotropin secretion. Then, as the endogenous estradiol level increases exponentially, it provides positive feedback to give an

LH/FSH surge that reproduces the hormonal events occurring in a spontaneous ovulatory cycle.

TREATMENT PROTOCOL

Beginning Regimen

Before beginning treatment, the patient should be investigated to rule out ovarian failure, any serious cause of anovulation, associated endocrinopathies such as a pituitary tumor or thyroid or adrenal disorder, and any contraindications to pregnancy. Coincident with the first course of therapy, a semen analysis should be obtained to rule out azoospermia or severe oligospermia. Clomiphene is administered beginning on day 5 following a spontaneous or induced menstrual period, beginning with a dose of 50 mg/day for 5 days. If ovulation will occur, it will usually do so within 3-14 days (mean, 7 days) following the last clomiphene tablet.

Documenting Ovulation

Ovulation should be documented in each cycle of treatment. This is best done by the use of a basal body temperature (BBT) record. If a classic biphasic shift occurs, ovulation may be presumed. Ovulation may also be presumed if the serum progesterone level is in excess of 3 ng/ml 2 weeks after the last clomiphene tablet. The level of progesterone determined at the time of peak production will usually be higher than 15 ng/ml.

An endometrial biopsy may also be used, as well as urinary pregnanediol excretion, to confirm that ovulation has occurred. For ease and convenience, as well as expense, BBT is obviously the method of choice and should be employed if it yields satisfactory results. In addition, the BBT provides information about the timing of ovulation, so that the frequency of coitus may be increased during this period.

Ovulatory Cycle

If menstrual bleeding does not occur within 4 weeks after the last clomiphene tablet and the cycle was ovulatory, an examination and pregnancy test should be performed. In each treatment cycle, the patient should be re-examined in the luteal phase or following a spontaneous menstrual period. If bleeding has occurred, if the cycle was ovulatory, and if the pelvic examination is completely within normal limits, the patient should be retreated with the same dose of clomiphene beginning on the fifth day after the onset of bleeding.

Anovulatory Cycle

If the cycle was anovulatory, whether or not bleeding occurred, the dose of clomiphene should be increased. If there was no bleeding, give 100 mg progesterone in oil or oral medroxyprogesterone acetate (Provera) to induce withdrawal bleeding. On the fifth day of spontaneous or induced bleeding, clomiphene treatment should begin with 100 mg/day for 5 days. If this course of therapy produces ovulation, the same dose should be continued, preceded by monthly examinations. These examinations serve to exclude the presence of pregnancy as well as ovarian enlargement, which would delay further therapy until the ovarian enlargement has regressed.

If ovulation does not occur at the 100-mg dosage, the amount of clomiphene should be increased, in 50-mg/day increments, up to five tablets, or 250 mg/day, for 5 days. If this dose is not successful in inducing ovulation, a maximal dose of 250 mg of clomiphene daily for 5 days, followed 4-8 days later by 10,000 IU of human chorionic gonadotropin (hCG) IM in a single dose to simulate the LH surge, should be given. The ideal day for hCG administration should be determined by following estrogen production. A marked increase in cervical mucus production (the semiquantitative cervical score is very helpful) may be used to improve timing.

Recent research has demonstrated that occasional patients who fail to ovulate with 250 mg/day for 5 days will ovulate when 250 mg is given daily for 8 days. However, if ovulation does not occur in these patients, they should be considered for therapy with either bromocriptine (Parlodel), if they have hyperprolactinemia, or human menopausal gonadotropins (hMG, Pergonal).

The clomiphene regimen outlined includes treatment above the 100-mg/day dosage, which is the maximum recommended in the physician's product brochure. However, approximately 25% of patients who ovulate and conceive with clomiphene citrate will do so only when these higher doses have been employed. In addition, treatment should be extended beyond the recommended three ovulatory cycles. Studies at many medical centers have proven the safety and efficacy of exceeding the manufacturer's recommendation. Once an ovulatory dose is reached, treatment should be continued on a regular basis until either conception occurs, other infertility factors are discovered that would preclude pregnancy, serious side effects occur, or the couple wishes to discontinue therapy.

Estrogen Deficiency/Androgen Excess

Approximately 95% of oligomenorrheic patients will ovulate. If the woman has secondary amenorrhea and evidence of endogenous estrogen production as shown by uterine withdrawal bleeding following the IM administration of progesterone in oil, she should be advised that her chance of ovulating during therapy is approximately 75%. An estrogen-deficient amenorrheic woman—that is, one who does not have uterine bleeding following progesterone administration and who has a normal or low level of gonadotropins—rarely has an ovulatory response to clomiphene citrate. She should be treated with human menopausal gonadotropins. However, since there is a slight chance that clomiphene will induce ovulation, she should be treated for one cycle with a high dose of clomiphene, i.e., 250 mg/day for 5 days, followed by 10,000 IU of hCG. If ovulation does occur, the same regimen should be continued monthly. If the patient remains anovulatory, treatment with other agents should be instituted.

Some hyperandrogenic anovulatory women who do not respond to this treatment regimen will be found to have elevated serum levels of the adrenal androgen dehydroepiandrosterone sulfate (DHEA-S). If the DHEA-S level exceeds 2.8 μg/ml, treatment with dexamethasone 0.5 mg HS should be started. After 2 weeks, menses should be induced, the dexamethasone continued, and clomiphene 250 mg/day given on days 5-9 of the cycle. With this combined regimen, a few more anovulatory patients may be made to respond.

FURTHER INFERTILITY WORK-UP

Of all patients who conceive during therapy, three-quarters will do so within the first three ovulatory cycles. For this reason, extensive infertility studies should be delayed until after ovulation is induced three times. Following these three ovulatory cycles, a fractional postcoital test should be performed to verify the presence of normal sperm transport. An endometrial biopsy should be obtained to ascertain whether the endometrial response is normal. If this study is normal, the next step would be investigation of the uterine and tubal factors by means of hysterosalpingography. The final infertility study would be investigation of the pelvic factor by laparoscopy.

At the initial interview with the couple, prior to induction of ovulation, the physician should explain that this regimen may be expected to induce ovulation in over 90% of patients who have oligomenorrhea. The overall incidence of pregnancy during treatment with clomiphene citrate is approximately 45%. However, if patients with other infertility factors have been eliminated, more than 85% of those who ovulate when treated with clomiphene will conceive.

RISKS OF CLOMIPHENE THERAPY

Congenital Anomalies

There is no increased risk of congenital anomalies during clomiphene treatment, nor is there an increased risk of spontaneous abortion. However, early studies showed that when clomiphene was administered inadvertently during the first 6 weeks of pregnancy, the incidence of birth defects was 5.1%. Although this frequency is not significantly higher than the 2.4% observed in patients to whom the drug was given prior to conception, the increase is of concern. Therefore, it is important that clomiphene be administered only when a patient has had normal withdrawal bleeding.

Ovarian Cysts

The risk of ovarian cyst formation during therapy is increased to 5-10%. If a cyst forms, it will regress spontaneously in less than a month provided that clomiphene is withheld during that time. Cysts may occur at any dose and during any course of therapy. The risk of multiple gestations, nearly all twins, is also between 5% and 10%.

SUGGESTED READING

Gysler M, March CM, Mishell DR Jr, Bailey EJ: A decade's experience with an individualized clomiphene treatment regimen including its effect on the post-coital test. *Fertil Steril* 37:161, 1982

Lobo RA, Gysler M, March CM, Goebelsmann U, Mishell DR Jr: Clinical and laboratory predictors of clomiphene response. *Fertil Steril* 37:168, 1982

Lobo RA, Paul W, March CM, Granger L, Kletzky OA: Clomiphene and dexamethasone in women unresponsive to clomiphene alone. *Obstet Gynecol* 60:497, 1982

March CM, Davajan V, Mishell DR Jr: Ovulation induction in amenorrheic women. *Obstet Gynecol* 53:8, 1979

March CM, Israel R, Mishell DR Jr: Pregnancy following twenty-nine cycles of clomiphene citrate therapy: A case report. *Am J Obstet Gynecol* 124:209, 1976

93

Ovulation Induction With Human Menopausal Gonadotropins

CHARLES M. MARCH, M.D.

The use of gonadotropins for ovulation induction has been limited by insufficient knowledge regarding the indications, administration, results, and side effects of therapy. The limited availability of rapid estrogen assays and high drug cost have also been deterrents. The effects of various urinary and pituitary sources of gonadotropins, which have varying LH/FSH (luteinizing hormone/follicle-stimulating hormone) ratios, are similar. Therefore, this chapter will discuss only human menopausal gonadotropins, the preparation available in the United States.

Human menopausal gonadotropins (hMG, Pergonal) are extracted from the urine of postmenopausal women. Each ampule of the preparation contains 75 IU of FSH and 75 IU of LH. Although hMG has been used for treatment of luteal phase defects and for the timing of ovulation in conjunction with artificial insemination, its use is accepted universally only for ovulation induction. This chapter will be limited to that indication.

SELECTION CRITERIA

Candidates for ovulation induction must have ovarian follicles. This criterion will include patients with oligomenorrhea or amenorrhea who have uterine bleeding following the administration of progesterone in oil. These patients have normal circulating estrogen levels and, therefore, functioning follicles.

Women with either primary or secondary amenorrhea who do not have uterine bleeding after progesterone administration are estrogen-deficient. These patients should have measurements of serum FSH levels. Elevated levels are diagnostic of ovarian failure. These women are sterile and should not be considered for treatment with ovulatory drugs.

The estrogen-deficient, amenorrheic woman who has normal or low serum levels of FSH should be completely investigated to rule out a hypothalamic or pituitary tumor. If the investigation is negative, these patients may be considered for ovulation induction.

Candidates for treatment with gonadotropins are anovulatory women who do not ovulate when treated with clomiphene citrate (Clomid, Serophene) followed by human chorionic gonadotropin (hCG), administered according to the regimen outlined in Chapter 92. These patients should be considered clomiphene failures. This term applies only to patients who fail to ovulate when treated with clomiphene, not to those who ovulate but fail to conceive. The use of hMG in the latter group of patients is not indicated. Anovulatory women with hyperprolactinemia who fail to respond to bromocriptine are also hMG candidates, as are patients developing serious side effects during clomiphene or bromocriptine therapy.

PRETREATMENT STUDIES AND COUNSELING

Pretreatment studies should include semen analysis to rule out oligospermia, azoospermia, or other gross abnormality in the male partner. Uterine and tubal factors should be investigated by hysterosalpingogram and laparoscopy with chromopertubation. If a hysteroscope is available, hysteroscopy (together with laparoscopy) may be substituted for the hysterosalpingogram. These procedures will ensure that multiple causes of infertility are not present. Although multifactorial infertility is not a contraindication to therapy with hMG, the chance of a full-term gestation is markedly reduced, and the couple should be afforded a realistic prognosis.

Extensive pretreatment counseling of both members of the couple is mandatory. They should have a stable relationship. Therapy with hMG is inconvenient and stressful for both partners, and each must provide support for the other. They should be advised of the likelihood of success: The chance of conceiving in any one course of therapy is about 25%, a rate similar to that in spontaneous ovulatory cycles. Among patients conceiving during therapy, the average number of treatment courses needed to achieve a pregnancy is three. Of all patients treated with hMG, 60% conceive. These data, in addition to a thorough explanation of the risks and sequelae of multiple gestations and hyperstimulation, will ensure that both partners are well informed before the therapy begins.

TREATMENT PROCEDURE

Three different regimens are used for hMG administration: hMG only, sequential clomiphene-hMG, and sequential estrogen-hMG. In all instances, hCG is added to cause ovum release.

Patients with oligomenorrhea and amenorrheic patients who have withdrawal bleeding following progesterone in oil should receive pretreatment with clomiphene citrate for 5 days. On day 6, hMG is administered. In this group of patients, duration of treatment and hMG dosage will be reduced by one-half compared to the hMG-only regimen.

Hypogonadotropic, estrogen-deficient, amenorrheic women will not benefit from clomiphene pretreatment, but should receive two treatment courses of sequential estrogen-progestin. This regimen will prime the endometrium and endocervix for response to the endogenous estradiol that will be secreted during gonadotropin therapy.

The hMG treatment should mimic as closely as possible the follicular development of a spontaneous cycle. Since an index of this development is the rising serum level of estradiol, treatment should be undertaken only in centers where daily estrogen levels may be obtained rapidly.

Individuality in response is the hallmark of therapy with gonadotropins. The dosage required to induce adequate follicular development, as well as the duration of therapy, vary greatly not only from one patient to another, but also from one course of treatment to another in the same patient. However, as a general rule, progesterone-negative amenorrheic patients require significantly more medication than progesterone-positive patients who do have withdrawal bleeding. Therefore, the treatment must be individually tailored to each patient.

Patients are divided into two groups: those with normal estrogen status and those who are estrogen-deficient. In the former group, withdrawal uterine bleeding is induced by administration of progesterone in oil (100 mg IM). On the fifth day of withdrawal bleeding, clomiphene citrate (200 mg/day PO) is begun and continued for 5 days. hMG (one or two ampules/day) is begun on day 6. In these patients, who are usually more sensitive to hMG, clomiphene will induce partial follicular maturation. Monitoring (described below) is begun on the first day of hMG administration.

The hypoestrogenic patients are first treated with two courses of sequential estrogen-progestin. Conjugated estrogens (1.25 mg/day) is administered for 25 days, and medroxyprogesterone acetate (10 mg/day) is added on days 20-25. Following the end of the second withdrawal bleeding, hMG is begun.

On the first day of hMG administration, patients in both groups are seen in the morning, a serum sample is obtained for estradiol (E_2) measurement, and a real-time ultrasound examination of the ovaries is performed to assess the number and size of ovarian follicles. A pelvic examination is performed to calculate the cervical score (quantity of cervical mucus, extent of ferning, spinnbarkeit, and size of external os) as well as to palpate the ovaries to rule out enlargement or tenderness. Then hMG is given. Treatment is usually initiated with a dose of two ampules and is continued daily.

The serum E_2 level, pelvic examination, and ultrasound are repeated in 3 or 4 days. If the E_2 concentration remains unchanged, the dose of hMG is increased by a factor of 0.5 and continued for another 3 or 4 days. This stepwise increase every 3-4 days by a factor of 0.5 is continued until the dose is found that will initiate a rise in serum E_2 levels. Then this "ideal dose" is maintained.

When the serum E_2 level rises above 400 pg/ml, E_2 determinations are performed daily and patients are seen in both morning and afternoon. In the morning, the pelvic examination is performed and the serum sample obtained. But hMG is not administered until the patient returns in the afternoon. By then, the results of the E_2 assay are known and either more hMG or hCG is given, depending on the E_2 level. These twice-daily visits are usually required only one or two times.

The optimal serum E_2 level is between 500 and 1,000 pg/ml. This would be comparable to 50-100 μg of total estrogens in a 24-hour urine specimen. This level is higher than the preovulatory estrogen peak of a normal menstrual cycle because more than one follicle is stimulated.

More recently, the monitoring process has been streamlined dramatically by the use of a real-time sector scanner to assess follicular development. Scanning becomes most important after one or more follicles begin to develop, as evidenced by an increased serum E_2 level. At this point, provided adequate visualization of both ovaries can be achieved, E_2 determinations may be eliminated and further treatment guided solely by the changes in number and size of follicles. When a follicle reaches 14 mm, all further monitoring can usually be by ultrasound. When a single dominant follicle (or at most two) reaches 18-22 mm in maximal diameter, ovulation may be induced with hCG.

The correlation between total follicular volume and serum E_2 levels is excellent. But the advantages of ultrasound monitoring are immediate results, obviating twice-daily visits, assurance that there are not too many mature follicles, and verification that at least one follicle has matured (has reached preovulatory size). Because of the many uses of ultrasound, this monitoring technique will probably become more common than rapid serum E_2 assays and thus make hMG treatment more widely available than at present.

A subgroup of anovulatory women are exquisitely sensitive to hMG. These patients have normal E_2 levels and either normal LH/FSH levels or elevated LH levels consistent with polycystic ovarian disease. They do not ovulate when treated with clomiphene, but develop very many small follicles during hMG stimulation. Hyperstimulation frequently occurs, and these follicles may not reach preovulatory size when hCG is given. This supposition is supported by the low pregnancy rate in this group. Some of these women have a normal response to hMG following pretreatment with oral contraceptives for one cycle. The endogenous LH/FSH levels are lowered and thus ovarian stimulation is reduced. When hMG is begun, all follicular development is controlled by the exogenous gonadotropins. Further studies are needed before the value of this regimen can be assessed fully.

As an adequate degree of follicular development is achieved, the rapidly rising estrogen levels will stimulate cervical mucus production. When there is an increase in the amount of cervical mucus, as well as an increase in spinnbarkeit and ferning, a fractional postcoital test is performed. In this way, the adequacy of the sperm transport is verified. If sperm transport is abnormal, a cervical cup insemination using the husband's semen is performed 24-36 hours following the injection of hCG.

When optimal levels of estrogen are reached, provided the ovaries are not tender or enlarged, 10,000 IU of hCG are given 24-36 hours after the last injection of hMG. The couple is instructed to have intercourse at least every other day including the last day of hMG therapy, as well as 24-36 hours after the hCG injection. On days 4 and 8 following the first injection of hCG, 3,000 IU of hCG are given to maintain the corpus luteum *only* in hypogonadotropic and estrogen-deficient patients or those who have had a short luteal phase during prior treatment cycles. The supplemental hCG is withheld if the ovaries are enlarged or tender.

Eight days after the first injection of hCG, a serum sample is obtained for measurement of progesterone concentration. After an estrogen-deficient patient has been treated for one cycle, her clinical response (cervical mucus production, ferning and spinnbarkeit, and changes in cervical configuration) is correlated with her daily E_2 levels. If the clinical changes were able to predict the rising E_2 levels, the frequency of serum samples may be markedly reduced during subsequent courses of treatment.

Using this protocol, we have been able to achieve ovulation in 99% of our courses of therapy. This high rate surpasses other published reports and reflects careful patient selection as well as strict adherence to the protocol. Only 6% of our pregnancies have been multiple gestations, and these have all involved either twins or triplets. Minimal ovarian enlargement (5-10 cm), which resolved spontaneously, occurred in 7% of our treatment cycles. We also attribute these excellent results to strict adherence to our protocol.

SUMMARY

Treatment with hMG is complex. In the absence of a carefully planned protocol and strict adherence to it, and in the absence of careful monitoring techniques, treatment with hMG may lead to complications. However, with an appropriate protocol and monitoring techniques, almost all patients treated may expect to ovulate safely. Pregnancy rates of 60% with a very low rate of multiple gestations and other complications may be expected. Although the rate of spontaneous abortion is increased to about 25-50%, no increase in the incidence of congenital anomalies has been reported.

SUGGESTED READING

March CM: Complications of gonadotropin therapy. *J Reprod Med* 21:208, 1978

March CM: Therapeutic regimens and monitoring techniques for human menopausal gonadotropin administration. *J Reprod Med* 21:198, 1978

March CM, Davajan V, Mishell DR Jr: Ovulation induction in amenorrheic women. *Obstet Gynecol* 53:8, 1979

March CM, Tredway DR, Mishell DR Jr: Effect of clomiphene citrate upon amount and duration of human menopausal gonadotropin therapy. *Am J Obstet Gynecol* 125:699, 1976

Marrs RP, March CM, Mishell DR Jr: A comparison of clinical and laboratory methods in monitoring human menopausal gonadotropin therapy. *Fertil Steril* 34:542, 1980

94

Male Factor in Infertility

GERALD S. BERNSTEIN, Ph.D., M.D.

Anyone who evaluates or treats the female member of the infertile couple must have some knowledge of male as well as female reproductive physiology, particularly the relationship between semen quality and fertility. About one-third of cases of infertility are due to an abnormality of the male, and in other instances combined male and female factors must be evaluated.

Initial assessment of an infertile couple should always include some evaluation of the male. A semen analysis is essential. A postcoital test also provides information about semen quality as well as the interaction between spermatozoa and cervical mucus.

SEMEN ANALYSIS

Semen analysis should be done in a reliable laboratory by an experienced technician. The specimen should be collected in a wide-mouthed container by masturbation after 2-5 days of sexual abstinence. It should be examined within 1 hour, if possible, and never later than 2 hours after collection; sperm motility usually begins to decline after 2 hours. If the male has frequent emissions, a specimen should also be obtained without a period of abstinence. The patient may have a normal semen analysis following abstinence but a decreased count under his normal conditions of sexual activity.

If the specimen is collected at home, it should be protected against cold during transport to the laboratory. To keep the specimen at body temperature in cold weather, the patient can place the sample container in the waistband of his trousers.

Several semen samples should be studied, as semen quality may vary over a period of time. If the analysis is abnormal, at least three specimens collected at monthly intervals should be evaluated.

Standard values for semen quality, as defined by the International Committee of Andrology, are volume: 2-6 ml; sperm count: 40-250 million/ml; sperm motility: at least 60% motile initially, with good progressive motility; sperm morphology: normal in at least 60%. But these values do not define the limits of fertility. Although, by definition, a man with a sperm count under 40 million has oligospermia, essentially normal fertility can be expected with counts between 20 and 40 million if motility is normal. Pregnancy rates as high as

50% have been obtained over a period of time for couples in which the male's sperm count is consistently under 10 million.

The most important aspect of semen quality in relation to fertility seems to be the number of morphologically normal sperm with good motility. Motility is important because nonmotile and poorly motile sperm usually do not penetrate into and migrate through the cervical mucus. Therefore, such sperm do not enter the upper female reproductive tract.

Morphology is also important. Some morphologically abnormal sperm are excluded from the cervix. Those with large or misshapen heads do not usually fit into the channels formed by the macromolecules within the cervical mucus. Sperm with very small or round rather than oval heads are able to enter the cervical mucus, but lack acrosomes that permit sperm to penetrate and fertilize ova.

CAUSES OF SEMEN ABNORMALITIES

A number of etiologic factors can cause semen to be abnormal. These include:

1. Anatomic factors, including varicocele and cryptorchidism
2. Endocrine factors
3. Genetic factors, such as Klinefelter's syndrome, other manifestations of the 47,XXY karyotype, and various types of translocations
4. Inflammatory disease, such as prostatitis (frequently asymptomatic) and epididymitis
5. Autoimmune phenomena, leading to the formation of autoantibodies against spermatozoa
6. Ejaculatory dysfunction, including retrograde ejaculation, occurring in some diabetics or following bladder neck surgery; and ejaculatory failure, occurring after sympathectomy or use of ganglionic-blocking drugs
7. Psychological factors, such as impotence and premature ejaculation
8. Faulty coital technique
9. Exogenous factors, including drugs, radiation, chemicals, and alcohol
10. Factors of unknown etiology, including absence of germinal epithelium in the testes (Sertoli-cell-only syndrome), abnormalities of spermatogenesis (maturation arrest and hypospermatogenesis), and disorganization of the germinal epithelium.

The following relationships between specific causes and abnormalities have been noted:

- A low sperm count may be caused by an endocrine disorder, varicocele, prostatitis or other genital infection, or exogenous agents. Sometimes the diagnostic evaluation is normal except for idiopathic changes in the germinal epithelium.
- Absence of sperm in the ejaculate may result from genetic disorder, Sertoli-cell-only syndrome, testicular failure, endocrinopathy, or inflammatory or congenital obstruction of the male genital tract.
- Orgasm without production of ejaculate may be due to retrograde ejaculation or ejaculatory failure.

- Low semen volume may be due to partial retrograde ejaculation, obstruction of the ejaculatory ducts, or malfunction of the prostate or seminal vesicles.
- Poor sperm motility may be caused by autoantibodies, infection, or varicocele. The presence of white blood cells or erythrocytes in the semen may also be due to infection.
- Autoagglutination of the sperm may be the result of either infection or autoantibodies.
- Abnormal sperm morphology may be caused by a number of factors, including varicocele, stress, infection, and exogenous factors.

THE POSTCOITAL TEST

The semen analysis must be considered in relation to the postcoital test. If the postcoital test is consistently good, it may not matter that the semen quality is subnormal. If the postcoital test is poor and the semen contains at least 2 million sperm/ml with good motility, artificial insemination with the husband's semen (AIH) can be attempted.

ARTIFICIAL INSEMINATION

The husband's semen sample should be examined just prior to use and then placed against the cervix in an insemination cup. A postcoital test should be done 1-2 hours after insemination. If AIH improves the postcoital test, insemination should be done in at least 4-6 cycles.

An alternative method is intrauterine insemination. In our opinion, it is preferable to avoid inserting seminal plasma into the endometrial cavity; uterine cramping and an immune reaction to seminal antigens are possible. Instead, we dilute the semen with Ham's solution and sediment the sperm by centrifugation. The sperm are resuspended in Ham's solution and the centrifugation is repeated. Then the cells are resuspended in approximately 0.5 ml of Ham's solution, and the suspension of washed sperm is instilled into the endometrial cavity by means of a catheter. Since the reservoir capacity of the cervix is bypassed, better results may be obtained if recipients are monitored by ultrasound and the insemination is done near the time of ovulation.

EVALUATING THE MALE WITH ABNORMAL SEMEN

When the semen is abnormal, the male should be evaluated, even if AIH is used for therapy. Infertility may be the presenting complaint in cases of pituitary tumor, chronic genitourinary infection, or other problems that may require treatment. Some types of male infertility—varicocele, infection, and certain endocrine disorders—can be successfully treated. Others are difficult to treat due to the still-limited knowledge of male reproductive physiology.

The work-up should be done by a physician competent in andrology. This may be a urologist, internist, or, in some cases, a gynecologist with a special interest in male reproductive disorders. The evaluation may include endocrine, microbiologic, immunologic, and genetic studies, depending on the results of the semen analysis, history, and physical examination. The andrology consultant and the gynecologist should work in close cooperation.

FUTURE DEVELOPMENTS

Current research in male reproduction will improve our ability to diagnose and treat disorders that are still poorly understood. Some areas of interest include endocrine disorders that may not be detected by current routine testing, such as qualitative or quantitative defects in androgen and gonadotropin receptors, and abnormalities in androgen metabolism; ultrastructural defects in normal-appearing sperm that may affect motility or fertilizing capacity; biochemical abnormalities of seminal plasma that may influence sperm motility and ability to penetrate and activate ova; and identification of substances in the environment and workplace that may adversely affect semen quality and male fertility.

SUGGESTED READING

Amelar RD, Dubin L, Walsh PC: *Male Infertility*. Philadelphia: Saunders, 1977

Bardin CW, Paulsen CA: The testis. In Williams RH, ed: *Textbook of Endocrinology*. Philadelphia: Saunders, 1981, p 293

Bernstein GS: Male factor. In Mishell DR Jr, Davajan V, eds: *Reproductive Endocrinology, Infertility and Contraception*. Philadelphia: FA Davis, 1979, p 351

Eliasson R: Standards for investigation of human semen. *Andrologia* 3:49, 1971

Frajese G, Hafez ESE, Conti C, Fabbrini A, eds: *Oligozoospermia: Recent Progress in Andrology*. New York: Raven, 1981

Greenberg SH: Varicocele and male fertility. In Wallach EE, Kempers RD, eds: *Modern Trends in Infertility and Conception Control*, vol 1. Baltimore: Williams & Wilkins, 1979, p 302

Hafez ESE, ed: *Techniques of Human Andrology*. New York: North-Holland, 1977

MacLeod J, Wang Y: Male fertility potential in terms of semen quality: A review of the past. A study of the present. In Wallach EE, Kempers RD, eds: *Modern Trends in Infertility and Conception Control*, vol 2. Baltimore: Williams & Wilkins, 1982, p 361

Mann T, Lutwak-Mann C: *Male Reproductive Function and Semen*. Berlin: Springer-Verlag, 1981

Nachtigall RD, Faure N, Glass RH: Artificial insemination of husband's sperm. In Wallach EE, Kempers RD, eds: *Modern Trends in Infertility and Conception Control*, vol 2. Baltimore: Williams & Wilkins, 1982, p 404

Shulman S, et al: Immune infertility and new approaches to treatment. *Fertil Steril* 29:309, 1978

Steinberger A, Steinberger E, eds: *Testicular Development, Structure, and Function*. New York: Raven, 1980

Steinberger E: The etiology and pathophysiology of testicular dysfunction in man. In Wallach EE, Kempers RD, eds: *Modern Trends in Infertility and Conception Control*, vol 1. Baltimore: Williams & Wilkins, 1979, p 273

Troen P, Nankin HR, eds: *The Testis in Normal and Infertile Men*. New York: Raven, 1977

95

Tubal Factor in Infertility

ROBERT ISRAEL, M.D.

Fallopian tube abnormalities, adhesive pelvic disease, and endometriosis, along with the male factor, account for the majority of infertility. In most clinics, the pelvic factor is the etiology in 30-40% of infertility cases. With indigent populations, tubal disease and pelvic adhesions may account for even a higher percentage of infertility. Although the diagnosis of tubal or pelvic disease is relatively straightforward, surgical correction of tubal obstructions does not yield satisfying results.

Diagnostic techniques for evaluating tubal function, and the pelvis in general, have become more sophisticated. However, they still indicate only patency, obstruction, or distortion—not the degree of physiologic impairment. Reproductive function remains unmeasured.

UTEROTUBAL INSUFFLATION (RUBIN'S TEST)

In 1920, Rubin described a nonoperative method of determining tubal patency by instilling a gas, initially oxygen, via a transvaginal-transuterine route. To eliminate the possibility of air embolism, carbon dioxide (CO_2) soon replaced oxygen. Uterotubal insufflation should be carried out in the follicular phase of the menstrual cycle, after the menses and before ovulation. Any investigation of tubal patency is contraindicated in the luteal phase because it may damage or delay implantation of a fertilized ovum. Also, the thicker secretory endometrium may occlude the tubal ostia at the tubal-endometrial cavity junction and yield a false result. Other contraindications are pregnancy, uterine bleeding, pelvic infection, recent curettage, and inadequate equipment.

Numerous instruments are available for uterotubal insufflation. Requirements include a constant source of CO_2, a flowmeter, a pressure gauge, and a kymograph for recording the degree of peristaltic activity that presumably arises from tubal contractions. A cervical obturator that fits the cervix in leakproof fashion must be used. After inserting the cannula into the cervical canal, the operator should wait at least 1 minute before instilling the CO_2. This pause helps the uterus adapt to the intrusion of the cannula and relax, thus reducing the incidence of cornual spasm, which falsely indicates tubal obstruction. A slow, even flow rate of 50-60 cc/minute is recommended. The total volume of CO_2 utilized should be 100 cc or less.

The kymograph tracing is helpful in determining whether there is tubal patency or occlusion. In a normal study, the pressure rises to 80-120 mm Hg and subsequently falls to 40-80 mm Hg when the CO_2 enters the peritoneal cavity. Tubal occlusion, or presumed occlusion, exists with pressures of 200-250 mm Hg, excessive uterine cramping, and no fall in pressure. Additionally, auscultation over the lower abdomen by an assistant will reveal a characteristic gurgling sound as the CO_2 rushes from the fimbriated end of the tube into the wide expanse of the peritoneal cavity.

At the conclusion of the study, when the patient sits up, she may experience shoulder pain if the CO_2 has reached the abdominal cavity. If at least 100 cc of CO_2 are utilized, the phrenic nerve, running from the diaphragm to the shoulder, will be irritated. However, *right* shoulder pain does not mean that one can assume the *right* tube is patent, the left tube is patent, or both tubes are patent, but only that patency or partial patency is present in one or both of the tubes.

In fact, interpretation of uterotubal insufflation must be tempered with a great deal of caution. Cornual spasm can mimic occlusion, and indications of tubal patency can be misleading. The test gives no assurance that both tubes are open, that one tube is open, or that partial patency exists. Obviously, pelvic adhesions cannot be diagnosed. Therefore, the value of uterotubal insufflation must be questioned. If used as a quick office screening study, its limitations must be considered and the results must not be utilized as a definitive evaluation of the tubes and pelvis.

The therapeutic benefit of repeated insufflation, or "blowing out the tubes," in three successive cycles has not been proven by any prospective study. Following certain types of tubal surgery, it can be utilized to maintain patency. However, hydrotubation appears to be more efficacious. The most important consideration in analyzing uterotubal insufflation is the realization that it does not depict the actual condition of the fallopian tubes. The decision whether to perform conservative tubal surgery must not be made on the basis of a Rubin test.

HYSTEROSALPINGOGRAPHY (HSG)

A more definitive study of the fallopian tubes involves transuterine dye instillation under x-ray visualization. The contraindications to HSG are the same as for uterotubal insufflation. The study is performed after the menses, in the follicular phase, prior to ovulation. Exactness and care are essential.

The instrumentation can be the same as for uterotubal insufflation, but utilizing a Malmström-Westman vacuum cannula reduces cervical trauma and patient discomfort. If a radiologist is going to perform the HSG, the gynecologist should be in attendance or, at the very least, review the x-rays. Preferably, the dye instillation should be set up and administered by the gynecologist. Image intensification fluoroscopy adds to the interpretation of the final x-rays and should be part of the procedure. However, it must be carried out by a radiologist skilled in the technique. If 1 minute of fluoroscopy is utilized during an HSG, the patient receives a radiation dose equal to that of one conventional film.

Two types of contrast media are available for HSG: oil-based and water-soluble. Although the oil-based solutions outline the uterine and tubal surfaces very sharply, they have distinct disadvantages. For example, the stagnation inherent in oil media can lead to foreign-body reactions, causing granulomas and dangerous intravascular dissemination that can create possibly fatal pulmonary emboli. These adverse reactions are even more likely in the presence of tubal obstruction. With the advent of laparoscopy, the advantage of taking a 24-hour-delay film after oil HSG has lost its importance. As a greater amount of water-soluble medium than oil-based medium is necessary for an HSG, uterine cramps may be a greater problem. However, using a solution of extremely low viscosity, e.g., diatrizoate meglumine and iodipamide meglumine (Sinografin), and warming it, will reduce uterine cramping, thus improving patient acceptance and study accuracy. In summary, water-soluble media are preferable.

In patients with a history of pelvic inflammatory disease (PID), the HSG should be deferred until the white blood count and erythrocyte sedimentation rate have returned to normal. Antibiotic coverage before and after HSG may provide additional protection. A flare-up of acute salpingitis after an HSG is a poor prognostic sign regarding the success of any subsequent reparative surgery. If even attempted, surgery should be deferred at least 3 months.

The HSG is extremely valuable in the work-up of the infertile patient. In a population with a high incidence of salpingitis, an HSG should be obtained relatively early in the infertility investigation. In some pathologic conditions, an HSG can be the definitive study. As noted by Klein and co-workers in our clinic, the HSG in pelvic tuberculosis is diagnostic. In salpingitis isthmica nodosa, an HSG defines the extent of the process even with patent tubes.

The discovery of extensive tubal disease may alter, and certainly speed up, the other infertility studies. Multifactor infertility does not have a very good prognosis. An abnormal HSG will hasten the time of laparoscopy and, possibly, bring the investigation to an early conclusion. In addition, according to studies in our institution, unsuspected intrauterine pathology will be demonstrated in 10% of HSGs obtained for infertility. Confirmatory hysteroscopy should be done whenever an intrauterine defect is found on HSG.

The illuminated hysterosalpingogram must be present in the operating room at the time of surgery. Although, in some series, discrepancies between HSG and definitive laparoscopy have occurred as much as 25% of the time, HSG is still a valuable study. Its technical problems can be overcome by endoscopy. For example, occasionally a tube that seemed to be blocked on HSG can be proven to be patent at laparoscopy by occluding the other tube at the uterine cornu with a probe while continuing to instill the dye transcervically. If several months have elapsed between the HSG and surgery, advancing disease or a reaction to the HSG may explain tubal occlusion found at laparoscopy and not present on an earlier HSG.

On occasion, mechanical problems with laparoscopic chromopertubation can occur, and the illuminated HSG can provide evidence of patency. As mentioned by Ozaras, if the patient has a history of PID, the HSG can provide helpful prognostic information for the physician-patient discussion concerning the proposed surgery. The reality of a cornual (interstitial) block seen at laparoscopy is made more convincing if the same finding was present on an earlier HSG. Only a patient with definitively proven, bilateral proximal interstitial blocks should be subjected to reimplantation surgery.

If an HSG is obtained either as the "final" evaluation in the infertility work-up or only, as in repeated uterotubal insufflations, for its "therapeutic" benefit, its continuing value must be questioned. However, as an adjuvant to laparoscopy and infertility surgery, the HSG can be of significant benefit.

LAPAROSCOPY

The panoramic view of the pelvis provided by the laparoscope is far superior to that provided by the culdoscope. Sources of pelvic pain can be pinpointed to a pelvic structure or confidently referred to another specialty. Tubal sterilization has become a 1-day, outpatient procedure. An intra-abdominal IUD can be removed without major surgery. For the infertility patient, laparoscopy has become an integral part of the entire investigation.

An ovulatory infertile patient with a normal postcoital test and semen analysis first undergoes hysterosalpingography. If the HSG is abnormal, laparoscopy should follow in the next cycle. As previously noted, discrepancies have been reported between HSG and laparoscopy up to 25% of the time. Therefore, if the HSG is entirely normal, 3 months should elapse before laparoscopy is undertaken. Although the therapeutic value of HSG is debatable, reports by Horbach and co-workers and Kletzky and Halbrecht indicate that a patient should be given some time to conceive after tubal flushing. If an abnormal parameter is found during the infertility work-up, e.g., a poor postcoital test, that abnormality should be treated. However, an HSG should be obtained so that pelvic status is illuminated somewhat before extensive time and therapy are devoted to correcting a cervical problem.

An anovulatory infertile patient should be evaluated and have ovulation therapeutically induced before an extensive infertility work-up is undertaken. Although a postcoital test should be deferred until ovulatory cycles have been achieved, an early semen analysis and HSG will rule out or rule in other significant pathology. If more than one factor exists to account for the infertility, pregnancy becomes even more difficult and the entire situation should be reviewed. But if all studies have been normal and clomiphene (Clomid, Serophene)-induced ovulatory cycles have been achieved for at least 6 months, laparoscopy should be performed to eliminate the possibility of unsuspected pelvic pathology. Even in an asymptomatic patient with unexplained infertility, laparoscopy can reveal significant disease 44-75% of the time.

In addition to its value in diagnosing unsuspected pelvic pathology, laparoscopy is an essential primary step when conservative infertility surgery is contemplated. The laparoscope can reveal a normal pelvis, thus eliminating the need for further surgery. With the laparoscope, the infertility surgeon can begin to define and categorize the degree of pelvic disease and distortion. In some instances, surgery can be deferred and the medical work-up and/or therapy continued on a more solid basis—the accurate laparoscopic view of the pelvis. In other cases, laparoscopy can reveal such extensive pelvic destruction that a laparotomy is avoided and the patient can be advised to abandon further infertility studies and consider alternatives such as adoption and/or in vitro fertilization. In view of its importance in determining the degree of pelvic pathology and the necessity for conservative infertility surgery, laparoscopy in the infertile patient should be carried out only by a gynecologic surgeon who is prepared to make endoscopic judgments and perform the required surgery.

As with any study of tubal function, laparoscopy should be performed in the follicular phase of the menstrual cycle. A thorough examination of the pelvis must be carried out, utilizing the accessory probe to lift, move, and feel all areas of the pelvis. Since the manipulations are extensive and adhesive disease is often encountered, a double-puncture technique under general endotracheal anesthesia is preferred. Prior pelvic surgery is usually not a deterrent to an adequate laparoscopic examination. In a study from this institution, 38 of the 155 infertility patients (25%) who underwent uneventful laparoscopy had a history of previous pelvic surgery, usually a salpingectomy for an ectopic pregnancy. During laparoscopy, chromopertubation is carried out with a dilute indigo carmine solution instilled via an Eder-Cohen cannula placed in the uterine cavity.

The decision to proceed with conservative infertility surgery is made at the time of laparoscopy. Therefore, prior to laparoscopy, all possible pelvic findings and surgical risks are explained to the patient and her husband. If pelvic pathology is confirmed, or unsuspected pathology found, the patient is prepared to undergo definitive tubal or pelvic surgery immediately following laparoscopy, utilizing the same anesthetic. Occasionally, minimal filmy adhesions can be lysed through the laparoscope. However, the laparoscope should not be considered a primary surgical tool in infertility. If surgical correction is found to be necessary, only a laparotomy provides the needed space and exposure to perform the job properly.

The presence or absence of additional infertility factors plays a prognostic role when combined with the laparoscopic findings. When laparoscopy reveals a normal pelvis, the presence of an infertility factor that has responded to treatment is an encouraging sign. Continuing to treat that problem may result in pregnancy. On the other hand, the patient who has minimal or unilateral disease at laparoscopy has a more favorable outlook for pregnancy if the pelvic pathology is not compounded by an additional infertility factor. In view of the generally poor results achieved with conservative tubal surgery, the laparoscope must be used very critically in order to select the best candidates for reparative operations.

SUGGESTED READING

Corson SL: Use of the laparoscope in the infertile patient. *Fertil Steril* 32:359, 1979

Drake TS, et al: Unexplained infertility—A reappraisal. *Obstet Gynecol* 50:644, 1977

Drake TS, Grunert GM: The unsuspected pelvic factor in the infertility investigation. *Fertil Steril* 34:27, 1980

Horbach JGM, Mattheis JB, Van Hall EV: Factors influencing the pregnancy rate following hysterosalpingography and their prognostic significance. *Fertil Steril* 24:15, 1973

Israel R, March CM: Diagnostic laparoscopy: A prognostic aid in the surgical management of infertility. *Am J Obstet Gynecol* 125:969, 1976

Israel R: Tubal factor. In Mishell DR Jr, Davajan V, eds: *Reproductive Endocrinology, Infertility and Contraception*. Philadelphia: FA Davis, 1979, pp 405-424

Klein TA, Richmond JA, Mishell DR Jr: Pelvic tuberculosis in an infertility clinic. *Obstet Gynecol* 48:99, 1976

Kletzky OA, Halbrecht JG: Hydrotubation in the treatment of the tubal factor. *Acta Eur Fertil* 2:31, 1970

Musich JR, Behrman SJ: Infertility laparoscopy in perspective: Review of five hundred cases. *Am J Obstet Gynecol* 143:293, 1982

Ozaras H: The value of plastic operations on the fallopian tubes in the treatment of female infertility. A clinical and radiological study. *Acta Obstet Gynecol Scand* 47:489, 1968

Stumpf PG, March CM: Febrile morbidity following hysterosalpingography: Identification of risk factors and recommendations for prophylaxis. *Fertil Steril* 33:487, 1980

96

Treatment of the Tubal Factor in Infertility: Salpingolysis and Salpingostomy

ROBERT ISRAEL, M.D.

Following the laparoscopic decision to perform conservative surgery, the surgeon and patient are faced with end results that leave much to be desired. In most instances, subsequent pregnancy rates do not exceed 50% and include abortions and ectopics as well as term gestations. With tubal closure, surgical correction can achieve patency in the majority of cases. However, a postoperative patent tube is no guarantee that pregnancy will ensue. Prior involvement of the endosalpinx, or its distortion by the surgery itself, may disturb the reproductive physiology of the fallopian tube to such an extent that pregnancy will never occur.

It is difficult to compare the results of conservative infertility surgery among surgeons or even among the patients of a single surgeon. The variability of pelvic pathology makes prospective, randomized studies virtually impossible. Are pelvic adhesions present or absent? If present, to what degree and in what areas? With distal tube disease, what degree of tubal abnormality exists? Are the tubes dilated and, if so, to what extent? Are intraluminal adhesions present? Do fimbrial remnants remain? What is the condition of the endosalpinx? Even in the available retrospective studies, many of these questions are never answered.

Another complexity is the fact that many surgeons view conservative surgery of the oviduct as very simple in comparison with other forms of abdominopelvic surgery. Extirpative surgery is more daring and demonstrative, but the judgment, skill, and patience required by the reconstructive surgeon are usually less well appreciated.

As the remote chance of a pregnancy is eliminated and the pelvis in general is less vascular, reparative surgery should be performed in the follicular phase of the cycle. Meticulous technique is a must, including excellent hemostasis. Appropriate magnification, either by a microscope or with loupes, is utilized to delineate fine fimbrial adhesions and approximate the tubal segments end to end. Tissue irrigation during surgery via a syringe containing physiologic lactated Ringer's solution with heparin added (mixed as 5,000 units in 1,000 ml of lactated Ringer's) is invaluable in identifying small bleeders and preventing clot formation. Sharp dissection of adhesions will produce fewer raw surfaces, and peritonealization of all denuded areas should be accomplished without anatomic distortion.

Delicate instruments are another must. Because of their minimal tissue reactivity, polyglycolic or polyglactic suture, 5-0, 6-0, or 7-0, should be utilized in and around the fallopian tubes. Alan Grant's advice should always be kept in mind: ". . . in tubal plastic surgery most extensive and complicated operations for infertility are followed by extensive and complicated adhesions. Sterility surgery should be as simple as possible for successful results. The surgeon who works on the sterile pelvis will get the best results from the operation that produces at least *one* good tube next to *one* good ovary, with the minimum of surgical trauma, and the minimal number of stitches."

Four basic operative procedures are utilized in conservative tubal surgery: (1) lysis of peritubal adhesions (salpingolysis), (2) opening of the occluded distal tube (salpingostomy), (3) correction of midsegment occlusions (end-to-end anastomosis), and (4) repair of cornual (interstitial) occlusions (cornual implantation). This chapter covers the first two operations; the other two are discussed in Chapter 97.

SALPINGOLYSIS

The most successful type of "tubal" surgery involves the lysis of peritubal and/or pelvic adhesions and does not involve primary tubal surgery. Ovum pickup is impeded by adhesions isolating the tubes and ovaries. The tubes may spill dye into isolated pockets of adhesions, but the fimbriated ends are open and endosalpinx is intact. Ultimate success depends on the extent and type of adhesions encountered, and whether they re-form postoperatively. In reported series, the overall pregnancy rate varies from 40% to 60%, with 70-95% of the pregnancies going to term.

In order to prevent the tubes and ovaries from falling back into areas of recently denuded adhesions, a uterine suspension should be part of the operative procedure. This is particularly important if the uterus is not in an anterior position at the conclusion of the surgery. Because it utilizes the distal, weaker portions of the round ligaments in the suspension, leaving the proximal, stronger areas for support, the Gilliam uterine suspension is preferred.

Various techniques are reported to reduce adhesions postoperatively. Although valid statistical support regarding their efficacy is lacking, most of these ancillary measures are strongly (perhaps emotionally) advocated by their proponents. A broad-spectrum antibiotic can be given prophylactically and should be started preoperatively to achieve an adequate tissue level at the time of surgery. In an effort to dissolve any fibrinous exudate postoperatively and delay fibroblast and collagen formation, Replogle et al suggested a medical regimen employing high doses of promethazine (25 mg) and dexamethasone (20 mg) administered IM in separate syringes 2-3 hours preoperatively and leaving a similar dose in the cul-de-sac at the time of peritoneal closure. Beginning 4 hours postoperatively, the same dose is given IM every 4 hours for 12 doses. As wound healing is delayed, the fascia should be closed with permanent suture material and the skin sutures left in place 10-14 days.

This therapy was utilized in conservative infertility surgery by a collaborative study group. A final 3-year follow-up report was published by Horne et al in 1973. The 240 patients underwent a variety of conservative operations for pelvic adhesions, tubal obstruction, and endometriosis. The amount of pelvic pathology encountered was not quantitated by individual cases or groups of cases. The overall pregnancy rate was 52%, with 73% of the pregnancies ending in term deliveries. However, when broken down by operative procedures, the results do not justify the expensive, relatively risky promethazine-dexamethasone treatment.

In an NIH study, diZerega and Hodgen compared adhesion formation in monkeys subjected to fimbrial trauma and subsequently exposed to the promethazine-dexamethasone protocol outlined above (with the addition of ampicillin) or a 10% solution of dextran 40 (Rheomacrodex) or a 32% solution of dextran 70 (Hyskon), both administered intraperitoneally. Only dextran 70 retained tubal patency in all animals, with only a minimal, unilateral peritubal adhesion noted in one monkey. Dextran 70 was still present in the pelvis 5 days following instillation, by which time significant tubal repair had occurred. Physiologically, dextran may act to separate the surfaces of recently traumatized tissues by increasing the peritoneal colloid osmotic pressure, thereby inducing an influx of fluid into the abdominal cavity. Additionally, it covers the peritoneal surfaces with a very fine, silicon-like film, which could hinder adhesion formation. However, the results of ongoing prospective, comparative studies of adhesion formation following infertility surgery in women are needed before diZerega and Hodgen's encouraging work can be confirmed.

SALPINGOSTOMY

Opening distal tubal occlusions is the least successful type of tubal surgery. A hydrosalpinx is the end stage of generalized tubal disease. Although the surgeon may be able to open the tube, and have it remain open, residual anatomic and physiologic damage to the rest of the tube is usually sufficient to disrupt the reproductive processes necessary to achieve an intrauterine pregnancy. The fimbria are often gone, the endosalpinx is denuded partially or totally, the tubal musculature is nonfunctional, and various degrees of tubal dilation may be present. Additionally, distal tubal closure is often associated with pelvic adhesions varying from minimal and filmy to extensive and thick.

To compound the salpingostomy problem, some surgeons include lesser degrees of fimbrial pathology in this surgical category. Fimbrial "agglutination" and "phimosis" are two of the favorites. Teasing apart filmy strands between the fimbria or "dilating" the fimbriated end of the tube with small bougies does not represent salpingostomy surgery. If they can be considered "indicated" forms of conservative infertility surgery, they should be classified in a subcategory under salpingolysis.

Surgically, distal tubal occlusion has been approached by two different methods. In both, the hydrosalpinx is opened through its central dimple with iris scissors or needle electrocautery. Utilizing electrodissection, the distal tubal scars are excised and any fimbrial bridges lysed. In locating and eliminating fimbrial adhesions, magnification with a microscope or loupes is helpful. Repeat chromopertubation should be carried out and the lumen investigated for adhesions with fine metal probes or, preferably, retrograde instillation of lactated Ringer's solution. At this point, the operation can proceed in one of two directions: with or without a prosthetic device to maintain patency.

If a prosthetic device is used, the oldest and best known is the Rock-Mulligan hood, a Silastic implant that is slid over the newly created ostium and secured to the serosomucosal junction by three stay sutures of 5-0 Mersilene. The hood requires removal at a second laparotomy 4-5 months later. More recently, Roland has introduced a modified hood device that has a "tail" to be brought out to the anterior abdominal wall. At a later date, traction on the tail removes the entire prosthesis without the necessity for a second laparotomy. Results with Roland's spiral Teflon splint have been limited. As adhesion formation has been reported to occur around these devices, and they do not improve postoperative patency/pregnancy rates, their use today does not seem justified.

If a prosthetic device is not used, a cuff salpingostomy is performed by turning back the mucosal edges of the fimbriated end of the tube and suturing them to the serosa overlying the ampulla. Either 6-0 or 7-0 polyglycolic or polyglactic suture should be used in creating the cuff, and no more than four to six interrupted sutures should ever be necessary. Utilizing lactated Ringer's solution with heparin for irrigation, small bleeders on the mucosal edge should be specifically identified and gently fulgurated with a hand-controlled, bipolar forceps or needle electrocautery.

In addition to the ancillary procedures—antibiotics, dextran, and uterine suspension—already discussed, postoperative hydrotubation should be carried out via a No. 8 or No. 10 intrauterine Foley catheter or Jarcho cannula, utilizing 50 ml of dextran 40. Although dextran 70 may be preferable, it is too viscous to instill transcervically through small-bore equipment. Broad-spectrum antibiotic coverage, e.g., doxycycline (Vibramycin) 100 mg PO bid, should be given 2 days before, the day of, and 2 days after hydrotubation.

Routinely, hydrotubation is performed once while the patient is still hospitalized and is repeated 1 week after discharge. It is continued once per cycle in the midfollicular phase for 6 months. A hysterosalpingogram should replace one hydrotubation between the third and sixth postoperative months. Although hydrotubation may improve the postoperative tubal patency rate, there is no evidence that tubal flushing improves the pregnancy rate. However, with antibiotic coverage and meticulous performance, the benefit of hydrotubation outweighs any potential risks.

From published reports, cuff salpingostomy with postoperative hydrotubation yields overall pregnancy rates of 10-40%, with term pregnancies ranging from 5% to 50%. As noted, the ultimate results depend on the anatomic and physiologic condition of the remainder of the tube rather than on the specific operative method. If tubal patency were the only necessary end point, postoperative pregnancy rates would be much higher. After cuff salpingostomy, the percentage of patent tubes varies from 50% to 90%. Usually, the surgeon can open the pipeline, but he cannot restore proper function.

The increased incidence of ectopic pregnancies in postsalpingostomy tubes reinforces the concept that tubal closure is not the only problem in these cases. With an indigent population prone to pelvic inflammatory disese, postsalpingostomy tubal pregnancies occur with disturbing frequency. In 27 patients who underwent cuff salpingostomy with postoperative hydrotubations at this institution, 10 pregnancies occurred in seven patients during a 5-34-month (mean, 15-month) follow-up period.

Superficially, a 26% pregnancy rate coupled with a 60% tubal patency rate may seem acceptable. As suggested by Umezaki et al, salpingostomy-treated tubes may require a longer healing time, so results could improve with continued follow-up. However, of the 10 pregnancies, only two culminated in term gestations and six tubal ectopics occurred. Since 60% of the salpingostomy pregnancies resulted in tubal implantations, the risk/benefit ratio of this type of tubal surgery must be seriously considered. Although the significant amount of pelvic disease found in a clinic population may explain the high tubal-to-intrauterine gestation ratio, Swolin, despite meticulously performed surgery utilizing microdissection techniques, has reported comparable findings from a Scandinavian population exhibiting less extensive pelvic pathology. If an alternative fertility approach, such as in vitro fertilization, ever achieves a successfully repetitive pregnancy rate of 25-30%, the first tubal reparative surgery it will replace is distal salpingostomy.

SUGGESTED READING

diZerega GS, Hodgen GD: Prevention of postoperative tubal adhesions. *Am J Obstet Gynecol* 136:173, 1980

Grant A: Infertility surgery of the oviduct. *Fertil Steril* 22:496, 1971

Horne HW Jr, et al: The prevention of postoperative pelvic adhesions following conservative operative treatment for human infertility. *Int J Fertil* 18:109, 1973

Kistner RW, Patton GW Jr: Surgery of the oviduct. In *Atlas of Infertility Surgery*. Boston: Little, Brown, 1975

Patton GW Jr: Pregnancy outcome following microsurgical fimbrioplasty. *Fertil Steril* 37:150, 1982

Replogle RL, Johnson BA, Gross RD: Prevention of postoperative intestinal adhesions with combined promethazine and dexamethasone therapy. *Ann Surg* 163:580, 1966

Roland M: Spiral Teflon splint for tuboplasty involving fimbria. *Obstet Gynecol* 36:359, 1970

Swolin K: Electromicrosurgery and salpingostomy, long-term results. *Am J Obstet Gynecol* 121:418, 1975

Umezaki C, Katayama KP, Jones HW Jr: Pregnancy rates after reconstructive surgery on the fallopian tubes. *Obstet Gynecol* 43:418, 1974

97

Treatment of the Tubal Factor in Infertility: End-to-End Anastomosis and Cornual Implantation

ROBERT ISRAEL, M.D.

END-TO-END ANASTOMOSIS

The most successful primary tubal surgery is the correction of midtubal occlusion secondary to previous tubal sterilization. The remainder of the tube, proximally and distally, is normal and the pelvis is free of adhesions. Additionally, the patient has proven her fertility and is infertile only because of tubal sterilization.

As has been stressed with any form of conservative surgery, laparoscopy should precede laparotomy to confirm the normal status of the pelvis and to decide that adequate tubal segments exist for anastomosis. If the sterilization was performed by laparoscopic fulguration, with or without tubal transection, a hysterosalpingogram should be obtained prior to diagnostic laparoscopy to determine the extent of the interstitial-isthmic fill. At laparoscopy, the most proximal portions of the tubes often are difficult to visualize even when they fill with dye.

Ideally, for end-to-end reconstruction, the prior tubal sterilization should have been a small, midtubal (Pomeroy) segmental resection. If a satisfactory end-to-end anastomosis can be performed in the isthmus, success should be extremely high. In a young woman, sterilization by segmental midtubal resection or laparoscopic sterilization with a band or clip should be considered the technique of choice. With these procedures, if the future brings a change of mind, reanastomosis success will be high.

Unfortunately, reversal of laparoscopic tubal fulguration, especially if it was performed with unipolar equipment, is often impossible because insufficient tubal segments remain. If no proximal tube can be located, even with shaving back of the uterine cornu, or if the proximal segments are abnormal as a result of poststerilization changes, implantation of the distal tube into the uterine wall is the only alternative. For implantation surgery, the distal tubal segments must be at least 5 cm long. Fimbriectomy represents even worse reversal odds than laparoscopic tubal fulguration. With removal of the distal tube, only cuff salpingostomy is available as a reversal procedure, and even this approach requires a residual tube extending into the midampulla.

The technique of end-to-end anastomosis requires excision of the scarred site of the previous tubal sterilization and approximation of the distal and proximal segments. Loupe magnification or the use of an operating microscope, especially in isthmic-isthmic or isthmic-interstitial anastomoses, has improved the subsequent pregnancy rates by 10-15% compared with surgery done without magnification. The tubal ends are pulled together with three or four interrupted 7-0 or 8-0 polyglycolic or polyglactic sutures placed through the muscularis, but not including the mucosa. The serosa is closed over the anastomotic site with interrupted 6-0 sutures of the same material. When the operating microscope is used, nonabsorbable monofilament 9-0 or 10-0 nylon sutures are preferred.

The pregnancy rate following microsurgical end-to-end anastomosis should be in the 60-75% range. Gomel's 80% pregnancy rate remains the highest reported. At USC, in our private population, I continue to achieve a 72-78% pregnancy rate following end-to-end anastomosis. The vast majority of these pregnancies are term births. The spontaneous abortion rate is unchanged from a normal obstetric population. However, the tubal pregnancy rate following end-to-end reanastomosis increases to 5%.

CORNUAL IMPLANTATION

The least frequently performed, and technically most complex, reparative tubal surgery is the correction of cornual (interstitial) occlusion. The anatomic site of obstruction includes at least the proximal segment (adjacent to the endometrium) of the interstitial portion of the tube, so that an end-to-end anastomosis, even with the use of cornual shaving, is impossible. Usually the patient has a history of "uterine invasion"—D&C, pregnancy with sepsis, IUD insertion, and so forth. In many instances, these events were not accompanied by any clinical evidence of pelvic sepsis, yet interstitial occlusion was the end result. Additionally, salpingitis isthmica nodosa, a condition unique to the interstitial and isthmic portions of the tube, may create blockage.

As the cornual segment of the tube is very important in reproduction and impossible to duplicate surgically, it is imperative that an interstitial block be proven definitively before surgical correction is undertaken. At least two tubal evaluation studies, one of which is laparoscopy, must indicate clearly that cornual occlusion exists bilaterally or in the only remaining fallopian tube. In addition, laparoscopy must demonstrate that the rest of the tube(s) is perfectly normal and sufficiently long (5 cm or greater) and that the pelvis is free of adhesions. As the chance of subsequent pregnancy is remote, conservative tubal surgery is contraindicated in the presence of proximal and distal blocks existing in the same tube. Occasionally, even laparoscopy does not indicate the extent of intraluminal disease, and probing of the tubal lumen at laparotomy will reveal that the block actually extends out into the ampulla even though the external tube and fimbria appear normal. With this degree of pathology, reconstructive surgery is impossible and alternative methods (in vitro fertilization, adoption) must be recommended.

Following definitive diagnosis, the surgical technique involves reimplantation of the normal distal tube into the uterus. Tubal implantation can be performed in the classical manner by isolating each cornu, resecting the area, and implanting the patent distal tube(s) into the resected space. Alternatively, the distal tubes can be implanted into the posterior uterine wall at the level of the utero-ovarian ligaments.

Initially, in both techniques, the tube is explored through the fimbriated end into the isthmus, utilizing a fine lacrimal duct probe or retrograde irrigation. If patency is present into the isthmus and cornual implantation is planned, the most proximal isthmus and cornu are excised by securing the blood supply in the proximal mesosalpinx and suturing the ascending branch of the uterine artery on the lateral uterine wall. To achieve even better hemostasis, 20 units of vasopressin (Pitressin) can be diluted in 20 ml of saline and injected in and around the cornual areas.

The cornual segment is wedged out, starting with an elliptical incision around the tube and continuing down through the myometrium to the endometrial cavity. The latter is easy to identify, as it has been stained blue by prior dye instillation. The endometrial cavity opening is smaller in diameter than the one on the serosal surface of the uterus. It is unnecessary to open the entire fundus between the areas of cornual resection. If an intrauterine-intratubal splint is utilized, it can be pushed through one cornu and positioned well by manipulating it with a clamp through the other open cornu. Avoiding a large fundal incision keeps the uterus more intact and secure during a subsequent pregnancy.

Before the isolated, distal tubal segment is implanted, its proximal end is split for a distance of 1-2 cm and single "U-sutures" of 4-0 polyglycolic or polyglactic are placed through each flap, not tied, and held long. When the proximal portion of the tubal segment is drawn into the cornual opening, these sutures are used to secure the tube by passing them from the endometrial cavity out to the serosal surface of the uterus, where they are tied. At the conclusion of the implantation, any defects in the myometrium and uterine serosa are closed with interrupted 4-0 polyglycolic or polyglactic sutures, but the serosal surface of the tube is not attached to any of these sutures, as any limitation of tubal motility may be detrimental to its subsequent function. Defects in the mesosalpinx are also closed.

The majority of conservative infertility surgeons favor the use of an intra-uterine-intratubal splint in cornual implantation surgery. A Silastic ring prosthesis with a stainless steel core and double limbs, one of which splints each implantation site, is available. However, a simple prosthesis can be constructed utilizing a stringless IUD with a length of Silastic tubing tied to the upper segment of the IUD to splint the reimplanted tubes. Transcervical removal of the splint is carried out 5-6 weeks postoperatively, using an IUD removal hook. Following splint removal, hydrotubation or an HSG should be used to determine tubal patency.

Following the article by Peterson, Musich, and Behrman in 1977 espousing posterior uterine wall tubal implantation for reversal of sterilization in the absence of proximal tubes, this simpler form of tubal-uterine implantation has gained favor. With short distal segments, a transverse incision in the posterior uterine wall at the level of the ovarian ligaments permits easy placement of one or both tubal segments. The technique is similar to classical cornual implantation, except that after isolation of the patent distal segments, vasopressin is injected into the posterior uterine wall and the transverse incision is made into the endometrial cavity. No intrauterine-intratubal splint is utilized. With the distal tubes prepared for implantation, they are pulled in side by side through the uterine incision and secured similarly to tubes reimplanted in the cornual areas. Postoperatively, pregnancy is avoided for 6 months and a hysterosalpingogram with lateral views is obtained at 3-4 months.

The vast majority of studies composed of more than 20 cornual implantations report overall pregnancy rates between 35% and 50%. However, spontaneous abortions and a 10-12% rate of tubal pregnancies are included in the total figure. As with other forms of conservative tubal surgery, postoperative tubal patency rates are at least double the pregnancy rates. Although pregnancy and patency rates do not differ significantly with or without tubal splinting, most recent reports suggest that an intrauterine-intratubal splint be used. However, as in many areas of conservative infertility surgery, no prospective, randomized study exists comparing the use and nonuse of splints. In the two published reports concerning posterior uterine wall tubal implantation, the term pregnancy rates have been reported to be 50% (in a study group of 16 patients) and 60% (in a group of 35 patients).

When intrauterine pregnancy follows uterotubal implantation, uterine rupture occurs as an occasional, but potentially disastrous, complication. Any patient agreeing to implantation surgery should be aware that any subsequent pregnancy will require careful antenatal supervision and should be terminated by cesarean section. Even though the incidence of uterine rupture following uterotubal implantation is less than 1%, most obstetricians will not permit these patients to undergo labor, but, rather, select cesarean section for delivery.

MICROSURGERY/LASER SURGERY

Although relatively crude eyeglass magnification had been used for many years by some tubal surgeons, only in the last few years has "microsurgery" become popular and successful in reconstructive pelvic surgery. Although gynecologic microsurgery includes magnification with an operating microscope or binocular lenses ($\times$3-6), its definition encompasses ophthalmic-type instrumentation, gentle tissue handling, well-controlled hemostasis, extremely fine (7-0 through 10-0) sutures, and the ancillary techniques already described to reduce postoperative adhesion formation.

Although all of these surgical techniques have enhanced conservative reproductive surgery, magnification by itself seems to have improved the pregnancy rates in only one form of reconstructive tubal surgery. Following end-to-end tubal reanastomosis utilizing an operating microscope or binocular lens magnification, pregnancy rates have improved by 10-20% over conventional, nonmagnified end-to-end anastomosis. However, there is no evidence that magnification is associated with higher pregnancy rates in other forms of tubal surgery, such as salpingostomy or salpingolysis.

It is difficult to compare the results of any type of conservative infertility surgery when the operations are performed by different surgeons. Ideally, variations in surgical skills could be controlled by having the same surgeon alternately perform macro- and microsurgical repairs. However, encountering varying pelvic conditions could skew even this approach. Perhaps the ultimate contribution of microsurgical principles will be their impact on gynecologic surgery in general. With the emphasis on gentle tissue handling and well-controlled hemostasis, routine gynecologic surgery, especially when it involves preservation of the uterus and adnexa, will be carried out with more care and attention to detail, so that future reproductive potential will not be compromised.

If the role of microsurgery is still being discussed and analyzed, the value of the carbon dioxide laser in tubal surgery must be considered totally undefined. Despite the proliferation of publicity, the gynecologic literature lacks any prospective or reasonably large retrospective studies analyzing the results of conservative tubal surgery performed with the laser. Potentially, the major advantage of laser surgery is the hemostasis obtained when tissue is vaporized. In addition, the operative time should be shortened and surgical precision enhanced. However, Baggish and Chong, utilizing a CO_2 laser for tubal reanastomosis in a small group of rabbits and an even smaller group of humans, found that substituting laser welding for reanastomotic site sutures did nothing to hold the anastomosis together structurally. Whether patency and/or pregnancy rates are improved following reconstructive laser surgery remains to be shown. At the moment, the laser stands where microsurgery did several years ago. It would benefit by less sound and fury and more scientific precision and evaluation.

SUMMARY

It is difficult to analyze the reported results of conservative tubal surgery. Great variation exists between the number of operative procedures performed per series, the degree of tubal and adhesive disease encountered, the specific surgical techniques utilized, and the ancillary therapeutic measures employed. In addition, many series mention only the total pregnancy rate and fail to break this figure down into spontaneous abortions, ectopic pregnancies, and term gestations. Although the total pregnancy rate may satisfy the surgeon, the couple considering conservative surgery is interested primarily in the expected outcome of pregnancy. Postoperatively, the only happy outcome

TABLE 97-1. RANGE OF REPORTED PREGNANCY OUTCOMES FOLLOWING
SURGICAL CORRECTION OF THE TUBAL FACTOR IN INFERTILITY

Operation	Outcome (%)			
	Pregnancy rate	Spontaneous abortion	Ectopic pregnancy	Term gestation
Salpingolysis	40-60	10-20	1-2	70-90
Salpingostomy	10-40	10-20	15-40	45-55
End-to-end anastomosis	60-75	10-20	5-10	60-70
Implantation	35-55	10-20	10-15	50-60

for the infertile patient is a term gestation. A review of the literature yields the ranges of pregnancy outcomes summarized in Table 97-1 for the four surgical procedures discussed in this chapter and in Chapter 96.

In view of their frequent involvement in the etiology of infertility, evaluation of the fallopian tubes will remain an extremely important part of the infertility investigation. Until in vitro fertilization or tubal replacement (transplant or prosthetic) becomes a consistent reality, reparative tubal surgery will continue to be the only avenue of potential success open to the woman with a positive tubal factor.

SUGGESTED READING

Baggish MS, Chong AP: Carbon dioxide laser microsurgery of the fallopian tube. *Obstet Gynecol* 58:111, 1981

Fayez JA, Suliman SO: Infertility surgery of the oviduct: Comparison between macrosurgery and microsurgery. *Fertil Steril* 37:73, 1982

Gomel V: Microsurgical reversal of female sterilization: A reappraisal. *Fertil Steril* 33:587, 1980

Israel R: Tubal factor. In Mishell DR Jr, Davajan V, eds: *Reproductive Endocrinology, Infertility and Contraception*. Philadelphia: FA Davis, 1979, pp 405-424

Kistner RW, Patton GW Jr: Surgery of the oviduct. In *Atlas of Infertility Surgery*. Boston: Little, Brown, 1975, pp 95-171

Levinson CJ: Implantation procedures for intramural obstruction. *J Reprod Med* 26:347, 1981

Peterson EP, Musich JR, Behrman SJ: Uterotubal implantation and obstetric outcome after previous sterilization. *Am J Obstet Gynecol* 128:662, 1977

98

Endometriosis: Diagnostic Evaluation

ROBERT ISRAEL, M.D.

In 1921, J.A. Sampson described endometriosis as "the presence of ectopic tissue which possesses the histological structure and function of the uterine mucosa." Although the occurrence of aberrant endometrium had been described by various individuals in the 19th century, it was not until Sampson's classic contribution that there was any appreciation of the frequency, pathology, and clinical characteristics of this enigmatic gynecologic disorder.

INCIDENCE AND DISTRIBUTION

Since endometriosis is dependent on the ovarian steroids for its existence and proliferation, its occurrence and clinical importance are confined generally to the reproductive years. Although Kempers et al have reported active postmenopausal endometriosis *without* exogenous hormone use, the peak incidence is in the fourth decade. The "typical" patient is nulliparous, in her late 20s or early 30s, intelligent, egocentric, overanxious, and a perfectionist. Marriage and childbearing have often been deferred.

Whether the emergence and widespread use of steroidal contraceptives over the past 20 years have reduced the incidence of endometriosis by reducing menstrual flow, thereby preventing tubal reflux, remains an unanswered question. However, if operative statistics from predominantly private-practice hospitals are used, endometriosis continues to be a significant gynecologic entity. Gross or microscopic endometriosis was noted in 14-21% of all laparotomies performed for gynecologic disease between 1950 and 1970. Depending on the population being investigated, endometriosis has been noted in 30-40% of laparoscopies performed for the investigation of infertility.

Although in many instances the endometriosis does not appear to be interfering with the normal reproductive process, 30-40% of patients with endometriosis have concomitant infertility. Sperm ascension, ovulation, and ovum pickup and transport can all take place, but the presence of even minimal pelvic endometriosis seems to be the causative infertility factor.

SITES

The most frequent pelvic locations for endometriosis are the ovaries, uterine ligaments (round, broad, uterosacral), pelvic peritoneum, and rectovaginal septum. Other sites include the umbilicus, laparotomy scars, hernial sacs, appendix, small intestine, rectum, sigmoid, bladder, ureters, vulva-vagina-cervix, lymph nodes, extremities, pleural cavity, and lung. The multiplicity and widespread distribution of these sites makes acceptance of any *one* histogenetic theory difficult. Possibly histochemical and immunologic investigations will provide some definitive clues to the many unanswered questions raised by the presence of endometriosis.

GROSS PATHOLOGY

Like everything else connected with endometriosis, the gross pathology is characterized by variability. With mild involvement, the adnexa will be free of adhesions, and a variable number of reddish-blue (raspberry) or brown, fibrin-like implants will be present on the ovaries and/or peritoneal surfaces. With progressive disease, the older implants will have coalesced and "burnt out," leaving scarred, retracted areas that may involve peritoneal surface *only* or include peritubal and periovarian involvement and fixation.

More significant ovarian involvement means the formation of single or multiple, unilateral or bilateral endometrial cysts (endometriomas, "chocolate" cysts). Even when quite small, the cysts show a strong tendency to perforate, with escape of menstrual blood and subsequent ovarian adherence to any adjacent structure, usually the posterior surface of the broad ligament or uterus. If early perforation does not occur, larger endometriomas form with thicker walls and few surrounding adhesions. When the uterine ligaments are involved, especially the uterosacrals, endometriotic nodules form that can often be palpated on bimanual or rectovaginal examination. Endometrial islands may occur on any part of the pelvic peritoneum, involving the serosal surface of any pelvic structure. Occasionally, invasion and penetration occur in the sigmoid so that progressive submucosal scarring results in luminal constriction. Mucosal involvement with associated rectal bleeding is a late phenomenon in bowel endometriosis.

MICROSCOPIC PATHOLOGY

Definitive diagnosis requires microscopic demonstration of endometrial tissue, preferably both glands and stroma. However, a wide range of patterns may occur. Some specimens reveal endometrium that histologically and functionally cannot be distinguished from normal uterine epithelium. In others, the endometrium has been completely denuded due to repeated menstrual bleeding and desquamation. Hemorrhage and pigment-laden macrophages may be the only microscopic clues. No specific pathologic diagnosis can be made definitively in one-third of clinically typical endometriosis cases.

Endometriomas, when *lacking* endometrial glands and stroma, can often be identified by a broad surrounding zone rich in large phagocytic cells laden with blood pigment (hemosiderin). These pseudoxanthoma cells have a superficial resemblance to lutein cells. When *present*, the endometrial glands usually have a proliferative or cystic hyperplastic appearance, containing low-lying and inactive cells. Accompanying, and often surrounding, the endometrial reaction may be a zone of hyalinized fibrous tissue.

Malignant changes occurring in endometriomas are very rare and always of low grade (adenoacanthoma). Although 10% of endometrioid ovarian carcinomas are associated with ovarian endometriosis, it is unusual for malignant transformation of the endometriosis to be demonstrable. However, endometriosis has a cancer-like characteristic in the insidious, invasive way it spreads, terminating in fibrosis and scarring of any, and all, pelvic structures.

DIAGNOSIS

The symptomatology associated with endometriosis can be as variable as anything else connected with the disease. Dysmenorrhea, dyspareunia, and dyschezia may be present as a symptom complex or individually. However, even with extensive endometriosis, pain may not be a significant clinical entity. Unless rupture occurs, ovarian endometriomas can expand painlessly. On the other hand, incapacitating dysmenorrhea and pelvic pain may be associated with minimal amounts of active peritoneal surface endometriosis. Thus, the degree of endometriotic involvement and spread bears no constant relationship to the presence or absence of subjective discomfort.

Over 50% of patients with endometriosis complain of dysmenorrhea. Usually, it is the secondary or acquired variety, although if primary dysmenorrhea is present, endometriosis can worsen it. The dysmenorrhea can be attributed to secretory changes in the endometriotic islands with subsequent miniature menstruation and bleeding in areas encapsulated by fibrous tissue or to the release of prostaglandins from the aberrant endometrium. With involvement of the rectovaginal septum or uterosacral ligaments, the dysmenorrhea is often referred to the rectum or lower sacrococcygeal area, and dyspareunia is a common complaint. Dyschezia results from endometriotic bleeding in the rectosigmoid muscularis or serosa with subsequent fibrosis. Occasionally, abnormal uterine bleeding, e.g., premenstrual spotting, may occur.

Although the diagnosis may be suggested by the history, it cannot be made with any certainty based on symptoms alone. Even a pelvic examination, which, at times, can be quite distinctive, *cannot* be considered pathognomonic. Tender, nodular uterosacral ligaments combined with a fixed, retroverted uterus are findings highly suggestive of endometriosis, but inflammation and cancer cannot be ruled out by bimanual examination.

For definitive diagnosis, endoscopic visualization of the pelvis must be carried out prior to institution of therapy. When lesions are identified and doubt still remains, confirmatory transendoscopic biopsy should be performed. Although culdoscopy was the diagnostic procedure of choice from 1945, when it was introduced, to the early 1970s, it has now been replaced by laparoscopy. In addition to providing a panoramic view and more operative mobility, the laparoscope can be used regardless of the extent of endometriotic spread. Culdoscopy, however, is contraindicated in the presence of a fixed, nodular cul-de-sac—not an uncommon feature in moderate or severe endometriosis.

Double-puncture laparoscopy should be utilized so that a careful, complete pelvic inspection can be carried out. Additionally, one of several available instruments for uterine manipulation should be secured in the cervical canal. Preferably, it should have a central cannula for subsequent transuterine-tubal dye instillation.

The procedure requires a transabdominal operation under general anesthesia; to make it worthwhile, the surgeon must be compulsively thorough in his inspection and investigation of the peritoneal cavity. The palpating probe, placed through the accessory trocar, can be used as an examining finger running over various structures, e.g., the uterosacral ligaments, to detect subperitoneal implants. Each ovary must be lifted up to visualize the undersurface adjoining the broad ligaments. The appendix and the serosa of any bowel in the pelvis should be carefully inspected for endometriotic implants.

Until Acosta et al proposed a classification in 1973, the extent of pelvic endometriosis was described by individual cases. Although it may seem a small step forward, uniformity in classification has helped categorize and analyze the success or failure of the various therapeutic modalities used in the treatment of endometriosis.

The most recent and widely accepted classification is that of the American Fertility Society (AFS), published in the December 1979 issue of *Fertility and Sterility*. It uses four categories: stage I (mild), stage II (moderate), stage III (severe), and stage IV (extensive), based on the degree of involvement of the peritoneum, ovaries, and tubes. Involvement is categorized as active endometriosis and/or adhesions. Points are assigned based on dimensional spread in three categories: <1 cm, 1-3 cm, and >3 cm. The AFS* provides copies of its classification system, for a nominal fee, in the form of individual tear-off sheets. They can be used in the operating room to immediately stage the extent of disease.

*The American Fertility Society
 1608 13th Avenue South
 Birmingham, Ala. 35205

SUGGESTED READING

Acosta AA, et al: A proposed classification of pelvic endometriosis. *Obstet Gynecol* 42:19, 1973

American Fertility Society: Classification of endometriosis. *Fertil Steril* 32:633, 1979

Buttram VC Jr, Betts JW: Endometriosis. *Curr Prob Obstet Gynecol* II:11, 1979

Drake TS, O'Brien WF, Ramwell PW, Metz SA: Peritoneal fluid thromboxane B_2 and 6-keto-prostaglandin $F_{1\alpha}$ in endometriosis. *Am J Obstet Gynecol* 140:401, 1981

Israel R: Endometriosis. In Mishell DR Jr, Davajan V, eds: *Reproductive Endocrinology, Infertility and Contraception*. Philadelphia: FA Davis, 1979, pp 425-438

Kempers RD, et al: Postmenopausal endometriosis. *Surg Gynecol Obstet* 111:348, 1960

Peterson EP, Behrman SJ: Laparoscopy of the infertile patient. *Obstet Gynecol* 36:363, 1970

Ridley JH: The histogenesis of endometriosis. *Obstet Gynecol Surv* 23:1, 1968

Sampson JA: Perforating hemorrhagic (chocolate) cysts of the ovary. *Arch Surg* 3:245, 1921

99

Endometriosis: Treatment

ROBERT ISRAEL, M.D.

The therapeutic approach to endometriosis must be individualized according to the patient's desired reproductive status. There are three categories: therapy for infertility, symptomatic therapy that preserves reproductive capacity, and therapy following completion of childbearing.

THERAPY FOR INFERTILITY

Hormonal suppression and/or conservative surgery constitute the available therapeutic modalities. Diagnosis and stage (mild, moderate, severe) are established by laparoscopy and become the basis for selection of subsequent therapy.

Mild Endometriosis

This is the most unsettled therapeutic area in endometriosis. Satisfactory pregnancy rates (50-75%) have been reported with laparoscopic observation only, laparoscopic fulguration only, fulguration and danazol (Danocrine) therapy, or danazol alone.

If fulguration is used, it should be limited to areas not immediately adjacent or contiguous to bowel or bladder. The presence of nonvisible, microscopic implants must be considered. Common sense would suggest that unless the endometriosis is extremely minimal (scattered dots), postlaparoscopic danazol (200 mg qid × 6 months) seems reasonable. It is not known whether danazol can be used at a lower dose and/or for a shorter period in cases of infertility. As continuous oral contraceptive therapy is associated with post-therapy pregnancy rates of only 20-40%, contraceptive drugs should not be used in the treatment of infertility.

Moderate Endometriosis

With more extensive pathology (ovarian endometriomas, adhesions), conservative surgery becomes the therapeutic choice. With moderate endometriosis, there is no evidence that preoperative danazol therapy improves the postoperative pregnancy rate, but it may make surgery less difficult technically. The laparoscope should be used as an operative instrument only in minimal degrees of moderate endometriosis, e.g., small (<1 cm) endometriomas and/or filmy adhesions. Since complication rates rise with "endoscopic gymnastics," extensive laparoscopic surgical manipulations are contraindicated. If the patient has been prepared for all diagnostic possibilities, laparotomy can follow laparoscopy under the same anesthesia.

Endometriosis surgery must be performed with meticulous care and excellent hemostasis. The uterus and adnexa must be mobilized and carefully inspected. The serosa of the large and small bowel either in or contiguous to the pelvis must be visualized for any endometriotic involvement. If the appendix is an endometriotic site, an appendectomy is indicated. All areas of endometriosis should be excised and reperitonealized as well as possible.

The ovaries must be palpated carefully and cystic areas punctured or incised so that small endometriomas are not missed. Ovarian endometriomas should be excised; a major portion of one or both ovaries may have to be resected. Pregnancy can still occur following unilateral oophorectomy and resection of three-quarters of the contralateral ovary. In reconstructing an ovary, the cortical surfaces should be approximated as closely as possible using nonreactive 5-0 polyglycolic or polyglactic suture in order to reduce the chance of subsequent adhesions.

If secondary dysmenorrhea is part of the symptomatology, presacral neurectomy and resection of the uterosacral ligaments at their uterine insertion are indicated. If the uterus is not anterior and/or the cul-de-sac is scarred, a uterine suspension should be performed, preferably a Gilliam type.

Although there is no evidence that postoperative danazol therapy improves the pregnancy rate or reduces recurrences, if residual endometriosis exists, a short course (200 mg qid × 3 months) seems reasonable. Prophylactic antibiotic treatment started preoperatively and high-molecular-weight dextran (dextran 70, 200-300 ml) left in the pelvis at the conclusion of surgery may be of benefit. With moderate endometriosis, pregnancy rates after reconstructive surgery should be in the area of 50%.

Severe Endometriosis

With extensive pathology attributable to endometriosis, the postsurgical pregnancy outlook will be 25-30% at best. In addition to massive pelvic adhesions, the fallopian tubes can be involved to the point of closure. Reconstructive or ablative surgery for severe degrees of endometriosis can be the most difficult gynecologic surgery encountered, more difficult than even end-stage salpingitis or oncology operations.

In the presence of extensive and/or deep-seated rectovaginal septum endometriosis, preoperative therapy with danazol (200 mg qid × 4-6 weeks) may enhance the surgery by reducing and/or softening the active areas of endometriosis. As a corollary, with similar surgical findings, postoperative short-term (2-3 months) danazol therapy may suppress any residual macroscopic or microscopic endometriosis. Whether this therapy improves the pregnancy rate remains to be proven. In any case, following conservative surgery, endometriosis recurs in 5-25% of patients.

THERAPY THAT PRESERVES REPRODUCTIVE CAPACITY

For the woman with pelvic endometriosis who is not interested in fertility now, but wishes to retain her reproductive potential, hormonal suppression is the therapeutic choice. If at all possible, conservative surgery should be avoided, to be utilized later if infertility becomes a problem. After laparoscopy has established the diagnosis, the hormonal choices include either an oral contraceptive or danazol, with medroxyprogesterone acetate (Depo-Provera) indicated in certain clinical situations.

Oral Contraception

Although pregnancy rates following the use of oral contraceptives are low, this relatively inexpensive form of therapy retains a front-line place in the suppression of endometriotic symptoms and signs. Any low-dose preparation (containing 50 μg or less of ethinylestradiol) with a high progestin/estrogen ratio can be selected, e.g., Ovral or Lo/Ovral. As it creates a pseudopregnancy state, the drug should be used *continuously* (daily) for nine months.

A single tablet per day is sufficient. If breakthrough bleeding occurs, the dose can be doubled or tripled. The increased dosage should be continued only until the bleeding has stopped. Then the dose can be dropped in stepwise fashion back to the original. However, if bleeding recurs, the increased dosage necessary to stop it should be continued. Breakthrough bleeding may also be controlled by the short-term addition of 20 μg of ethinylestradiol to the original regimen.

Obviously, any contraindications to oral contraceptives should be ascertained prior to the start of therapy. In addition, the patient should be informed that the hormonal therapy of endometriosis is suppressive rather than curative, and, after an interval of nontreatment, repeat therapy may be indicated with increasing symptomatology.

Danazol

Prior to its FDA approval and release, danazol, a synthetic derivative of 17α-ethinyltestosterone, had numerous clinical trials. As with most new drugs, the initial therapeutic results, in terms of symptom relief and disappearance of minimal amounts of endometriotic implants, were good and the investigators enthusiastic. Continued studies have confirmed that danazol has a significant role in the management of endometriosis. However, unlike its unique role in infertility, danazol must share equal billing with oral contraceptives when it comes to symptomatic therapy only. It provides an alternative choice, albeit an expensive one, when oral contraceptives are contraindicated or complicated by side effects. In addition, when danazol is used to treat symptoms or physical findings, an increasing body of data supports its use in lower doses, e.g., 200 mg tid or bid. Whatever dose creates and maintains an amenorrheic state seems sufficient.

Danazol is an antigonadotropin that appears to act on the cyclic LH center, thus inhibiting the LH surge. However, tonic LH and FSH are not significantly depressed, so danazol appears to block ovulation in a manner similar to the action of oral contraceptives. It also acts at the level of the ovary, altering estrogen synthesis by competing for receptor sites. Although danazol does not suppress serum estrogen below follicular phase values, it creates an atrophic endometrium within the first month of treatment.

As with oral contraceptives, side effects can be a problem. In addition to cost, androgenic changes (acne, deepening of voice, increased hair growth), skin rashes, and weight gain can be troublesome enough to cause discontinuation of therapy. Like oral contraceptives, danazol is, for the most part, suppressive rather than curative. Repetitive 6-month courses may be necessary after drug-free intervals.

Medroxyprogesterone Acetate

As an alternative in deep-seated (rectovaginal) endometriosis or when symptoms persist despite treatment with oral contraceptives and danazol, intramuscular medroxyprogesterone acetate can be used (100 mg/week × 4 doses, then 100 mg bimonthly × 2 doses, then 100 mg/month × 10 doses). Side effects include weight gain, breakthrough bleeding (25-30%), and post-therapy amenorrhea (20-25%). The patient who wishes immediate resumption of fertility upon completion of therapy should be cautioned that ovulatory medication may be necessary if amenorrhea follows treatment.

THERAPY FOLLOWING COMPLETION OF CHILDBEARING

For the woman with moderate or severe pelvic endometriosis who has completed her family, a total abdominal hysterectomy is the therapeutic choice. *If the ovaries are involved* or other endometriotic areas remain, a bilateral salpingo-oophorectomy should be performed. Any remaining endometriosis will become fibrotic and scar without ovarian stimulation. *If the ovaries must be preserved*, e.g., in a young woman or by patient desire, and residual endometriosis is present, postoperative hormonal suppression must be used for 6-9 months depending on the agent selected.

After hysterectomy and bilateral salpingo-oophorectomy, estrogen replacement therapy can be used. However, as low a dose as possible should be prescribed. If residual endometriosis remains *after* removal of the uterus and ovaries, progestogen therapy or medroxyprogesterone acetate, rather than estrogen alone, should be given for 6 months. Otherwise, the estrogen-only therapy could activate any residual disease.

SUGGESTED READING

Biberoglu KO, Behrman SJ: Dosage aspects of danazol therapy in endometriosis: Short-term and long-term effectiveness. *Am J Obstet Gynecol* 136:645, 1981

Daniell JF, Christianson C: Combined laparoscopic surgery and danazol therapy for pelvic endometriosis. *Fertil Steril* 35:521, 1981

Dmowski WP: Endocrine properties and clinical application of danazol. *Fertil Steril* 31:237, 1979

Dmowski WP, Cohen MR: Antigonadotropin (danazol) in the treatment of endometriosis. *Am J Obstet Gynecol* 130:41, 1978

Moore EE, Harger HH, Rock JA, Archer DF: Management of pelvic endometriosis with low-dose danazol. *Fertil Steril* 36:15, 1981

Schenken RS, Malinak CR: Conservative surgery versus expectant management for the infertile patient with mild endometriosis. *Fertil Steril* 37:183, 1982

Sulewski JM, Curcio FD, Bronitsky C, Stenger VG: The treatment of endometriosis at laparoscopy for infertility. *Am J Obstet Gynecol* 138:128, 1980

Wheeler JM, Malinak CR: Postoperative danazol therapy in infertility patients with severe endometriosis. *Fertil Steril* 36:460, 1981

100

Luteal Phase Defects

CHARLES M. MARCH, M.D.

Virtually every aspect of the topic of luteal phase defects remains controversial. The definition, incidence, pathophysiology, effects, methods of diagnosis, and modes of therapy all have yet to be completely clarified.

A luteal phase defect is currently defined as abnormal corpus luteum function associated with insufficient progesterone production. The deficiency may be in the amount of progesterone produced per day and/or in the duration of progesterone production. Estrogen production usually remains normal. Classically, there are two types of luteal phase defects: the short luteal phase and the inadequate luteal phase.

THE SHORT LUTEAL PHASE

Women with a short luteal phase (SLP) have short ovulatory menstrual cycles, due entirely to a reduction (to less than 10 days) in the interval between the luteinizing hormone (LH) peak and the onset of menses. In SLP patients, the patterns of follicle-stimulating hormone (FSH) and LH secretion during the menstrual cycle are normal, but the mean FSH levels and the FSH/LH ratios are reduced. The peak serum concentrations of progesterone are lower and occur earlier. If an endometrial biopsy is performed and the histology of the endometrium is correlated with the LH peak or the basal body temperature (BBT) shift, the endometrial response will be in phase.

Strott and associates demonstrated that this defect occurs commonly in young women and may represent insufficient maturation of the hypothalamic-pituitary-ovarian axis. It is uncertain if the SLP plays a significant role in infertility. But if this defect were severe, follicular development and corpus luteum function would be grossly abnormal and infertility would result.

Treatment should be directed toward increasing the extent of FSH stimulation very early in the menstrual cycle. Clomiphene citrate (Clomid, Serophene) should be prescribed as discussed below. If this fails to restore normal luteal function, low doses (1-2 ampules/day) of human menopausal gonadotropins (hMG, Pergonal) should be given beginning on day 1 of the cycle. In milder forms of the SLP, the corpus luteum can probably be maintained by the endogenous human chorionic gonadotropin (hCG) produced by a recently implanted blastocyst, and therapy would not be indicated.

THE INADEQUATE LUTEAL PHASE

In contrast to the SLP, the inadequate luteal phase (ILP) does have a significant effect upon reproductive performance. It occurs in menstrual cycles of normal length in which progesterone production can be demonstrated. The diagnosis of the ILP is most difficult; various authors have used different, arbitrary criteria that do not correlate well.

The classical diagnosis of ILP depends upon the interpretation of a properly timed endometrial biopsy. There is little risk of interrupting a pregnancy if an endometrial biopsy is obtained in the luteal phase, provided that only a single anterior or lateral fundal sample is taken. The histologic pattern of the endometrium must be correlated with both the apparent date of ovulation (judged by the date of the BBT shift) and the first day of the patient's next menstrual period.

In cases of ILP, the histologic pattern should be 2 days or more behind the expected pattern. An out-of-phase endometrium has been reported to occur in one cycle in up to 20% of women. But if two cycles are examined, the incidence falls to less than 3%. Thus, since occasional lags in endometrial histology are frequent in normal women and since endometrial dating is imprecise and can vary depending on interpretations of different pathologists, the defect must be documented in two or more cycles.

To establish the diagnosis, the endometrial biopsy is best obtained 2 days prior to the expected onset of menses, i.e., on day 26 of an idealized 28-day cycle. At this time, almost the entire estrogen and progesterone secretion by the ovary has been completed. Therefore, the endometrium reflects most of the steroid production of that cycle.

Single, multiple, and even daily luteal phase progesterone assays have also been used to diagnose the ILP. If only histologic criteria are used, not all women with reduced luteal phase progesterone concentrations will be detected. Although total luteal phase progesterone production is reduced in women with retarded histologic patterns, the overlap with patients with normal biopsies is too great to permit easy discrimination. Thus, some investigators have rejected the biopsy criteria and have used a single peak luteal phase serum concentration of less than 10 or 15 ng/ml. Others use three pooled specimens from between days 4 and 11, and consider a level less than 15 ng/ml diagnostic. It is likely that a continuum of defects is being detected by these different techniques.

Atypical BBT charts showing a "stepladder" pattern or erratic shifts cannot be used to establish the diagnosis of ILP. The BBT does not reflect a specific serum progesterone concentration, and a maximal increase in BBT may occur with a serum progesterone level of only 3 ng/ml.

The incidence of the ILP is unknown. It probably occurs in only a very small percentage of infertile patients, perhaps less than 2%. However, the ILP is more commonly associated with recurrent abortion. Now that the more sensitive β-subunit and radioreceptor assays for hCG are available, the true incidence of occult abortions may become known. It is likely that the etiology in some cases of recurrent occult abortion involves a luteal phase defect. The cause of reproductive failure in women with luteal phase defects is uncertain. But progesterone deficiency may interfere with tubal transport mechanisms, uterine motility, and/or proper development of the nidation site.

ETIOLOGY

Luteal phase defects may be cerebral in origin or secondary to hypothalamic lesions or pituitary, ovarian, or endometrial causes. Since the roles of higher cerebral centers and the hypothalamus are poorly understood at this time, only pituitary, ovarian, and endometrial causes will be considered here.

Pituitary Causes

Four types of pituitary lesions may lead to luteal insufficiency: (1) inadequate or asynchronous FSH/LH stimulation during the follicular phase or, more important, during the luteal phase of the preceding menstrual cycle, (2) asynchronous or inadequate surges of LH at midcycle, (3) inadequate LH stimulation to maintain the corpus luteum during the luteal phase—primary, or (4) secondary to sustained hyperprolactinemia. It has been demonstrated that elevated prolactin levels interfere with progesterone synthesis by the corpus luteum. Additionally, a number of investigators have reported that some patients with luteal phase defects do have hyperprolactinemia. Treatment with the dopamine receptor agonist bromocriptine (Parlodel) has sometimes been successful.

Ovarian Causes

There are four possible ovarian causes of luteal phase defects: (1) chromosome abnormalities associated with reduced numbers of follicles and, therefore, inadequate steroidogenesis, (2) recruitment and development of an insufficient number of follicles during the early follicular phase of the menstrual cycle, (3) inadequate ovarian response to a normal gonadotropin stimulus, and (4) poor corpus luteum function secondary to defective or inadequate numbers of ovarian LH receptors.

Endometrial Causes

An endometrial lesion can cause apparent luteal insufficiency. Such a defect would not fall within the confines of the definition of an inadequate corpus luteum, but the histologic pattern would be the same. With a defect in endometrial receptors, the response to normal sex hormone stimulation would be reduced and recurrent abortion or infertility would result. Recently, Keller and associates reported a patient with pseudocorpus luteum deficiency due to a lack of endometrial receptors.

TREATMENT

Five therapy modalities have been recommended to treat the inadequate luteal phase: progesterone, hCG, clomiphene, hMG, and bromocriptine.

Progesterone therapy may be started with one 25-mg suppository inserted intravaginally bid beginning on the day of BBT rise and continuing until menses begin. (Standard infertility textbooks should be consulted for compounding information.) If pregnancy occurs, therapy should continue until the 10th week of gestation. This time period extends somewhat beyond the time when placental steroidogenesis replaces that of the corpus luteum. Or progesterone in oil may be used, 12.5 mg IM daily for the same duration as described for suppositories.

Parenteral *hCG* 2,500-5,000 IU may be administered every other day beginning on the date of BBT rise, for the same duration as described for progesterone. This therapy is less successful than progesterone substitution because it cannot maintain an abnormal corpus luteum. hCG can be used only for patients whose lesions are mild and central in origin. One successful end point of therapy is a normal endometrium. Therefore, the adequacy of therapy can be documented by repeating the endometrial biopsy after treatment has been initiated.

Although *clomiphene citrate* has been recommended by some authors for management of the ILP, it has also been incriminated as causing ovulatory cycles with luteal phase insufficiency. But the latter claim has not been well substantiated.

Treatment is begun with one 50-mg tablet on day 2 of the menstrual cycle and continued for 5 days. This is earlier than the conventional schedule (days 5-9) of clomiphene administration for ovulation induction. It is employed to provide an early FSH surge necessary for follicular recruitment and early development. If the diagnosis was established by a low luteal phase progesterone level, the progesterone assay should be repeated during the treatment cycle to verify correction. The daily dose of clomiphene should be maintained if normalcy has been restored. If the defect persists, the dose should be increased sequentially in 50-mg/day increments in each successive cycle until correction has been achieved.

Other luteal phase defects may respond to therapy with *hMG* in low doses. This therapy may be used if clomiphene treatment fails.

The use of *bromocriptine* should be restricted to patients with hyperprolactinemia. Although early work has been encouraging, more studies are needed. At present, bromocriptine is not approved for use in patients with luteal phase defects.

If luteal insufficiency is the sole cause of infertility, term gestations may be expected in up to 75% of patients properly treated by one of the regimens outlined in this chapter.

SUGGESTED READING

Goldstein D, Zuckerman H, Harpaz S, Barkai J, Geva A, Gordon S, Shalev E, Schwartz M: Correlation between estradiol and progesterone in cycles with luteal phase deficiency. *Fertil Steril* 37:348, 1982

Jones GS: The luteal phase defect. *Fertil Steril* 27:351, 1976

Jones GS, Aksel S, Wentz AC: Serum progesterone values in the luteal phase defects. Effect of chorionic gonadotropin. *Obstet Gynecol* 44:26, 1974

Keller DW, Wiest WG, Askin FB, Johnson LW, Strickler RC: Pseudocorpus luteum insufficiency: A local defect of progesterone action on endometrial stroma. *J Clin Endocrinol Metab* 48:127, 1979

McNatty KP, Sawyers RS, McNeilly AS: A possible role for prolactin in control of steroid secretion by the human Graafian follicles. *Nature* 250:653, 1974

Noyes RW, Hertig AT, Rock J: Dating the endometrial biopsy. *Fertil Steril* 1:3, 1950

Strott CA, Cargille CM, Ross GT, Lipsett MB: The short luteal phase. *J Clin Endocrinol Metab* 30:246, 1970

101

Intrauterine Adhesions

CHARLES M. MARCH, M.D.

ETIOLOGY

There are three common etiologies for the development of intrauterine adhesions (IUA, Asherman's syndrome). The most common antecedent factor is curettage of the pregnant or recently pregnant uterus. Almost 40% of the patients with intrauterine adhesions who have been referred to the University of Southern California Medical Center have had an elective termination of pregnancy. Patients may also develop synechiae following a curettage performed because of a spontaneous abortion. It appears that those women who have had a missed abortion are at the greatest risk among all patients in the abortion category. Finally, it has been reported that almost one-fourth of women who undergo curettage in the first 2 months postpartum develop adhesions. The second to fourth weeks postpartum are the most critical.

Another common etiology for IUA is endometritis. Endometritis may be the sole cause of IUA in patients who have tuberculous infection of the endometrium. However, other types of bacterial infection increase the risk of adhesive disease in patients who have had endometrial curettage or uterine surgery. A small percentage of patients develop IUA after a diagnostic D&C. Thus, routine D&C done at the time of laparoscopy on infertile women serves no purpose, may be harmful, and should be abandoned.

Although previous uterine surgery is an unusual antecedent of IUA, adhesions have been noted following cesarean sections, hysterotomies, myomectomies, and metroplasties.

The common denominator in the development of IUA in all of these conditions is excessive endometrial trauma, especially to the basalis layer. Additive factors in the patient who has been pregnant are tetanic uterine contractions, which maintain the anterior and posterior walls in close apposition, and the low levels of estradiol present immediately following pregnancy. Low levels of estradiol greatly decrease the stimulus to endometrial regeneration.

DIAGNOSIS

Patients with IUA may complain of menstrual abnormalities, infertility, or recurrent abortion, or they may be asymptomatic. Despite extensive adhesions, a woman may have normal, painless, spontaneous menses.

The relationship between recurrent abortion and adhesions is difficult to assess. Women with recurrent abortion may have the diagnosis of intrauterine adhesions established. However, this diagnosis may be made only after multiple curettages have been performed and the adhesions therefore may be the sequelae to treatment for, rather than the cause of, recurrent abortion. Moreover, these adhesions may have developed only after the last curettage.

The key to establishing the diagnosis is a high index of suspicion. All women who have menstrual complaints and/or infertility and who have a history of prior endometrial trauma should be investigated for IUA. Five diagnostic techniques are utilized to establish their presence:

1. Amenorrhea with evidence of luteal phase activity, such as a biphasic basal body temperature or elevated serum progesterone, is evidence of end organ failure. However, the same symptoms may occur in patients with cervical stenosis, even in the absence of cyclic abdominal pain.

2. Failure to have withdrawal uterine bleeding following combined or sequential estrogen-progestin treatment is also evidence of endometrial insufficiency. If this test is utilized, sequential estrogen-progestin therapy is preferable to the use of oral contraceptives, since the latter may cause hypomenorrhea or amenorrhea. However, because intrauterine adhesions may exist in patients with normal menses, neither regimen may be used to rule out the presence of intrauterine synechiae.

3. Difficulty in sounding the endometrial cavity, or the impression of an irregular or small cavity, also suggests the presence of adhesions.

4. A hysterosalpingogram under fluoroscopic control is the study most often utilized to establish the presence of adhesions. The finding of lacunar defects placed irregularly throughout the uterine cavity strongly supports the impression of intrauterine adhesions. Unfortunately, false-positive studies occur and neither the extent nor the exact location of the adhesions may be determined with certainty. However, patients with a normal hysterogram do not have adhesions.

5. The definitive diagnostic study is hysteroscopy, which permits the extent and location of the adhesions to be determined accurately by direct vision. These factors, together with the density of the adhesions, permit the disease to be classified. Because the symptoms of Asherman's syndrome are variable and because hysteroscopy is not available to all patients, the incidence of IUA is unknown.

TREATMENT

Therapy of IUA is directed toward four goals: restoration of normal uterine architecture, prevention of readherence, stimulation of endometrial regeneration, and verification that the uterus is normal before conception is attempted. Treatment should be instituted as soon as the diagnosis is established, whether or not the patient wishes to conceive at that time, in order to prevent possible complicated pregnancies. However, there is no information to suggest that the condition is progressive. If the patient does not wish to conceive, she must be cautioned that intrauterine adhesions cannot be used as a method of contraception, even if she is amenorrheic and a hysterosalpingogram suggests total obliteration of the cavity.

Restoration of Normal Architecture

The treatment of choice is transhysteroscopic lysis of adhesions. This is safer and easier than previously advocated methods of management. Under direct vision the surgeon may lyse all the adhesions and not traumatize normal endometrium. The medium utilized to distend the uterine cavity during hysteroscopy should be a viscous 32% solution of dextran with an average molecular weight of 70,000 in glucose and water (Hyskon). This medium is not miscible with blood and permits the surgeon to have a clear view of the cavity even after extensive surgery has been performed.

Hysteroscopy may be performed under paracervical block anesthesia with either meperidine (Demerol) or diazepam (Valium) for sedation. If the dissection is unusually difficult, the procedure should be discontinued and rescheduled using general anesthesia. If necessary, simultaneous laparoscopy may be performed by an assistant who guides the hysteroscopist and thereby reduces the risk of uterine perforation.

Prevention of Readherence

During hysteroscopy the uterine synechiae are visualized and the extent of the adhesions classified. The adhesions are considered to be extensive if more than three-fourths of the uterine cavity is obliterated, moderate if one-fourth to three-fourths is involved, and only minimal if less than one-fourth of the uterus is scarred. The adhesions are then divided with miniature scissors through the hysteroscope. Following complete dissection of the adhesions, a Lippes loop is inserted to reduce the chance of readherence of the recently dissected uterine surfaces.

Stimulation of Endometrial Regeneration

The third goal of therapy, endometrial regeneration, is achieved by the administration of conjugated estrogens, 2.5 mg bid for 60 days. On the last 5 days of this treatment, medroxyprogesterone acetate, 10 mg/day, is added. Following the withdrawal bleeding induced by this regimen, the intrauterine device is removed.

Verification That the Uterus Is Normal

One month later a hysterosalpingogram is obtained to verify that the normal uterine architecture has been maintained. If the first hysteroscopy was very difficult, or if recurrent or persistent adhesions are suspected, repeat hysteroscopy should be performed and any remaining adhesions lysed. Assessment of the uterus is mandatory prior to permitting pregnancy. It is likely that the poor gestational outcome from previous treatment regimens was secondary to persistent adhesions.

COMPLICATIONS

Normal menses should be expected following therapy. Before hysteroscopy became available, pregnancy rates were low and those patients who did conceive experienced high rates of spontaneous abortion, prematurity, intrauterine growth retardation, and fetal demise. Fewer than one-half of patients who conceived delivered an infant who survived. A very serious complication was an error of placental implantation, such as placenta previa, accreta, increta, or percreta, reported in 20% of patients who conceived following treatment of IUA by repeat D&C.

Following hysteroscopic therapy of IUA, pregnancies have occurred in about three-fourths of patients in whom other infertility factors were not identified. These pregnancies have generally been uncomplicated, and more than 85% of them have gone to term. As more centers gain experience with the hysteroscopic treatment of IUA, older methods of treatment will be abandoned. Finally, the use of the hysteroscopic classification of IUA will make it possible to compare dissection techniques and place the value of adjunctive therapy in proper perspective.

SUGGESTED READING

Bergquist CA, Rock JA, Jones HW: Pregnancy outcome following treatment of intrauterine adhesions. *Int J Fertil* 26:107, 1981

Jewelewicz R, Khalaf S, Neuwirth RS, Vande Wiele RL: Obstetric complications after treatment of intrauterine synechiae (Asherman's syndrome). *Obstet Gynecol* 47:701, 1976

March CM, Israel R: Gestational outcome following hysteroscopic lysis of adhesions. *Fertil Steril* 36:455, 1981

March CM, Israel R, March AD: The hysteroscopic management of intrauterine adhesions. *Am J Obstet Gynecol* 130:653, 1978

Sugimoto O: Diagnostic and therapeutic hysteroscopy for traumatic intrauterine adhesions. *Am J Obstet Gynecol* 131:539, 1978

102

Human In Vitro Fertilization

RICHARD P. MARRS, M.D.

INTRODUCTION

The first human birth resulting from in vitro fertilization occurred in England in 1978. Since then, pregnancies have been achieved with this technique in Australia and the United States as well. By 1982 over 100 women had become pregnant after in vitro fertilization procedures.

This type of procedure can benefit three categories of patients: (1) women who have irreparable tubal disease, (2) couples in which the male partner is oligospermic, and (3) couples with an undiagnosable etiology of infertility. Pregnancies have now been reported in all three categories.

PROCEDURE

Ovulatory Monitoring

Precise monitoring of ovulation is of utmost importance. Various factors have traditionally been used to predict the *approximate* time of ovulation. These include basal body temperature graphs, cervical mucus changes, vaginal cytology, and serum hormonal parameters. For in vitro fertilization, the time of ovulation must be exact, and more precise methods must be used.

In the early work in England and Australia, spontaneous ovulatory cycles were monitored by measurement of luteinizing hormone (LH), and a single oocyte was obtained laparoscopically. But the pregnancy rate with this type of system was less than 5%. Later studies in Australia demonstrated that multiple follicle development induced by either clomiphene citrate (Clomid, Serophene) or human menopausal gonadotropins (hMG, Pergonal) improves the rate of oocyte recovery, fertilization, and embryo growth. As a result, we use clomiphene (150 mg/day for 5 days) to stimulate multiple follicle development.

The day of initiation of clomiphene treatment depends upon the patient's overall average cycle length. For instance, if the patient has a cycle length of 32 days, clomiphene treatment will be initiated on day 5 of her cycle. With a cycle length of 24 days, clomiphene will be started on day 2 or 3. Using this type of regimen, two mature follicles have been found at laparoscopy in the majority of cycles monitored. To ensure recovery of mature oocytes, two major parameters are used to monitor ovulatory function: real-time ultrasound scanning and rapid estrogen determinations.

Real-time ultrasound scanning of ovarian follicle development has been shown to be a very good predictor of dynamic, day-to-day follicular changes. Therefore, we use a real-time sector scanner (ADR Model 2140) to monitor follicle growth daily.

The first ultrasound scan is performed 1 day following the cessation of clomiphene therapy. At that time, the dominant follicle or follicles visualized should be ≥14 mm in diameter. If follicle development is not adequate, clomiphene therapy will be extended an additional 1-3 days or hMG will be added. Ultrasound monitoring is performed daily until the follicle reaches 18-20 mm in diameter. At this point, twice-daily blood samples are obtained, and estradiol is assayed by a rapid radioimmunoassay. These estradiol measurements are used to monitor the appearance of the preovulatory estradiol peak.

Once the preovulatory surge of estradiol has occurred, 4,000 IU of human chorionic gonadotropin (hCG) is given. Laparoscopy is performed precisely 36 hours following hCG administration. This timing is necessary since spontaneous ovulation will occur about 38-39 hours after hCG is given.

With this method of monitoring, mature oocytes have been obtained in 60 of 62 treatment cycles. This combined method of monitoring follicle growth by ultrasound and estradiol measurement ensures that the aspirated oocyte is mature and capable of being fertilized.

Laparoscopic Oocyte Recovery

To ensure that spontaneous ovulation has not been initiated, a blood sample is obtained immediately prior to the hCG injection, and LH is measured by a rapid radioimmunoassay. (Baseline LH levels are determined for each patient using the samples obtained for estradiol measurement.) If LH levels are basal, the laparoscopy is performed. If an increase in LH is found in the final blood sample, the laparoscopic attempt at oocyte recovery is aborted, since ovulation will occur at an unpredictable time prior to the scheduled 36 hours.

Oocyte recovery by laparoscopic techniques has been described in the literature. It is performed in a manner similar to other laparoscopic procedures, except that a special oocyte recovery system developed specifically for follicle aspiration is used. Under direct laparoscopic visualization, the oocyte aspiration needle is placed in the follicle, and the intrafollicular contents are aspirated. If ovulatory monitoring has been precise, a mature oocyte should be found within the follicular fluid.

To ensure consistency in environment, the system used for collecting the follicular fluid is placed between prewarmed IV bags so that the follicular contents will be brought into the collecting tube at body temperature. The follicular fluid is immediately taken to the laboratory, which should be located in the operating room area. The oocytes are rapidly identified, removed from the follicular fluid, and placed in a previously prepared culture medium.

Oocyte culture is currently being performed in a solution of Ham's F-10 medium that is supplemented with calcium lactate, sodium and potassium bicarbonate, as well as the patient's preovulatory serum (10%). The serum has been heat-inactivated and filtered prior to addition to the culture medium. The Ham's F-10 medium is prepared on a weekly basis. Prior to use in the human oocyte cultures, it is tested to ensure that it supports mouse embryo growth as well as human sperm survival. Only batches that have been tested and proven are used in human oocyte culturing.

The oocytes are placed in 1 ml of Ham's medium in a 12 × 75 mm tissue culture tube and cultured in an environment of 5% oxygen, 5% carbon dioxide, and 90% nitrogen gas mixture, with 100% humidity at 37°C. The medium is adjusted to a pH of 7.4 and an osmolarity of 280.

The oocytes are preincubated in the culture medium for approximately 7-8 hours prior to addition of washed spermatozoa. The exact duration of the preincubation interval is determined after oocyte maturity is judged according to the following criteria: (1) volume of follicular fluid, (2) appearance of cumulus mass and corona radiata, and (3) estimated maturity of the granulosa cells as judged grossly by low-power magnification. The use of a variable preincubation interval in combination with the ovulatory monitoring system described above has resulted in a 95% fertilization rate in our clinic.

Oocyte Fertilization and Embryo Growth

A semen sample is provided by the husband by masturbation approximately 5 hours after successful oocyte recovery. A rapid estimation of sperm count and motility is performed. If these parameters are adequate (at least 20 million/ml and 40% motility), a 0.5-ml aliquot of semen is washed in Ham's F-10 solution in a two-wash technique. After removal of the seminal plasma, the spermatozoa are incubated at 37°C for an additional 40 minutes to allow capacitation to occur. Then half a million motile sperm are added to each oocyte culture dish, and each mixture is cultured for a total of 18 hours. At the end of that period, the oocytes are transferred into fresh growth media containing 20% patient serum and left for an additional 20 hours.

At this point (38 hours after the sperm were added to the oocyte cultures), the corona, which is usually still surrounding the fertilized oocyte, is removed by microdissecting needles under dissecting microscope visualization. Without removal of the corona, visualization of embryo development is very difficult. The average time for development of a two-cell embryo is approximately 33 hours from sperm addition. A range of up to 47 hours is considered normal.

If an embryo of two cells or more can be seen at 38-47 hours, the patient is brought back into the hospital for embryo transfer. If abnormal cleavage (fragmentation) has developed, the embryo will not be placed in the uterus. If two oocytes have been fertilized and have developed into embryos, both will be inserted into the uterus. It has been shown that double-embryo transfers appear to increase overall pregnancy success with this system.

Embryo Transfer

Once normal embryo development has been observed, the patient is returned to the operating room adjacent to the laboratory, where she is given 10 mg of diazepam (Valium). If the patient has an anterior uterus, she is placed in the knee-chest position; with a retroverted uterus, the lithotomy position is used. The transfer is performed by a transcervical approach after the embryo or embryos have been loaded into a No. 5 French Teflon catheter with a 3-mm side opening. After the catheter is passed through the cervical canal into the uterine fundus, the embryo(s) are deposited by injecting 0.05 ml of Hepes buffer solution through the catheter.

The patient is placed in the Trendelenburg position for 8 hours. Then she is discharged to be maintained on bed rest for the next 36 hours.

PREGNANCY SUCCESS

Prior to 1981, overall pregnancy success with in vitro fertilization ranged from 1% to 8%. In 1981, five centers reported pregnancies following in vitro fertilization. At Bourn Hall in England, Edwards and Steptoe reported between 40 and 50 pregnancies in approximately 300 stimulated cycles. At Royal Women's Hospital in Melbourne, Australia, 17 pregnancies occurred in approximately 200 attempts, but only four attained viability. Queen Victoria Hospital in Melbourne reported approximately 40 pregnancies in 300 attempts. In the United States, eight pregnancies were initiated in 1981. Seven occurred in 44 embryo transfers at the Eastern Virginia Medical Center, while one occurred in the first 14 embryo transfers at the University of Southern California Medical Center. In 1982, after adjustments of technique, an additional three pregnancies were established in six embryo transfers at USC, for a total of four viable pregnancies in 20 embryo transfers. The worldwide pregnancy success rate for in vitro fertilization in 1982 was 15-20%, a vast improvement over what it was 18 months previously.

The factors that have led to improvement in pregnancy statistics include better and more precise monitoring of the ovulatory process, which has resulted in obtaining more mature oocytes; and multiple follicle development using clomiphene and hMG, which has improved oocyte recovery rates and fertilization success. Multiple-embryo transfer has also helped improve the overall pregnancy statistics.

FUTURE DEVELOPMENTS

The use of in vitro fertilization to overcome human infertility is now a reality. Increasing numbers of pregnancies will result from this type of procedure in the future. As more centers are involved, it is conceivable that the overall success rate will eventually exceed the expected pregnancy rate of 25% per in vivo attempt. Fertilization, embryo growth, and entrance of the cleaving embryo into the uterine cavity can be controlled with the in vitro system (in contrast to the in vivo system). Failure of one of these three steps accounts for part of the high rate of wastage observed with in vivo attempts at pregnancy.

If future success rates with in vitro fertilization reach and exceed 50% per attempt, this technique should eventually replace oviductal surgery for distal tubal disease, with its relatively high rate of ectopic gestation and low rate of success. The in vitro fertilization process is currently reserved for patients with infertility factors that are untreatable by conventional therapy. For the select population of patients requiring the in vitro fertilization process, the future looks much brighter.

SUGGESTED READING

Chang MC: Fertilization of rabbit ova *in vitro*. *Nature* 184:877, 1959

Edwards RG, Purdy JM, Steptoe PC, Walters DE: The growth of human preimplantation embryos *in vitro*. *Am J Obstet Gynecol* 141:408, 1981

Hackeloer BJ, Fleming R, Robinson HP, Adam AH, Coutts JRT: Correlation of ultrasonic and endocrinologic assessment of human follicular development. *Am J Obstet Gynecol* 135:122, 1979

Kreitmann O, Nixon WE, Hodgen GD: Induced corpus luteum dysfunction after aspiration of the preovulatory follicle in monkeys. *Fertil Steril* 35:671, 1981

Lopata A, Johnston IWH, Hoult IJ, Speirs AI: Pregnancy following intrauterine implantation of an embryo obtained by *in vitro* fertilization of a preovulatory egg. *Fertil Steril* 33:117, 1980

Marrs RP, March CM, Vargyas JM, Mishell DR Jr: Correlation of ultrasonic and endocrinologic measurements in human menopausal gonadotropin therapy. *Am J Obstet Gynecol* (in press)

Steptoe PC, Edwards RG, Purdy JM: Clinical aspects of pregnancies established with cleaving embryo grown *in vitro*. *Br J Obstet Gynecol* 87:757, 1980

Vargyas JM, Marrs RP, Kletzky OA: Correlation of human follicular development with peripheral concentrations of serum estradiol. *Am J Obstet Gynecol* 144:569, 1982

Wood C, Trounson A, Leeton J, Talbot JM, Buttery B, Webb J, Wood J, Jessup D: A clinical assessment of nine pregnancies obtained by *in vitro* fertilization and embryo transfer. *Fertil Steril* 35:502, 1981

103

Müllerian Anomalies

WILLIAM E. GIBBONS, M.D.

Müllerian duct malformations constitute an interesting group of clinical problems. Many müllerian anomalies are asymptomatic and are never detected. Gynecologic complaints include amenorrhea, oligomenorrhea, dysmenorrhea, menorrhagia, metrorrhagia, and dyspareunia. Menstrual outflow obstruction may lead to endometriosis, hematometra, and hematocolpos. But it is in the area of pregnancy wastage that uterine anomalies have generated the most attention. Fetal wastage is increased in all trimesters. Second-trimester abortion of a normal fetus, premature labor, and abnormal fetal presentation are conditions classically associated with müllerian anomalies. For instance, the incidence of breech presentation is increased from the normal 3.7% to 20%. Abdominal delivery and postpartum complications, including retained placenta, subinvolution, and hemorrhage, are more frequent. Müllerian malformations may present as surgical emergencies, such as rupture of a gestation in a rudimentary uterine horn.

EMBRYOGENESIS

The müllerian ducts (paramesonephric ducts) arise in the seventh week of embryologic life as infoldings and then closings off of the coelomic mesothelium of the lateral walls of the urogenital ridge. The ducts grow caudally and then medial to the wolffian (mesonephric) duct to abut the urogenital sinus at the end of the eighth week. The place where the ducts contact the urogenital sinus is called the müllerian tubercle. Fusion of paired müllerian ducts proceeds to the level of the round ligaments, forming the uterovaginal primordium. Fusion is followed shortly by disappearance of the septum between the ducts. It is failure of fusion and disappearance of the septum that leads to the continuum of anomalies that are observed clinically.

INCIDENCE

Anomalies of müllerian development occur in approximately 1-2% of females. The difficulties in detection place the actual incidence at variance with the estimated incidence. As techniques such as hysterosalpingography and ultrasonography have become more widely used, the incidence of genital tract anomalies has increased; however, physician awareness also plays a key role in diagnosis. In 1931, Smith observed the incidence change from 1:7,040 obstetric patients to 1:1,453 patients—only because of his personal interest in malformations. In 1962, Zabriskie reported a change in müllerian anomaly incidence from 1:321 to 1:109, depending on the physician's desire to evaluate patients with suggestive histories. Complicating this process is the observation by Rock and Jones that only 20-50% of patients with a double uterus have reproductive difficulty—the clinical evidence most likely to arouse suspicion.

The incidence of uterine anomalies diagnosed by hysterography varies in the literature from 1% to 3.5% and averages around 2%. The relative frequency of the different types of anomalies is difficult to ascertain because of variations in classification. Also, many series depend on hysterosalpingographic data alone to establish the diagnosis. This can be confusing, since the hysterogram cannot distinguish between bicornuate and septate uteri. It is often necessary to employ some form of pelvic visualization, such as laparoscopy, laparotomy, or cesarean section, to fully evaluate the extent of malformation.

ASSOCIATED URINARY TRACT ANOMALIES

Because of their close relationship embryologically, urinary and reproductive system anomalies frequently coexist. Approximately 20% of patients with unilateral renal agenesis will also have major genital anomalies. Likewise, two-thirds to three-fourths of patients with unicornuate uteri will have an absent kidney. These examples underline the importance of evaluating the urinary tract in a patient in whom a müllerian anomaly is diagnosed. Women with abnormalities of the urinary tract are more susceptible to kidney disease, such as pyelonephritis. In some cases, gynecologic therapy may be affected by an associated urinary tract malformation, such as a pelvic kidney.

Müllerian anomalies may be divided into six classes. Examining each of the müllerian anomaly types individually will give an appreciation of the diversity of their clinical presentations.

CLASS I

Vaginal Agenesis

Class I malformations (segmental müllerian agenesis/hypoplasia) include pure and mixed vaginal agenesis and cervical and fundal agenesis. They generally result from abnormal development of the caudal portion of the uterovaginal primordium. Vaginal occlusion with obstruction of the vagina outflow tract may take the form of a transverse membrane or various degrees of agenesis or hypoplasia. The presenting symptoms are similar: primary amenorrhea with or without cryptomenorrhea.

A complete or partial transverse membrane is usually located in the distal third of the vagina. With vaginal agenesis, the uterus usually is absent or is represented by rudimentary muscular buds (Rokitansky-Küster-Hauser syndrome, or Mayer-Rokitansky-Küster syndrome). The ovaries and secondary sexual characteristics are normal. The diagnosis of testicular feminization must be distinguished from congenital absence of the uterus because of its malignant potential. Urinary malformations are common. In 8% of cases of vaginal agenesis, the uterus is normally developed. The presentation may be a pelvic mass secondary to hematocolpos, hematometra, and/or hematosalpinx.

Endometriosis is a serious consequence of menstrual outflow obstruction and may lead to pain and adhesion formation. Schifrin, Erez, and Moore noted 15 cases of endometriosis in patients between the ages of 12 and 20 years. Six were accompanied by obstructive lesions.

The classical treatment of vaginal agenesis has been the McIndoe procedure. A cavity is surgically created between the urethra and anus, and into it is placed a vaginal mold containing a split-thickness skin graft. McIndoe reported on 63 patients, 50 of whom had "excellent" results. Successful therapy is judged to be a functional vaginal length of 12 cm or more. Poor results are vaginal lengths of 7 cm or less.

The Williams vulvovaginoplasty has also been recommended and offers some benefits in terms of simplicity, reduced operative time, and decreased risk to bowel and bladder. A U-shaped incision is made in the introitus between the urethra and anus. The medial mucosal edges are sutured together, and then the lateral mucosal edges are sutured together in the midline, thus creating a mucosal pouch, which can then be lengthened with intercourse or dilator therapy.

Vaginal dilator therapy alone has been successful in creating and maintaining a functional vagina, but requires a high degree of motivation on the part of the patient. When there is a functional uterus with vaginal agenesis, the proximal and distal vaginal mucosal ends can be joined. Several pregnancies have been reported following this procedure.

Cervical and Fundal Agenesis

There have been 17 reported cases of congenital absence of the cervix in the literature. Presenting symptoms are similar to those of the other obstructive lesions. Various procedures have been devised to establish a menstrual outflow tract and preserve reproductive potential. Farber reported two cases in which a fistulous tract was created and a T-tube was inserted to maintain patency and allow egress of blood. Zarou, using a similar technique, reported a subsequent term pregnancy. However, pregnancies are rare and infection and reoperation are common. Therefore, except under optimal conditions, hysterectomy is often the therapy of choice.

CLASS II

In class II anomalies, unicornuate uteri, the abnormal shape and reduced uterine volume available for the developing fetus result in an increased incidence of premature labor and abnormal presentations. Reported spontaneous first-trimester abortion rates vary from 15% to 85%. No surgical therapy is recommended for the unicornuate uterus without a rudimentary horn unless an incompetent cervix is suspected. If second-trimester loss occurs, cervical cerclage is indicated in subsequent pregnancies.

Whether the presence of a rudimentary horn is conducive to pregnancy wastage is unclear. In the largest single reported series of patients with a unicornuate uterus, reproductive performance was routinely poor whether or not a rudimentary horn was present. The presence of an endometrial cavity in a rudimentary horn increases the risk of morbidity, whether secondary to endometriosis or due to a pregnancy in the rudimentary horn. Communication between the two cavities is uncommon, and pregnancy occurs by transperitoneal migration of sperm and/or ova. O'Leary and O'Leary found 327 reported cases of gestation in a rudimentary horn. Eighty-nine per cent of the abnormal uteri ruptured by the end of the second trimester, and only 1% of the pregnancies resulted in live term births.

When a unicornuate uterus has a rudimentary horn with a functional endometrial cavity, and hysterosalpingography suggests the presence of endometriosis or menstrual egress from the ipsilateral fallopian tube, the horn should be excised. There is currently no information to suggest that excision of a rudimentary horn without an endometrial cavity increases fetal salvage.

CLASS III

Class III, or uterus didelphys malformations, presents a striking form of uterine malfusion. Urinary tract abnormalities are common. Premature labor is a particular problem in this classification. Green and Harris reported on 15 patients, of whom 14 delivered prematurely (average, 36 weeks). Musich and Behrman observed a 43% fetal wastage rate, but noted that the 57% survival rate was higher than for any other untreated anomaly group. Because of the "acceptable" fetal salvage rate and the difficulty of uteroplasty, surgical therapy is rarely performed. For patients with multiple fetal wastage, some recommend a modified Strassman procedure or cervical cerclage.

CLASS IV

The bicornuate uterus, the class IV anomaly, is associated with a 20% incidence of premature labor, breech presentation, and cesarean section. The incidence of first-trimester abortion is also increased, but the exact incidence is difficult to estimate since many reported series have failed to separate patients with bicornuate uteri from those with septate uteri. In series reporting fetal wastage rates for bicornuate uteri, the rates vary from 40% to 90%. Green and Harris did not notice a significant reduction in length of gestations that continued into the last trimester, but observed an increased incidence of retained placental fragments. The recommended therapy for bicornuate uterus is the Strassman procedure, which has the advantage of not requiring excision of uterine tissue and thus of not reducing the potential uterine space.

CLASS V

The most impressive feature of class V malformations, septate uteri, is the fetal wastage noted in the first half of pregnancy. In the series of Buttram and Gibbons, 88% of pregnancies associated with a complete septum ended in abortion, as did 70% associated with an incomplete septum. It is possible that the more complete the septum, the greater the probability of abortion. Jones has for many years classified the "double uterus" (bicornuate and septate) into two groups: those not treated, usually because of adequate reproductive performance, and those requiring therapy. In 1969, Jones and Wheeless reported that of 22 patients requiring surgical therapy, only one did not have a septate uterus. They observed that the septate uterus was more apt to present serious reproductive difficulty. The recommended therapy is the Tompkins procedure.

Although not common, müllerian malformations may be one of the more successfully treatable forms of pregnancy wastage. The septate uterus is the most common anomaly associated with early fetal wastage. Fetal wastage decreases from 85-88% prior to therapy to 12-15% after therapy. Before surgical therapy, a complete infertility work-up should be performed to rule out other infertility factors. And as with other fertility therapies, multiple adverse factors may be present.

Some authors have used cervical cerclage to treat pregnancy wastage associated with various müllerian anomalies, achieving fetal salvage rates comparable to those due to more complicated surgical procedures. Indeed, cervical cerclage may be the therapy of choice in cases involving unicornuate or didelphys anomalies, where previous premature delivery often resulted and more time for fetal maturation is needed. Cervical cerclage will rarely benefit the patient with a septate uterus, whose fetal wastage occurs most commonly in the first trimester.

CLASS VI

The class VI anomalies, which arise secondary to diethylstilbestrol (DES) exposure in utero, will represent one of the most common müllerian malformations during the 1980s. Kaufman and Adam reported that intraluminal uterine changes—i.e., T-shaped uterine cavities—occurred in 44 of 66 DES-exposed women. Ninety per cent of patients who had DES cervical changes, such as cervical hood, had hysterosalpingographic abnormalities, versus 18% of women with normal cervices. DES-exposed women also have a slightly decreased likelihood of carrying a pregnancy to term. Because of this, it is recommended that DES-exposed women be observed for cervical effacement and dilation during the first half of pregnancy and, if these changes are noted, that cervical cerclage be performed. DeCherney et al observed at surgery that the fallopian tubes of DES-exposed women had abnormal fimbriae and convolutions that might explain the increased tendency toward ectopic pregnancy and reduced fertility noted in these patients.

Nevertheless, the chance that a DES-exposed woman will have at least one viable pregnancy is not decreased relative to women who were not exposed to DES in utero, and it is not recommended that routine hysterosalpingography or cerclage be performed unless the patient has demonstrated some form of reproductive failure.

SUGGESTED READING

Buttram VC, Gibbons WE: Müllerian anomalies: A proposed classification (an analysis of 144 cases). *Fertil Steril* 32:40, 1979

Capraro VJ, Gallego MB: Vaginal agenesis. *Am J Obstet Gynecol* 124:98, 1976

DeCherney AH, Cholst I, Naftolin F: Structure and function of the fallopian tubes following exposure to diethylstilbestrol during gestation. *Fertil Steril* 36:741, 1981

Farber M, Marchant DJ: Congenital absence of the uterine cervix. *Am J Obstet Gynecol* 121:414, 1975

Green LK, Harris RE: Uterine anomalies. Frequency of diagnosis and associated obstetric complications. *Obstet Gynecol* 47:427, 1976

Jones HW Jr, Wheeless CR: Salvage of the reproductive potential of women with anomalous development of the Müllerian ducts: 1868-1968-2068. *Am J Obstet Gynecol* 104:348, 1969

Kaufman RH, Adam E: Genital tract anomalies associated with *in utero* exposure to diethylstilbestrol. *Isr J Med Sci* 14:353, 1978

McIndoe AH: The treatment of congenital absence and obliterative conditions of the vagina. *Br J Plast Surg* 2:254, 1950

Moore LL: *Before We Are Born*. Philadelphia: Saunders, 1974, p 148

Musich JR, Behrman SJ: Obstetric outcome before and after metroplasty in women with uterine anomalies. *Obstet Gynecol* 52:63, 1978

O'Leary JL, O'Leary JA: Rudimentary horn pregnancy. *Obstet Gynecol* 22:371, 1963

Rock JA, Jones HW Jr: The clinical management of the double uterus. *Fertil Steril* 28:798, 1966

Schifrin BS, Erez S, Moore JG: Teen-age endometriosis. *Am J Obstet Gynecol* 116:973, 1973

Semmens JP: Congenital defects of the reproductive tract: Clinical implications. *Contemp Ob/Gyn* 5(3):95, March 1975

Smith FR: The significance of incomplete fusion of the müllerian ducts in pregnancy and parturition, with a report on 35 cases. *Am J Obstet Gynecol* 22:714, 1931

Strassman ED: Fertility and unification of double uterus. *Fertil Steril* 17:165, 1966

Zabriskie JR: Pregnancy and the malformed uterus. Report of 92 cases. *West J Surg* 70:293, 1962

Zarou GS, Acken HS, Brevetti RC: Surgical management of congenital atresia of the cervix. *Am J Obstet Gynecol* 82:923, 1961

104

Recurrent Abortion

CHARLES M. MARCH, M.D.

Recurrent abortion is the occurrence of three consecutive spontaneous terminations of pregnancy before the 20th week of gestation. The incidence of habitual abortion is not certain, but it is approximately 0.1-0.2% of all clinically diagnosed pregnancies. If occult pregnancies—that is, pregnancies that are diagnosed only by the detection of human chorionic gonadotropin in a serum sample obtained late in the luteal phase and that terminate before a "missed period"—are included, the incidence is at least twice as high. The risk of recurrent abortion in a woman who has lost her two preceding pregnancies is approximately 25%. After three consecutive abortions, the rate of recurrence has been reported to be between 27% and 32%. These rates are slightly higher than the overall incidence of abortion, which is 20%.

Because the incidence of recurrent abortion is quite low, and because the chance that a pregnancy following three consecutive abortions will go to term is high (70-75%), empirical treatment of women who have had repeated abortions is not indicated. Empirical regimens used in the past include progestins or estrogens alone as well as in combination. When diethylstilbestrol (DES) was used to treat threatened abortion, vaginal adenosis and adenocarcinoma have occurred in female offspring, and urethral abnormalities in males. In addition, DES-exposed women have a high incidence of uterine anomalies and have themselves been shown to have a high incidence of pregnancy wastage. These regimens were advocated although there were few or no scientific data to support their use. Their efficacy was supported by incorrect estimates of the risk of recurrent abortion. These estimates were derived from inaccurate mathematical models, which have been disproven.

In evaluating the patient with recurrent abortion, a complete history and examination are extremely important. A careful history will frequently discover an infertile woman with oligomenorrhea who has infrequent, heavy, anovulatory periods and who has been diagnosed as having recurrent first-trimester abortions. This patient should be treated with clomiphene citrate (Clomid, Serophene) and not undergo a work-up for pregnancy wastage. If the history does support the diagnosis of recurrent abortion, appropriate laboratory studies should be done to determine the etiology of the losses, and specific therapy should be initiated in order to reverse the defect.

ETIOLOGY

Chromosomal Abnormalities

Chromosomal defects may follow abnormalities that occur during meiotic divisions in either oogenesis or spermatogenesis, or during mitosis. Chromosomal defects are detected most often in very early abortions, and the incidence declines steadily with increase in gestational age. Between 50% and 60% of first-trimester abortuses have chromosomal abnormalities, whereas the incidence of these defects falls to less than 25% when the abortion occurs in the second trimester.

The most common type of chromosomal defect in the abortus is autosomal trisomy. Of all abortuses with karyotype defects, trisomy is detected in 50-60%. Approximately 25% of abortuses with chromosomal abnormalities have deletion of one sex chromosome, with the resultant 45,X karyotype. Most fetuses with this karyotype are aborted, and those who survive present with the stigmata of Turner's syndrome. Polyploidy occurs in about 20-25% of karyotype defects and is usually of the triploidy type.

Most defects are random events; however, in some instances chromosomal defects in fetuses occur because a parent has a balanced translocation and transfers unbalanced genetic material to the offspring. Although approximately 1:250 phenotypically normal persons has a balanced translocation, the frequency of such defects is at least 10-fold higher among couples who experience recurrent abortion. Over the past few years, chromosomal banding techniques have been utilized to study genetic material. These methods are more sensitive and should replace older techniques. By utilizing banding methods, minor chromosomal abnormalities have been identified in up to 8% of couples who have recurrent abortions, compared with less than 3% of the general population. If a karyotype abnormality is detected in the husband, donor insemination may be considered.

Faulty Intrauterine Environment

The other major class of causes of recurrent abortion is a faulty maternal environment. Congenital anomalies of the uterus may be found in 10-15% of women with recurrent abortions. Although all types of anomalies may be detected, septate uterus is the anomaly most commonly associated with recurrent abortion. Abortion rates of up to 90% have been reported in patients with this defect. It is mandatory to make a complete investigation before attempting surgical correction of this lesion, to rule out other causes of abortion.

In women with submucous leiomyomas infertility, first- and second-trimester abortion, and premature labor have been reported. The mechanism of first-trimester abortion is most likely a poor implantation site secondary to poor endometrial nutrition. The relationship to second-trimester abortion is unclear, although the myomas may impair uterine enlargement, thereby causing premature labor. Intrauterine exposure to DES has been associated with upper genital tract anomalies. Approximately two-thirds of these women have a T-shaped uterus, pretubal bulges in the cornual regions, constriction bands, a lower uterine segment bulge, or combinations of these. The rates of ectopic pregnancy, spontaneous abortion (especially in the second trimester), and premature deliveries are increased among DES-exposed women. In addition, the term gestation rate is significantly lower in DES-exposed women with an abnormal hysterosalpingogram (HSG) compared with DES-exposed women with a normal HSG. The ideal method of treatment is unknown at present, but a cerclage should be performed in those who have had a second-trimester loss.

Intrauterine adhesions have also been associated with recurrent abortion, but the relationship is uncertain. Although adhesions may be an etiologic factor in recurrent abortion, they may be merely the sequelae of multiple curettages. An incompetent cervical os is also associated with recurrent abortion. Not all patients with this defect have the classical history of spontaneous rupture of membranes followed by painless delivery of the living fetus. However, some elements of this history are usually present and are sufficient to establish the diagnosis. The incompetent cervical os is unique in that this diagnosis is established by history, not by any laboratory studies. An inadequate corpus luteum may be associated with both infertility and repeated early abortions. Many of these abortions are subclinical and may be detected only with the use of the more sensitive β-subunit or radioreceptor assays for hCG.

Other Factors

Increasing maternal and paternal age is also associated with an increased risk of abortion. Other possible etiologies include subclinical hypothyroidism, immunologic factors, and infection with toxoplasmosis, *Ureaplasma urealyticum,* or *Listeria monocytogenes*. Absolute evidence of a cause-and-effect relationship between these etiologies and recurrent abortion is lacking at this time. The effect of a prior elective termination of pregnancy on the outcome of a subsequent pregnancy is uncertain. In many studies, an increase in both first- and second-trimester abortion among women who have had a prior elective abortion has been reported. However, other studies have not confirmed these findings.

Finally, immunologic factors have been implicated in recurrent abortion. Couples in whom tests for serum agglutination antibodies (Kibrick and Franklin-Dukes tests) and sperm-immobilizing antibodies (Isojima test) are positive have a higher abortion rate than couples whose tests are negative. In addition, couples who share multiple HLA antigens are at increased risk for pregnancy wastage. This is the newest area of research into the problem of recurrent abortion, and many problems remain unsolved.

MANAGEMENT

Investigation and therapy of the patient with recurrent abortion depend on the history and examination. However, investigation should be undertaken in any patient who has had even one second-trimester abortion. Such a history suggests a faulty maternal environment. At the time of the pregnancy loss, the uterine cavity should be carefully explored. If this has not been done, the cavity should be investigated by hysterosalpingography or hysteroscopy following the first spontaneous menstrual period. There is no benefit to be gained by delaying work-up or therapy until multiple second-trimester losses have occurred.

For a patient who has a history of cervical incompetence, a McDonald cervical cerclage should be performed at 14 weeks' gestation. An ultrasound scan should be performed before cerclage to rule out a gross fetal defect. If uterine enlargement or menorrhagia is present in addition to recurrent abortion, submucous leiomyomas should be suspected and hysteroscopy and/or hysterosalpingography performed. If submucous myomas are detected, myomectomy should be performed.

Because most abortions occurring in the first trimester are due to chromosomal defects, a woman with early pregnancy wastage who has submucous myomas should not undergo surgery unless more than one first-trimester abortion has occurred.

In those who have hypomenorrhea or amenorrhea, intrauterine adhesions should be suspected. However, even if the menstrual history is normal, adhesions may be present and such a diagnosis should be considered in patients who have a history of intrauterine instrumentation. Hysteroscopy should be employed for both diagnosis and therapy. Treatment consists of division of the adhesions using miniature scissors, placement of an intrauterine device, which is left in place for 2 months, and high-dose estrogen therapy for 2 months.

In the absence of a specific etiology, endometrial biopsy should be performed on day 26 or 27 of an idealized 28-day cycle to assess the adequacy of the luteal phase. Serum progesterone levels cannot be utilized to make this diagnosis unless specimens are obtained daily throughout the luteal phase. Luteal-phase inadequacy is best treated by either progesterone supplementation or clomiphene citrate as described in Chapter 92. Subclinical hypothyroidism may be detected by obtaining a serum TSH level. A karyotype should be obtained in both husband and wife, especially if the complaint is primary habitual abortion. However, this study is also mandatory if the couple has had only one abortion but has also had a child with a congenital defect.

SUMMARY

The causes of recurrent abortion may be genetic, uterine, or endocrinologic. Data supporting infectious etiology and wastage secondary to immunologic causes are less convincing. The investigation should be guided by the history. All patients with recurrent abortion should have a TSH level, cultures for *Ureaplasma urealyticum*, and an HSG. Couples with first-trimester losses should have a karyotype with banding and the woman should have a late luteal-phase endometrial biopsy. If one abnormality is detected, e.g., a uterine anomaly, the work-up should be completed before planning a treatment regimen, as a second cause might be found.

SUGGESTED READING

Beer AE, Quebbeman JF, Ayers JW, Haines RF: Major histocompatibility complex antigens, maternal and paternal immune responses, and chronic habitual abortions in humans. *Am J Obstet Gynecol* 141:987, 1981

Carr DH: Cytogenic aspects of induced and spontaneous abortions. *Clin Obstet Gynecol* 15:203, 1972

Hertig AT, et al: Thirty-four fertilized human ova, good, bad and indifferent, recovered from 210 women of known fertility. A study of biologic wastage in early human pregnancy. *Pediatrics* 23:202 (suppl), 1959

Husslein P, Huber J, Wagenbichler P, Schnedl W: Chromosome abnormalities in 150 couples with multiple spontaneous abortions. *Fertil Steril* 37:379, 1982

Jones GS, Madrigal-Castro V: Hormonal findings in association with abnormal corpus luteum function in the human: The luteal phase defect. *Fertil Steril* 21:1, 1970

Jones HW, Jones GS: Double uterus as an etiological factor in repeated abortion: Indications for surgical repair. *Am J Obstet Gynecol* 65:325, 1953

Warburton D, Fraser FC: On the probability that a woman who has a spontaneous abortion will abort in subsequent pregnancies. *J Obstet Gynaecol Br Commonw* 68:784, 1961

105

Evaluation of Pregnancy Tests

SUBIR ROY, M.D.

The evaluation of pregnancy tests requires an understanding of the normal production of human chorionic gonadotropin (hCG) in a pregnancy cycle. With this as background, it then becomes possible to choose the most appropriate pregnancy test based on the interval between the onset of the last menstrual period and the time of the test. Sensitivity, specificity, accuracy, requirements for special equipment, speed, availability, and cost are some of the factors to consider in choosing the most suitable pregnancy test for a given clinical situation.

PRODUCTION OF HCG IN A PREGNANCY CYCLE

β-hCG has been detected in the serum of pregnant women as early as 8-11 days after the luteinizing hormone (LH) peak, or 7-9 days after ovulation. The trophoblast production of hCG has been estimated to increase two-fold every 2 days, reaching a serum concentration of approximately 100 mIU/ml about 2 days after the expected menses would have begun.

SENSITIVITY

If we assume a 28-day cycle length, then a 200 mIU/ml level would be reached by 32 days after onset of the last period. This is the sensitivity level of the radioreceptor assay for hCG, commercially available as Biocept-G. β-Neocept, Sensi-Tex, and UCG-Beta Stat are three newer urine tube tests also claimed to have approximately this level of sensitivity.

The Pregnosticon tube test, the UCG-Wampole, Placentex, and In-Home Early Pregnancy Test (e.p.t.) can detect a 36-38-day pregnancy, equivalent to approximately 1,000 mIU/ml. Between days 36 and 40, the hCG level should be between 1,600 and 3,200 mIU/ml. The Pregnosticon Dri-Dot, Pregnosis, DAP, and Gravindex slide tests have this level of sensitivity.

The hCG values stated above are based on an ideal 28-day cycle. As is well known, the follicular phase of the menstrual cycle may be variable. When the follicular phase is prolonged, ovulation is delayed and the levels of hCG are lower than would be expected at each interval from onset of the last menstrual period. A pregnancy test, therefore, might give false-negative results because of the delayed ovulation.

SPECIFICITY

Generally speaking, serum tests are more specific than urine tests for the detection of hCG. Substances such as proteins, blood, some drugs, metabolites of drugs such as phenothiazines and methadone, soaps, and detergents may interfere with agglutination in latex pregnancy tests and give false-positive results. (This limitation applies more to slide than to tube tests.) This is why prior centrifugation or filtration of the specimen is sometimes necessary.

The radioreceptor assay cannot distinguish hCG from LH. It may, therefore, give a false-positive result at midcycle during the LH peak or in a perimenopausal patient. For this reason, the radioreceptor test uses a quantitative hCG level of 200 mIU/ml, a level not reached in either condition described above, to denote a positive test.

False-negative results usually occur with tests that are not sufficiently sensitive. However, bacterial contamination, heat, extreme pH shifts, metabolic inactivation in the body, and dilute urine can all lead to negative tests. (A concentrated first-voided specimen of morning urine more nearly approximates the serum concentration of hCG.)

ACCURACY

The accuracy of a urine test for pregnancy can be checked by comparing its results with β-hCG levels in a serum sample drawn at the same time the urine was obtained. However, this has not been done for every available test. Therefore, the accuracy of some tests (as a function of number of days from onset of last period) is not known.

Negative results with the Pregnosticon Dri-Dot slide test do not necessarily rule out pregnancy, even in excess of 42 days after onset of the last period. But if positive, it is *almost* always an accurate indication of pregnancy.

When used less than 42 days after the last menstrual period, the Pregnosticon and UCG-Wampole tube tests are not completely accurate if negative, but are 100% accurate if positive.

In theory, in a normal pregnancy cycle, the radioreceptor assay for hCG will be positive a few days after the time of the expected menses. But in practice, it is not 100% accurate when negative until after 42 days. If positive at any time, it is 100% accurate provided the patient is not perimenopausal.

Tests with positive and negative controls provide an internal standard for easier comparison of end points.

CHARACTERISTICS OF REPRESENTATIVE TESTS

The qualitative agglutination-inhibition tests (AITs), whether slide or tube, have similar features. The test kit contains purified hCG bound to a carrier (either latex particles or sheep red blood cells), plus antibody against hCG (produced by injecting hCG into an animal) and a control solution. In the presence of inadequate or no hCG in the urine, the anti-hCG binds to the hCG carrier and agglutination occurs. Detection of particles in the slide test or a diffused sediment in the tube test indicates an absence of hCG in the test specimen. In the presence of hCG in the urine, the anti-hCG binds to it and not to the hCG carrier; hence, no agglutination occurs. The absence of particles in the slide test or a ring comprised of hCG carrier alone in the tube test indicates inhibition of agglutination and a positive test.

A variant method has been recorded that may be more sensitive. In the direct agglutination test (DAT), anti-hCG, instead of hCG, is bound to the carrier. When a test sample containing hCG is added, agglutination of the hCG with the anti-hCG carrier complex occurs. Thus, in contrast to the test described above, agglutination indicates the *presence* of hCG.

The presence of *some* hCG in the test specimen can cause partial binding to the anti-hCG and, consequently, an incomplete lack of agglutination in the AIT or incomplete agglutination in the DAT. This may be difficult to distinguish from specimens that have been disturbed during the test. If this situation occurs, the test should be repeated.

Serum tests for the diagnosis of pregnancy include the radioreceptor assay (RRA) for hCG and the radioimmunoassay (RIA) for hCG or the more specific β-subunit of hCG (β-hCG). The RIA tests, until recently, were research tools not ordinarily used as pregnancy tests. Now, clinical laboratories are able to use β-hCG kits with sensitivity levels varying from 5 to 30 mIU/ml, which require less than an hour of laboratory time. It is possible, therefore, to diagnose pregnancy even before the missed menstrual period.

The RRA has been used as both a qualitative pregnancy test and (when used with a standard curve) a quantitative hCG assay. It employs bovine corpora lutea membrane receptors in place of anti-hCG. Radioactive iodine-labeled hCG and a gamma counter are required. The RRA does not distinguish LH from hCG; this could lead to false-positives in perimenopausal women.

Requirements for Special Equipment

The Sensi-Tex requires a heating block to accelerate the kinetics of the reaction. The RRA for hCG or RIA for β-hCG are laboratory (not office) tests requiring capabilities for handling radioactive materials and a gamma counter. Many pregnancy tests recommend that the specimen be centrifuged or filtered (with specific filter paper) prior to performance of the test.

Speed

The slide tests require 2 minutes to perform, while the tube tests require from 90 minutes to 2 hours. The radioreceptor assay and the β-hCG kit tests require about an hour of laboratory time, but in practice are available from most commercial laboratories only twice a day.

Availability

All the slide and tube tests are available as kits and can be used in the office or at home. The Biocept-G and the β-hCG RIA kit tests are commercially available through almost all diagnostic laboratories.

Cost

The slide test may cost a couple of dollars; the tube test costs about $10; and the RRA for hCG and the RIA kit for β-hCG cost from $10-15.

CONCLUSION

The earlier the pregnancy needs to be detected, the more sophisticated and time-consuming will be the test. This review should enable the clinician to decide which test to use in a given situation. Not all available pregnancy tests have been mentioned by name here, but some of the more common ones have been used as examples of the basic types. The use of pregnancy tests in suspected ectopic gestations is discussed in Chapter 57.

SUGGESTED READING

Landesman R, Saxena BB: Results of the first 1000 radioreceptorassays for the determination of human chorionic gonadotropin: A new, rapid, reliable and sensitive pregnancy test. *Fertil Steril* 27:357, 1976

Mishell DR Jr, Nakamura RM, Barberia JM, Thorneycroft IH: Initial detection of human chorionic gonadotropin in serum in normal human gestation. *Am J Obstet Gynecol* 118:990, 1974

Roy S, Klein TA, Scott JZ, Kletzky OA, Mishell DR Jr: Diagnosis of pregnancy with a radioreceptor assay for hCG. *Obstet Gynecol* 50:401, 1977

Vaitukaitis JL, Braunstein GD, Ross GT: A radio-immunoassay which specifically measures human gonadotropin in the presence of human luteinizing hormone. *Am J Obstet Gynecol* 113:751, 1972

Wide L: An immunologic method for the detection of human chorionic gonadotropin. *Acta Endocrinol* 41 (suppl 70):1, 1962

106

Precocious Puberty

PAUL F. BRENNER, M.D.

Precocious puberty has been defined as the presence of breast budding prior to age 8, or appearance of the first menstrual flow prior to age 9.

In evaluating patients with precocious puberty, first determine by history and physical examination whether the secondary sex characteristics agree or disagree with the genetic sex. A girl who feminizes early is defined as having *isosexual precocious puberty*; her secondary sex characteristics are in agreement with her genetic sex. A girl who virilizes early is defined as having *heterosexual precocious puberty*; her secondary sex characteristics are in disagreement with her genetic sex. Girls with heterosexual precocious puberty should be evaluated like all patients who present with androgen excess and will not be considered further in this chapter.

INCOMPLETE PRECOCIOUS PUBERTY

Precocious puberty is incomplete if only one pubertal change is clinically apparent without any evidence of a systemic estrogen effect. Absence of superficial cells desquamated from the vaginal mucosa or failure of the roentgenologic bone age to exceed the chronologic age has been accepted as evidence for the absence of a systemic estrogen effect. Incomplete forms of precocious puberty include premature thelarche, premature adrenarche, and premature pubarche.

Premature Thelarche

Premature thelarche is the clinical presentation of only breast development, usually incomplete. There are no other pubertal changes or systemic effects of estrogen on the maturation index or bone age. This condition is benign, and the breast development usually regresses spontaneously within 6 months. Therapy is not required.

Premature Adrenarche

Premature adrenarche is the clinical presentation of only axillary hair. Again, there are no other pubertal changes or systemic evidence of estrogen or androgen effects accompanying this condition. Premature adrenarche is also benign and therapy is not required.

Premature Pubarche

Premature pubarche is the clinical presentation of only pubic hair. Axillary hair growth, breast development, menarche, and systemic estrogen effects do not occur. Some series report that approximately one-half of all patients with premature pubarche have organic brain disease. The reason for this association is unknown.

At the initial visit, if the patient has only one clinical pubertal change, it may be difficult to determine whether it is an incomplete form of precocious puberty or the first evidence of a progressive spectrum of pubertal changes. Tests to detect a systemic estrogen effect (advancement of bone age, maturation index) may be necessary in order to distinguish clearly between the two possibilities.

COMPLETE ISOSEXUAL PRECOCIOUS PUBERTY

Isosexual precocious puberty has been classified as either *true* or *pseudo*. Ninety per cent of all patients with precocious puberty have the true form, which has also been called the cerebral form because all its causes have been located in the central nervous system. In the true form there is normal cyclic adult function of the reproductive axis. Cyclic secretion of gonadotropins and estrogen occurs, and the negative and positive feedback mechanisms of sex steroids on the hypothalamus and pituitary develop early. The cyclic patterns of hormone production result in the appearance of secondary sex characteristics, maturation of ovarian follicles, ovulation, and the potential for fertility. Constitutional and organic brain disease are the two causes of true isosexual precocious puberty.

The remaining cases of isosexual precocious puberty have been classified as pseudo because cyclic function of the hypothalamic-pituitary-ovarian axis does not occur, gonadotropin secretion does not increase, and follicle maturation and ovulation are absent. There is an increase in estrogen, resulting in the precocious development of secondary sex characteristics, but these patients are not fertile. The causes of pseudo isosexual precocious puberty include ovarian, adrenal, or iatrogenic factors, hypothyroidism, Albright's syndrome, and hemihypertrophy syndrome.

ETIOLOGY

True Isosexual Precocious Puberty

Constitutional. The most common cause of true isosexual precocious puberty is constitutional, or idiopathic. The etiology of this premature attainment of adult function of the reproductive axis is unknown. The premature pubertal changes do not affect patients' general health but can represent emotional crises to patients and their families. The increased estrogen levels result in premature distal epiphyseal closure of the long bones. While patients are initially taller than their peers, their growth spurt lasts for a short time and ultimately they are short in stature. The earlier in life the disease begins, the shorter will be the patient's final height.

These patients are fertile. Constitutional precocious puberty may occur at any age, and the progression of pubertal changes varies greatly. The sequence of pubertal changes may be rapid or slow and may or may not mimic the events of normal puberty. Rare spontaneous remissions have been reported. Approximately half the patients have diffuse electroencephalographic abnormalities. There are no specific laboratory parameters or group of tests that establish the diagnosis of constitutional precocious puberty. The diagnosis is one of exclusion.

Organic brain disease. Patients with various types of organic brain disease, including tumors, congenital defects, obstructive lesions, and infection, sometimes manifest precocious pubertal development. It is rare for the practitioner to see these patients prior to the development of the signs and symptoms of their brain disease. A neurologic examination will identify the cause of their precocious development.

Pseudo Isosexual Precocious Puberty

Ovarian tumors. The most common cause of pseudo isosexual precocious puberty is an ovarian tumor that produces estrogen. Granulosa-theca-cell tumors secrete estrogens, which in female children may result in precocious pubertal development. These tumors are palpable on rectal-abdominal examination. Most granulosa-theca-cell tumors are benign, and the treatment of choice is unilateral oophorectomy. A very rare cause is a choriocarcinoma, which originates either in an ovary or in an extragonadal teratoma. Choriocarcinomas elaborate human chorionic gonadotropin, which may stimulate the ovary to secrete estrogen.

Adrenal tumors. An adrenal tumor that secretes estrogen is an extremely rare cause of isosexual precocious puberty. In the infrequent case reports of this tumor, virilizing symptoms and signs have preceded the clinical manifestations of excess estrogen.

Iatrogenic causes. Iatrogenic agents are increasing in importance as causes of precocious puberty. Cosmetics, cleansing creams, creams for diaper rash, and medications containing estrogens have all been implicated as causes of isosexual precocious puberty. A complete history and careful review of all possible sources of estrogen in the home are the only available means of identifying iatrogenic sources of this sex steroid.

Hypothyroidism. A girl who is markedly hypothyroid has diminished thyroid hormone production and a decreased negative feedback of thyroxine on the hypothalamus and pituitary. As the output of thyroid-stimulating hormone is increased by the pituitary, there is also an indiscriminate increase in gonadotropins. The increase in gonadotropins produces clinical precocious puberty and may stimulate the growth of ovarian cysts. The treatment of these cysts is not surgical extirpation, but thyroid replacement. As the patient becomes euthyroid, the cysts will disappear. Children with hypothyroidism are short and their bone age is retarded. Hypothyroidism as a cause of precocious puberty is limited almost entirely to girls.

McCune-Albright syndrome. This syndrome consists of sexual precocity, multiple areas of fibrous dysplasia of bone, and café-au-lait spots on the skin. The diagnosis can be entertained from the characteristic skeletal deformities and facial asymmetry. This syndrome is identified more frequently in girls.

Hemihypertrophy syndrome. The hemihypertrophy syndrome of Wilkins is the appearance of both unilateral sexual precocity and vascular anomalies in the same individual. The diagnosis of this very rare condition is made by physical examination.

DIAGNOSIS

The evaluation of girls with evidence of precocious sexual development includes a careful history, physical examination, and selection of adjunctive diagnostic tests, ordered in a logical sequence. Heterosexual precocious puberty, organic brain disease, iatrogenic sources, granulosa-theca-cell tumors, hypothyroidism, McCune-Albright syndrome, and hemihypertrophy syndrome can be diagnosed largely as the result of the history and physical examination, including a neurologic examination, rectal-abdominal exam, and the pediatrician's sequential recordings of the patient's height.

A bone age study is the first diagnostic procedure ordered. Only patients with marked hypothyroidism have retarded bone age and retarded height. Patients with incomplete sexual precocity (premature thelarche, premature adrenarche, premature pubarche) have a normal bone age and their observed height agrees with their chronologic age, denoting an absence of systemic estrogen effects. Repeated observations several months apart may be necessary, particularly to establish the diagnosis of incomplete sexual precocity.

Advancement of bone age and observed height beyond the 95th percentile for the individual's corresponding chronologic age indicates an estrogen effect. Whether the estrogen is derived from a true or a pseudo source (hypothyroidism having previously been excluded) can be determined by ordering a serum follicle-stimulating hormone (FSH) level. In the true forms of isosexual precocious puberty, the hypothalamic sensitivity to circulating estrogen decreases and gonadotropin secretion rises to adult levels. An abnormal neurologic exam may suggest organic brain disease. Constitutional precocious puberty is a diagnosis reached by exclusion of all other causes.

In pseudo forms, the hypothalamus remains exquisitely sensitive to the negative feedback of estrogen, whether endogenous or exogenous, and FSH concentrations are very low. The specific causes can be separated by the history and physical examination. A serum human chorionic gonadotropin concentration below the level of sensitivity of the assay will exclude a choriocarcinoma. Serum dehydroepiandrosterone sulfate will be elevated if the condition is due to an adrenal cause.

TREATMENT

The ideal treatment for constitutional precocious puberty would cause the regression of secondary sex characteristics, the suppression of ovulation and menstruation, and the prevention of premature epiphyseal closure. This therapy has not been found. Antiandrogens recommended in Europe are not available in this country. Danazol (Danocrine) was used in a small series of patients, but resulted in virilization and has been discarded as a treatment of constitutional precocious puberty for girls.

Medroxyprogesterone acetate (Provera) has been used in the treatment of constitutional precocious sexual development. Even in very high doses, however, this agent does not prevent premature fusion of the distal epiphyses of the long bones. It has an unpredictable effect on the regression of secondary sex characteristics, although it does suppress both ovulation and menstruation. Depot medroxyprogesterone acetate (Depo-Provera) has been administered in doses of 100-200 mg every 2-6 weeks. We have recently used this agent in a titration dosage sufficient to keep the patient's serum estradiol levels below 20 pg/ml. This usually results in less frequent administration of the drug.

The long-term effects of medroxyprogesterone acetate given during puberty and the possible prolonged suppression of the hypothalamic-pituitary axis when the medication is discontinued must be weighed very carefully. The decision to use this agent is a very serious one and must be individualized for each patient. Luteinizing hormone-releasing hormone agonists are being tested clinically in the treatment of precocious puberty, with encouraging results.

SUGGESTED READING

Crowley WF, Comite F, Vale W, Rivier J, Loriaux DL, Cutler GB Jr: Therapeutic use of pituitary densensitization with long-acting LHRH agonist: A potential new treatment for idiopathic precocious puberty. *J Clin Endocrinol Metab* 52:370, 1981

Madden JD, MacDonald PC: Origin of estrogen in isosexual precocious pseudopuberty due to a granulosa theca-cell tumor. *Obstet Gynecol* 51:210, 1978

Richman RA, Underwood LE, French FS, Van Wyk JJ: Adverse effects of large doses of medroxyprogesterone (MPA) in idiopathic isosexual precocity. *J Pediatr* 79:963, 1971

Riddlesberg MM Jr, Kuhn JP, Munschauer RW: The association of juvenile hypothyroidism and cystic ovaries. *Radiology* 139:77, 1981

Werder EA, Murset G, Zachman M, Brook CGD, Prader A: Treatment of precocious puberty with cyproterone acetate. *Pediatr Res* 8:248, 1974

Wohltman H, Mathur RS, Williamson HO: Sexual precocity in a female infant due to a feminizing adrenal carcinoma. *J Clin Endocrinol Metab* 50:186, 1980

107

Hormone Replacement Therapy After the Menopause

DANIEL R. MISHELL JR., M.D.

In the United States, the mean age at menopause is 50 years. A woman's life expectancy is now nearly 80 years; therefore, more than one-third of her life span will be spent in the postmenopausal years. After the menopause, ovarian production of estrogen ceases and circulating levels fall dramatically, with estrone levels becoming greater than estradiol levels. Extraglandular conversion of circulating androstenedione accounts for almost all estrone production. After the menopause, about 85% of androstenedione comes from adrenal secretion and about 15% from the ovaries. The conversion of androstenedione to estrone takes place mainly in the fatty tissue; therefore, obese women have higher levels of estrone and are less likely to be estrogen-deficient.

GENITOURINARY SYMPTOMS

As a result of the decreased circulating estrogen levels, estrogen-dependent target tissues usually atrophy. The vaginal mucosa becomes thin, pale, and almost transparent. In some instances, atrophic vaginitis may develop, with vaginal bleeding, itching, and burning. Coitus may be extremely painful or impossible for women with marked atrophy of the vaginal vault.

The urethral mucosa is also estrogen-dependent, and it becomes thinner as the amount of estrogen in the circulation falls. Atrophic urethritis may develop and produce dysuria, frequency, and urinary incontinence. Shrinkage of the vulva may produce vulvitis with pruritus.

The best treatment for postmenopausal vaginal atrophy is estrogen. It is best to administer estrogen systemically to treat atrophic vaginitis, as estrogen administered locally is adsorbed into the circulation to varying degrees in different patients and thus produces variable systemic effects. With oral estrogen the dosage can be regulated better. Atrophic changes of the urethra producing urge incontinence and dysuria may also be reversed with estrogen.

EXTRAGENITAL SYMPTOMS

Extragenitally, the most common symptom is the hot flush. Hot flushes may persist for seconds or last up to several minutes, and may occur as frequently as every 10-30 minutes or only once every few days. They are more common at night and frequently awaken the woman.

It is estimated that three-quarters of all women develop hot flushes during the menopausal transition and half these women seek medical attention. The flushes persist for more than 1 year in 85% of women and for more than 5 years in 25%. Almost half of the women experiencing hot flushes have at least one episode per day. The exact mechanism causing hot flushes is not known, but it is thought to be due to a decline in estrogen levels with increased hypothalamic activity.

There is excellent scientific evidence that estrogens are beneficial in relieving hot flushes. In a double-blind cross-over study in which half the subjects received estrogen and the other half a placebo for 3 months, after which the preparations were reversed, both groups reported a significant decrease in the frequency of flushes in response to both estrogen and placebo, but the decrease in number of flushes was much greater with the estrogen therapy than with the placebo. When subjects who were taking estrogen were changed to placebo, the number of flushes increased, while subjects changing from placebo to estrogen had a further reduction in the number of flushes. This study indicated that estrogen therapy does result in marked clinical improvement in vasomotor symptoms, and also demonstrated a placebo effect.

Women who have a contraindication to estrogen therapy, such as a carcinoma of the breast, are best treated with progestins. Best results have been obtained with the use of 20 mg of medroxyprogesterone acetate (Provera) orally daily or 150 mg of depot medroxyprogesterone acetate (Depo-Provera) every 3 months. These doses of progestins relieve hot flushes as well as estrogens, but progestins do not have the beneficial effects of estrogen on the vagina and uterus.

It has not been proven that estrogen therapy is of benefit in relieving other common symptoms of the climacteric, such as irritability, anxiety, nervousness, depression, and fatigue, but relieving the hot flushes allows the postmenopausal woman to sleep better, which in turn often reduces the frequency of these other symptoms.

CARDIOVASCULAR EFFECTS

The incidence of atherosclerosis is increased in women after the menopause. Although this increase has not been demonstrated to be due to estrogen deficiency, a recent epidemiologic study indicated that exogenous estrogen has a beneficial effect in the retardation of atherosclerotic heart disease. The doses of exogenous estrogen used in oral contraceptives, which are several times as potent as those generally used for replacement therapy, have been shown to increase the risk of myocardial infarction in premenopausal women over 35 who smoke. However, several studies indicate that the doses of estrogen generally used to treat postmenopausal women—i.e., 2.5 mg of conjugated equine estrogen or less per day—do not increase the incidence of heart attacks, stroke, or hypertension in postmenopausal women, even if they smoke.

OSTEOPOROSIS

Osteoporosis is a disorder in which bone mass is reduced. It occurs in both men and women after the age of 40, but women experience a three-fold greater loss than do men. This loss of bone mass can cause fractures of the vertebral bodies, the distal radius, and the neck of the femur. It is estimated that about 700,000 postmenopausal women have osteoporotic fractures in the United States each year. Since the process of osteoporosis proceeds slowly for many years, by the time a fracture occurs the osteoporotic process is well advanced. Blacks, men, and tall or obese women have greater than average bone mass and, therefore, a lower incidence of osteoporotic fractures. Osteoporosis cannot be detected on routine x-rays until a large percentage of the bone mass is lost, so the process may progress without signs or symptoms until a fracture occurs, usually beginning about 10 years after the menopause.

Many studies indicate that osteoporosis is related to a decline in ovarian function. After the menopause, women lose about 1.5% of their bone mass each year. Bilateral oophorectomy prior to age 45 increases the likelihood of developing osteoporosis, while oophorectomy after the age of 45 does not increase this risk. Because of the difficulty in diagnosing osteoporosis and the necessity for prolonged follow-up, there is a paucity of good clinical studies involving the use of exogenous estrogen for the prevention and treatment of osteoporosis. Nevertheless, a few long-term studies indicate that estrogen prevents the development of osteoporosis as well as stabilizes the process once it has developed. Several epidemiologic studies show that estrogen reduces the incidence of fractures in postmenopausal women. It has recently been demonstrated that the equivalent of 0.625 mg of conjugated estrogens per day is necessary to prevent osteoporosis. Estrogen has not been shown to produce a sustained increase in bone mass in osteoporotic patients, as it does not stimulate new growth but only decreases bone resorption.

There is no evidence that ingestion of a small amount of calcium supplement or vitamin D prevents or retards osteoporotic loss of bone. It is recommended that nonobese white women should ingest adequate amounts of calcium—the equivalent of 1.5 gm/day—in the diet, along with a calcium supplement of 500 mg/day in addition to estrogen. Since lack of exercise is a factor in osteoporosis, women should be encouraged to continue or start exercising daily after the menopause.

ADVERSE EFFECTS

There are some theoretical and actual adverse effects of estrogen replacement therapy. The adverse metabolic changes associated with the use of oral contraceptives—hypertension, thromboembolism, and altered glucose tolerance—have not been demonstrated in postmenopausal women receiving estrogen replacement. This difference is due to the fact that the pharmacologic doses of estrogen in oral contraceptives are more potent than the amount of estrogen usually given for hormone replacement. Estrogen doses equivalent to 0.625 mg/day of conjugated estrogens do not produce the same alteration of serum proteins as do the equivalent of higher doses of conjugated estrogens or the amount of ethinylestradiol found in oral contraceptives. Therefore, 0.625 mg/day of conjugated estrogens can be considered a physiologic replacement dose, while higher doses may be considered pharmacologic.

Several recent retrospective studies have shown that women receiving supplemental estrogen have an increased risk of developing adenocarcinoma of the endometrium. Although the increased risk is reported to vary from three- to eight-fold, the annual incidence of adenocarcinoma is relatively low, 30:100,000 and 50:100,000 women at ages 50 and 60, respectively. Therefore, the increased risk of developing adenocarcinoma might change from 1:2,500 to 1:500. Furthermore, the risk of developing adenocarcinoma was noted only when high doses—i.e., 1.25 mg of conjugated estrogens or more—were ingested for more than 5 years. One study showed the risk of developing endometrial adenocarcinoma was not increased if the daily dose was 0.625 mg or less of conjugated estrogens. Other studies have shown that risk of adenocarcinoma is not increased if a progestogen is added to the estrogen regimen.

DOSAGE

The initial dosage should be the equivalent of 0.625 mg/day of conjugated estrogens, as this amount is required to prevent osteoporosis. The specific formulation is not critical. Orally the medication should be given discontinuously, with some medication-free days each month. We recommend that estrogen be given orally for the first 25 days of each month, with a gestagen such as 5.0 mg of medroxyprogesterone acetate added during the last 10 days of estrogen treatment to differentiate the endometrium and reduce the risk of adenocarcinoma. It is probably not necessary to give higher doses of this progestin. With these low doses of estrogen and progestin, regular uterine bleeding during the medication-free days is infrequent. Oral contraceptives should not be used in treatment of the menopause, as the dose of estrogen is excessive and associated with adverse metabolic effects.

It is not possible to correlate the degree of menopausal symptoms with the results obtained by measurement of endogenous estrogen levels or by use of vaginal smears. Postmenopausal women receiving exogenous estrogens should be examined 3 months after the therapy is initiated, and at least annually thereafter. At these examinations the breasts and pelvis should be examined and blood pressure, weight, and height measured. There is no evidence to date that estrogen therapy induces breast cancer. However, since estrogen can stimulate growth of this malignancy, it is best to use mammography before starting estrogen therapy to rule out a small, nonpalpable lesion.

Prior to initiation of estrogen therapy, patients should be fully informed of its benefits and risks and a written informed consent obtained. If abnormal bleeding develops during therapy, an endometrial biopsy should be done; otherwise, an annual biopsy is unnecessary. Since osteoporosis will develop at any age following cessation of estrogen therapy, treatment of nonobese white or Oriental women should continue until age 75 to 80.

SUGGESTED READING

Collins J, Donner A, Allen LH, Adams O: Oestrogen use and survival in endometrial cancer. *Lancet* 2:961, 1980

Gambrell RD Jr: The prevention of endometrial cancer in postmenopausal women with progestogens. *Maturitas* 1:107, 1978

Lindsay R, Hart DM, Forrest C, Baird C: Prevention of spinal osteoporosis in oophorectomised women. *Lancet* 2:1151, 1980

Mack TM, Pike MC, Henderson BE, et al: Estrogens and endometrial cancer in a retirement community. *N Engl J Med* 294:1262, 1976

Morrison JC, Martin DC, Blair RA, et al: The use of medroxyprogesterone acetate for relief of vasomotor symptoms. *Am J Obstet Gynecol* 138:99, 1980

Ross RK, Paganini-Hill A, Mack TM, Arthur M, Henderson BE: Menopausal oestrogen therapy and protection from death from ischaemic heart disease. *Lancet* 1:858, 1981

Whitehead MI, Townsend PT, Prys-Davies J, et al: Effects of estrogens and progestins on the biochemistry and morphology of the postmenopausal endometrium. *N Engl J Med* 305:1599, 1981

SEVEN

FAMILY
PLANNING

108

Management of Common Problems With Oral Contraceptives

DANIEL R. MISHELL JR., M.D.

In addition to preventing ovulation and affecting the female genital tract in various ways, both the estrogen and gestagen components of oral contraceptive pills have many actions that affect nearly every organ system of the body. As a result of these metabolic changes, patients taking oral contraceptives frequently experience undesirable symptoms.

COMMON SIDE EFFECTS

Although unwanted symptoms associated with oral contraceptive therapy are not infrequent, serious complications are relatively rare. Furthermore, with the newer, low-dose formulations, both mild symptoms and serious complications occur with much less frequency. The most common undesirable symptoms are nausea, breast tenderness, breakthrough bleeding, failure of withdrawal bleeding (amenorrhea), fluid retention (edema), weight gain, acne, nervousness, headaches, and mood changes, particularly depression.

Nausea, breast tenderness, fluid retention, and mood changes are due mainly to the estrogenic components of the formulations. If these symptoms persist for more than 3 months, a formulation with less estrogen should be used. Weight gain, acne, and nervousness are due to the androgenic type of gestagens, which are present in all of the currently marketed formulations. Thus, if an individual gains more than 10 lb annually or develops or has worsening of acne or nervousness, she should be switched to a formulation with a less potent gestagen and a higher estrogen/gestagen potency ratio. Breakthrough bleeding and failure of withdrawal bleeding are caused by insufficient estrogen or excessive progestogen and can be ameliorated by increasing the amount of estrogen in relation to the amount of gestagen by temporarily adding 20 μg of ethinylestradiol per day of active pill intake to her existing formulation for three consecutive cycles.

AMENORRHEA

The development of amenorrhea during oral contraceptive use is of concern because the diagnosis of pregnancy must be considered. The periodic appearance of menstrual bleeding provides a signal to the woman that she is not pregnant. Therefore, it is best to induce regular withdrawal bleeding in women who have amenorrhea while taking oral contraceptives, and are not pregnant, by increasing the estrogenic component or using a less potent gestagen. If a woman experiences gradual decreases in withdrawal bleeding followed by amenorrhea, the endometrium can be built up by adding 20 μg of ethinylestradiol per day of active pill intake to the oral contraceptive formulation for about 3 months. Withdrawal bleeding will usually be reinstated. If a woman taking an oral contraceptive with regular withdrawal bleeding suddenly fails to have withdrawal bleeding, the oral contraceptive should be stopped, a barrier method used, and a sensitive pregnancy test performed.

CEREBROVASCULAR PROBLEMS

If an individual develops a greater frequency of headaches, especially of the migraine type, her oral contraceptive should be stopped, as these symptoms may be prodromal for a stroke, a rare but serious complication of oral contraceptives. Other prodromal symptoms include fainting, paresthesias, and loss of vision. Depression and other mood changes in women ingesting oral contraceptives are physiologic changes caused by the effect of the estrogenic component on tryptophan metabolism, which in turn lowers brain serotonin levels. Women who develop depressive symptoms should be switched to another method of contraception or perhaps to a daily oral contraceptive containing a progestin without estrogen.

Development of hypertension is another result of the estrogenic component of oral contraceptives. The estrogen increases the amount of circulating angiotensinogen, which in turn causes hypertension to develop in fewer than 5% of oral contraceptive users after 5 years of use. This incidence is about twice the incidence in a control population of similar age. Thus, blood pressure should be monitored at each visit and if hypertension develops, the medication should be stopped.

POSTPILL AMENORRHEA

Postpill amenorrhea is estimated to occur in about 0.2-0.8% of women who stop oral contraceptives. This disorder is a hypothalamic effect and is not related to the occurrence of amenorrhea while taking the steroids, which is an endometrial effect. The incidence of postpill amenorrhea is higher in patients who had oligomenorrhea or amenorrhea prior to starting oral contraceptives than in those with regular menses. About 35-45% of women who develop amenorrhea after taking oral contraceptives have a history of prior menstrual irregularity. Postpill amenorrhea is not caused by continued suppression of the hypothalamic-pituitary axis; instead, the periodic withdrawal bleeding produced by an oral contraceptive serves to mask an amenorrheic state that would have existed without the steroids.

In any event, the use of any oral contraceptive steroid is contraindicated in patients who have oligomenorrhea or amenorrhea unless they have a diagno-

sis of polycystic ovarian disease. If individuals with amenorrhea or oligomenorrhea desire regular menses, treatment with a gestagen alone for 5 days each
month is usually sufficient to induce menses without suppressing hypothalamic function or masking the development of amenorrhea associated with low
estrogen production. If these women desire contraception, it is best for them
to use a method other than hormonal steroids, preferably a barrier method, as
they ovulate infrequently, if at all.

EFFECTS ON FERTILITY

There is no evidence that women who discontinue oral contraceptives have a
higher incidence of infertility than women who discontinue other methods of
contraception, although there is a delay of 2-3 months after stopping oral contraceptives before conception rates are similar to those of women who stop
mechanical methods of contraception. There is no increased risk of abortion
or congenital defects in infants born to women who conceive after stopping
oral contraceptives, even if they conceive in the first cycle after stopping the
pills. It is best to wait one cycle before trying to conceive after stopping an oral
contraceptive so that the date of conception can be estimated more accurately, as ovulation is delayed in the first cycle after pills are discontinued.

SUGGESTED READING

Fisch IR, Frank J: Oral contraceptives and blood pressure. *JAMA* 237:2494, 1977

March CM, Mishell DR Jr: A ten-year comparison of post oral contraceptive amenorrhea with amenorrhea
unrelated to use of drugs. In *Endocrinology of Human Infertility: New Aspects*. London: Academic Press,
1981, pp 207-219

*Oral Contraceptives and Health: An Interim Report From the Oral Contraceptive Study of the Royal College
of General Practitioners*. New York: Pitman, 1974

Oral contraceptives—Update on usage, safety, and side effects. *Popul Rep* ser A(5):January 1979

Vessey MP, Wright NH, McPherson K, et al: Fertility after stopping different methods of contraception. *Br
Med J* 1:265, 1979

109

Serious Complications of Oral Contraceptives

DANIEL R. MISHELL JR., M.D.

Patients are concerned about the increased risk of the rare but serious complications associated with oral contraceptive use, such as thromboembolism, stroke, myocardial infarction, diabetes mellitus, and liver adenoma. In addition, they are concerned about developing postpill amenorrhea and infertility and cancer, especially cancer of the breast. There is no evidence that oral contraceptives produce sterility or increase the incidence of spontaneous abortion or congenital abnormalities when conception occurs after these agents have been stopped. However, a temporary period of infertility, usually less than 6 months, may occur.

RISK OF CANCER

There is no evidence at present that oral contraceptives cause an increased incidence of any type of human carcinoma, including cancer of the breast, cervix, or endometrium. The gestagenic component of the formulation actually acts to prevent the mitogenic action of the estrogenic component on target tissues by decreasing the synthesis of estrogen receptor protein, and therefore reduces the incidence of cancer of the endometrium and benign breast disease in oral contraceptive users. Although oral contraceptives probably do cause an increased incidence of benign liver adenomas, these are very rare tumors and are estimated to occur in only about 1:50,000 oral contraceptive users. These tumors, which are palpable when large, but do not alter liver function tests, are more common in women who have used oral contraceptives for more than 5 years and regress when oral contraceptive ingestion ceases. They do not become malignant.

THROMBOEMBOLIC DISEASE

Although oral contraceptives have been reported to increase the incidence of thromboembolism, stroke, and myocardial infarction about three-fold, the baseline incidence of these disorders is extremely low in women in the reproductive age group. Thus, despite the several-fold increased risk, the actual chance that an individual will develop one of these serious problems while taking oral contraceptives is small. Furthermore, recent studies with the lower-estrogen-dose formulations indicate that the risk of vascular problems is much less than with the higher-estrogen-dose formulations used by women in most of the epidemiologic studies.

Mortality from thromboembolic disease associated with the use of hormonal contraceptives is estimated to be about 3:100,000 women per year. Development of thromboembolic disease is related to age but not to parity, smoking, or duration of oral contraceptive use. The increased incidence of thromboembolism is related to the amount of estrogen, and formulations containing more than 50 μg of the estrogen component are associated with a higher incidence of thromboembolic phenomena. Therefore, it is best not to prescribe oral contraceptives containing more than 50 μg of estrogen.

Patients receiving oral contraceptives need not have clinical evidence of deep vein thrombophlebitis of the lower extremities prior to the development of pulmonary thromboembolism. There is no evidence that the incidence of thromboembolism is increased in women with varicosities of the lower extremities. Individuals who develop chest pain while taking contraceptive steroids should discontinue therapy as well as have further diagnostic studies, including a lung scan. Finally, several reports have linked use of oral contraceptives immediately prior to surgical procedures with about a two-fold increased incidence of postoperative venous thromboembolism. For this reason, oral contraceptives should be discontinued at least 1 month prior to any elective surgical procedure.

STROKE

There is a strong correlation between increasing blood pressure and relative risk for developing thrombotic or hemorrhagic stroke in oral contraceptive users as well as nonusers. Therefore, oral contraceptives should not be used by women with hypertension. Heavy cigarette smoking is correlated with an increased risk of hemorrhagic stroke in oral contraceptive users.

MYOCARDIAL INFARCTION

The incidence of myocardial infarction in oral contraceptive users is significantly increased only if they are over 35 years of age and certain risk factors are present. The major risk factor is heavy cigarette smoking. Cigarette smoking acts synergistically with oral contraceptives to increase the risk of myocardial infarction. It is now believed that the etiology of myocardial infarction in oral contraceptive users is a thrombotic, not atherogenic, phenomenon, since the increased risk does not persist in former users and is unrelated to duration of use. Thus, nicotine narrows the vessels and allows a thrombus to occur.

Other risk factors include hypertension, hypercholesterolemia, and possibly diabetes. With these antecedent risk factors—especially in cigarette smokers—the use of oral contraceptives increases the chance of dying from myocardial infarction about three-fold, or to about 1:4,000 annually for women aged 35-39 and 1:1,000 annually for women aged 40-44.

Increased mortality from all cardiovascular diseases combined occurs predominantly in oral contraceptive users over 35 who smoke or have other risk factors. It is now recommended that women over 35 who smoke should discontinue oral contraceptives, and that women under 35 with hypertension, diabetes, or hyperlipidemia not use oral contraceptives.

AGE

With advancing age, the risk of mortality with use of oral contraceptives increases, the risk of death with IUDs declines, and the risk of death with tubal sterilization remains low. Because of the increasing risk of death in older women using oral contraceptives, as well as the increased incidence of systemic disease among older women, oral contraceptives should be used mainly by young, healthy women for the purpose of family spacing. Once childbearing is complete, alternative forms of contraception—mainly the IUD or a barrier method—can be used or sterilization performed for either partner.

Women who wish to continue using oral contraceptives after their families are complete may do so up to about 40 years of age with careful monitoring, if they have no associated risk factors. Oral contraceptive use after the age of 40 should be discouraged.

CONTRAINDICATIONS

Women of any age should not take oral contraceptives if they have any contraindication to their use. Absolute contraindications include (1) a history of vascular disease, including thromboembolism, thrombophlebitis, atherosclerosis, or stroke, (2) hypertension, (3) diabetes, (4) hyperlipidemia, (5) cancer of the breast or endometrium, (6) pregnancy, (7) heart disease, and (8) active liver disease. Relative contraindications include (1) undiagnosed amenorrhea, (2) migraine headache, and (3) depression.

PRECAUTIONS

All patients should have a history and physical examination, including weight, blood pressure, and Pap smear, before starting oral contraceptives, and should be seen 3 months later to determine whether any problems have occurred. At this visit, the blood pressure should be measured. Patients should be seen annually thereafter, at which time, in addition to the history, a breast, pelvic, and abdominal examination should be performed and weight and blood pressure measured. Women over 35 or those of any age with a family history of diabetes or early development of atherosclerosis should have a fasting lipid profile and 2-hour postprandial blood sugar measured. If any of these parameters is abnormally elevated, the oral contraceptive should be stopped.

SUGGESTED READING

Oral Contraceptives and Health: An Interim Report From the Oral Contraceptive Study of the Royal College of General Practitioners. New York: Pitman, 1974

Royal College of General Practitioners' Oral Contraception Study: Further analyses of mortality in oral contraceptive users. *Lancet* 1:541, 1981

Vessey M, Doll R, Peto R, Johnson B, Wiggins P: A long-term follow-up study of women using different methods of contraception. An interim report. *J Biosoc Sci* 8:373, 1976

Vessey MP, Doll R, Jones K, McPherson K, Yeates D: An epidemiological study of oral contraceptives and breast cancer. *Br Med J* 1:1757, 1979

Vessey MP, Wright NH, McPherson K, Wiggins P: Fertility after stopping different methods of contraception. *Br Med J* 1:265, 1979

Walnut Creek Contraceptive Drug Study: *A Prospective Study of the Side Effects of Oral Contraceptives,* NIH publication 81-564. Washington, DC: Government Printing Office, January 1981

Weiss NS, Sayvetz TA: Incidence of endometrial cancer in relation to the use of oral contraceptives. *N Engl J Med* 302:551, 1980

110

Intrauterine Devices:
Benefits and Risks

DANIEL R. MISHELL JR., M.D.

The main benefits of IUDs are their lack of associated systemic metabolic effects and their excellent effectiveness. These two characteristics account for a very high continuation rate. In contrast to other types of contraception, there is no need for the frequent motivation needed to ingest a pill daily or consistently use a coitus-related method. The method effectiveness and use effectiveness rates for IUDs are similar. Although first-year failure rates are generally reported to range from 2% to 3%, the annual incidence of accidental pregnancy decreases steadily after the first year. After 6 years, the cumulative annual failure rate is less than 1% per year for the loop. The incidence of adverse events with IUDs, such as pregnancy, expulsion, or removal for bleeding and/or pain steadily decreases with increasing age. Thus, the IUD is especially suited for older parous women who wish to delay or prevent further pregnancies and do not wish to be sterilized.

BLOOD LOSS

Risks associated with IUDs include excessive blood loss, uterine and cervical perforation, pregnancy-related complications, and pelvic infection. Women wearing IUDs lose a significantly greater amount of blood in each menstrual cycle than do nonwearers. Normal blood loss is about 35 ml/cycle. This rises to 70-80 ml/cycle in women wearing a coil or loop, and to about 50-60 ml/cycle in those wearing a copper-bearing IUD.

In patients who develop increased frequency or an excessive amount of vaginal bleeding with an IUD, ancillary therapeutic formulations such as an antiprostaglandin or ϵ-aminocaproic acid (EACA, Amicar) have been used with success. Excessive bleeding the first few months after IUD insertion should be treated with reassurance and supplemental oral iron, since the bleeding frequently diminishes with time as the uterus adjusts to the presence of the foreign body. Increased bleeding due to an IUD rarely causes anemia when the diet contains adequate iron.

If women develop menorrhagia after using an IUD for several months or years, their hemoglobin levels should be measured. If hemoglobin is low, iron supplementation and one of the antiprostaglandins or ϵ-aminocaproic acid should be given.

Excessive bleeding that continues with use of these agents or develops several years after IUD insertion is best treated by removal of the device. After 1 month, if the patient still wishes to use an IUD, another device may be inserted. If the original device was plastic, a copper IUD should be substituted, as copper IUDs produce less blood loss than the larger plastic devices.

Copper-bearing IUDs need to be replaced at intervals of 3-4 years and can be removed and replaced at the same visit. The large plastic IUDs do not have to be periodically replaced unless adverse symptoms develop.

PERFORATION

Although uncommon, one of the potentially serious complications associated with use of IUDs is perforation of the uterine fundus. Fundal perforation at the time of insertion can best be prevented by straightening the uterine axis with a tenaculum and then probing the cavity with a uterine sound before IUD insertion. An IUD inserted entirely within the uterine cavity does not enter the peritoneal cavity unless there has been at least partial myometrial perforation at the time of insertion. Perforation rates with the loop, Cu-7, and T devices have been reported to be about 1:1,000-2,000 insertions. The physician should always suspect perforation if a patient states she cannot feel the appendage ("strings") but did not actually see the expelled device. The physician should not assume that an unnoticed expulsion has occurred.

In this situation, after pelvic examination is performed and the possibility of pregnancy excluded, the uterine cavity should be probed. If the device cannot be felt with a uterine sound or biopsy instrument, an x-ray or sonogram should be obtained. With x-rays, it is best to take both anteroposterior and lateral views with contrast medium or a uterine sound inside the uterine cavity, as the IUD may be located in the cul-de-sac and the diagnosis missed with only an anteroposterior film. Ultrasound equipment with good resolution can also be used to locate an IUD.

If the IUD is found to be outside the uterus, it should be electively removed, as complications such as adhesions and bowel obstruction have been reported to occur with all types of IUDs. Both the copper IUDs and shields have been found to produce severe peritoneal reactions. Therefore, it is best to remove these devices as soon as possible after the diagnosis of perforation is made. Unless severe adhesions have developed, most extrauterine IUDs can be removed by means of laparoscopy rather than laparotomy.

PREGNANCY-RELATED COMPLICATIONS

Spontaneous Abortion

Pregnancies that occur with an IUD in the uterine cavity show no evidence of an increased incidence of congenital anomalies, even with copper IUDs. But if the IUD is not removed, the incidence of spontaneous abortion is about 55%, approximately three times greater than would occur without an IUD.

If, after conception, the IUD is spontaneously expelled or if the appendage is visible and the IUD is removed by traction, the incidence of spontaneous abortion is significantly reduced, to about 20%. Thus, if a woman conceives with an IUD in situ and she wishes to continue the pregnancy, the IUD should be removed if the appendage is visible in order to reduce the chance of spontaneous abortion. If the appendage is not visible and the patient does not wish the pregnancy terminated, the endometrial cavity should not be probed.

Sepsis

If the IUD cannot be easily removed or the appendage is not visible, the risk of septic abortion is increased if the IUD is the shield type. Thus, if a patient conceives with a shield IUD in utero and wishes to continue the pregnancy and the device cannot be removed without entering the uterine cavity, she should be fully informed about the increased risk of sepsis. Because of the increased incidence of death due to sepsis in pregnancy reported with the shield, it is advisable that it be removed and the pregnancy terminated.

Although there is no conclusive evidence that the incidence of severe sepsis is increased if conception occurs with an IUD other than the shield, the patient should be informed of the possibility of sepsis and, if she wishes to continue the pregnancy, of the need to report symptoms of infection promptly. If intrauterine infection does occur with an IUD in the pregnant uterus, the endometrial cavity should be evacuated after a short interval of appropriate antibiotic treatment, similar to the treatment of uterine sepsis without an IUD in place.

Ectopic Pregnancy

The IUD does not produce ectopic pregnancy, but it prevents intrauterine pregnancy more effectively than it prevents ectopic pregnancy. Thus, if pregnancy occurs with an IUD in place, the chance that it is ectopic is 10-fold greater (5% incidence) than if no IUD were used. Patients having an elective abortion due to IUD failure should have the evacuated uterine contents examined histologically to be certain villi are present. If they are not, laparoscopy is indicated if the pregnancy test remains positive.

If it is not possible to remove the IUD and the patient wishes to continue her gestation, she should be warned of a possibly increased risk of premature labor (although this is not well documented) in addition to the increased risk of spontaneous abortion. She should also be informed about an increased risk of ectopic pregnancy and possibly septic abortion, and warned to report the first signs of pelvic pain and fever.

PELVIC INFECTION IN THE NONPREGNANT PATIENT

Although bacteriologic and epidemiologic studies with the loop IUD, performed in the 1960s, indicated that it did not increase the risk of salpingitis more than 30 days after insertion, results of retrospective studies in the 1970s indicated that there was a three- to five-fold increased risk of developing clinical salpingitis in certain women who use an IUD. These studies overestimated the risk because the diagnosis of salpingitis was based on clinical criteria (which are frequently erroneous), the controls were using a method of contraception that reduced the risk of salpingitis, and the shield type of IUD was used by a large percentage of the IUD-wearing subjects.

A recent multiclinic study in the United States revealed that there was no significant increased risk of salpingitis in users of the Cu-7 and loop types of IUD more than 4 months after insertion, while the risk in users of the shield was about 18 times greater in long-term users. Nevertheless, at present it is best to avoid the use of an IUD in a young, nulliparous woman because of the risk of impairing future fertility from acute salpingitis developing soon after insertion. Since there is no conclusive evidence that the incidence of clinical salpingitis is increased more than 4 months after IUD insertion in women using IUDs other than the shield type, parous women who wish to use an IUD should be counseled accordingly.

If a patient develops symptomatic salpingitis with an IUD in place, it can usually be successfully treated by antibiotics without removing the IUD until the patient becomes asymptomatic. In patients who have clinical evidence of a tubo-ovarian abscess or who have a shield in place, the IUD should be removed after a good serum level of appropriate parenteral antibiotics has been reached, and preferably after a clinical response has been observed.

An alternative method of contraception should be used in patients who develop salpingitis with an IUD in place or in those with a past history of salpingitis. All IUD users should have Pap tests annually, and if actinomycosis is seen on the smear, the device should be removed. Antibiotic therapy is not necessary unless the patient has symptoms of uterine infection.

SUGGESTED READING

Alvior GT Jr: Pregnancy outcome with removal of intrauterine device. *Obstet Gynecol* 41:894, 1973

Burkman RT, Women's Health Study: Association between intrauterine device and pelvic inflammatory disease. *Obstet Gynecol* 57:259, 1981

Cates W Jr, Ory HW, Rochat RW, Tyler CW Jr: The intrauterine device and deaths from spontaneous abortion. *N Engl J Med* 295:1155, 1976

Mishell DR Jr: Oral contraception: Facts and fallacies. *Female Patient* 6(1), 1981

Mishell DR Jr, Bell JH, Good RC, Moyer DL: The intrauterine device—Bacteriologic studies of the endometrial cavity. *Am J Obstet Gynecol* 96:119, 1966

Ory HW, Women's Health Study: Ectopic pregnancy and intrauterine contraceptive devices: New perspectives. *Obstet Gynecol* 57:137, 1981

Tatum HJ, Schmidt FH, Jain AK: Management and outcome of pregnancies associated with the copper T intrauterine contraceptive device. *Am J Obstet Gynecol* 7:869, 1976

111

Contraception in the Teen-ager

DANIEL R. MISHELL JR., M.D.

ORAL CONTRACEPTIVES

Benefits

Use of oral contraceptives by teen-agers should be encouraged, as they are the most effective method of contraception. Since unplanned sexual intercourse is more frequent among young teen-agers, all coitus-related methods, such as the condom, diaphragm, contraceptive foams, or suppositories, have a higher failure rate than use of these same methods by older women.

In addition to their excellent contraceptive effectiveness, oral contraceptives provide teen-agers with many noncontraceptive health benefits. These include regular, predictable menstrual cycles with a significantly decreased incidence of premenstrual tension and dysmenorrhea. In addition, there is a lessened incidence of abnormal bleeding episodes and less total blood loss, reducing the incidence of iron-deficiency anemia. And because ovulation is inhibited, teen-agers using oral contraceptives have a lessened incidence of functional ovarian cysts and also less benign cystic breast disease. Finally, oral contraceptives protect women from development of salpingitis when they are infected with pathogenic organisms such as the gonococcus. Thus, use of these agents will prevent some individuals from becoming infertile.

Physician Concerns

Clinicians have voiced some concerns about the use of oral contraceptives in young teen-agers. One concern is that ingestion of these steroids might cause premature closure of the epiphyses. This concern is unwarranted because by the time menarche has occurred, the process of epiphyseal closure has already been initiated by endogenous estrogen production and cannot be accelerated by exogenous sex steroids.

Another concern is that use of these potent steroids in young teen-agers will cause permanent hypothalamic-pituitary dysfunction. This concern is also unwarranted, provided the patient has already established regular cyclic menses. Use of contraceptive steroids by teen-agers does not cause a higher frequency of ovulatory problems after their discontinuation than in women of older age, provided they both have regular menstrual cycles prior to starting the steroids. Oligomenorrhea prior to starting oral contraceptives is associated with a higher rate of postpill amenorrhea no matter what the patient's age. Therefore, in general, oral contraceptives should not be prescribed for patients of any age with hypothalamic-pituitary dysfunction who are not having regular cyclic menses.

A young woman should have at least three regular, spontaneous menstrual periods occurring at intervals of less than 35 days before starting an oral contraceptive. Teen-agers with oligomenorrhea have a low risk of conceiving because of infrequent or absent ovulation, and thus should be advised to use a barrier method of contraception to avoid the increased possibility of developing postpill amenorrhea. However, there is no evidence that oral contraceptives cause permanent sterility in any woman, even one with oligomenorrhea, although a period of infertility may ensue after these agents are stopped.

Patient Concerns

Older patients are more concerned about the rare but serious adverse effects associated with oral contraceptive use, such as thromboembolism, heart disease, and stroke. Because these disorders are extremely rare in teen-agers, no increased cardiovascular risk associated with oral contraceptive use in this age group has been documented. Most teen-agers are not concerned about these problems, but are concerned about the frequent, but less serious, side effects, such as nausea, weight gain, edema, breast tenderness, breakthrough bleeding, failure of withdrawal bleeding, and skin changes, especially the development or worsening of acne.

Adolescent girls are very conscious of their physical image and are very disturbed about weight gain, edema, and skin changes. Development of such side effects frequently causes young girls to stop taking oral contraceptives and results in unwanted pregnancies. To increase the rate of compliance, it is important to inform patients about the possibility of these effects and assure them that many of the minor side effects, such as nausea, breast tenderness, and breakthrough bleeding, decrease in incidence with increasing duration of oral contraceptive use. Young patients should be seen after three cycles of oral contraceptive treatment to inquire about their symptoms, answer their questions, and give them reassurance.

Most teen-agers are healthy and have no medical contraindications to use of oral contraceptives, but the same contraindications that occur in older women, such as any type of vascular disease, thromboembolism, and active liver disease, can also be present in the teen-ager. When medical contraindications exist, alternative methods of contraception should be used. If no contraindications exist, women can take these agents continuously until at least age 35.

Optimal Formulation

All combined oral contraceptives are equally effective, and no significant differences in the incidence of breakthrough bleeding or failure of withdrawal bleeding have been demonstrated among the various formulations, although comparative studies have not been done. In deciding which formulation to prescribe initially for teen-agers, it is best to use one with less than 50 μg of ethinylestradiol, as the estrogenic component accounts for most of the undesirable metabolic effects.

Estrogens decrease sebum production, while the androgenic progestogens used in oral contraceptives increase sebum production. Since acne is common in this age group, it is best to avoid formulations with the most androgenic progestogen, norgestrel, as they may cause a greater incidence and severity of acne than those with less potent progestogens.

Use of a daily progestogen that contains no estrogen avoids many of the estrogenic symptoms, such as fluid retention and nausea. However, these formulations produce a higher frequency of irregular bleeding and a higher failure rate, especially if the pill is not taken exactly at the same time every day. Therefore, it is best not to prescribe daily progestogens for teen-agers.

To decrease the chance of the patient's extending the medication-free interval for more than 1 week, it is best to give a teen-ager one of the formulations containing packages of 28 pills instead of 21. In this way a pill is taken every day and there is less chance that the patient will forget to resume medication after an interval without ingestion of pills.

THE INTRAUTERINE DEVICE

The IUD has certain advantages for teen-agers. It requires only one act of motivation and it does not cause the systemic effects that occur with oral contraceptives. The IUD also has a high rate of effectiveness, although slightly less than that of oral contraceptives. Annual pregnancy rates with the Cu-7 in nulliparous women are in the range of 1-2%.

The disadvantages of the IUD are increased and irregular bleeding and pain. Furthermore, there is evidence of an increased risk of pelvic infection in IUD users if they are nulliparous and younger than 25. Many teen-agers have more than one sexual partner and thus run a higher risk of acquiring gonococcal infection than older, married women. As the IUD may increase the chance of symptomatic salpingitis in women infected with the gonococcus, use of the IUD in teen-agers with multiple sexual partners may increase the incidence of subsequent infertility from tubal damage. At present, until more definitive data are available, it would appear prudent to avoid the use of an IUD in a nulliparous woman unless other methods are contraindicated and she has a single sexual partner and a negative culture for gonococcus.

ABORTION

Finally, it is necessary to state that abortion is not the answer to the problem of teen-age pregnancy. It is much safer to prevent a pregnancy than to disrupt one after it occurs. Abortion, even when done by vacuum aspiration, is associated with a certain incidence of infection, perforation, intrauterine synechiae, and subsequent infertility. Also, many teen-agers with unwanted pregnancies do not elect to have abortions, and if they do, they frequently delay the procedure until the second trimester. Termination of pregnancy in the second trimester has greater medical and psychological problems than first-trimester termination and is more difficult to obtain. Finally, many teen-agers do not have access to abortion services. For these reasons, every effort should be made to encourage sexually active teen-agers to use effective contraceptives, particularly the oral steroids, to decrease the extremely high numbers of unwanted teen-age pregnancies.

SUGGESTED READING

Ryden G, Fahraeus L, Molin L, et al: Do contraceptives influence the incidence of acute pelvic inflammatory disease in women with gonorrhea? *Contraception* 20:149, 1979

Senanayake P, Kramer DG: Contraception and the etiology of pelvic inflammatory disease. New perspectives. *Am J Obstet Gynecol* 138:852, 1980

Tyrer LB, Josimovich J: Contraception in teenagers. *Clin Obstet Gynecol* 20:651, 1977

Zelnik M, Kantner JF: Contraceptive patterns and premarital pregnancy among women aged 15-18 in 1976. *Fam Plann Perspect* 10:135, 1978

Zelnik M, Kantner JF: First pregnancies of women aged 15-19: 1976 and 1971. *Fam Plann Perspect* 10:11, 1978

Zelnik M, Kantner JF: Sexual and contraceptive experience of young unmarried women in the United States, 1976 and 1971. *Fam Plann Perspect* 9:55, 1977

112

Postcoital Contraception/Interception

PAUL F. BRENNER, M.D.

There are women who for a variety of reasons are unable to anticipate the need for adequate contraception until after coitus has occurred. This may be the result of the failure of a contraceptive method, sexual assault, or, most commonly, both partners' neglect to practice contraception. Pregnancy may result from the first sexual encounter if the coital experience was either unprotected or inadequately protected. The risk of pregnancy from one coital exposure at any time during the menstrual cycle, irrespective of the regularity of the patient's cycles and at any age in the reproductive years, has been estimated to be 2-4%. The risk of pregnancy from one coital exposure at midcycle has been estimated to be 25-30%. Thus there is a need for reversible pregnancy prevention that can be administered after coitus has occurred. These methods are referred to as postcoital contraception, interception, or morning-after estrogen therapy.

DIETHYLSTILBESTROL

The first hormonal formulation used for postcoital contraception was the synthetic estrogen diethylstilbestrol (DES). This agent was administered to women of childbearing age who requested treatment within 72 hours after a single unprotected or inadequately protected coital experience since the onset of the last menses. The therapeutic regimen consisted of 25 mg of DES administered by mouth twice a day for 5 days.

A dual mechanism of action was suggested for DES: The estrogen affects tubal physiology and hastens the transport of the ovum through the fallopian tube, at the same time making the endometrial environment unfavorable for implantation.

The DES regimen proved to be highly effective. The University of Michigan Health Service reported a series of 1,410 women who received DES; of this group, complete follow-up was obtained from 1,298 women. No pregnancies occurred in the 1,217 women who had a single coital exposure within 72 hours before receiving DES. In this group, approximately 90% used no method of contraception and coitus was judged to have occurred at midcycle in 70%. Eighty-one women had multiple coital exposures and/or sought medical advice more than 72 hours after coitus, and six of this group became pregnant.

Fewer than half the women (45%) reported the absence of side effects. Approximately half complained of nausea and vomiting. The incidence of all other side effects (headaches, dizziness, diarrhea, bloating, breast discomfort, leukorrhea, mild lower abdominal cramping pain, weight gain, irritability, darkening of the breast areola, rash, increased libido, anorexia, leg cramps, and depression) was 1% or less. The timing and character of the menstrual flow following the administration of DES were not greatly altered.

The observation that maternal ingestion of DES in the first trimester of pregnancy increases the risk of vaginal adenosis and adenocarcinoma years later in female progeny of these pregnancies and is associated with other untoward effects on fetuses of either sex has led to the recommendation that DES not be used as a postcoital contraceptive when the patient does not agree to an abortion should the method fail. A comprehensive informed consent should be obtained from all women electing to use postcoital contraception.

OTHER ESTROGENS

The possibility of teratogenic and other serious side effects in babies of either sex born to women treated with DES in the first trimester of pregnancy, as well as the high incidence of gastrointestinal side effects, provided the stimulus to investigate other agents for use as postcoital contraceptives. Under the same criteria as for the use of DES, ethinylestradiol 2-5 mg daily for 5 days and conjugated estrogen 30-50 mg daily for 5 days have been used for postcoital contraception. The results for more than 9,000 women with midcycle coital exposures treated with postcoital estrogen indicate there were 29 pregnancies, for a failure rate of 0.3%. When women were excluded who did not take the estrogen as directed, had multiple coital exposures in the same cycle, or failed to begin treatment within 72 hours after coital exposure, there were only three pregnancies, for a failure rate of 0.03%. The concomitant use of an antiemetic with postcoital estrogens greatly reduces the nausea and emesis frequently reported with these formulations.

COMBINED THERAPY

Because compliance with the 5-day estrogen regimen is not optimal, a combination of norgestrel 1 mg and ethinylestradiol 100 μg, with a second, identical dose repeated 12 hours after the first, has been used as a postcoital contraceptive regimen. The initial dose must be given within 72 hours after a single unprotected coital exposure. Eleven pregnancies occurred in a multicenter study of 692 women treated with this regimen, for an overall failure rate of 1.7%. Four pregnancies occurred in women who failed to satisfy the study's inclusion criteria.

This combined regimen produces lesser gastrointestinal side effects than the high-dose estrogen-only regimens, but it affects the length of the menstrual cycle. If treatment is given at or before midcycle, that cycle tends to be shorter than normal; if the treatment is given after midcycle, that cycle tends to be prolonged. At present, this regimen is preferred.

GESTAGENS

Gestagen-only formulations have been investigated for use as postcoital contraceptives. Quingestanol acetate 0.5, 0.8, and 1.5 mg, levonorgestrel 0.15, 0.25, 0.3, 0.35, and 0.4 mg, clogestone acetate 1.0 mg, retroprogestogen 30 and 40 mg, norgestrienone 0.5 mg, and ethynodiol diacetate 0.5 mg have been studied as immediate postcoital contraceptives. In general, failure rates of 2.2-4.5 pregnancies per 100 woman-years of use were observed in these investigations.

These regimens must be initiated soon after coitus, usually within 1-3 hours. Therefore, they are not used strictly for postcoital emergency contraception and should be classed with the gestagen-only oral contraceptives.

THE INTRAUTERINE DEVICE

The IUD has also been used for postcoital contraception. It has the advantage that once inserted, it can serve not only as a postcoital contraceptive modality but also as an ongoing form of contraception. However, the IUD's association with a possible increased risk of pelvic inflammatory disease in young, nulliparous women with multiple sexual partners limits its suitability in the group of women who may have the greatest need for postcoital contraception.

SUMMARY

Postcoital contraception should be considered emergency therapy only, not a primary method of ongoing, long-term contraception. DES, ethinylestradiol alone or in combination with norgestrel, and conjugated estrogens on a short-term basis can be used safely and effectively for the purpose of achieving postcoital contraception. The currently preferred regimen is two doses of norgestrel 1 mg with ethinylestradiol 100 μg, 12 hours apart. The closer to the time of coitus the method is initiated, the more effective it is. Therapy should be started as early as possible and no later than 72 hours following coitus. If the expected menstrual period is 2 weeks late following the use of a postcoital contraceptive regimen, a pregnancy test should be done.

SUGGESTED READING

Haspels AA: Interception: Post-coital estrogens in 3,016 women. *Contraception* 14:375, 1976

Herbst AL, Ulfelder H, Poskanzer DC: Adenocarcinoma of the vagina. Association of maternal stilbestrol therapy with tumor appearance in young women. *N Engl J Med* 284:878, 1971

Kuchera LK: Postcoital contraception with diethylstilbestrol. *JAMA* 218:562, 1971

Tietze C: Probability of pregnancy resulting from a single unprotected coitus. *Fertil Steril* 11:485, 1960

Yuzpe AA, Smith RP, Rademaker AW: A multicenter clinical investigation employing ethinyl estradiol combined with dl-norgestrel as a postcoital contraceptive agent. *Fertil Steril* 37:508, 1982

113

Management of Complications of First-Trimester Pregnancy Termination

CHARLES A. BALLARD, M.D., and PAUL F. BRENNER, M.D.

EARLY COMPLICATIONS

The complications of first-trimester pregnancy termination may be divided into two groups: early and late. Early complications occur at the time of evacuation of the products of conception and consist of uterine perforation, bleeding, inability to dilate the cervix, failure to obtain tissue, and underestimation of uterine size.

Uterine Perforation

Uterine perforation is a potentially serious complication. Its management depends on the site of perforation, the instrument that caused the perforation, and the likelihood of injury to the bowel.

If a midline perforation occurs during sharp curettage, the procedure should be terminated and the patient observed overnight. During this time the patient's vital signs should be taken at least every 2 hours and her peripheral hematocrit determined every 4 hours. Signs of peritonitis or hemorrhage indicate the need for immediate laparotomy.

If a midline perforation occurs with a suction cannula, with the suction turned off, the management is similar to that of a perforation during sharp curettage. If a midline perforation occurs with a suction cannula, with the suction turned on and without obvious injury to the omentum or bowel, the surgeon has two options: The patient may be closely observed for peritoneal signs and/or blood loss, or the surgeon may proceed immediately to laparotomy to assess potential injury to the abdominal organs. The latter alternative is recommended.

A lateral perforation requires, at the minimum, a laparoscopy to evaluate the possibility of uterine vessel damage and development of a broad ligament hematoma. Quite frequently a broad ligament hematoma expands rapidly and can be evaluated with a pelvic examination.

Perforations occur most frequently in severely anteverted or retroverted uteri or in patients with uterine anomalies such as a bicornuate uterus. If perforation occurs with a large instrument, such as a dilator, the surgeon should not proceed to suction curettage. If the membranes are intact, the procedure may be terminated and the patient may return in 2 weeks for the evacuation of her pregnancy. If the membranes are ruptured and the procedure is to be continued after perforation of the uterus with a dilator, sharp curettage may be performed with simultaneous laparoscopic visualization. A small midline perforation with a uterine sound is usually managed by continuing the procedure.

A perforation in which bowel or omental tissue is obtained requires laparotomy and repair of the damaged structures. Perforation with a suction cannula, with the suction turned on, may lead to injury of the bowel and/or omentum. The most serious perforations are lateral perforations, perforations with a suction cannula with the suction turned on, and perforations causing injury to the bowel and/or omentum.

Uterine Bleeding

Heavy vaginal bleeding is a rare complication of pregnancy termination. When it does occur, the pregnancy has usually progressed to the end of the first trimester or beyond. Causes such as incomplete evacuation, uterine perforation, and laceration of the uterine vessels must be considered. Carefully sound the uterine cavity to determine whether a perforation has occurred. If there is no evidence of a perforation, dilate and aspirate the endometrial cavity with a larger cannula. If this does not control the bleeding, perform a sharp curettage of the uterine cavity. If the vaginal bleeding persists, the management is intravenous oxytocin (Pitocin) 20 units/l of 5% dextrose in water with or without the addition of intramuscular ergonovine (Ergotrate) 0.2 mg. Should the uterine bleeding continue, one-half ampule (10 units) of vasopressin (Pitressin) mixed with 20 ml of saline can be injected into the cervix.

Inability to Dilate the Cervix

Inability to dilate the cervix occurs most frequently in primigravidas. This condition may be alleviated by the insertion of *Laminaria* and delaying the evacuation of the products of conception for at least 6-24 hours.

Failure to Obtain Tissue

If no tissue is obtained, the surgeon should repeat the pregnancy test. Occasionally, uterine fibroids or adenomyosis may mimic a pregnant uterus. Other diagnostic possibilities include a complete abortion that occurred prior to the surgery, ectopic pregnancy, a uterine anomaly (bicornuate uterus), and uterine perforation.

Underestimation of Uterine Size

Under anesthesia, the uterus may be found to be considerably larger than was anticipated. The diagnostic possibilities include advanced gestational age, multiple gestation, associated gynecologic pathology (leiomyomata uteri, adenomyosis), and trophoblastic disease. If the uterus is larger than a 12-week gestational size, the operator should not proceed until the precise diagnosis is obtained and adequate blood replacement is available.

If the correct diagnosis is a second-trimester intrauterine pregnancy and the membranes have not been ruptured, the surgeon can elect to stop the procedure and instead terminate the pregnancy by standard second-trimester abortion methods. If the abortion has proceeded to a stage where the membranes are ruptured, the evacuation of the products of conception must be completed.

LATE COMPLICATIONS

Late complications are those occurring anytime after the evacuation procedure is terminated. Late complications of first-trimester pregnancy termination consist of infection, bleeding, retained tissue, continuation of pregnancy, ectopic pregnancy, persistent amenorrhea, and postabortion pain syndrome.

Infection

Infection frequently occurs when the products of conception are incompletely evacuated from the uterus, but it may occur even without retained tissue. If the patient has developed a postabortal infection, appropriate antibiotic therapy should be instituted. If her temperature is less than 101°F and the physical findings indicate a diagnosis of postabortal endometritis, she may be treated with a 10-day course of ampicillin 0.5 gm 4 times a day.

If the patient's temperature exceeds 101°F and/or there are findings suggestive of parametritis or peritonitis, she should be hospitalized and given nothing by mouth. Her vital signs should be monitored at frequent intervals, and daily fluid intake and output measured. Initial laboratory evaluation includes complete blood count, total platelet count, serum fibrinogen, and prothrombin time. Supine and upright x-rays of the abdomen should be taken. Two units of blood should be cross-matched for transfusion. Samples for a culture of the cervix, gonorrhea culture of the cervix, and aerobic and anaerobic blood cultures should be obtained.

An intravenous infusion of 1,000 ml of 5% dextrose with lactated Ringer's solution should be initiated. Antibiotic therapy should include aqueous penicillin G 5 million units IV over 30 minutes every 6 hours, clindamycin (Cleocin) 300-600 mg IV over 30 minutes every 6-8 hours, and gentamicin (Garamycin) 80 mg over 30 minutes every 8 hours. Once the patient has been afebrile for 48 hours, she can be switched to oral doses of ampicillin 0.5 gm 4 times a day and clindamycin 300 mg 4 times a day for a total course of 10 days of antibiotics.

Any remaining products of conception should be evacuated from the uterus by dilation, if necessary, and curettage after therapeutic levels of antibiotics are attained (2 hours). The primary treatment entails removal of the focus of infection. If the patient fails to respond to antibiotic therapy and no retained tissue is found, or if she develops a pelvic abscess, the possibility of uterine perforation and bowel injury must be considered.

Bleeding

Bleeding frequently follows an incomplete abortion, although it can occur without tissue being left behind. Bleeding less than the patient's normal menstrual flow can occur up to 6 weeks postabortion. If bleeding is more than the normal menstrual flow, retained tissue, cervical vessel injury, uterine vessel injury, or trophoblastic disease should be considered. If the bleeding exceeds normal menstrual flow, if the cervix is dilated, if the uterus is still enlarged, or if tissue is present in the cervix or vagina, a repeat curettage is advocated.

Retained Tissue

Infection and/or bleeding frequently signal that evacuation of the uterus was incomplete and that some tissue was left in the uterus. The uterus may still be enlarged. If there is retained tissue, another curettage should be performed.

Continuation of Pregnancy

The initial menstrual cycle following a first-trimester abortion is usually an ovulatory one and occurs 4-6 weeks after the abortion. Patients who fail to menstruate within 6 weeks after an abortion should be evaluated with a pregnancy test and pelvic exam to determine whether the pregnancy is continuing. Continuation of pregnancy is more likely when only decidua has been obtained on the initial curettage, but it has also been known to occur even when some villi have been obtained. When a pregnancy has continued after abortion, uterine anomalies must be strongly considered. The surgeon must always be aware of the possibility of a blind horn when it is impossible to complete the procedure vaginally. Continuation of pregnancy is managed by another attempt to evacuate the products of conception from the uterus.

Ectopic Pregnancy

After each abortion, the surgeon must confirm the presence of fetal tissue. Absence of fetal tissue indicates either that the attempted termination of pregnancy failed, that the pregnancy was aborted prior to the surgical procedure, or that the patient has an ectopic pregnancy. An ectopic pregnancy should be considered in any patient whose pathologic specimen was reported as decidua only or exhibits the Arias-Stella reaction. Finally, the rare possibility of coexisting intrauterine and ectopic pregnancies must be considered.

Persistent Amenorrhea

Patients with persistent amenorrhea following a first-trimester abortion usually have a continuing pregnancy or Asherman's syndrome. These patients are best managed by repeating the pregnancy test. If the test is positive, another curettage should be performed. If the uterus is normal in size and the pregnancy test is negative, intrauterine synechiae should be suspected. Inability to sound the uterine cavity, a biphasic basal body temperature, or one of four weekly progesterone determinations exceeding 3 ng/ml (indicating an ovulatory cycle) further suggests the diagnosis of Asherman's syndrome. Hysteroscopy is recommended for accurate diagnosis and treatment of this syndrome (see Chapter 101).

Postabortion Pain Syndrome

Infrequently a postabortion pain syndrome occurs, in which the patient develops cramping abdominal pain several hours to even days after her abortion. In association with the pain, the uterus is large and boggy. Postabortion pain syndrome is best managed by a repeat suction curettage to remove retained blood clots. This syndrome is usually prevented by the use of intravenous oxytocin administered at the time of the original curettage.

SUGGESTED READING

Atrash HK, Peterson HB, Cates W Jr, Grimes DA: The risk of death from combined abortion-sterilization procedures: Can hysterotomy or hysterectomy be justified? *Am J Obstet Gynecol* 142:269, 1982

Ballard CA: Therapeutic abortion. In Quilligan EJ, ed: *Current Therapy in Obstetrics and Gynecology.* Philadelphia: Saunders, 1980

Brenner PF, Mishell DR Jr: Abortion—Therapy. In Conn HF, ed: *Current Therapy 1979.* Philadelphia: Saunders, 1979

Cates W Jr: Abortion myths and realities: Who is misleading whom? *Am J Obstet Gynecol* 142:954, 1982

Manabe Y, Manabe A: Nelaton catheter versus laminaria for a safe and gradual cervical dilation. *Contraception* 24:53, 1981

Margolis AJ, Greenwood SB: Aspiration abortion in an office setting. In Glass RH, ed: *Office Gynecology.* Baltimore: Williams & Wilkins, 1981

Niloff JM, Stubblefield PG: Low-dose vaginal 15 methyl prostaglandin $F_{2\alpha}$ for cervical dilatation prior to vacuum curettage abortion. *Am J Obstet Gynecol* 142:596, 1982

Selik RM, Cates W Jr, Tyler CW Jr: Behavioral factors contributing to abortion deaths: A new approach to mortality studies. *Obstet Gynecol* 58:631, 1981

114

Female Sterilization:
Choice of Technique

ROBERT ISRAEL, M.D.

Sterilization is the final step in preventing procreation. As it plays such a prominent role in fertility termination, sterilization must be an integral part of any family planning program. Over the past decade, voluntary sterilization has emerged from public unawareness and medically restrictive guidelines to become a widely used method throughout the world, and one that continues to offer exciting, new methodology for simplifying female sterilization.

Of the 900,000 sterilizations performed in 1972, male operations accounted for 60% of the total. Parity was achieved in 1973, and the male/female ratio was subsequently reversed. Since 1977, over 1 million sterilizations per year have been carried out in the United States and women have undergone 60% of these procedures. In addition, according to the 1965-1975 National Fertility Study published in 1977, sterilization was selected as a family planning method by 44% of couples in 1975, compared with only 14% in 1965.

REVERSIBILITY

Along with increased public acceptance of sterilization, a better understanding of the physiologic and psychological changes connected with such surgery has developed. With the wider use of sterilization, new operative techniques have been, and continue to be, devised. Although sterilization is utilized as a final, permanent contraceptive technique by individuals concluding their reproductive potential, reversible sterilization may become a "family-spacing" technique of the future. Male and female sterilization methods that permit reversibility are under investigation in a very preliminary fashion. However, the most effective techniques owe their success to their high degree of *nonreversibility*. A reliably reversible technique must retain the maximum pregnancy prevention associated with currently available sterilization methods.

METHODOLOGY

Postpartum Tubal Ligation

The Pomeroy and Irving tubal ligations performed through a small subumbilical incision remain the procedures of choice in the immediate postpartum period. They can be performed on the delivery table, often utilizing the same anesthesia; they are simple and rapid with an "acceptable" failure rate—well below 1:1,000 for the Irving; and they do not prolong the postpartum hospital stay. Although the modified Irving tubal sterilization (the proximal stump buried in the myometrium, the distal stump tied off but not buried in the broad ligament) requires more time than the Pomeroy, it is worth the extra effort, as only one pregnancy is documented in the literature. Cesarean hysterectomy should not be performed unless removal of the uterus is indicated medically by multiple myomas, cancer, or irreparable uterine damage. Excessive blood loss and an increased incidence of ureteral/bladder injury preclude cesarean hysterectomy as a routine method of female sterilization.

Vaginal Hysterectomy
In the past, although vaginal hysterectomy was often performed for sterilization, this primary operative indication was often camouflaged by convenient secondary diagnoses often found in parous women—e.g., pelvic relaxation. Although vaginal hysterectomy is associated with greater blood loss, higher morbidity, and a longer hospital stay than tubal sterilization, these are short-term disadvantages and must be balanced against the long-term benefits seen with vaginal hysterectomy: the guarantee of absolute sterility, the ability to correct concomitant pelvic relaxation problems often found in the over-30 multipara, and the prevention of future uterine disease. Gynecologic disorders following tubal ligation may be quite frequent, necessitating further pelvic surgery 25% of the time, and hysterectomy could make up 50% of these operations. It seems apparent that sterilization may be the sole indication for vaginal hysterectomy, and in the properly selected, properly prepared patient, it would be the procedure of choice. Today, however, in cases where governmental funding is the payment source for sterilization, hysterectomy is prohibited as a method of sterilization.

Classical methods of tubal ligation or standard gynecologic operations offer reliability but little innovation in the rapidly expanding field of female sterilization. Laparoscopic, transvaginal, and, in the future, transuterine methods of sterilization represent new approaches that highlight current concepts in female sterilization.

Laparoscopy
Laparoscopic sterilization is a combination of two procedures—laparoscopy and tubal sterilization—both devised for different purposes, but combined in this century and improved in the past decade by new technologies and new enthusiasms.

Technique. There are wide variations in preoperative preparation, the majority of which are not crucial to the success of the operation. Unless there are significant medical problems (diabetes, hypertension, etc.) or excessive obesity (200 lb or over), or both, there is no reason why laparoscopic tubal sterilization cannot be performed as an outpatient (1-day) procedure. The operation should take place in an operating room equipped and staffed for general anesthesia—and for exploratory laparotomy if it proves necessary. Although a crossmatch would seem to be an expensive extra, blood bank accessibility is a necessity.

Although the proponents of local anesthesia for laparoscopic sterilization have been vociferous, most laparoscopists continue to favor a short-acting general anesthetic with endotracheal intubation and controlled ventilation. It is unnecessary to shave either the abdomen or the perineum. The bladder is catheterized, but an indwelling catheter is unnecessary. At laparoscopy, it is often helpful to be able to elevate and rotate the uterus via a vaginal "handle." Various instruments can be utilized.

The creation of a satisfactory pneumoperitoneum is the keystone to any successful laparoscopic procedure. A Veress needle should be used to insufflate the peritoneal cavity, as its spring action combines a sharp outer point for penetrating tissue planes and a retractable, blunt inner stylet for peritoneal puncture and intra-abdominal safety. With the laparoscope in place, a brief overview of the pelvis should confirm the normal structures visualized in almost all sterilization procedures.

Various instruments and methods for tubal occlusion are available. Whatever tubal occlusion technique is utilized, tissue destruction should be confined to the midisthmus. In this way, if sterilization reversal is subsequently requested, enough proximal and distal tubal segments will remain for end-to-end reanastomosis.

Fulguration, usually with transection, remains the most widely used technique. Before transection, fulguration must be complete and must include a portion of the adjacent mesosalpinx to avoid bleeding at the transection site. After transection, each cut tubal stump (especially both proximal ends) should be recoagulated briefly to prevent tubal fistulas or recanalization.

Utilizing bipolar equipment for fulguration eliminates the electrical hazards associated with unipolar coagulation, in which the current must pass through the patient to the grounding plate. In bipolar conduction, the electrical current passes in and out through the forceps, thus eliminating electrical "scatter" within the abdominal cavity and avoiding bowel burns. The introduction of the Falope ring, whereby a Silastic band is used to occlude the tube, as well as the spring-loaded clip, has provided alternatives to electrocoagulation, thus eliminating electrical hazards. Postoperative abdominal discomfort is experienced for 24-48 hours in 20-25% of the patients undergoing occlusive ring or clip tubal sterilization. However, both these methods destroy less tube than laparoscopic fulguration and thus may offer better potential for reversibility.

Laparoscopic sterilization can be performed through a single-incision technique utilizing the operating laparoscope and, most commonly, local anesthesia. The accessory instrument for performing the tubal sterilization is inserted in the laparoscope itself. Therefore, the forceps moves only when the laparoscope moves and cannot move separately. Pelvic manipulation, e.g., for identification of tubal fimbria, is more restricted with the operating laparoscope than with an accessory instrument inserted at a second puncture site. If used at all, the single-incision technique should be attempted only after the laparoscopist has become thoroughly familiar with the two-incision approach.

Pregnancy rate. When laparoscopic tubal sterilization is correctly performed, either by fulguration or by fulguration and transection, the risk of subsequent pregnancy is approximately 1:1,000. This pregnancy rate does not include luteal-phase failures, where the patient was already pregnant at the time of surgery, or surgical errors, such as coagulating the round ligament. To avoid luteal pregnancies, sterilization can be limited to the follicular phase of the menstrual cycle or a curettage can accompany the laparoscopy. If effective contraception precedes the sterilization request, it is unnecessary to restrict surgery to a particular phase of the cycle or add an extra operative procedure (D&C) to laparoscopy. Pregnancies secondary to surgical errors can be eliminated by properly identifying the fallopian tubes.

Although fewer Silastic band sterilizations than laparoscopic fulgurations have been performed, the pregnancy rates seem comparable. However, the failure rates published in preliminary studies utilizing the spring-loaded clip have been much higher. Design modifications may eventually improve the efficacy of tubal sterilization.

Any pregnancies occurring after tubal sterilization must be carefully evaluated to rule out ectopic gestations. Published reports indicate that 15% of pregnancies following all types of tubal sterilization procedures will be ectopic. However, following laparoscopic fulguration, the risk that any subsequent pregnancy will be ectopic rises to 25%, with a literature range of 9-67%.

Colpotomy

Transvaginal (colpotomy) tubal ligation still has its proponents. It can be performed between pregnancies (interval) or following a curettage for abortion in patients with a normal or 6-8-week-sized, mobile uterus without known or palpable adnexal masses. Usually general anesthesia is used, although conduction anesthesia (spinal or epidural) can be utilized. Each tube is secured and ligated by means of a standard technique, usually the Pomeroy or fimbriectomy approach. Fimbriectomy seems to have variable success rates, from total pregnancy prevention up to a failure rate as high as 3%. Perhaps careful attention to surgical technique accounts for the better success rates in some series. However, fimbriectomy should not be performed for sterilization. It destroys an essential area of the tube and can rarely be reversed.

Colpotomy tubal ligation has a postoperative complication rate of 5%, of which 20% can be classed as major. Pelvic infection with abscess formation is reported in most series. As laparoscopy has so many advantages over the transvaginal route, colpotomy tubal ligation today has little justification.

Transuterine Approach

To bring absolute safety and simplicity to female sterilization, penetration of the abdominal cavity must be avoided. Laparoscopy has provided the gynecologist with a sophisticated endoscopic technique, but as an instrument of tubal sterilization, it is not the final answer. The transuterine approach to the fallopian tubes may be the ultimate solution, but at the moment it represents a good idea in search of the right technique.

Hysteroscopy has permitted direct visualization of each tubal orifice. An electrode can be threaded through the operating channel of the hysteroscope and guided under visual control to the tubal ostium. Unfortunately, too many failures have occurred to consider hysteroscopic tubal fulguration a satisfactory technique of female sterilization. Even bilateral cornual occlusion 3 months postoperatively may represent only unilateral or bilateral cornual spasm, not true closure. In addition to subsequent pregnancies, including some cornual ectopics, bowel burns have been reported due to the varying degrees of myometrial thickness present at the time of ostial fulguration.

To eliminate electrocoagulation, some investigators have turned their efforts toward developing a Silastic tubal plug that would be placed as liquid silicone rubber in each orifice under hysteroscopic guidance. The liquid silicone would "cure" to form a soft plug conforming to the oviductal lumen. Tubal plugs must remain in place and provide complete blockage, which may prove difficult over time because of the known contractile strength of tubal and uterine musculature. The Silastic tubal plug is currently being tested at several locations in the United States and Europe. Tubal plugs, like tubal clips, offer the possibility of reversible sterilization. However, absolute effectiveness of sterilization is more important than potential reversibility, and the former must be demonstrated in any new sterilization technique before the latter can even be considered.

Chemical Sterilization

The ultimate goal in transuterine sterilization would be to eliminate instrumentation like hysteroscopy altogether. By means of a syringe, catheter, or specialized delivery system, a chemosterilant that acts on the mucosa of the fallopian tube could be instilled via the uterine cavity. Two groups of chemical agents are under investigation. One consists of nonspecific tissue adhesives or sclerosing agents that produce oviductal obstruction through scar formation. Methyl cyanoacrylate (MCA), the most promising of these compounds, polymerizes in the tubes and causes a local reaction leading to fibrotic occlusion over a period of 3 months, during which time the MCA is degraded and eliminated from the body. Spillage into the peritoneal cavity seems to have no deleterious effects. Bilateral tubal occlusion has been achieved over 80% of the time with a single application, and over 95% of the time with two applications. Clinical trials with pregnancy as an end point are planned.

The other chemosterilant group consists of highly specific chemical agents capable of inducing morphologic changes in the interstitial tubal epithelium. Quinacrine has been the most tested compound in this group, and from recent human studies by Zipper et al, utilizing three insertions of quinacrine pellets placed high in the endometrial cavity via an IUD inserter, the pregnancy rate at 12 months has been reduced to 1.5:100 women. In one respect, quinacrine sterilization is unique among all carefully studied sterilization procedures. No ectopic pregnancies have occurred in over 200 reported pregnancies in women who have had one or more quinacrine instillations. The possibility of developing a nonsurgical sterilization technique with a chemical agent of low toxicity, which can be employed by paramedical personnel without sophisticated delivery equipment, opens exciting perspectives in the expanding area of female sterilization.

CONCLUSION

Female sterilization has become an accepted, integral part of family planning. Laparoscopic sterilization techniques have simplified the surgery and suggested new approaches to the fallopian tubes. The future is represented by transuterine sterilization that promises to avoid anesthesia, complicated instrumentation, and penetration of the peritoneal cavity. When evaluated against the comparable standard criteria for contraception (acceptability, safety, effectiveness, and cost), surgical sterilization, even as it is performed today, appears to be one of the best family planning methods available.

SUGGESTED READING

Brenner WE: Evaluation of contemporary female sterilization methods. *J Reprod Med* 26:439, 1981

Chi I-C, Laufe LE, Gardner SD, Tolbert MA: An epidemiologic study of risk factors associated with pregnancy following female sterilization. *Am J Obstet Gynecol* 136:768, 1980

Kessel E, Mumford SD: Potential demand for voluntary female sterilization in the 1980s: The compelling need for a nonsurgical method. *Fertil Steril* 37:725, 1982

Neuwirth RS, Richart RM, Stevenson T, et al: An outpatient approach to female sterilization with methylcyanoacrylate. *Am J Obstet Gynecol* 136:951, 1980

Westoff CF, Jones EF: Contraception and sterilization in the United States, 1965-1975. *Fam Plann Perspect* 9:154, 1977

Zipper J, Cole LP, Goldsmith A, et al: Quinacrine hydrochloride pellets: Preliminary data on a nonsurgical method of female sterilization. *Int J Gynaecol Obstet* 18, 275, 1980

115

Vasectomy

GERALD S. BERNSTEIN, Ph.D., M.D.

Vasectomy is one of the few methods currently available for the control of male fertility. It is a popular procedure; several hundred thousand men are sterilized each year. The operation is simple, can be performed as an office procedure under local anesthesia, and does not involve invasion of the peritoneal cavity. The failure rate in the past was generally about 0.5%, or 1:200 procedures. However, use of techniques that involve separating the two ends of the severed vas by enclosing one within the sheath of the vas deferens and leaving the other free has reduced the failure rate to zero in the hands of some surgeons. Some physicians performing vasectomies no longer excise a segment of the vas. Whether or not a segment is removed, the ends of the divided vas must be sealed by ligatures, electrocautery of the lumen using a fine cautery tip, or various types of clips.

COMPLICATIONS

The complications of vasectomy are usually minor and consist of pain, swelling, ecchymoses, and superficial wound infections. More severe complications include epididymitis, excessive bleeding with hematoma formation, and the development of a sperm granuloma at the proximal end of the vas that may cause pain in the scrotum. There have been no deaths due directly to vasectomy in the United States. Deaths have been reported in some of the underdeveloped countries, where the facilities for sterilizing instruments have not been adequate or patients have neglected to practice adequate postoperative hygiene.

REVERSAL

Progress has also been made in reversing vasectomy in order to restore fertility. The success of the surgery depends partly on how the original surgery was performed and the degree of inflammatory reaction that followed. If a long segment of the vas was excised, or a segment was removed from the convoluted portion of the vas, near the epididymis, the reconstruction is less likely to be successful. With conventional surgical techniques, sperm are restored to the ejaculate in 80% of cases, but only about 35% of all patients who have had the reversal procedure impregnate their wives.

Better results have been obtained with microsurgical techniques, and it is possible to restore sperm to the ejaculate in as many as 90% of cases if the surgery is done within 10 years after the vasectomy was performed. The pregnancy rate has also improved with microsurgery, but pregnancy does not result in all cases.

There is some controversy as to why the pregnancy rate is less than the success of restoring continuity of the vas deferens, but there is inadequate information at this time to resolve it. The follow-up data do not always include a complete evaluation of both partners in order to determine the factor responsible for failure to conceive.

RISKS

Immunization

One aspect of vasectomy has attracted considerable attention in the past few years. In the late 1950s and early 1960s, two groups of investigators reported that some men whose vas deferens had been obstructed, by surgery or natural causes, developed circulating antibodies against spermatozoa. A number of investigators have subsequently shown that up to 70% of vasectomized men develop circulating antibodies that can agglutinate or immobilize spermatozoa. The antibodies usually can be found in the serum within the first 3 months after the surgery. In some cases, the antibodies can no longer be detected 2 years following the operation.

Initially this immunologic reaction was considered to be only an interesting laboratory phenomenon without any clinical significance. In 1968, however, Roberts described seven young men who developed various medical problems after they had been vasectomized. One had multiple sclerosis, three had thrombophlebitis, and three had a variety of diseases and systemic symptoms. Roberts felt that these disorders resulted from the activation of the immune system caused by the vasectomy, and he suggested that vasectomy may be more dangerous than had previously been thought.

Although these cases were anecdotal, Roberts's paper created a great deal of interest. There have been numerous animal and clinical studies in the intervening years. These investigations have shown that rabbits that develop high titers of sperm antibodies following vasectomy may also develop autoimmune orchitis and have immune complexes deposited in their kidneys. Other rodents also may have marked immunologic reactions following vasectomy.

Atherogenesis

In 1978 it was reported that monkeys fed a high-fat, atherogenic diet and then vasectomized developed more extensive atherosclerosis than control animals fed the same diet but not vasectomized. This study was conducted because there is some evidence that immune complexes can damage the arterial intima and thereby initiate changes that can lead to the development of atheromas. There may be a similar difference between vasectomized and nonvasectomized monkeys not fed an atherogenic diet.

Comparative Safety

These various studies and observations have raised some questions about the safety of vasectomy, but it is not clear whether they are clinically relevant. It is not possible to extrapolate from animal work to man, nor can one generalize from anecdotal clinical reports. There have been controlled, prospective studies of the health of vasectomized men, but these have involved relatively small numbers of subjects who were followed for only a few years. Such studies have revealed no changes in pituitary-gonadal endocrine function over a period of several years following vasectomy. Recent epidemiologic studies have not shown any increase in morbidity among vasectomized men, compared with controls, or any relationship between vasectomy and nonfatal myocardial infarctions. Other studies of general health and cardiovascular disease among vasectomized and nonvasectomized men are now in progress.

The consensus at this time is that there is little if any risk that vasectomy will cause significant alterations in human health. If there are any men at special risk, they remain to be defined. Furthermore, any risk due to vasectomy is probably less than the surgical risk of tubal ligation or hysterectomy, and there is no rationale for discouraging a healthy man from having a vasectomy if he wishes to use this method of fertility control.

SUGGESTED READING

Alexander NJ, Clarkson TB: Vasectomy increases the severity of diet-induced atherosclerosis in *Macaca fascicularis*. *Science* 201:538, 1978

Bernstein GS, Chopp R, Cosgrove M, et al: A controlled, prospective study of the effects of vasectomy. In Lepow IH, Crozier R, eds: *Vasectomy: Immunologic and Pathophysiologic Effects in Animals and Man*. New York: Academic Press, 1979, pp 473-489

Bigazzi PE: Immunologic effects of vasectomy in men and experimental animals. In Gleicher N, ed: *Reproductive Immunology*. New York: Alan R Liss, 1981, pp 461-476

Clarkson TB, Alexander NJ: Vasectomy: Effects on the occurrence and extent of atherosclerosis in rhesus monkeys. *J Clin Invest* 65:15, 1980

Goebelsmann U, Bernstein GS, Gale JA, et al: Serum gonadotropin, testosterone, estradiol, and estrone levels prior to and following bilateral vasectomy. In Lepow IH, Crozier R, eds: *Vasectomy: Immunologic and Pathophysiologic Effects in Animals and Man*. New York: Academic Press, 1979, pp 165-181

Goldacre MJ, Vessey M, Clarke JA, Heasman M: Record linkage study of morbidity following vasectomy. In Lepow IH, Crozier R, eds: *Vasectomy: Immunologic and Pathophysiologic Effects in Animals and Man*. New York: Academic Press, 1979, pp 567-575

Lepow IH, Crozier R, eds: *Vasectomy: Immunologic and Pathophysiologic Effects in Animals and Man*. New York: Academic Press, 1979

Petitti DB, Klein R, Kipp H, Kahn W, Siegelaub AB, Friedman GD: Survey of habits, symptoms of illness, and histories of disease in men with and without vasectomies. *Am J Public Health* 72:476, 1982

Roberts HJ: Delayed thrombophlebitis and systemic complications after vasectomy: Possible role of diabetogenic hyperinsulinism. *J Am Geriat Soc* 16:267, 1968

Schmidt SS: Prevention of failure in vasectomy. *J Urol* 109:296, 1973

Silber SJ: Vasectomy & vasectomy reversal. In Wallach EE, Kempers RD, eds: *Modern Trends in Infertility and Conception Control*, vol 1. Baltimore: Williams & Wilkins, 1979, pp 286-301

Special Programme of Research, Development, and Research Training in Human Reproduction: Sequelae of vasectomy. *Contraception* 25:119, 1982

Walker MW, Jick H, Hunter JR, et al: Vasectomy and non-fatal myocardial infarction. *Lancet* 1:13, 1981

Wortman J: Vasectomy. What are the problems? *Populat Ser D* 25, 1975

116

Fetal Demise

CHARLES A. BALLARD, M.D.

Fetal demise may be separated into two groups: missed abortion and intrauterine fetal demise. The classical definition of missed abortion is fetal demise in the first or second trimester without expulsion of the fetus for a minimum of 8 weeks. But it would seem more logical to consider any fetal demise in the first or second trimester a missed abortion.

DIAGNOSIS

A diagnosis of fetal demise may be suspected in any patient in whom there is no fetal growth or cessation of fetal movement. The patient may also complain of loss of breast tenderness, nausea, frequency of urination, and lassitude.

After 20 weeks' gestation, fetal heart sounds may be listened for with a DeLee stethoscope or fetoscope. After 12 weeks' gestation, an office Doppler device may be used. Neither procedure is diagnostic and may yield a small rate of false-negative results. Serial 24-hour urinary estriols would be highly significant if a fall greater than 30% in two or more specimens occurred, but sample collection and analysis would necessitate several days' delay in making a diagnosis. The urinary pregnancy test is unreliable because even though the fetus may have expired, the placenta may still function, resulting in a persistent positive pregnancy test.

An x-ray can be extremely helpful, but only when fetal demise has occurred several days previously, and only after 18-20 weeks' gestation. The diagnostic radiologic signs to look for are intravascular fetal gas, overlapping of the cranial bones, or "halo sign," and an abnormal increase in width of the cranial soft tissues as a result of maceration. Also, with the loss of fetal muscle tone, the fetal spine may collapse. A more rapid, reliable means of determination of fetal demise is the use of ultrasound. A Doppler device may be used to determine loss of fetal heart tones, and a real-time B-scan sonogram may be used to determine the presence or absence of fetal movement.

MANAGEMENT

Expectant Waiting

Management of fetal demise consists of expectant waiting or active intervention. Previously, expectant management was the more frequent modality for management of fetal demise because of complications of active intervention. The assumption with expectant waiting was based on the rationale that 75% of patients would deliver spontaneously within 2 weeks and all but 7% would deliver by 3 weeks.

Since 93% of patients would deliver within 3 weeks, the major complication of hypofibrinogenemia was of significance only in a small percentage of patients. Furthermore, it usually did not occur before 5 weeks after demise, and then in only approximately 25-40% of patients. It is important to obtain a weekly fibrinogen level for patients who are being observed for spontaneous onset of labor. Fortunately, if a drop in fibrinogen occurs, it is gradual.

Active Intervention

With modern means of pregnancy termination, active intervention becomes more attractive as therapy for patients with fetal demise. In fact, in a very small percentage of patients the emotional impact of carrying a dead fetus is overwhelming to the point of severe depression.

In patients at less than 12 weeks' gestation, active surgical intervention is the treatment of choice; whether by sharp curettage or suction curettage is up to the individual operator. Routine preoperative laboratory tests must include a hematocrit and fibrinogen level. If either or both are below normal, typing and crossmatching the patient for several units of blood are imperative.

Major difficulty in termination may occur after 12 weeks' gestation. In the past, high doses of estrogen were suggested, but were found to be ineffective in inducing labor. Oxytocin has frequently been used for patients in the second and third trimesters. At least in the second trimester, however, the pregnant uterus resists oxytocin stimulation. Serial attempts at induction over several days are often necessary, with the concomitant risk of water intoxication and even a possibility of uterine rupture. To increase the success rate, a combination of amniotomy and continuous intravenous oxytocin has been recommended, but if the patient fails to abort, she runs an increased risk of uterine infection with prolonged ruptured membranes.

To prevent these problems in patients after 12 weeks' gestation, hysterotomy has been suggested. This carries all the inherent risks of general anesthesia, the risk of uterine rupture in subsequent pregnancies, and the likelihood of repeat cesarean section.

An alternative in pregnancies after 16 weeks' gestation has been the use of intra-amniotic hypertonic saline or prostaglandin $F_{2\alpha}$. Intra-amniotic saline probably should not be used because of its risk of causing hypofibrinogenemia—which may be accelerated in a patient with an already low fibrinogen level. Also, there frequently is not much amniotic fluid, and this increases the difficulty of obtaining a successful tap.

Recently, 20-mg prostaglandin E_2 suppositories have been released for use in patients at less than 29 weeks' gestation. They are administered intravaginally at 3-5-hour intervals, depending on the frequency of uterine contractions. These suppositories have been shown to be highly effective in more than 95%

of patients, with a mean of 10-12 hours from installation to delivery. In patients at less than 13 weeks' gestation, the success rate has been poor; in fact, prostaglandin suppositories offer no advantage over D&C.

COMPLICATIONS

Complications depend on the length of demise and the mode of termination. Patients with prolonged demise risk hypofibrinogenemia. Intravenous oxytocin places the patient at risk of uterine rupture and hyponatremia, possibly leading to water intoxication. D&C increases the risk of hemorrhage and uterine perforation. Uterine instillation of either prostaglandin or saline carries the risk of infection.

The use of vaginal suppositories produces a high incidence of gastrointestinal side effects, such as vomiting and diarrhea; patients may develop temperatures as high as 104°F and frequently may experience chills. Rarely, uterine rupture may occur, especially in patients in the third trimester and those with an abnormal fetal lie. Vaginal suppositories probably should not be used after 28 weeks' gestation in patients who have had a cesarean section or hysterotomy, or in patients with an abnormal fetal lie. These patients may be managed expectantly or delivered by cesarean section.

SUGGESTED READING

Bailey DH, Newman C, Ellinas SP, Anderson GG: Use of prostaglandin E_2 vaginal suppositories in intrauterine fetal death and missed abortion. *Obstet Gynecol* 45:110, 1975

Dippel AL: Death of foetus in utero. *Johns Hopkins Med J* 54:24, 1934

Pritchard JA, Ratnoff OD: Studies of fibrinogen and other hemostatic factors in women with intrauterine death and delayed delivery. *Surg Gynecol Obstet* 101:467, 1955

Ruthland A, Ballard CA: Vaginal prostaglandin E_2 for missed abortion and intrauterine fetal death. *Am J Obstet Gynecol* 128:5, 1977

Southern EM, Gutknecht GD: Management of intrauterine fetal demise and missed abortion using prostaglandin E_2 vaginal suppositories. *Obstet Gynecol* 47:602, 1976

Tricomi V, Kohl SG: Fetal death in utero. *Am J Obstet Gynecol* 74:1092, 1957

INDEX

Benemid. *See* Probenecid
Benzathine penicillin G (Bicillin), 24
Benzodiazepines, 4
Betamethasone, 99, 153, 154, 155
Beta receptors. *See* Receptors, *β*
Betke, K., 29
Bevis, D. C. A., 29
Bicillin. *See* Benzathine penicillin G
Bicornuate uterus, 456
Bilateral cystic ovarian tumor, 234
Bilateral groin lymphadenectomy, 269, 270
Bilateral salpingo-oophorectomy, 304, 327
Bilirubin, 52, 129, 148
  amniotic fluid, 29, 30, 33, 34
Biopsy
  cervical, 287
  cone, 288
  endometrial, 213, 226, 228, 230, 292, 302, 387, 388, 389, 402
  excision, 269, 288
Biparietal diameter (BPD), 71, 94, 148, 151
Biphasic infections, 202
Birth
  See also Delivery
  anoxia at, 73, 102
  breech. *See* Breech presentation
  cesarean. *See* Cesarean section
  injury at, 101
  premature. *See* Prematurity
  trauma at, 73
Birth defects, 2
  See also Congenital anomalies
Bladder
  capacity of, 256
  injuries to, 259-260
  and repair of ureteral injury, 265
  unstable, 256
Bleeding, 105, 106, 113
  See also Blood loss
  acyclic, 230
  antepartum, 141
  concealed, 111-112
  cyclic, 230
  external (revealed), 111
  fetomaternal, 140, 141
  following incomplete abortion, 501
  intracranial, 129
  intraperitoneal, 238
  maternal, 75
  time, 227
  uterine. *See* Uterine bleeding
  vaginal. *See* Vaginal bleeding
Blenoxane. *See* Bleomycin
Bleomycin (Blenoxane), 300, 317, 327, 332
Blood
  See also Plasma; Serum
  clotting factors in pregnancy, 38
  crossmatch of, 112

fetal scalp, 120, 129, 169-172, 183
  impaired flow of, 178
Blood count, 387
Blood dyscrasias, 227
Blood gases
  analysis of, 170
  arterial, 40
Blood glucose. *See* Blood sugar
Blood loss
  See also Bleeding
  anemia from, 15
  and IUDs, 487-488
Blood pressure
  control of, 65-66
  high. *See* Hypertension
  low. *See* Hypotension
Blood smear, 227
Blood sugar
  excess. *See* Hyperglycemia
  fasting, 387
  low. *See* Hypoglycemia
  post-Glucola, 148
Blood type, 112
Bone age, 471
Bone scan, 313
Boronow, R. C., 309
Bowe, E. T., 171
Bowman, J. M., 30
Boyes, D. A., 282
BPD. *See* Biparietal diameter
Bradycardia, 113, 158, 162, 163, 167, 173, 175, 177, 180
Brain
  CSF accumulation in, 10
  damage, 182
  organic disease of, 470
"Brain-sparing." *See* "Head-sparing"
Breast
  examination of, 332
  manipulation of, 362
Breast-feeding, 364
Breech presentation, 101-104, 128
Breen, J. L., 116, 118
Brenner tumors, 373
Brethine. *See* Terbutaline
Bricanyl. *See* Terbutaline
British Columbia Screening Program, 282
Bromocriptine (Parlodel), 134, 135, 136, 359, 360, 364, 366-369, 389, 405
  and luteal phase defects, 442
  and PMS, 223
  side effects of, 367
Bromoergocryptine. *See* Bromocriptine
B-scans. *See* Ultrasound
Burch procedure, 210, 257, 258
Burke, J. F., 209
Butazolidin. *See* Phenylbutazone
Buttram, V. C., 456

C

Calcium gluconate, 76
Caldeyro-Barcia, 143
Calymmatobacterium granulomatis, 197
Canadian Task Force on Cervical Cancer Screening Programs, 282, 283
Cancer. *See* Carcinoma; Sarcoma; specific types of cancer
Candida, 186, 187, 188, 192-193
Carbon dioxide, 169
Carbon dioxide laser, 288
Carcinoma
  See also Adenocarcinoma
  cervical. *See* Cervical cancer
  of cervical stump, 297-298
  clear-cell, 274-280
  embryonal, 328
  endometrial. *See* Endometrial cancer
  of fallopian tube, 320-324
  invasive, 289-301
  microinvasive, 270
  oral contraceptives and, 483
  ovarian epithelial, 330-333
  preinvasive, of cervix and vagina, 286-288
  squamous-cell. *See* Squamous-cell carcinoma
  staging of, 272
  urethral, 268-270
  vaginal, 271-273
  vulvar, 268-270
Cardiac arrest, fetal, 180
Cardiac asystole (heart block), 167
Cardiac disease. *See* Heart disease
Cardiotachometer, 157
Cardiovascular changes
  in menopause, 474
  in pregnancy, 22-23
Casey, J., 371
Castor oil, 244
Catecholamines, 164
Catheters, catheterization
  intrauterine pressure, 125
  ovarian venous, 377
  transcervical, 73
  ureteral, 262
CCCLA. *See* Community Cancer Center of Los Angeles
Cefazolin (Ancef, Kefzol), 209
Cefotaxime (Claforan), 204, 205, 209
Cefoxitin (Mefoxin), 204, 205, 207, 209, 261
Cellulitis
  pelvic, 208
  streptococcal, 270
Centers for Disease Control (CDC), 206-207
Cephalhematoma, fetal, 129
Cephalometry, 148
Cephalopelvic disproportion, 125, 131

Cephalosporins, 204, 205, 206, 209
  in pyelonephritis, 53
  in urinary tract infection, 49, 52
Cephalothin (Keflin), 209
Cephradine (Anspor, Velosef), 205,
  206, 209
Cerclage, 7-8, 462
Cerebral irritability, 129
Cerebrospinal fluid (CSF)
  accumulation in brain, 10
Cerebrovascular problems with
  oral contraceptives, 481
Cervical cancer, 260
  chemotherapy for, 299-300
  invasive, 289-301
  preinvasive, 286-288
  radiation for, 295, 298
  radical hysterectomy for, 295-
    297
  recurrent, 299
Cervical cup insemination, 397,
  407
Cervical incompetence, 6-9, 462
  diagnosis of, 6-7
  Hegar test in, 6
  hysterogram in, 6
  spontaneous abortion in, 6
  surgical management of, 7-8
Cervical intraepithelial neoplasia
  (CIN), 282-283, 289
Cervical stump carcinoma, 297-298
Cervicitis, 195, 226, 253
Cervix
  avulsion of, 129
  barrel-shaped, 292, 297
  biopsy of, 287
  carcinoma of and pregnancy, 297
  cerclage of, 7-8, 462
  congenital absence of, 455
  dilation of, 123, 218, 499
  Gram stain of mucus of, 228
  inability to dilate, 499
  stenosis of, 395
Cesarean section, 8, 73, 77, 84,
  102, 113, 124, 128, 130, 157,
  158, 200, 478
  indications for, 131
  in placenta previa, 109
  vaginal delivery following, 131-
    133
Chancroid (soft chancre), 197
Chan, W. Y., 218, 219
Chart recorder, 157
Chemical irritants and
  vulvovaginitis, 195
Chemical sterilization, 507-508
Chemotherapy, 273, 324
  in cervical cancer, 299-300
  in endometrial cancer, 312
  in fallopian tube cancer, 323
  in metastatic trophoblastic
    disease, 339
  in nonmetastatic trophoblastic
    disease, 336
  in ovarian cancer, 332

  in recurrent endometrial cancer,
    316-318
Chest
  pain in, 79
  trauma to, 362
  x-ray of, 234
Chicago Lying-In Hospital, 279
Chlamydia, 196, 198, 203, 204,
  206, 207, 392
Chlorambucil (Leukeran), 316,
  329, 339
Chloramphenicol, 205, 206
  in lactation, 4
  in pregnancy, 4
Chloroquine, 4
Chlorotrianisene (TACE), 135
Chlorpromazine (Thorazine), 360
Chorioamnionitis, 72, 82-85, 98-99,
  105
Choriocarcinoma, 139, 329, 340
  See also Trophoblastic disease
  metastatic, 338
Chromic phosphate therapy, 323,
  331
Chromosomal abnormalities, 460
Chung, W. S., 294
Cigarette smoking, 93
Cimetidine (Tagamet), 380
CIN. *See* Cervical intraepithelial
  neoplasia
Cisplatin (Platinol), 300, 317, 318,
  324, 327, 331
Claforan. *See* Cefotaxime
Clear-cell carcinoma, 274-280
  See also Adenocarcinoma,
  vaginal
Cleocin. *See* Clindamycin
Clindamycin (Cleocin), 194, 205
Clinoril. *See* Sulindac
Clomid. *See* Clomiphene citrate
Clomiphene citrate (Clomid,
  Serophene), 72, 135, 232,
  355, 356, 358, 367, 372, 383,
  384, 385, 389, 396, 399-403,
  405, 407, 448, 459
  in luteal phase defects, 442
  risks of, 402
Clostridium perfringens, 17
Clotrimazole (Gyne-Lotrimin,
  Mycelex-G), 193
Coagulation
  disseminated intravascular, 83,
    113, 114
  factors in pregnancy, 38
  failure of, 112, 113-115
  and heparin, 42
Coital technique and infertility,
  397
Colistimethate (Coly-Mycin M),
  253
Collins, C. G., 261
Colon bacilli, 194
Colporrhaphy, 211
  posterior, 257
Colposcopy, 287

Colpotomy, 214
Colpotomy (transvaginal) tubal
  ligation, 506
Coly-Mycin M. *See* Colistimethate
Community Cancer Center of Los
  Angeles (CCCLA), 291
Complement fixation tests, 196,
  198
Computerized tomography (CT)
  scan, 293, 328, 362, 364, 377
Concealed hemorrhage, 111-112
Conduction anesthesia, 66
Condyloma acuminatum, 194
Condyloma latum, 196
Condyloma virus, 290
Cone biopsy, 288
Congenital absence of cervix, 455
Congenital adrenal hyperplasia
  (CAH), 343, 346, 373, 376,
  377-378, 380
Congenital anomalies, 88, 402
  See also Birth defects
  in breech presentation, 101
Congenital infection, 84, 200
Congenital nephrosis, 140
Congestion
  pelvic, 217
  vascular, 213
Conization-associated infertility,
  288
Contraception
  See also specific types
  in heart disease, 25
  oral. *See* Oral contraceptives
  postcoital, 495-497
  in teen-agers, 491-494
Contractions
  premature ventricular, 158
  uterine. *See* Uterine contractions
Contraction stress test (CST), 58,
  87, 89, 90, 144, 145
Convulsion prevention, 63
Cord. *See* Umbilical cord
Cornual implantation of fallopian
  tube, 425-427
Corpus luteum cysts, 233
Corticosteroids, 17, 79, 156, 188,
  374, 380
  fetal secretion of, 87
  and uterine bleeding, 227
Cortisol, 148, 153
Corynebacterium vaginale, 190
  See also *Gardnerella vaginalis*
Cosmegen. *See* Dactinomycin
Coumadin. *See* Warfarin
Coumarins, 4
Coupling gel, 159
Couvelaire uterus, 113, 114
Creasman, W. T., 309
Creatinine, 148
  serum levels of, 205
CRL. *See* Crown-rump length
Crossmatch of blood, 112
Crown-rump length (CRL), 94
Cruse, P. J. E., 211

Intravesicular pressure, 256
Intrinsic (primary) dysmenorrhea,
216
In vitro fertilization, 448-452
Iodides, 4
Iodophor douche, 210
Iron-binding capacity, 14
Iron-deficiency anemia, 14, 15
Iron therapy, 15
Irradiation. *See* Radiation
Irritability, cerebral, 129
Irritants and vulvovaginitis, 195
Irving, F. C., 116
Irving tubal ligation, 504
Isoimmunization, 31, 36, 149, 151,
165, 179
Isojima, S., 397, 461
Isosexual precocious puberty, 468,
469-471
Isoxsuprine (Vasodilan), 77, 79, 80,
164, 174
IUA. *See* Intrauterine adhesions
IUD. *See* Intrauterine device
IUGR. *See* Intrauterine growth
retardation
IVP. *See* Intravenous pyelogram

J
Jobst stockings, 42
Johnson, J. W. C., 154
Johnson, M. L., 10
Jones, H. W., Jr., 458

K
Kallmann's syndrome, 348
Kanamycin (Kantrex), 197
Kantrex. *See* Kanamycin
Karyotype, 10, 460
Kaufman, R. H., 458
Keflin. *See* Cephalothin
Kefzol. *See* Cefazolin
Kelly, R. M., 314
Kempers, R. D., 430
Kernicterus of newborn, 29
17-Ketosteroids, 376, 461
Kibrick test, 461
Kidney disease, 93
and anemia, 15
chronic, 15
Kidney failure, 83, 113
Killian nasal speculum, 187
Klebsiella, 49
Kleihauer-Betke technique, 30,
109
Kleihauer, E., 29
Kletzky, O. A., 416
Klinefelter's syndrome, 343
Knox, G. E., 87
Kobayashi extractor, 128, 130
Krebs classification, 342
Kremer capillary tube method, 398
Krukenberg tumors, 373
Kubli, 143

L
Labor
abnormal, 123-127
active management of, 125
active phase of, 123, 124, 125-
126
advanced, 78
anesthesia during, 22
arrest of, 125
inhibition of, 174
latent phase of, 123, 125
premature, 72, 78-81, 97, 149,
156, 456
preterm, 75-77
prolonged, 105
Labor curve, 123
Lacerations, 129
vulvar, 247
Lactation
and drugs, 4-5
postpartum, 134-136
suppression of, 134-135, 368-369
Lactobacillus acidophilus
(Döderlein's bacillus), 190,
194
LAC/USC. *See* Los Angeles
County/University of
Southern California
Laminaria, 395, 499
Landes, R., 254
Landsteiner, K., 29
Laparoscopic fulguration, 434
Laparoscopic oocyte recovery, 449-
450
Laparoscopic sterilization, 504-506
Laparoscopy, 204, 214, 216, 235,
321, 390-391, 405, 416-417
Laparotomy, 234, 294, 321, 327,
332
Laser
carbon dioxide, 288
surgery, 427-428
Lash procedure, 7
Late decelerations, 113, 121, 143,
145, 163, 168, 178, 182
Latent phase of labor, 123, 125
Latzko's technique, 262
Lecithin, 148, 151
Lecithin palmitate/stearate ratios,
151
Lecithin-sphingomyelin (L/S) ratio,
73, 147, 149, 151, 152, 155,
297
Leiomyomas, 226, 237, 499
See also Fibroids; Myomas
submucous, 228, 460
Leukemia, 227
Leukeran. *See* Chlorambucil
Leukocytosis, 83
Leukopenia, 17
Leukorrhea, 186, 188
Lewis, C. G., 309
LH. *See* Luteinizing hormone
Liddle, G. W., 376
Ligament varicosities, 213

Ligation
arterial, 106
tubal, 504, 506-507
Liggins, G. C., 154, 155
Liley, A. W., 30, 33, 35
Lithium
in lactation, 4
and PMS, 223
in pregnancy, 4
Liver, 94, 227
function, 228
scan, 313
tenderness of, 204
Liver disease, 140, 227
Los Angeles County/University of
Southern California
(LAC/USC) Medical Center,
89, 102, 116, 117, 118, 153,
294, 357, 358, 363, 395
Low-birth-weight infants, 71
L/S ratio. *See* Lecithin-
sphingomyelin ratio
LSD, 4
Lugol's solution staining, 287
Lung
maturation of, 95, 147-152
scan of, 41
Lung profile (phospholipid profile),
99, 151, 152
Luteal phase
defects, 439-443
inadequate, 392-393, 440-441
short, 439
Luteinizing hormone (LH), 238,
348, 353, 354, 355, 367, 385,
399, 407, 439, 448, 464
Lymphadenectomy, 269, 270
Lymphangiography, 293, 328
Lymphatic buboes, 198
Lymphatic metastases, 275, 322
Lymphedema, 270
Lymphocysts, 269
Lymphogranuloma venereum,
196, 198

M
Macrosomia, 87, 105
Magnesium, 222
Magnesium sulfate, 73, 76, 155
administration of, 63-64
infusion of, 66
mode of action of, 64
toxicity of, 64
Male factor in infertility, 409-412
Male offspring, effects of DES on,
280
Male pseudohermaphroditism,
343, 344-345
Malignant melanoma, 269
Malmström extractor, 128, 129,
130
Malmström-Westman vacuum
cannula, 414
Malnutrition, 105

Placental fragments, 105
Placental perfusion, 95
Placental rupture, 112
Placental transfer, 3
Placenta percreta, 116
Placenta previa, 108-110, 113
Placentex test, 464
Plasma
    See also Blood; Serum
    estriols in, 94
Plasminogen activator, 39
Platelets, 112, 227
Plethysmography, 40
PMS. *See* Premenstrual syndrome
Pneumocyte, 147
Pneumography, 241
Pneumogynography, 214
Podophyllin, 194
    in pregnancy, 4
Polycystic ovarian disease (PCO),
    226, 235, 354, 355, 376, 377-
    378, 385
    treatment of, 383-386
Polycythemia, 95
Polyps, 217, 228, 230
Pomeroy tubal ligation, 504
Ponstel. *See* Mefenamic acid
Porphyria, 374
Port-A-Cul transport medium, 203
Porta-Pap program, 291
Posé, 143
Poskanzer, D. C., 274
Postabortion pain syndrome, 502
Postcoital contraception, 495-497
Postcoital test (PCT), 394-398
    abnormal, 395-398
    fractional, 402
Postdatism (post-term pregnancy),
    86-91, 144
Postmaturity syndrome (fetal
    dysmaturity), 86, 88, 89
Postmenopausal palpable ovary
    (PMPO), 234
Postoperative infection, 208-211,
    244
Postpartum endoparametritis, 83
Postpartum lactation suppression,
    134-136, 368-369
Postpill amenorrhea, 357-359, 481-
    482
Post-term pregnancy, 86-91, 144
Potter, E. L., 325
Povidone-iodine solution, 200
Precocious puberty, 468-472
Preeclampsia, 66, 78, 173
Pregnancy
    alcohol in, 4
    anemia in, 13-17
    anesthetics in, 4
    anticoagulants in, 44
    anticonvulsants in, 19-20
    appendicitis in, 68-70
    and carcinoma of cervix, 297
    cardiovascular changes in, 22-23
    circulating clotting factors in, 38

complications of, 226-227
continuation of, after abortion,
    501
diabetic, 56-60, 152
drugs in, 2-5, 52
ectopic. *See* Ectopic pregnancy
growth parameters, 87
hCG in, 464
and heart disease, 22-25
hematologic change in, 13
hypothyroidism in, 26-28
intrauterine, 230
and in vitro fertilization, 451
IUD complications in, 488-489
molar, 334-337
multiple, 71-74, 140, 141, 405,
    408
myomas in, 243
occult, 459
physiologic alterations in, 13
post-term (postdatism, postdate
    pregnancy, prolonged
    pregnancy), 86-91, 144
pulmonary embolism in, 38-41,
    42-46
radiography in, 49
refractory anemia of, 15
seizure disorders in, 18-21
sulfa drugs in, 52
teratogenic effects in, 2
thrombophlebitis in, 38-41, 42-
    46
urinary tract infections in, 47-51,
    52-55
urine collection in, 48
virilization in, 374-375
Pregnancy-induced hypertension
    (PIH), 61-67, 72, 73, 175
    diagnosis of, 61-62
    treatment for, 63
Pregnancy termination
    See also Abortion
    in fetal death, 513
    first-trimester, 498-502
    infection in, 500
    retained tissue after, 501
Pregnancy tests, 234
    agglutination inhibition, 237, 465
    evaluation of, 464-467
Pregnosis test, 464
Pregnosticon Dri-Dot test, 464
Preinvasive cancer of cervix and
    vagina, 286-288
Premarin. *See* Estrogen cream
Premature adrenarche, 468
Premature labor, 72, 78-81, 97,
    149, 156, 456
Premature ovarian failure, 354
Premature pubarche, 469
Premature rupture of membranes,
    75, 97-99
Premature thelarche, 468
Premature ventricular
    contractions, 158

Prematurity, 71, 72, 83, 162, 179
    fetal, 128
    and perinatal mortality, 101
    rate of, 101
Premenstrual molimina, 230
Premenstrual syndrome (PMS),
    221-224
Presacral neurectomy, 214, 218
Preterm labor and delivery, 75-77
Primaquine, 16
Primary amenorrhea, 348-351
Primary (intrinsic) dysmenorrhea,
    214, 216, 217-220
Pritchard's method of eclampsia
    management, 64
PRL. *See* Prolactin
Probenecid (Benemid), 204, 207
Progesterone, 13, 218, 222, 349,
    384, 388, 389
    for luteal phase defects, 442
    and PMS, 222
    serum concentration of, 228
Progesterone challenge test, 358
Progestins, 3, 231, 302, 316, 324,
    325, 350, 383
    for endometrial cancer, 314-316
    19-nortestosterone-derived, 374
    in pregnancy, 4
Proglycem. *See* Diazoxide
Prolactin (PRL), 148, 153, 359,
    360, 364, 367-368
    excess of. *See*
        Hyperprolactinemia
    levels of, 222, 362
    serum, 363
Prolactin-inhibiting factor (PIF),
    360
Prolapse
    genital, 270
    of ovaries, 214
    of umbilical cord, 73, 102, 178,
        179, 182
    urethral, 270
    uterine, 105
Prolonged (post-term) pregnancy,
    86-91, 144
Prophylactic antibiotics, 208-210,
    244
    and abdominal hysterectomy,
        208
    and pelvic cellulitis, 208
    and pregnant cardiac patient, 24
    and premature membrane
        rupture, 98
    and urinary tract infection, 208
    and vaginal hysterectomy, 208
Propranolol (Inderal), 162, 173, 175
Propylthiouracil, 4
Prostaglandin, 218, 223, 229, 335
    inhibitors of, 217, 218, 219, 232
    intramyometrial, 114
Prostate gland, 253
Protein, 148
Proteinuria, 93
Proteus, 49

Other Titles of Related Interest From
MEDICAL ECONOMICS BOOKS

Managing Ob/Gyn Emergencies, Second Edition
Edited by John T. Queenan, M.D.
ISBN 0-87489-344-5

Management of High-Risk Pregnancy
Edited by John T. Queenan, M.D.
ISBN 0-87489-221-X

Protocols for High-Risk Pregnancies
Edited by John T. Queenan, M.D., and John C. Hobbins, M.D.
ISBN 0-87489-275-9

Drugs Used With Neonates and During Pregnancy, Second Edition
Ina Lee Stile, Pharm.D., Thomas Hegyi, M.D., and Mark Hiatt, M.D.
ISBN 0-87489-342-9

Drug Interactions Index
The late Fred Lerman, M.D., and Robert T. Weibert, Pharm.D.
ISBN 0-87489-266-X

Sports Medicine for the Athletic Female
Edited by Christine E. Haycock, M.D.
ISBN 0-87489-212-0

Managing Sexual Dysfunction: A Basic Guide
John F. O'Connor, M.D.
ISBN 0-87489-217-1

For information, write:
Customer Service Manager
MEDICAL ECONOMICS BOOKS
Oradell, New Jersey 07649